Epilepsy Surgery: An Issue of Neurosurgery Clinics

Epilepsy Surgery: An Issue of Neurosurgery Clinics

Editor: Elias Gilbert

AMERICAN
MEDICAL PUBLISHERS
www.americanmedicalpublishers.com

AMERICAN
MEDICAL PUBLISHERS
www.americanmedicalpublishers.com

Cataloging-in-Publication Data

Epilepsy surgery : an issue of neurosurgery clinics / edited by Elias Gilbert.
p. cm.
Includes bibliographical references and index.
ISBN 979-8-88740-097-6
1. Epilepsy--Surgery. 2. Nervous system--Surgery. 3. Surgery, Operative.
4. Brain--Diseases--Treatment. 5. Developmental disabilities--Treatment.
I. Gilbert, Elias.
RD594 .E65 2023
617.481--dc23

American Medical Publishers,
41 Flatbush Avenue,
1st Floor, New York,
NY 11217, USA

ISBN 979-8-88740-097-6 (Hardback)

Contents

Preface

A seizure is a sudden, uncontrolled electrical activity between the brain's nerve cells. It can lead to changes in behavior, feelings, and in levels of consciousness, muscle control, etc. Epilepsy surgery is a surgical method concerned with the treatment of the brain. It is used to remove the part of the brain where seizures take place. There are several types of epilepsy surgeries and factors such as the site of the neurons that start the seizure and the age of the patient determine the type of surgery that should be performed. Resective surgery is the most common type of epilepsy surgical method. It involves the removal of a small portion of the brain. It is often performed in an area that controls language comprehension, visual memory and emotions, known as temporal lobe. Corpus callosotomy is another type of epilepsy surgery that involves complete or partial removal of the corpus callosum. This book is compiled in such a manner, that it will provide in-depth knowledge about epilepsy surgery. It will serve as a valuable source of reference for neurosurgery students.

Significant researches are present in this book. Intensive efforts have been employed by authors to make this book an outstanding discourse. This book contains the enlightening chapters which have been written on the basis of significant researches done by the experts.

Finally, I would also like to thank all the members involved in this book for being a team and meeting all the deadlines for the submission of their respective works. I would also like to thank my friends and family for being supportive in my efforts.

Editor

1

Treatment of Multi-Focal Epilepsy with Resective Surgery Plus Responsive Neurostimulation (RNS): One Institution's Experience

Diem Kieu Tran[1*], *Demi Chi Tran*[2], *Lilit Mnatsakayan*[2], *Jack Lin*[2], *Frank Hsu*[1] *and Sumeet Vadera*[1]

[1] *Department of Neurological Surgery, University of California, Irvine, Irvine, CA, United States,* [2] *Department of Neurology, University of California, Irvine, Irvine, CA, United States*

***Correspondence:**
Diem Kieu Tran
ktt967@gmail.com

Objective: Patients with medically refractory focal epilepsy can be difficult to treat surgically, especially if invasive monitoring reveals multiple ictal onset zones. Possible therapeutic options may include resection, neurostimulation, laser ablation, or a combination of these surgical modalities. To date, no study has examined outcomes associated with resection plus responsive neurostimulation (RNS, Neuropace, Inc., Mountain View, CA) implantation and we describe our initial experience in patients with multifocal epilepsy undergoing this combination therapy.

Methods: A total of 43 responsive neurostimulation (RNS) devices were implanted at UCI from 2015 to 2019. We retrospectively reviewed charts of patients from the same time period who underwent both resection and RNS implantation. Patients were required to have independent or multifocal onset, undergo resection and RNS implantation, and have a minimum of six-months for follow-up to be included in the study. Demographics, location of ictal onset, location of surgery, complications, and seizure outcome were collected.

Results: Ten patients met inclusion criteria for the study, and seven underwent both procedures in the same setting. The average age was 36. All patients had multifocal ictal onset on video electroencephalogram or invasive EEG with four patients undergoing subdural grid placement and four patients undergoing bilateral sEEG prior to the definitive surgery. Five patients underwent resection plus ipsilateral RNS placement and the remainder underwent resection with contralateral RNS placement. Two minor complications were encountered in this group. At six months follow up, there was an average of 81% $\pm$ 9 reduction in seizures, while four patients experienced complete seizure freedom at 1 year.

Conclusion: Patients with multifocal epilepsy can be treated with partial resection plus RNS. The complication rates are low with potential for worthwhile seizure reduction.

Keywords: epilepsy, lobectomy, temporal, surgery, robotic, responsive neurostimulation (RNS)

INTRODUCTION

Approximately one-third of epilepsy patients have seizures that are refractory to antiepileptic medications (1, 2). Left untreated, patients are at risk of developing multiple comorbidities, and potentially death (3). For this reason, patients with medically refractory focal epilepsy should be referred to a Level 4 NAEC (National Association of Epilepsy Centers) center to be evaluated for surgical candidacy. The best outcomes are seen with temporal lobectomy for mesial temporal sclerosis (MTS) or other lesional resections, with 68% of patients with MTS becoming seizure free and 50% of neocortical extratemporal resections becoming seizure free at 2 years (4).

After being diagnosed with medically refractory epilepsy, pre-surgical evaluation includes video electroencephalography (EEG) monitoring to localize the ictal onset zone(s). If ictal onset is difficult to localize, or if bilateral or eloquent area ictal onset is suspected, the patients move on to have invasive monitoring studies including stereoelectroencephalography (sEEG) or subdural grids (SDG) to better delineate the ictal onset zone(s). Depending upon the location of the onset zone, subsequent resection, neurostimulation, or laser ablation might be performed.

However, there are limitations associated with performing resections including the inability to perform bilateral resection of the same lobe and the unfavorable functional outcomes associated with resecting eloquent regions. Therefore, patients with medically refractory epilepsy which involve multiple independent ictal onset zones or eloquent areas can be very difficult to treat surgically. Historically, when there is bilateral or multifocal ictal onset, palliative procedures such as callosotomy or neuromodulation have been performed (5–9). Unfortunately, these rarely result in complete seizure freedom. The authors describe their experience with resection of primary ictal onset zone as well as RNS implantation for additional ictal onset areas. This combination approach provides the ability to expand the treatment area outside of what is possible with resection alone. The authors demonstrate their early series of patients who underwent resection and RNS as part of their surgical management.

METHODS

Patient Selection

A total of 43 responsive neurostimulation (RNS) were placed at UCI from 2013 to 2019. To be included in the study, patients must have independent multifocal ictal onset which was demonstrated with video encephalography (vEEG) or invasive monitoring (sEEG or SDG) and undergone resection plus RNS implantation. Resection and RNS implantation were not required to be performed during the same surgical setting. Subjects must also have at least six months of follow up. Between February 2015 to January 2019, 10 patients met inclusion criteria and underwent responsive neurostimulation implantation as well as a resective procedure. Eight out of ten patients underwent phase two invasive monitoring with either SDG placement and sEEG or bilateral sEEG, while two patients underwent definitive treatment without undergoing invasive monitoring (**Tables 1, 2**). This study was approved by the University of California, Irvine's Institutional Review Board (IRB).

Presurgical Workup

All patients completed neuroimaging, neuropsychological testing, and non-invasive vEEG as part of their phase one evaluation. They were then presented and discussed at our institution's multidisciplinary epilepsy management conference. Epileptologists, neuroradiologists, and neuropsychologists as well as the senior author (SV) were present during these conferences. The subjects were presented by their treating epileptologist, and all relevant imaging studies, vEEG clips, and

TABLE 1 | Patient characteristic.

Pt No	Age at onset, Sex	No baseline seizures/month	Invasive EEG type	No of clinical seizures/month at 6 months follow up	No of clinical seizures/ month at 1 year	No of clinical seizures/ month at 2 years
JA	1, M	Daily	SDG	8.2	7.8	0
VO	22, M	6	sEEG	0.16	0.08	0
RR	42, F	12	sEEG	2.6	6.8	3
JH	23, F	Daily	sEEG, then SDG*	7.5	7.1	1
MC	19, F	Daily	SDG with sEEG	6.8	6.1	1
JR	19, F	5	sEEG	1.2	1.2	
JW	8, F	Daily	sEEG, then SDG*	0.16	0.08	
EA	39, F	9	No invasive EEG done initially, then sEEG**	2.2	2.1	
SL	5, F	6	sEEG	1.2	0.08	
MM	0, F	8	No invasive EEG done	2.1	0.04	

**Patients initially underwent bilateral sEEG, which lateralized to one side, then were taken back to surgery for SDG on the side that sEEG lateralized to.*
***Patient initially underwent vEEG that showed left temporal ictal onset. Patient continued to have seizures after left anterior temporal lobectomy, so she was taken back for contralateral sEEG.*

TABLE 2 | Clinical data.

Pt	Semiology	MRI results	Neuropsychiatric testing	AEDs tried	Current AEDs
JA	Begins with staring and unresponsiveness, progressing to pursing of his lips, followed by repetitive opening and closing hands	Left encephalomalacia in left insula/parietal region	Deficits in bilateral fine motor coordination, working memory, selective attention, visuomotor and verbal processing speed, confrontation naming, verbal fluency, visuospatial processing, contextual verbal learning and memory, visuomotor set-shifting, and complex reasoning	Lamotrigine, Levetiracetam, Topiramate XR, Lacosamide	Levetiracetam, Lamotrigine, Lacosamide
VO	Arousing from sleep or rest, shifting in bed, kicking his legs, picking and grabbing at his blanket, wiping face and nose with his right and at times left hand	Encepholomacia in b/l frontal lobes, corpus collosum, and left anterior temporal region	Diffuse cognitive impairment including impaired attention, processing speed, executive function, and expressive language abilities	Topiramate, Vimpat, Brivaracetam	Brivaracetam
RR	1. Aura, twitching of lips, which spread to right hand 2. Bilateral upper extremity tonic extension and posturing with repetitive movements	Mild bilateral MTS	Diffuse deficits across language, graphomotor, reasoning, processing, speed, attention, executive functioning, memory ability	Topiramate, Clonazapam, Lacosamide, Phenobarbital	Topiramate, Brivaracetam
JH	Started with strange behavior, confusion, followed by a febrile illness leading to a convulsive status epilepticus, now semiology is tingling, burning sensation in the right lower extremity ascending to the right upper extremity at times also face for a few second duration	Non lesional	Mild cognitive and memory impairment	Levetiracetam, Lacosamide, Clonazapam	Levetiracetam
MC	Confusion and speech difficulty followed by loss of awareness with secondary generalization	Left temporal cyst, which was resected, leaving empty cavity	Severe impairments in memory and learning, sustained and divided attention, mental flexibility, bilateral fine motor speed and dexterity, receptive and expression language skulls, and reading comprehension	Zonisamide, Lamotrigine, Lacosamide, Perampanel	Zonisamide, Lamotrigine
JR	Aura: sometimes deja vu 1. Spaced out, arms clenched, head to the left, drooling 2. Generalized tonic-clinic activity, tongue biting	Moderate left MTS, mild right MTS	Mild cognitive and memory impairment	Levetiracetam, Lamotrigine, Eslicarbazepine, Lacosamide	Levetriacetam
JW	Touching her bilateral temporal head regions, followed by being confused and turning her body to the left side along the horizontal body axis	Non lesional	Impaired verbal working memory and naming	Carbamazepine, Oxcarbazepine, Topiramate, Clonazapam, Acetazolamide	Lamotrigine, Levetiracetam
EA	Arrest in behavior, gaze preference to the left with repetitive hand movements, more commonly with the right	Non lesional	Impaired expressive vocabulary, visual memory, bilateral fine motor speed, and verbal reasoning	Carbamazepine, Valproic Acid, felbamate, Lamotrigine, Phenyltoin, Topiramate, phenobarbital, Oxcarbamazepine, Lacosimide, Zonisamide	Levetiracetam, Eslicarbazepine

(Continued)

TABLE 2 | Continued

Pt	Semiology	MRI results	Neuropsychiatric Testing	AEDs Tried	Current AEDs
SL	Loud laughter followed by screaming, then progressed to rocking body back and forth	Right frontal encephalomalacia with ventricular dilation (patient had prior right frontal lobectomy from a different institution with persistent seizures)	Impaired fine motor speed and dexterity, working memory and verbal learning	Lamotrigine, Perampanel	Lamotrigine
MM	Aura of fear, anxiety, and impending doom, staring, unresponsiveness and seen walking around and repeating words	Left MTS	Impairments in mental flexibility, problem-solving, phonemic, fluency, and divided attention. Intact visual and recognition memory	Carbamazepine, Topiramate, Brivaracetam, Lacosimide	Lacosimide, Carbazmazepine

TABLE 3 | Surgical outcomes.

Pt No	Location of ictal onset	Location of RNS leads and resection	ECoG from RNS	Complications
JA	Left frontal with rapid spread to 3 left hippocampus	RNS strip electrodes in left frontal + left temporal lobectomy	Several areas of sharp waves, however, no clinical seizures seen	
VO	Right frontal, bilateral temporal	RNS depth electrodes in bilateral hippocampus + right frontal resection	Brief runs of sharp waves in right more than left temporal area, however, no clinical seizures	
RR	Bilateral temporal	RNS depth electrodes in right hippocampus + left temporal lobectomy	1-3 electroclinical seizures/month from right hippocampus, and runs of sharp waves seen in the same area	
JH	Left temporal	RNS strip electrodes in posterior left + left anterior temporal lobectomy	1-2 electroclinical seizures/month	
MC	Left temporal	RNS strip electrodes in posterior left + left anterior temporal lobectomy	3-5 electroclinical seizures/month, occasional prolonged runs of sharp waves	
JR	Left temporal, then right temporal	RNS depth electrodes in right hippocampus + left temporal lobectomy[β]	1-2 electrographic seizures from right hippocampus, runs of sharp waves from same area	
JW	Right frontal	RNS strip electrodes in anterior and posterior interhemispheric area + right frontal resection	1-2 brief electrographic seizures, but no clinical seizures	
EA	Left temporal, then right temporal	Right RNS depth electrodes in hippocampus + left temporal lobectomy[δ]	5-10 electrographic seizures from right hippocampus, and frequent runs of sharp waves	
SL	Right frontal	RNS strip electrodes in interhemispheric region near motor strip + right frontal resection	Several areas of sharp waves, no electroclinical seizure	CSF leak
MM	Bilateral temporal	RNS depth electrode into hippocampus + left temporal lobectomy[α]	Sharp waves from right hippocampus, no electroclinical seizures	EDH under RNS generator

[α] Patient only underwent vEEG which showed bilateral independent ictal onset. She later underwent WADA testing which showed language dominance on right side, therefore she underwent left temporal lobectomy and right RNS placement.

[β] Patient initially underwent RNS implantation into bilateral hippocampus, however, patient continued to have frequent seizure. ECoG data of RNS shows persistent left sided seizures, therefore she underwent left temporal lobectomy.

[δ] Patient initially underwent left temporal lobectomy, however, patient continued to have frequent seizures. She then underwent contralateral sEEG, which showed independent ictal onset, therefore she underwent right RNS placement.

Patient had electrographic seizures on ECoG that correlated with patient's seizure diary or magnet swipe.

neuropsychological tests were thoroughly discussed. A treatment consensus was reached amongst all members of the group. After invasive monitoring was complete, patients with complex seizure onset (i.e., bilateral, eloquent area, or multifocal ictal onset) were again discussed at epilepsy management conference and a treatment consensus was reached. Once treatment consensus

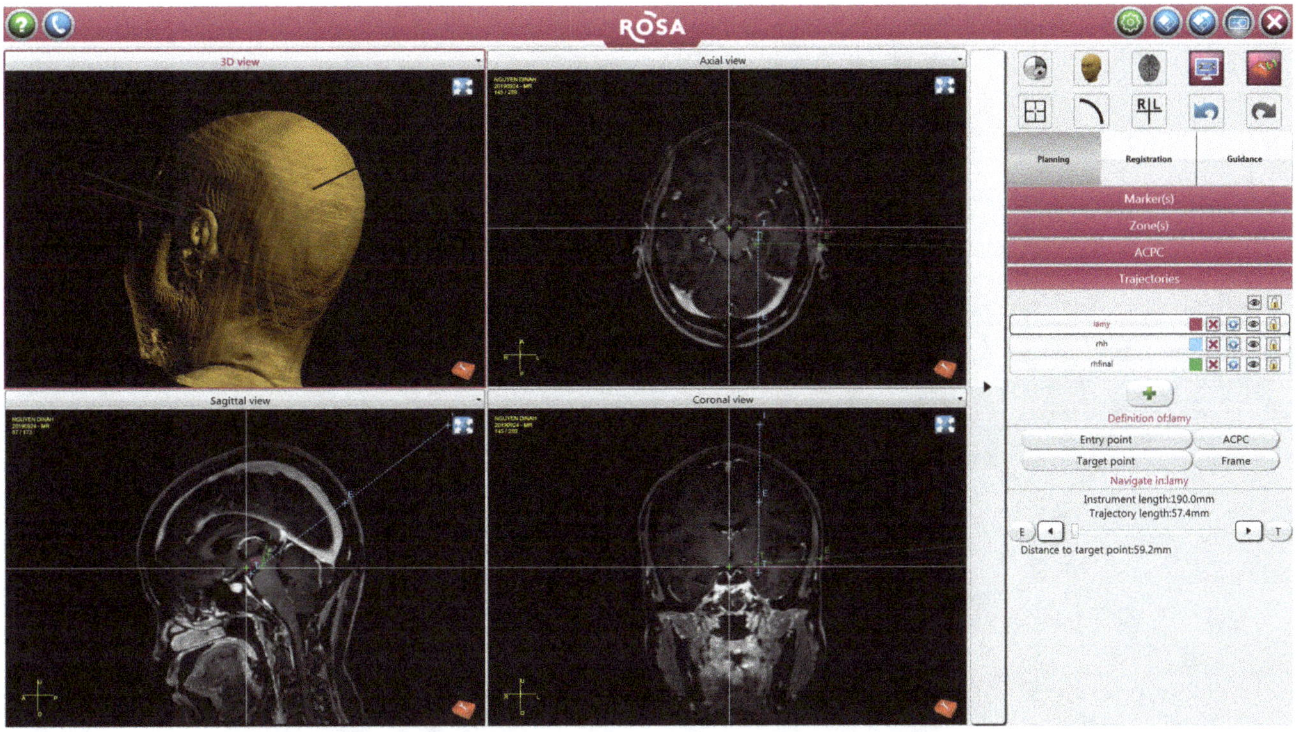

FIGURE 1 | Patient undergoing left sided RNS placement with right temporal lobectomy. The figure depicts trajectory and target points for the RNS leads.

was reached, the patient was scheduled for definitive surgery within two weeks. All patients in the study underwent resection plus RNS implantation, although these were not necessarily performed during the same surgery.

Surgical Technique

Patients first undergo either sEEG or SDG implantation to localize the ictal onset. If sEEG is performed and it is determined that they will require resection plus RNS, the patients are discharged home and brought back at a later date for the definitive surgery. If SDG is performed, the definitive surgery is performed upon removal of electrodes. Resections were performed after stereotactic RNS implantation to avoid risk of brain shift intraoperatively.

In patients that required depth electrode placement for RNS, stereotactic implantation of RNS was done using the Robotic Operating Surgical Assistant (ROSA) (Zimmer-Biomet, Warsaw, IN). A mayfield skull clamp was placed on the patient's head for immobilization. A curvilinear incision was marked in a location that was accessible to both leads and not interfere with reopening for future generator replacements, which served as the incision for placement of the RNS generator. The ictal onset zone identified by previously implanted sEEG electrodes were used to target RNS leads. All target and entry points were planned on the ROSA on the day of surgery (**Figure 1**).

The skull clamp was then attached to the robot with the patient in the correct position, and registration was performed using the robot's laser registration. Following registration, the robotic arm was used to identify the two entry points. A hand drill was utilized to access the cranial vault, and the dura was carefully opened with a dural probe. The robotic arm maintained a rigid trajectory to the target while an outer cannula and subsequently the RNS lead were passed. Each lead was secured in place using a dog bone-shaped plate from a cranial plating system, which has been previously described in a separate paper (10). The curvilinear incision was then opened, and a small craniectomy was created to hold the RNS generator. The device was then connected to the implanted leads.

For patients that required strip electrode placement for RNS, stereotactic implantation was done using the Stryker (Stryker Corporation, Kalamazoo, MI) neuro-navigation system. Again, a Mayfield skull clamp was applied and the images were uploaded onto the navigation system. Target areas were selected based on patient's SDG data. Patients requiring strip electrodes most commonly underwent temporal lobectomy and RNS placement on the ipsilateral side. The electrodes can be placed once the resection is completed and secured into place by anchoring it to the craniotomy site edges. The rest of the procedure is done in the similar way as described above.

In patients undergoing both resection and RNS placement, once the RNS is implanted successfully, the resection is performed based upon the area of interest with standard surgical techniques (**Figures 2A,B**).

An intraoperative CT is performed after the procedure and the image is fused with the planning MRI to confirm accurate placement of RNS leads.

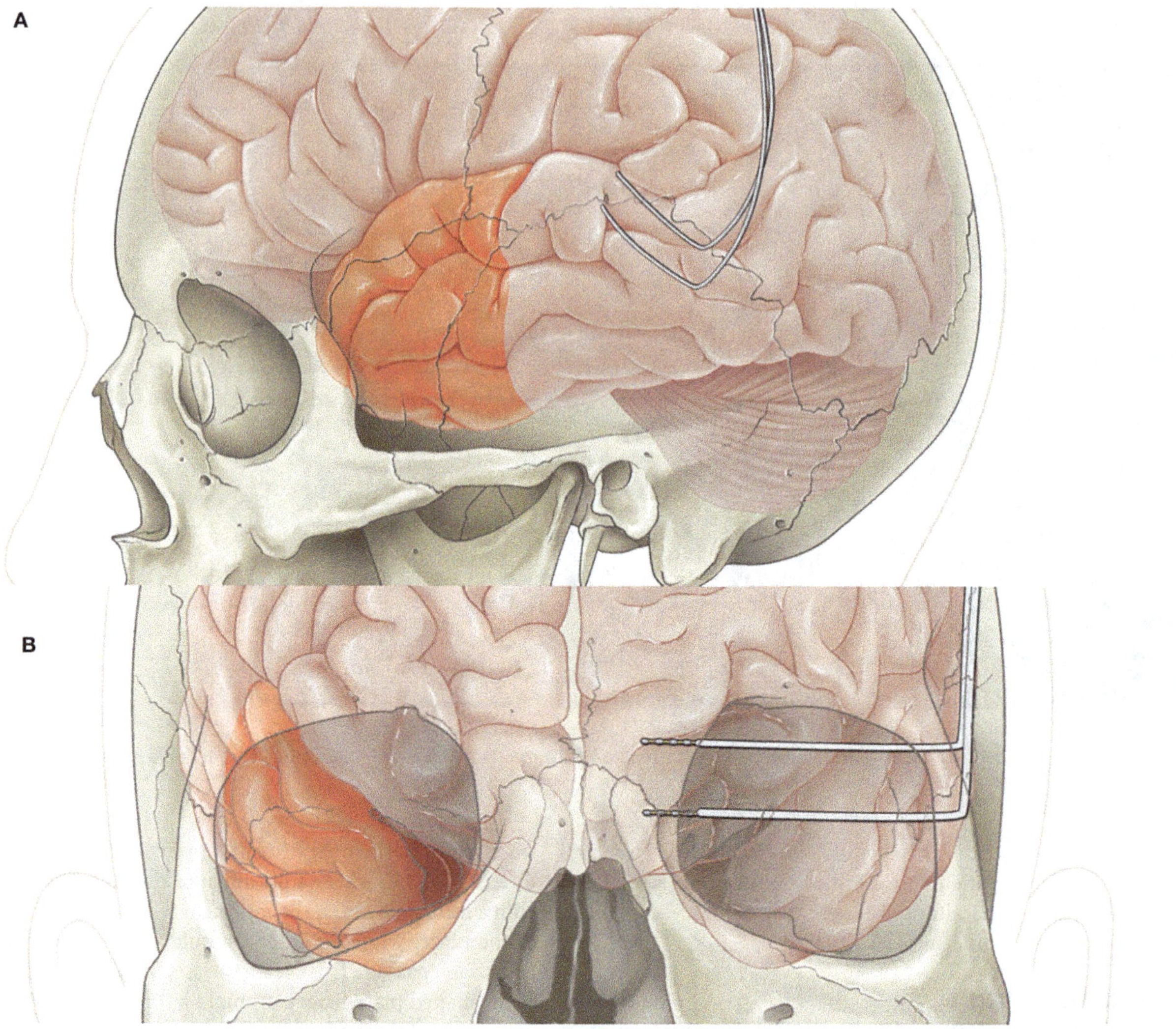

FIGURE 2 | (A) Lateral view of left anterior temporal lobectomy with RNS placement in posterior temporal area. **(B)** Coronal view of right temporal lobectomy with RNS placement in left mesial structures.

Data Collection

The clinical data of subjects who underwent resection plus RNS implantation from July 2015 to January 2019 was retrospectively collected and analyzed. Data for the following variables were collected: (1) age at seizure onset; (2) number of baseline seizures per month; (3) location of ictal onsets; (4) location of RNS leads and resection; (5) postoperative outcome; (6) ECoG from RNS; and (7) surgical complications.

RESULTS

The age range at the time of surgery was 27 to 53 years, with a mean age of 36 years (**Table 3**). There were two patients that underwent definitive treatment without first undergoing invasive monitoring because their vEEG showed clear independent bilateral ictal onset in one patient and left ictal onset in another patient. Four patients underwent SDG placement as part of the invasive monitoring, while the remainder underwent sEEG. Of the four patients that underwent SDG, two initially had sEEG that lateralized to one side and therefore patient returned for SDG implantation to better localize the onset zone. Five patients underwent RNS and ipsilateral resection and the remaining patients underwent contralateral RNS and resection. The patient with bilateral ictal onset later underwent wada testing which showed language dominance on the right, therefore she underwent left temporal lobectomy with right RNS placement. The patient that had only left ictal onset, underwent left temporal lobectomy but continued to have persistent seizures and therefore underwent bilateral sEEG, which showed right sided onset as well, therefore, she underwent right RNS placement. There were two minor postoperative

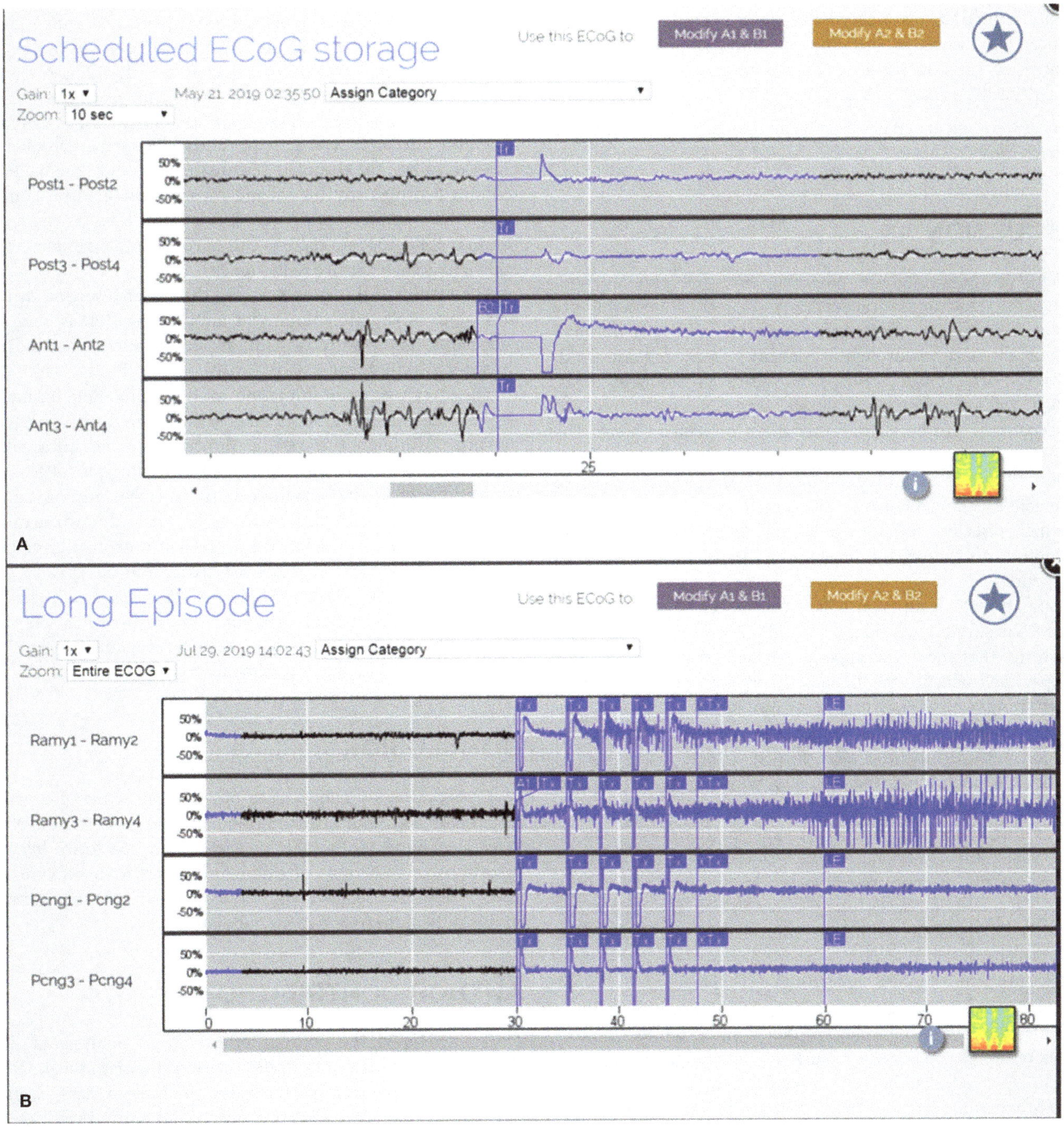

FIGURE 3 | (A) ECoG from patient JA showing epileptiform discharges from multiple areas. **(B)** ECoG from patient R.R. showing detection and treatment of another electrographic seizure from right amygdala.

complications; one patient developed an epidural hematoma under the RNS generator site requiring evacuation while the second had a cerebral spinal fluid leak that require lumbar drain placement (**Table 2**). No long-term sequela was noted and all patients returned to baseline. At six months of follow up, there was an average of 81% ± 9 decrease in seizure frequency, with two patients becoming seizure free. Four patients continued to remain seizure-free at their one year follow up with a total of 83% ± 17 seizure reduction in the study group. Two patients remained seizure free at 2 years follow up, while the rest have not had their 2 year follow ups yet. Seizure reduction was measured by subtracting the number of seizures per month at the time of follow up divided by the number of baseline seizures per month by the number one $\{[1 - (\frac{number\ ofseizure\ per\ month\ at\ time\ of\ follow\ up}{number\ ofseizures\ per\ month\ at\ baseline})] \times 100\}$. Baseline seizures were calculated based on number of seizures patients had for 6 months.

DISCUSSION

Epilepsy surgery offers a potential cure for patients with medically refractory focal epilepsy (6, 9). Resections are considered when the seizure focus can be removed with minimal risk of disabling neurological deficits. Thus, patients with multifocal ictal onset zones, ictal onsets in eloquent areas, or bilateral ictal onsets still pose a significant challenge and these patients can be significantly more difficult to treat. The RNS device provides us with the ability to treat patients with multifocal and eloquent region onset (5). In this case series, we were able to supplement resective surgery with RNS in patients in which resective surgery alone could not address the entire ictal onset zone, such as in eloquent areas or with bilateral onset zones.

Patients with multifocal epilepsy historically were thought to be poor surgical candidates (11–13). There have been a few case series that show that patients with bilateral temporal lobe epilepsy may benefit after unilateral surgery (14–16), however, determining which side to resect also poses a challenge. In patients that have bilateral temporal lobe epilepsy, the chance of good seizure outcome after surgery (Engel class I or II) (17) is still much lower than patients with unilateral temporal lobe epilepsy at about 25–45% depending on the study (12, 18, 19). In our patients with bilateral ictal onset, we were able to use invasive EEG to lateralize which side demonstrated greater seizure activity. Because resection has been shown to have the best seizure free outcomes (6), we chose to treat the most active region with resection, while the contralateral side underwent RNS placement.

Patients with eloquent area onset (i.e., language or motor regions) pose an even greater challenge for treatment. In these patients, the risk of neurological deficit in resecting eloquent cortex outweigh the benefits of surgery. In these patients, partial resection plus RNS on the ipsilateral side can be done. This allows us to broaden the scope of coverage from the safe margin of the resection to eloquent regions with the RNS, effectively allowing us to extend our treatment of ictal onset outside of what is safe with resection alone.

In our patient population, there was an overall reduction in clinical seizures post operatively. Despite this, at the most recent interrogation the RNS system recorded ongoing electrographic (**Figures 3A,B**) seizures in 60% of the patients and epileptiform discharges and patterns in all 10 patients from the remaining areas which were not able to be safely resected. Placement of the RNS system allowed for the detection and treatment of these residual activities. Partial resection of the seizure focus can help lessen the burden of ictal activities and reduce seizure frequency. However, when the complete seizure focus is not removed, there remains a propensity for seizure recurrences (6). The authors argue that supplementing resections with RNS to treat the residual epileptogenic regions can have a complementary effect and yield greater seizure reduction.

The results of this present study show that resection of ictal onset plus RNS implantation in another location is safe and efficacious. There were two minor complications that did not cause long-term deficits.

There are two main limitations of this study. One limitation is that the study group is not well powered with only 10 patients. Although our results provide valuable information regarding the safety and efficacy of resection plus RNS, the clinical outcomes data may not be statistically significant given the small sample. Additionally, there are only two patients included in the study who had long-term outcomes over one-year, and oftentimes, the clinical benefit from epilepsy surgery may take several years to fully manifest, especially in the setting of RNS placement. Nevertheless, neuromodulation often demonstrates improvements in seizure reduction over time, suggesting continued improvement in seizure control may be seen in this group in the future.

CONCLUSION

RNS plus resection allows us to broaden the scope of coverage in patients with multifocal or eloquent ictal onset zones. While resection alone is limited by inability to perform bilateral resections or resections of eloquent regions, RNS provides the ability to extend the coverage and aid with seizure management in this difficult to treat patient population.

AUTHOR CONTRIBUTIONS

DKT: developed the concept of the work, analysis of data, drafting the work, and critically revising the manuscript. DCT: developed the concept of the work, analysis of data, drafting the work, and critically revising the manuscript. LM, JL, and FH: revising the manuscript. SV: developed the concept of the work, analysis of data, drafting the work, critically revising the manuscript, and approved the manuscript for submission. All authors contributed to the article and approved the submitted version.

REFERENCES

1. Kwan P, Brodie MJ. Early identification of refractory epilepsy. *N Engl J Med.* (2000) 342:314–9. doi: 10.1056/NEJM200002033420503
2. Sillanpaa M, Schmidt D. Natural history of treated childhood-onset epilepsy: prospective, long-term population-based study. *Brain.* (2006) 129:617–24. doi: 10.1093/brain/awh726
3. Luoni C, Bisulli F, Canevini MP, De Sarro G, Fattore C, Galimberti CA, et al. Determinants of health-related quality of life in pharmacoresistant epilepsy: results from a large multicenter study of consecutively enrolled patients using validated quantitative assessments. *Epilepsia.* (2011) 52:2181–91. doi: 10.1111/j.1528-1167.2011.03325.x
4. Spencer SS, Berg AT, Vickrey BG, Sperling MR, Bazil CW, Shinnar S, et al. Predicting long-term seizure outcome after

resective epilepsy surgery: the multicenter study. *Neurology.* (2005) 65:912–8. doi: 10.1212/01.wnl.0000176055.45774.71

5. Ben-Menachem E. Neurostimulation-past, present, and beyond. *Epilepsy Curr.* (2012) 12:188–91. doi: 10.5698/1535-7511-12.5.188
6. Engel J Jr, McDermott MP, Wiebe S, Langfitt JT, Stern JM, et al. Early surgical therapy for drug-resistant temporal lobe epilepsy: a randomized trial. *JAMA.* (2012) 307:922–30. doi: 10.1001/jama.2012.220
7. Fisher R, Salanova V, Witt T, Worth R, Henry T, Gross R, et al. Electrical stimulation of the anterior nucleus of thalamus for treatment of refractory epilepsy. *Epilepsia.* (2010) 51:899–908. doi: 10.1111/j.1528-1167.2010.02536.x
8. Kasasbeh AS, Smyth MD, Steger-May K, Jalilian L, Bertrand M, Limbrick DD. Outcomes after anterior or complete corpus callosotomy in children. *Neurosurgery.* (2014) 74:17–28; discussion 28. doi: 10.1227/NEU.0000000000000197
9. Wiebe S, Blume WT, Girvin JP, Eliasziw M, Effectiveness, Efficiency of Surgery for Temporal Lobe Epilepsy Study G. A randomized, controlled trial of surgery for temporal-lobe epilepsy. *N Engl J Med.* (2001) 345:311–8. doi: 10.1056/NEJM200108023450501
10. Tran DK, Paff M, Mnatsakanyan L, Sen-Gupta I, Lin JJ, Hsu FPK, et al. A novel robotic-assisted technique to implant the responsive neurostimulation system. *Oper Neurosurg.* (2019) 18:728–35. doi: 10.1093/ons/opz226
11. Chung MY, Walczak TS, Lewis DV, Dawson DV, Radtke R. Temporal lobectomy and independent bitemporal interictal activity: what degree of lateralization is sufficient? *Epilepsia.* (1991) 32:195–201. doi: 10.1111/j.1528-1157.1991.tb05244.x
12. Holmes MD, Miles AN, Dodrill CB, Ojemann GA, Wilensky AJ. Identifying potential surgical candidates in patients with evidence of bitemporal epilepsy. *Epilepsia.* (2003) 44:1075–9. doi: 10.1046/j.1528-1157.2003.58302.x
13. Hufnagel A, Elger CE, Pels H, Zentner J, Wolf HK, Schramm J, et al. Prognostic significance of ictal and interictal epileptiform activity in temporal lobe epilepsy. *Epilepsia.* (1994) 35:1146–53. doi: 10.1111/j.1528-1157.1994.tb01781.x
14. Boling W, Aghakhani Y, Andermann F, Sziklas V, Olivier A. Surgical treatment of independent bitemporal lobe epilepsy defined by invasive recordings. *J Neurol Neurosurg Psychiatry.* (2009) 80:533–8. doi: 10.1136/jnnp.2008.155291
15. Hirsch LJ, Spencer SS, Spencer DD, Williamson PD, Mattson RH. Temporal lobectomy in patients with bitemporal epilepsy defined by depth electroencephalography. *Ann Neurol.* (1991) 30:347–56. doi: 10.1002/ana.410300306
16. Sirven JI, Malamut BL, Liporace JD, O'Connor MJ, Sperling MR. Outcome after temporal lobectomy in bilateral temporal lobe epilepsy. *Ann Neurol.* (1997) 42:873–8. doi: 10.1002/ana.410420608
17. Jr EJ. *Outcome With Respect to Epileptic Seizures, in Surgical Treatment of the Epilepsies.* New York, NY: Raven Press. (1987). p. 553–71.
18. Cukiert A, Cukiert CM, Argentoni M, Baise-Zung C, Forster CR, Mello VA, et al. Outcome after cortico-amygdalo-hippocampectomy in patients with severe bilateral mesial temporal sclerosis submitted to invasive recording. *Seizure.* (2009) 18:515–8. doi: 10.1016/j.seizure.2009.05.003
19. Holmes MD, Dodrill CB, Ojemann GA, Wilensky AJ, Ojemann LM. Outcome following surgery in patients with bitemporal interictal epileptiform patterns. *Neurology.* (1997) 48:1037–40. doi: 10.1212/WNL.48.4.1037

2

Accuracy and Workflow Improvements for Responsive Neurostimulation Hippocampal Depth Electrode Placement Using Robotic Stereotaxy

*Patrick J. Karas [1], Nisha Giridharan [1], Jeffrey M. Treiber [1], Marc A. Prablek [1], A. Basit Khan [1], Ben Shofty [1], Vaishnav Krishnan [2], Jennifer Chu [2], Paul C. Van Ness [2], Atul Maheshwari [2], Zulfi Haneef [2], Jay R. Gavvala [2] and Sameer A. Sheth [1]**

[1] Department of Neurosurgery, Baylor College of Medicine, Houston, TX, United States, [2] Department of Neurology, Comprehensive Epilepsy Center, Baylor College of Medicine, Houston, TX, United States

***Correspondence:**
Sameer A. Sheth
sameer.sheth@bcm.edu

Background: Robotic stereotaxy is increasingly common in epilepsy surgery for the implantation of stereo-electroencephalography (sEEG) electrodes for intracranial seizure monitoring. The use of robots is also gaining popularity for permanent stereotactic lead implantation applications such as in deep brain stimulation and responsive neurostimulation (RNS) procedures.

Objective: We describe the evolution of our robotic stereotactic implantation technique for placement of occipital-approach hippocampal RNS depth leads.

Methods: We performed a retrospective review of 10 consecutive patients who underwent robotic RNS hippocampal depth electrode implantation. Accuracy of depth lead implantation was measured by registering intraoperative post-implantation fluoroscopic CT images and post-operative CT scans with the stereotactic plan to measure implantation accuracy. Seizure data were also collected from the RNS devices and analyzed to obtain initial seizure control outcome estimates.

Results: Ten patients underwent occipital-approach hippocampal RNS depth electrode placement for medically refractory epilepsy. A total of 18 depth electrodes were included in the analysis. Six patients (10 electrodes) were implanted in the supine position, with mean target radial error of 1.9 ± 0.9 mm (mean $\pm$ SD). Four patients (8 electrodes) were implanted in the prone position, with mean radial error of 0.8 ± 0.3 mm. The radial error was significantly smaller when electrodes were implanted in the prone position compared to the supine position ($p = 0.002$). Early results (median follow-up time 7.4 months) demonstrate mean seizure frequency reduction of 26% ($n = 8$), with 37.5% achieving $\geq$50% reduction in seizure frequency as measured by RNS long episode counts.

Conclusion: Prone positioning for robotic implantation of occipital-approach hippocampal RNS depth electrodes led to lower radial target error compared to supine positioning. The robotic platform offers a number of workflow advantages over traditional frame-based approaches, including parallel rather than serial operation in a bilateral case, decreased concern regarding human error in setting frame coordinates, and surgeon comfort.

Keywords: hippocampal depth electrode, robotic stereotaxy, responsive neurostimulation (RNS), RNS workflow, robotic stereotaxy accuracy, NeuroPace

INTRODUCTION

Robotic stereotaxy is increasingly common both for the implantation of stereo-electroencephalography (sEEG) electrodes during phase 2 epilepsy monitoring and for the implantation of permanent therapeutic neuromodulation systems such as deep brain stimulation (DBS) and responsive neurostimulation (RNS) (1). Similar to frame-based stereotactic systems, robotic stereotaxy allows for submillimeter accuracy for the implantation of DBS electrodes (2, 3), which has broadened its application across the United States and Europe. Advances in computer planning software have also facilitated broader adoption.

In this paper we discuss our use of robotic stereotaxy for the placement of occipital-approach hippocampal depth electrodes for RNS therapy. We describe the evolution of our workflow, which started with the supine beach-chair semi-sitting positioning for implantation of depth electrodes and neurostimulator in one stage with evolution to prone implantation of hippocampal depth electrodes followed by supine implantation of the RNS neurostimulator in two stages. We present a technical note on our electrode implantation workflow, and our initial single center experience with electrode implantation accuracy and early seizure response rates.

MATERIALS AND METHODS

Subjects

Ten consecutive subjects (6 women and 4 men) who underwent unilateral or bilateral hippocampal RNS depth electrode implantation (**Figure 1A**) were included. The median age was 40 years (range 25–63), with median duration of epilepsy for 15 years (range 3–43 years). The subjects failed a median of 4 antiepileptic medications prior to RNS implantation (range 2–12 medications) and reported a median seizure frequency of 1–2 seizures weekly. Full demographic information is available in **Table 1**.

Procedure

Preoperative high-resolution CT and MRI scans are loaded into the ROSA (Zimmer Biomet, Warsaw, Indiana, USA) planning computer and merged. A preoperative CT is highly recommended, as intraoperative fluoroscopic CT imaging (O-arm O2, Medtronic, Minneapolis, MN, USA) merges best with CT; merging these images to MRI may result in suboptimal registration. The ROSA software automatic registration is used but must be checked carefully prior to proceeding with planning and implantation. The target trajectory length is set to 190 mm (based on cannula length; see below), and the intended electrode trajectory is planned based on the surgeon's standard procedure. We use an occipital approach and strive for a trajectory that spans the head and body of the hippocampus, often extending into the amygdala, with >25 mm of the trajectory within these structures. We use a T1 post-contrast MRI in order to identify and avoid traversing vascular structures and also try to avoid entering the occipital horn of the lateral ventricle in order to avoid deflection off the ependymal surface.

Prior to using robotic stereotaxy, we used a conventional frame for RNS depth electrode placement. For an occipital approach hippocampal depth electrode, we would position the patient supine in a slouched semi-sitting position with the neck flexed, such that the trajectory is approximately parallel to the floor. This position is not easily achieved with our preferred head fixation method using the robot (see below) because of the low occipital entry points and inferior-to-superior trajectory. We therefore evolved our approach to performing the electrode implant procedure prone, with a second stage for placement of the RNS generator. In some cases, the two stages were performed during the same procedure, but in others we separated them into separate admissions as is common in DBS surgery. The prone position during stage 1 facilitates placement of the hippocampal depth electrodes. The second stage, generator placement and connection to the depth leads, is performed supine with the head turned. This is the approach we describe in this report.

The patient is induced under general endotracheal anesthesia on the transport stretcher. The back of the stretcher can be easily raised to facilitate placement of the Leksell frame, which we use for both head fixation and robot registration. The Leksell frame is assembled "backwards" so that the short fixation posts are alongside the curved nasal front piece and the long fixation posts are along the straight portion of the frame (**Figures 2A,B**). The frame is still applied with the short posts on the occipital aspect and the front posts on the frontal aspect of the head, but the reverse assembly of the frame puts the curved nasal piece over the occipital aspect.

There are two types of Leksell frame pins available. We use the pins with a female head, as this socket allows for robot registration. The frame pins thus serve as skull fiducials, allowing the accuracy of skull fiducial-based registration without the need for placement of separate fiducials screws. The long fixation posts are placed at slightly different lengths creating non-coplanar registration points (**Figures 2A,B**). Non-coplanar registration points are important to ensure that the registration algorithm arrives at a unique (i.e., correct) solution. After applying the

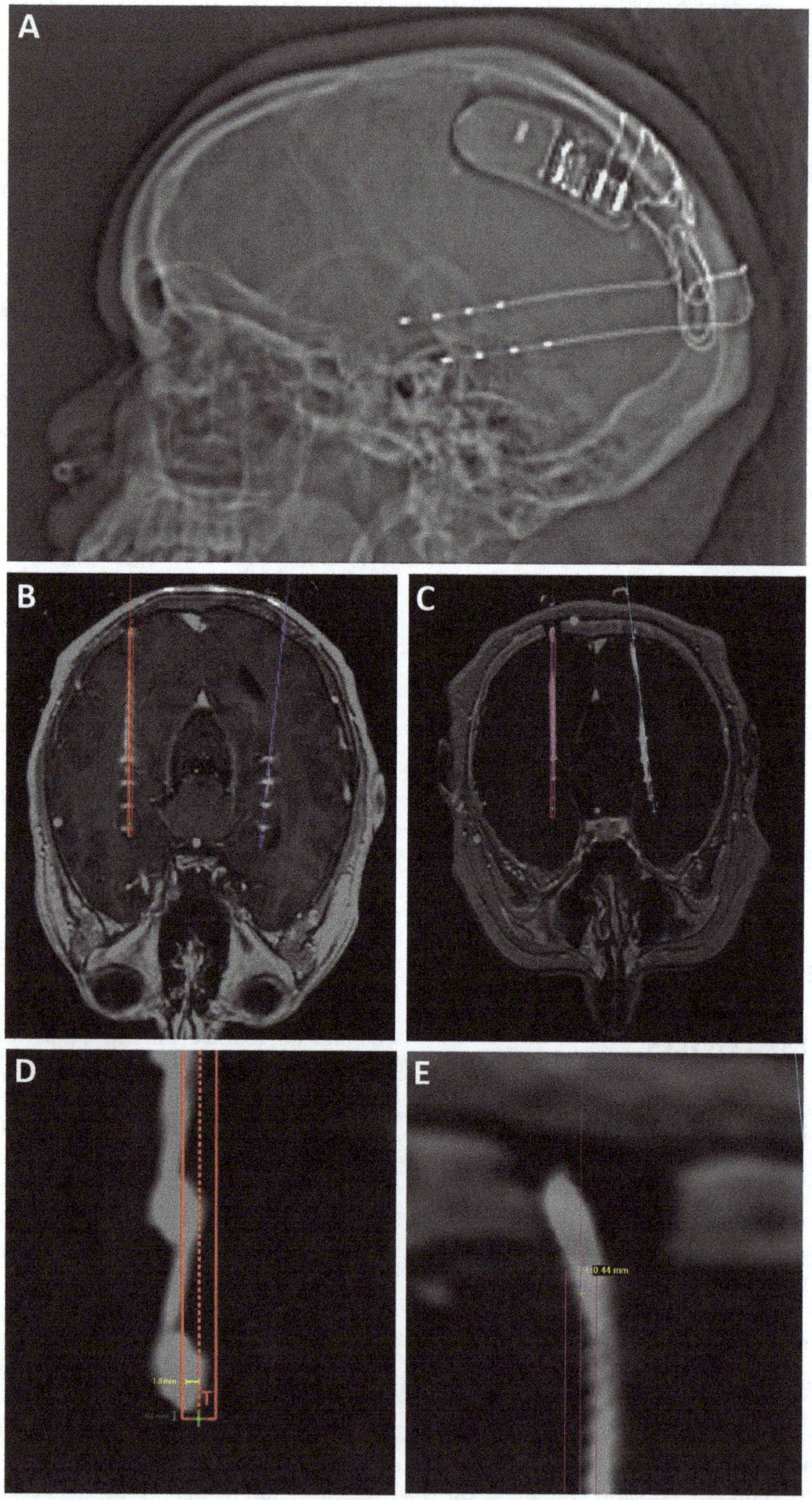

FIGURE 1 | (A) Scout x-ray showing lateral view after implantation of bilateral hippocampal RNS electrodes and RNS generator. **(B)** Intra-operative O-arm fluoroscopic CT projected over preoperative planning MRI is used to confirm target accuracy electrodes compared to operative plans (displayed in red and blue). **(C)** Post-operative CT projected over preoperative planning MRI was also used to confirm target accuracy in cases where O-arm fluoroscopic CT was not performed. **(D)** Radial target error (yellow line) was measured as the distance from the planned electrode target to the center of the actual electrode position. Depth target error (green) was measured as the difference in depth between the implanted electrode and the planned electrode tip measured along the trajectory of the implanted electrode. Positive values represent electrodes that were implanted past/deeper to target. Negative values represent electrodes that were implanted more shallow compared to target. **(E)** Radial entry point error was measured as the distance from the planned electrode entry point at the inner table of the skull to the center of the implanted electrode.

TABLE 1 | Patient demographics.

Patient number	Age	Duration of epilepsy (years)	Failed AEDs	Seizure frequency	Seizure onset zone	MRI findings	Aura	Semiology	Prior Surgery	RNS Implant
1	45–49	31	11	1–2/week	Left mesial temporal	L MTS	Fear, warmth	Staring, automatisms	Right ATL; VNS (removed)	L hippocampus; L temporal strip
2	60–64	43	4	1–3/week	Bilateral mesial temporal	Bilateral MTS	None	Slowed blinking; LOC; generalized convulsions	none	bilateral hippocampal
3	40–44	4	3	1–2/month	Left inferior temporal gyrus	L incomplete hippocampal inversion	Weird feeling	Alexia, aphasia, impaired awareness; GTC	none	L hippocampus; L anterior subtemporal strip
4	25–29	16	3	10–12/day	Left temporal	L MTS; tectal glioma	None	Left eye gaze, hand dystonia, amnesia, motor aphasia, oral automatisms	numerous surgeries for tumor and VP shunt	L hippocampus; L parahippocampus
5	30–34	4	4	1/week	Left mesial temporal	None	None	Loss of awareness, behavioral arrest	none	bilateral hippocampal
8	25–29	3	2	2/week	Bilateral mesial temporal	Possible small L temporal encephalocele	None	Growling noise; eyes roll back; body stiffening and shaking	none	bilateral hippocampal
6	60–64	23	12	1/week	Bilateral mesial temporal	None	Rotten meat smell	Salivation, behavioral arrest, lip smacking, confusion	none	bilateral hippocampal
7	55–59	37	5	1–2/week	Left mesial temporal	L MTS	Chills	Staring, right hand posturing, motor automatisms, head turn, LOC	none	bilateral hippocampal; L inferior temporal lobe strip
9	35–39	9	4	<1/month	Bilateral mesial temporal	L MTS	Bilateral arm tingling	Loss of awareness, vocalization, body shaking	none	bilateral hippocampal; L subtemporal strip
10	35–39	14	7	1–2/week	Bilateral mesial temporal	None	déjà vu	Staring, perseveration, bitter taste, altered awareness, orolingual automatisms	none	bilateral hippocampal

All patients had medically refractory epilepsy with seizure onset zone either in the left mesial temporal or bilateral mesial temporal regions. These patients were not considered to be candidates for resective or ablative surgeries after review at a multidisciplinary epilepsy conference. AED, antiepileptic drug; ATL, anterior temporal lobectomy; GTC, generalized tonic clonic; L, left; LOC, loss of consciousness; MTS, mesial temporal sclerosis; VNS, vagus nerve stimulator.

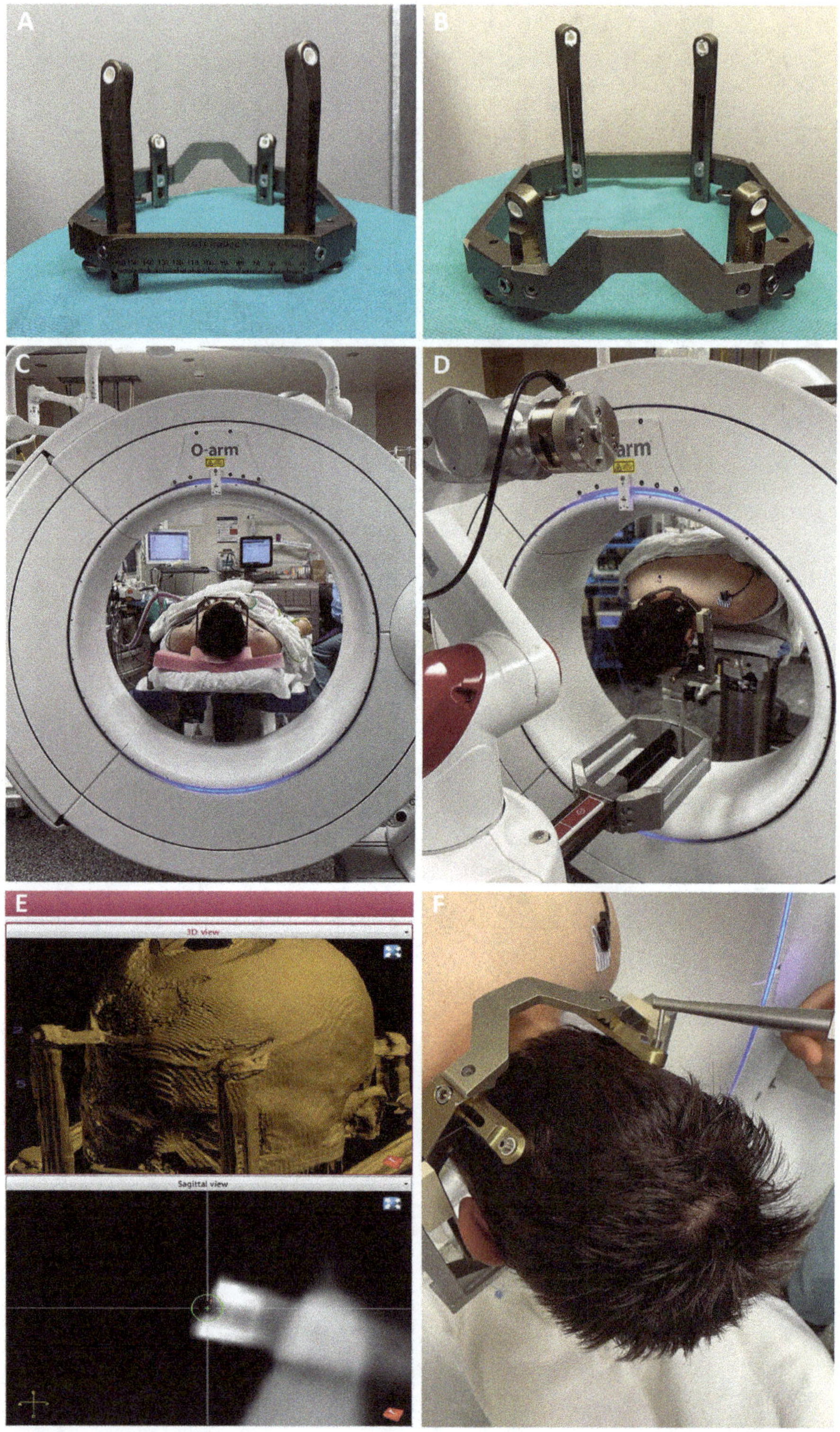

FIGURE 2 | (A,B) The Leksell frame is assembled opposite the traditional manner, with the short fixation posts flanking the curved nasal piece, and long fixation posts flanking the straight piece. Female fixation screws are used and serve as skull fiducials for robot registration after O-arm imaging. **(C)** After frame placement, the patient is initially positioned supine while still on the stretcher, with the head supported on a radiolucent plastic board, and a pre-operative O-arm image is obtained for registration to the pre-operative CT. **(D)** The patient is then flipped prone on gel rolls on the OR table, and the Leksell frame is affixed to the robot using the goalpost-shaped Leksell holder. The reverse orientation of the frame allows the three straight edges of the frame to fit within the beveled clamps of the Leksell holder, with the curved nasal piece over the occipital region. **(E)** Registration points are chosen on the merged fluoroscopic CT image including the frame. Four points are chosen, one for each frame pin, such that the registration marker sits in middle of the divot on the pin with its equator flush with the flat surface of the pin. **(F)** Registration is then performed using the ball-tip probe robot attachment.

frame, we place a radiolucent board under the stretcher mattress and slide the patient up so the head is on the board. The fluoroscopic CT system (O-arm O2, Medtronic, Minneapolis, MN, USA) is then positioned around the head, and we obtain the fluoroscopic CT including the frame in the field of view (**Figure 2C**). This process allows the acquisition of a suitable scan in the supine position, before flipping prone, and without metallic artifact. This fluoroscopic CT is then merged with the preoperative planning CT (1 mm axial cuts) on the ROSA robot.

The patient is then turned prone onto the OR table on gel rolls, and the frame is affixed to the "goalpost-shaped" ROSA Leksell holder (**Figure 2D**). This Leksell holder has fewer degrees of freedom than the Mayfield-style Leksell holder, making supine placement of occipital approach hippocampal depths difficult, but is extremely stable and sturdy. Once the frame is affixed, the OR table and robot are locked and should not be moved, as the head is affixed to the robot, and the body to the table. Ensuring that the bed control is off and the bed unplugged has been incorporated into our Time Out procedure.

Registration begins with choosing the registration points on the fluoroscopic CT (**Figure 2E**). The 3 mm diameter registration circle fits snugly within the divot of the frame pin, with little room for radial ambiguity. The depth ambiguity is reduced by choosing a depth that puts the equator of the registration circle at the flush surface of the frame pin. The surgeon then navigates the ball-tip registration attachment to each point and marks it (**Figure 2F**). Again, there is little room for laxity in the radial position for choosing this point given the close fit of the ball tip within the frame pin, and the depth position is chosen by placing the equator of the ball tip at the level of the surface of the pin. We strive for a registration error (root mean square, RMS) of <0.8 mm and are usually able to achieve <0.6 mm. After the subsequent verification step, we navigate to and mark the entry point(s). The fluoroscopic CT is then positioned over the patient to be draped in for intraoperative verification during the procedure. We plan for a $\sim$1 inch incision at each entry point and prep and drape these regions.

We create vertical linear incisions over the entry points and use a cutting burr to create small burr holes at each entry point. The burr hole can also be created with a twist-drill bit through the robot arm. If doing so, we recommend over-sizing the hole (e.g., with a 3.2 mm bit) in order to ensure that the cannula does not deflect off the bone edge. We use the 2.15 mm PEEK ROSA adapter attachment for the robot, which fits the slotted cannula (2.1 mm, Ad-Tech Medical Instrument Corporation, Oak Creek, WI, USA) that we use for electrode placement (**Figure 3A**). This slotted cannula is 190 mm in length, which is why each trajectory is defined as 190 mm long. In the "Axial Fast" mode within each trajectory, the robot arm and cannula can be quickly brought in and out to ensure that the burr hole is centered around the cannula as it is drilled. Because there are no frame coordinates to set and check between trajectories, a surgeon and assistant can work in parallel by handing the robot arm back and forth, thus greatly increasing efficiency in a bilateral case.

We pass monopolar cautery (set at 20) through the cannula to open the dura just around the cannula, thus minimizing CSF loss. With the robot arm at target, the slotted canula is advanced to full depth, placing it at target, and the inner stylet removed. Prior to placing the RNS (10 mm inter-contact spacing, NeuroPace Inc., Mountain View, CA, USA) depth lead, we mark it at three points: 190 and 200 mm, which flank the wide hub of the cannula, and the point corresponding to the outer table of the skull (measured on the robot, **Figure 3A**). Following placement of the lead into the cannula, the lead is bent out of the slot in the cannula, and the cannula is removed. The lead is held steady at the skull, visualizing the bottom pre-placed mark at the outer table. The lead stylet is then removed, and the robot arm is moved out of the way. At this point the only visual indication of depth is the mark at the outer table. The electrode is folded over and affixed to the skull with a "dog-bone" cranial plate, with a short cylinder of lead cap used as a shock absorber around the lead (**Figure 3B**). If using a smaller twist-drill burr hole, we recommend beveling the edge of the hole to prevent the sharp edge from damaging the lead over time. After placement of both leads, we obtain an intraoperative fluoroscopic CT, register it to the preoperative CT on the stereotactic plan, and verify lead location relative to the planned trajectory (**Figure 1B**). If accuracy is acceptable, we place temporary caps on the leads, mark them with our conventional marks to maintain laterality, and tunnel them subgaleally to the planned location of the RNS generator. The incisions are then irrigated and closed.

The stage 2 surgery is performed supine with the head turned. The RNS generator is placed using standard technique, typically in the right parietal area. Once the craniectomy is performed and the ferrule is secured, the previously tunneled leads are exposed and connected to the generator (**Figures 3C,D**). In some cases in our series, this stage 2 surgery followed immediately after the stage 1 surgery after re-positioning and re-prep/draping. In other cases, we separated the two stages with a 1 week interval, allowing the patient to go home between the stages, similar to the approach for DBS. In either case, we obtain a stereotactic head CT after stage 1 (if staged) or the whole procedure (if combined).

For comparison, we also briefly mention the supine method of placement used in our earlier cases. Notable differences are placing the Leksell frame in the usual front-facing orientation and using the Mayfield-style robot attachment to attach the frame to the robot. This arrangement allows better elevation and flexion of the head in order to produce an achievable angle for the occipital entry, but we found the operating position uncomfortable for drilling the burr hole and visualizing the cannula entry point on the dura. For these reasons we adopted the prone approach described above.

Analysis

Patient charts were retrospectively reviewed with institutional review board approval. Registration was performed using the automatic registration tool in the ROSA planning software and confirmed with manual inspection. All scans, including pre-operative planning MRI, intraoperative O-arm spins (**Figure 1B**), and post-operative CT scans (**Figure 1C**), were registered to a stereotactic pre-operative CT scan.

Radial target error (**Figure 1D**, yellow measurement) was measured as the distance from the planned electrode target to the

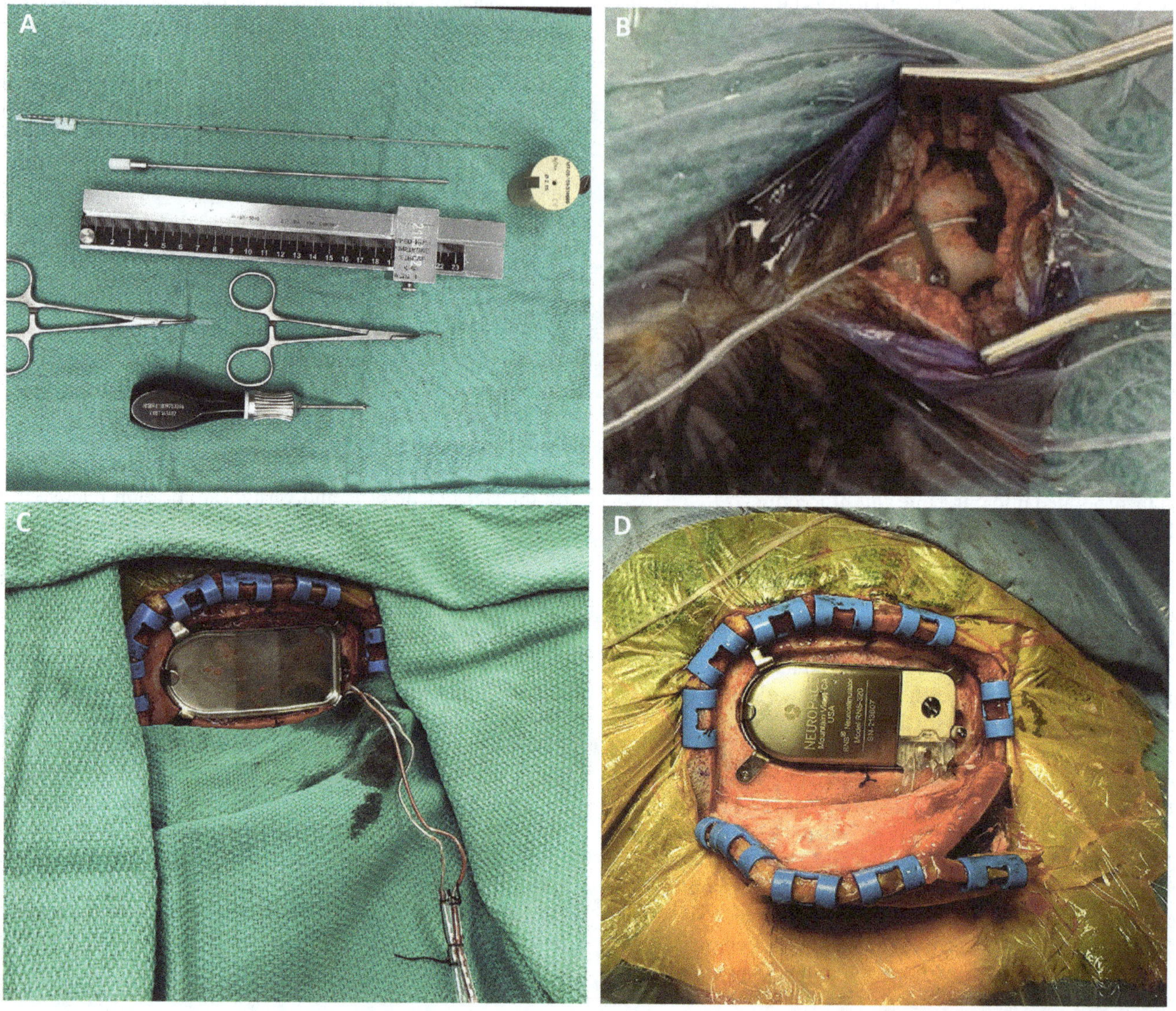

FIGURE 3 | (A) Required stereotactic equipment for the procedure: 2.15 mm PEEK ROSA adapter, 190 mm length slotted canula, RNS depth electrode, stereotactic ruler, bent cranial plate and cut segment of lead cap. The depth electrode is marked at three points: 190 and 200 mm, which flank the wide hub of the cannula, and the point corresponding to the outer table of the skull, measured on the stereotactic plan. This last point is important to mark, as it is the only one visible once the cannula is removed and the robot arm moved away. **(B)** After the electrode is inserted, a dog-bone cranial fixation miniplate is fastened to the skull to hold the electrode in place. We use the cut segment of the lead cap as a shock absorber around the lead. **(C)** After creating the craniectomy and securing the ferrule, the RNS leads are retrieved from their subgaleal position. **(D)** The RNS generator can be placed and connected to the depth electrodes. This can be performed either in the same prone position or after re-positioning the patient supine with the head turned.

center of the actual electrode position in the "Trajectory View" at the deepest point of the planned electrode trajectory. This measurement was confirmed on a "Cross-Sectional" view. Depth target error (**Figure 1D**, green measurement) was measured as the difference in depth between the actual electrode and the planned electrode tip, either deeper (positive) or more shallow (negative). Radial entry point error (**Figure 1E**) was measured as the distance from the planned electrode entry point at the inner table of the skull to the center of the actual electrode in the "Trajectory View." The trajectory length was measured as the distance from the inner table of the skull to the tip of the planned electrode position along the planned trajectory of the electrode.

Seizure outcomes were reported using proxy values obtained from the RNS recordings. We reviewed ECoG recordings and stimulations during the first month after the initial post-implantation detection stabilization. "Long events" identified by the RNS device were used as a proxy for seizure events, as home seizure diaries were not available for some of the patients implanted. All long events identified by the RNS were manually examined and only retained if they exhibited sustained rhythmic activity with epileptiform evolution. Daily activations were also recorded and averaged over the same month to calculate average daily activations. The same process was followed at 6 months after post-implantation detection stabilization and during the last month of available data (last follow-up). Responder rate was defined as the percentage of subjects with a 50% or greater reduction in seizure frequency.

All calculations were performed in Microsoft Excel. Reported errors were calculated using standard deviation. One-tailed unpaired t-test was used to determine statistical significance for comparisons of radial target error, radial entry point error, and CT vs. O-arm measurements. Two-tail unpaired t-test was used to determine statistical significance for the comparison of depth target error. We set statistical significance at $p < 0.01$ after Bonferroni correction for multiple comparisons ($p < 0.05/4$; $m = 4$). Linear correlation between trajectory length and radial target error was calculated using the Pearson correlation coefficient.

RESULTS

Ten consecutive patients who underwent robotic RNS hippocampal depth electrode implantation over 16 months were retrospectively included in this study. All ten patients' original implantation plans were available for review, totaling 18 depth electrodes. The locations of 8 electrodes (five patients) were measured with post-operative CT. The locations of 10 electrodes (five patients) were measured with intra-operative O-arm. Eight electrodes across four patients were implanted in patients positioned prone, and ten electrodes across six patients were implanted in supine procedures.

Electrode Placement

Electrode placement results are compiled in **Table 2**. The mean radial error across all patients was 1.4 ± 0.9 mm. Mean radial target error for the prone position was 0.8 ± 0.3 mm, significantly less than the 1.9 ± 0.9 mean radial target error in the supine position ($p = 0.002$). The mean depth error across all patients was past target by 2.9 ± 3.6 mm. There was no significant difference between the prone position (deep by 2.7 ± 2.3 mm) and the supine position (deep by 3.0 ± 3.8 mm, $p = 0.31$). The mean entry point radial error across all patients was 0.9 ± 0.7 mm with no significant difference between the prone position (0.8 ± 0.7 mm) and the supine position (0.9 ± 0.7 mm, $p = 0.39$). There was not a strong correlation between trajectory length and radial target error across all electrodes ($r = 0.26$). There was no significant difference between radial target error measured by intraoperative O-arm (1.2 ± 0.9 mm) vs. post-operative CT (1.6 ± 0.8 mm, $p = 0.14$).

Seizure Outcomes

Eight of ten patients had enough data after a baseline recording period to report seizure outcome based on RNS recordings and stimulations (**Table 3**). The two patients who did not have sufficient data recently had their detection parameters changed. Median time from implantation to stabilization of detection was 1.9 months (range 0.6–9.6 months). Median follow-up time after detection stabilization was 7.5 months (range 3.4–10.7 months).

Mean seizure frequency reduction at last follow-up was 26% (available in eight patients). Five patients (62.5%) had reduction in seizure frequency, and three of these (37.5%) had ≥50% reduction in seizure frequency at last follow-up. Mean reduction

TABLE 2 | Electrode measurements across all patients.

Patient number	Electrode number	Electrode location	Position	Electrode location confirmation	Radial target error	Depth error	Entry point radial error	Trajectory length
1	1	L HC	Supine	CT	2.7	0.0	0.5	92.6
2	1	R HC	Supine	CT	1.8	3.7	1.8	86.0
	2	L HC			2.4	3.3	0.4	88.9
3	1	L HC	Supine	CT	0.8	4.4	0.5	102.9
4	1	L HC	Supine	O-arm	3.0	5.8	0.1	97.4
	2	L para HC			2.7	−1.7	0.0	93.0
5	1	R HC	Supine	CT	0.4	−0.9	1.0	102.2
	2	L HC			2.1	−6.3	1.1	103.5
8	1	R HC	Supine	CT	1.0	−0.8	1.9	98.5
	2	L HC			2.0	−3.2	1.8	99.1
6	1	R HC	Prone	O-arm	0.7	−2	0.5	83.3
	2	L HC			0.9	−2.9	2.1	83.5
7	1	R HC	Prone	O-arm	0.3	5.3	0.2	85.7
	2	L HC			0.6	−1.2	0.9	87.7
9	1	R HC	Prone	O-arm	0.6	−1.8	0.5	89.8
	2	L HC			1.1	−7	0.0	92.9
10	1	R HC	Prone	O-arm	1.2	−0.4	0.8	83.1
	2	L HC			0.7	−1	1.5	81.9

All measurements in mm. Electrodes placed in the prone position had smaller radial target error compared to those placed in the supine position. HC, hippocampus.

TABLE 3 | Seizure outcomes at last follow-up.

Patient number	Monthly long episodes at first month	Average daily activations during first month	Monthly long episodes at last follow-up	% reduction in monthly long episodes at last follow-up	Average daily activations at last follow-up	% change in daily activations at last follow-up	Last follow-up (months)
1	19	1,300	16	16%	900	31%	10.7
2	32	2,000	41	−28%	2,100	−5%	7.4
3	4	1,250	2	50%	500	60%	7.6
4	43	1,000	52	−21%	1,500	−50%	9.0
5	1	240	0	100%	35	85%	9.4
8	0	800	3	N/A	500	38%	5.7
9	12	150	0	100%	200	−33%	4.6
10	9	1,000	12	−33%	1,250	−25%	3.4

In our preliminary short-term follow-up (median 7.5 months), mean seizure frequency reduction at last follow-up was 26%. Patients 6 and 7 had insufficient data for seizure outcome collection.

in the number of average daily activations at last follow-up was 9%. Four patients (50%) had a reduction in average daily activations at 6 months.

There were no complications, including no cases of intracranial hemorrhage, infection, or hardware failures.

DISCUSSION

This study describes the evolution and current details of our workflow for robotic stereotactic implantation and intraoperative image-guided verification of occipital approach mesial temporal depth electrode placement for RNS therapy. Robotic stereotaxy assists in accurate placement of hippocampal depth electrodes with submillimeter precision, especially when the patient is positioned prone, according to our data. Intraoperative image-based verification allows the surgeon to confirm that the electrode is in the intended target using volumetric imaging prior to leaving the OR.

Our initial robotic workflow, adopted from our frame-based workflow for both hippocampal RNS leads and for laser amygdalohippocampotomy (4, 5), used the slouched semi-sitting position for occipital-approach mesial temporal trajectories. As mentioned above, the Mayfield attachment of the robot allows this position, but it is fairly uncomfortable for the surgeon and also makes visualizing the full interior of the burr hole more difficult. This circumferential visualization is important for ensuring that the cannula is not deflecting off the edge of the burr hole or the edge of dura. Because the angle of the cannula is horizontal, it may also be more likely to deflect off trajectory due to gravity if there is any play in the adapter holding the cannula. All these factors may introduce errors in stereotactic accuracy. Additional errors in this position can be introduced secondary to cerebrospinal fluid egress since occipital burr holes are in a dependent position.

For all these reasons, we have shifted to the prone position. The setup requires the minor hassle of prone positioning, but the surgeon's comfort, easy view of the burr hole and dural entry point, and vertical trajectory relative to the ground are superior features. As we show here, this position also seems to produce better radial accuracy. Depth accuracy was worse than radial accuracy and did not differ between the positions. We suspect that the greater depth accuracy error is related to the method of securing the lead. Rather than clamping it in place *in situ*, as is typically done during DBS procedures using a lead securing system in the burr hole cover, we visualize a mark and secure the lead to the skull with a cranial miniplate. This method likely leads to slight depth movement of the lead and therefore the larger measured error. Our experience with robotic DBS demonstrates a significantly lower depth error, further implicating the lead securing technique as the cause of the increased error. The RNS depth electrode kit does provide a DBS-style burr hole cover that would allow *in situ* securing, should the surgeon want to try to reduce this depth error. We plan a trajectory spanning 26–30 mm of amygdala and hippocampal tissue, a distance that matches the 32 mm span of contacts across the wide-spaced (10 mm inter-contact distance) depth lead. Thus, a depth error of 2–3 mm is not critical. We feel that the much more important feature is a low radial error, which reduces the chance of being off trajectory enough to hit vascular structures that the trajectory was planned to avoid.

Prior reports of robotic stereotactic implantation for DBS devices have achieved submillimeter accuracy with average radial target errors of 0.86 mm (2, 3), suggesting that for DBS surgery robotic stereotaxy has at least equivalent accuracy compared to frame-based stereotaxy. Direct comparison of robotic *vs.* frame-based stereotaxy has also suggested that robotic stereotaxy has lower mean radial target error of 0.76 $\pm$ 0.37 mm compared to 1.11 $\pm$ 0.59 mm for frame-based implantation (6). Prior reports for robotic-assisted occipital-approach mesial temporal RNS depth electrode accuracy have not been as positive, with median radial error over 2.18 mm (7). We improved our initial mean radial target error of 1.9 $\pm$ 0.9 mm achieved in the supine position with better intraoperative ergonomics and positioning, decreasing it to 0.8 $\pm$ 0.3 mm with the prone technique described above.

The incorporation of intraoperative fluoroscopic CT also represents an important improvement in our workflow. It allows us to head fix and register the patient without leaving the OR for a CT scan, reducing procedural time and increasing efficiency. Draping the scanner into the field also allows easy and rapid acquisition of a volumetric image set to verify the location of the lead. Just as image verification prior to leaving the OR is becoming an essential feature of DBS procedures (8–10), we propose the same standard for other stereotactic procedures such as RNS depth electrode placement.

There are several advantages to robotic stereotactic procedures over using a conventional frame. Entry points can be easily marked prior to draping, allowing a smaller hair shave. Although setup may take slightly longer because of the registration process, the time savings during the procedure more than makes up for the setup time cost. The robot arm can move back and forth between the two trajectories of a bilateral implant, allowing the surgeon and assistant to work simultaneously. Resetting the five coordinates for a frame requires serial rather than parallel effort. Not having to set and check these coordinates also reduces the chance for human error and allows trainees to play a greater role, as the surgeon does not have to worry about coordinate errors. On top of these advantages, robotic procedures also do not sacrifice accuracy, as demonstrated here and by several others (2, 3).

One disadvantage to the prone lead placement is the slightly more awkward position for generator placement. It can either be placed in the same procedure, or the patient can be re-positioned supine with the head turned for a more comfortable position. In some cases, we staged the procedures, with prone lead placement in one procedure and supine generator placement and attachment to the leads in a separate procedure 1–2 weeks later. Logistical reasons such as OR time or equipment availability concerns usually drove the choice for staged procedures. The current additional burden of COVID-19 testing required before all elective surgical procedures favors a single-stage procedure.

Reported seizure outcomes are preliminary and include small sample size and relatively short follow-up duration. A 67.9% median reduction in seizure frequency, along with 64.5% responder rate, has been reported in patients with bilateral onset mesial temporal epilepsy observed 2–6 years after bilateral hippocampal RNS (11). Our observed median reduction in seizure frequency (26%) and responder rate (37.5%) are consistent with the 6–8 month outcomes in the RNS pivotal trial (12) and remain reassuring given observations that seizure reduction and response rates improve significantly over time with neurostimulation (13).

While most RNS outcomes are reported based on seizure diaries, we report results based on electrocorticographic "long events" that were detected and recorded automatically by the RNS device and then manually reviewed for accuracy. Long events were used for analysis because seizure diaries were not available for a few of the patients included in this study due to the short follow-up period. There is a strong correlation between reduction in patient-reported events and automatically recorded long events, however the relationship is not one-to-one (14). Long events generally overestimate patient-reported events. Large discrepancies between long events and patient-reported events have been reported (15), which introduces a degree of uncertainty in our results. However, it remains reassuring that our seizure response rates are consistent with other reported short-term results.

This study has limitations. The number of patients included is low, limiting the generalizability of the results. Furthermore, since our initial depth electrodes were placed in the supine position, with later electrodes placed in the prone position, a learning curve such as found by Faraji et al. (3) could account for some of the improvement in radial target error. Additionally, despite manual confirmation, errors in image registration and frame-robot registration could affect our analysis. The post-operative follow-up duration is relatively short, and we will continue to monitor these patients.

CONCLUSION

Robotic stereotaxy enables submillimeter radial target accuracy for implantation of occipital -approach hippocampal RNS depth electrodes. In our experience, accuracy is better when the patient is positioned prone compared to supine slouched semi-sitting positioning; However, more studies with larger cohorts of subjects are required before generalizing the findings reported in this study. In addition to its excellent accuracy, robotic placement of these depth leads improves ergonomic comfort, increases operative efficiency by allowing parallel bilateral operation, and reduces the chance for human error associated with frame coordinates.

AUTHOR CONTRIBUTIONS

PK and SS: drafted manuscript, critically revised manuscript, data collection, data analysis, and conceptualization. NG, JT, MP, AK, and BS: data collection, data analysis, conceptualization, and critically revised manuscript. JG, AM, ZH, PV, JC, and VK: data collection and analysis, conceptualization and interpretation of data, and critically revised manuscript. All authors contributed to the article and approved the submitted version.

ACKNOWLEDGMENTS

The authors would like to thank Stephen Cleboski for his help in the collection of seizure outcome data.

REFERENCES

1. Fomenko A, Serletis D. Robotic stereotaxy in cranial neurosurgery: a qualitative systematic review. *Neurosurgery.* (2017) 83:642–50. doi: 10.1093/neuros/nyx576
2. Liu L, Mariani SG, De Schlichting E, Grand S, Lefranc M, Seigneuret E, et al. Frameless ROSA® robot-assisted lead implantation for deep brain stimulation: technique and accuracy. *Oper Neurosurg.* (2019) 19:57–64. doi: 10.1093/ons/opz320
3. Faraji AH, Kokkinos V, Sweat JC, Crammond DJ, Richardson RM. Robotic-assisted stereotaxy for deep brain stimulation lead implantation in awake patients. *Oper Neurosurg.* (2020) 19:444–52. doi: 10.1093/ons/opaa029
4. Youngerman BE, Oh JY, Anbarasan D, Billakota S, Casadei CH, Corrigan EK, et al. Laser ablation is effective for temporal lobe epilepsy with and without mesial temporal sclerosis if hippocampal seizure onsets are localized by stereoelectroencephalography. *Epilepsia.* (2018) 59:595–606. doi: 10.1111/epi.14004
5. Karas PJ, Sheth SA, Yoshor D. Epilepsy: mesial temporal. In: Pouratian N,

Sheth SA, editors. *Stereotactic and Functional Neurosurgery: Principles and Applications.* Cham: Springer International Publishing (2020). p. 339–67.

6. Neudorfer C, Hunsche S, Hellmich M, El Majdoub F, Maarouf M. Comparative study of robot-assisted versus conventional frame-based deep brain stimulation stereotactic neurosurgery. *Stereotact Funct Neurosurg.* (2018) 96:327–34. doi: 10.1159/000494736
7. Chan AY, Mnatsakanyan L, Sazgar M, Sen-Gupta I, Lin JJ, Hsu FPK, et al. Accuracy and efficacy for robotic assistance in implanting responsive neurostimulation device electrodes in bilateral mesial temporal lobe epilepsy. *Oper Neurosurg.* (2017) 14:267–72. doi: 10.1093/ons/opx085
8. Burchiel KJ, McCartney S, Lee A, Raslan AM. Accuracy of deep brain stimulation electrode placement using intraoperative computed tomography without microelectrode recording. *J Neurosurg.* (2013) 119:301–6. doi: 10.3171/2013.4.JNS122324
9. Mirzadeh Z, Chapple K, Lambert M, Dhall R, Ponce FA. Validation of CT-MRI fusion for intraoperative assessment of stereotactic accuracy in DBS surgery. *Mov Disord.* (2014) 29:1788–95. doi: 10.1002/mds.26056
10. Mirzadeh Z, Chapple K, Lambert M, Evidente VG, Mahant P, Ospina MC, et al. Parkinson's disease outcomes after intraoperative CT-guided "asleep" deep brain stimulation in the globus pallidus internus. *J Neurosurg JNS.* (2016) 124:902–7. doi: 10.3171/2015.4.JNS1550
11. Geller EB, Skarpaas TL, Gross RE, Goodman RR, Barkley GL, Bazil CW, et al. Brain-responsive neurostimulation in patients with medically intractable mesial temporal lobe epilepsy. *Epilepsia.* (2017) 58:994–1004. doi: 10.1111/epi.13740
12. Heck CN, King-Stephens D, Massey AD, Nair DR, Jobst BC, Barkley GL, et al. Two-year seizure reduction in adults with medically intractable partial onset epilepsy treated with responsive neurostimulation: final results of the RNS system pivotal trial. *Epilepsia.* (2014) 55:432–41. doi: 10.1111/epi.12534
13. Nair DR, Morrell MJ. Nine-year prospective safety and effectiveness outcomes from the long-term treatment trial of the RNS® system. In: *American Epilepsy Society 2018 Annual Meeting (New Orleans, Louisiana), Abstract 2.075.* (2018). Available online at: https://www.aesnet.org/meetings_events/annual_meeting_abstracts/view/502690 (Accessed November 30, 2018).
14. Skarpaas TL, Tcheng TK, Morrell MJ. Clinical and electrocorticographic response to antiepileptic drugs in patients treated with responsive stimulation. *Epilepsy Behav.* (2018) 83:192–200. doi: 10.1016/j.yebeh.2018.04.003
15. Chen H, Koubeissi M. Seizure occurrences: patient report, scalp EEG, and RNS electrocorticography findings. *J Clin Neurophysiol.* (2020) 37:306–9. doi: 10.1097/WNP.0000000000000684

3

Phase Lag Analyses on Ictal Scalp Electroencephalography may Predict Outcomes of Corpus Callosotomy for Epileptic Spasms

Masayoshi Oguri[1], Tohru Okanishi[2,3], Sotaro Kanai[2,3], Shimpei Baba[3], Mitsuyo Nishimura[4], Kaoru Ogo[1], Takashi Himoto[1], Kazuo Okanari[5], Yoshihiro Maegaki[2], Hideo Enoki[3] and Ayataka Fujimoto[6]*

[1] Department of Medical Technology, Kagawa Prefectural University of Health Sciences, Takamatsu, Japan, [2] Division of Child Neurology, Faculty of Medicine, Institute of Neurological Sciences, Tottori University, Yonago, Japan, [3] Department of Child Neurology, Seirei-Hamamatsu General Hospital, Hamamatsu, Japan, [4] Department of Clinical Laboratory, University of Tsukuba Hospital, Tsukuba, Japan, [5] Department of Pediatrics, Faculty of Medicine, Oita University, Yufu, Japan, [6] Comprehensive Epilepsy Center, Seirei-Hamamatsu General Hospital, Hamamatsu, Japan

Correspondence:
Tohru Okanishi
t.okanishi@tottori-u.ac.jp;
okanishipediatrics@gmail.com

Objective: We aimed to clarify the patterns of ictal power and phase lag among bilateral hemispheres on scalp electroencephalography (EEG) recorded pre-operatively during epileptic spasms (ESs) and the correlation with the outcomes following corpus callosotomy.

Methods: We enrolled 17 patients who underwent corpus callosotomy for ESs before 20 years of age. After corpus callosotomy, seven patients did not experience further ESs (favorable outcome group), and the remaining 10 patients had ongoing ESs (unfavorable outcome group). We used pre-operative scalp EEG data from monopolar montages using the average reference. The relative power spectrum (PS), ictal power laterality (IPL) among the hemispheres, and phase lag, calculated by the cross-power spectrum (CPS) among symmetrical electrodes (i.e., F3 and F4), were analyzed in the EEG data of ESs from 143 pre-operative scalp video-EEG records. Analyses were conducted separately in each frequency band from the delta, theta, alpha, beta, and gamma range. We compared the means of those data in each patient between favorable and unfavorable outcome groups.

Results: Among all frequency bands, no significant differences were seen in the individual mean relative PSs in the favorable and unfavorable outcome group. Although the mean IPLs in each patient tended to be high in the unfavorable outcome group, no significant differences were found. The mean CPSs in the delta, theta, and gamma frequency bands were significantly higher in the unfavorable than in the favorable outcome group. Using the Youden index, the optimal cutoff points of those mean CPS values for unfavorable outcomes were 64.00 in the delta band (sensitivity: 100%, specificity: 80%), 74.20 in the theta band (100, 80%), and 82.05 in the gamma band (100, 80%). Subanalyses indicated that those CPS differences originated from pairs of symmetrical electrodes in the bilateral frontal and temporal areas.

Significance: Ictal power and laterality of the ictal power in each frequency band were not associated with the outcomes of CC; however, the phase lags seen in the delta, theta, and gamma frequency bands were larger in the unfavorable than in the favorable outcome group. The phase lags may predict outcomes of CC for ESs on pre-surgical scalp-ictal EEGs.

Keywords: corpus callosotomy, cross-frequency analysis, electroencephaloagraphy (EEG), epileptic spasms (ES), phase lag analysis, computer analysis, pre-surgical evaluation of epilepsy

INTRODUCTION

Epileptic spasms (ESs) are seizures leading to muscular contraction, typically involving the axial muscles and proximal limb segments (1); they appear mainly in patients with West syndrome. The patterns of electroencephalography (EEG) and electromyography (EMG) activity observed in these spasms are similar (2). Ictal EEG findings in these patients comprise three contiguous phases: (1) 15- to 20-Hz spindle-like fast activity in posterior areas, (2) diffuse polyphasic delta/theta waves, and (3) electrodecremental activity (1, 3). Diffuse polyphasic delta/theta waves occur in 100%, and electrodecremental activity occurs in 70% of patients with ESs (4). Ictal EMG findings in these patients have rhombus or diamond shapes. When electroencephalographic/video monitoring first came into clinical use, several studies investigated ictal EEG patterns of ESs, including isolated spindle-like activity, high-amplitude slow wave, the spindle-like activity followed by the slow wave, and decremental activity, which follows the slow wave (1). In recent studies, computer-based frequency analysis has been adapted to estimate the ictal-scalp EEG of ESs. The scalp EEG data of ESs showed components of wide frequencies from delta to high gamma bands, and the coupling of high gamma and slow wave EEG components associated with the response to medical treatment (5).

Corpus callosotomy (CC) is a valuable palliative surgical option for patients with generalized seizures with diffuse or multifocal epileptic discharges (6, 7). Some reports have indicated that CC exerts beneficial effects in patients with ESs (8–11). Taking the results of these studies collectively, ESs were eliminated after CC in 42 of 87 patients. Previous studies have attempted to elucidate the prognostic factors following CC for ESs, finding good prognostic factors to include the absence of imaging abnormalities, normal development at the time of surgery, no background etiology, and performance of total callosotomy (11–15). A developmental delay before the onset of epilepsy has been shown to be associated with the worst outcomes following CC for ESs in West syndrome (9). Although electrophysiological factors that predict the outcome of CC for ESs were previously unknown, we recently found symmetrical ictal slow waves during the emergence of ESs to be associated with good outcomes following CC (16). In this study, three asymmetrical indices were identified: interhemispheric delay of negative peaks, interhemispheric ratio of amplitude for the highest positive peak, and interhemispheric ratio of slow wave duration. However, the study did not include the analyses for ictal waves faster than alpha rhythms, and computer-based frequency analyses are necessary to identify more objective and detailed associations between interhemispheric brain activity and the effectiveness of CC.

The aim of the current ictal EEG study was to use computer-based quantitative analysis to clarify the power of ictal period, laterality of ictal power, and phase lag among bilateral hemispheres in the variable frequency bands.

MATERIALS AND METHODS

Patients

The studies involving human participants were reviewed and approved by the Seirei Hamamatsu General Hospital and Tottori University Hospital Clinical Research Review Committees. We retrospectively collected patients' clinical data from medical charts and reviewed the video-EEG recordings. Written informed consent to participate in this study was provided by the participants' legal guardian/next of kin.

Seventeen patients (female: 2; male: 15) with epilepsy were screened from patients admitted to the Seirei-Hamamatsu General Hospital between 2010 and 2017. The inclusion criteria for this study were the same as those in our previous study (16), which were as follows: (1) patients undergoing CC between January 2008 and December 2017 at the Seirei-Hamamatsu General Hospital, (2) CC performed before the age of 20 years, (3) the patient's main seizure type was ES, (4) the patient received ictal EEG recordings prior to CC, and (5) a follow-up period following CC of more than 6 months. We defined ES as a seizure (1) leading to contractions in axial muscles, (2) presenting with ictal EEGs containing polyphasic high-voltage delta/theta waves, and (3) presenting with an ictal electromyogram showing rhombus or diamond shapes. We excluded patients with inappropriate EEG recordings, such as those with misplaced EEG electrodes or serious surgical complications.

Clinical Profiles

We reviewed the patients' clinical profiles, including the sex, age at epilepsy onset, seizure types prior to CC, classification of epilepsy or epilepsy syndrome prior to CC, total number of antiepileptic drugs (AEDs) prescribed before CC, frequency of ESs, etiology, age at CC, procedures for CC, and follow-up period.

The seizure outcomes of ESs after CC were assessed based on the Engel's classification at the last follow-up. We classified the patients into a favorable outcome group (seizure free = Engel classification I) and an unfavorable outcome (residual seizures = Engel classifications II to IV).

Scalp Video-EEG Recordings

Scalp video-EEGs were performed using NicoletOne or BMSI6000 (Natus Medical Incorporated, WI) for patients 1–4, 6–9, and 11–16, and Neurofax (Nihon-Kohden, Japan) for patients 5, 10, and 17. EEG was sampled at 256 Hz (patients 3, 8, 12, and 16), 400 Hz (patients 1, 2, 4, 7, 11, 14, and 15), 500 Hz (patients 5, 10, and 17), 512 Hz (patients 6 and 13), and 1,024 Hz (patient 9). Electrodes were placed according to the international 10/20 system, using at least 16 EEG channels (Fp1, Fp2, F3, F4, C3, Cz, C4, P3, P4, O1, O2, F7, F8, T3, T4, T5, and T6). The ground electrode was set attached to the frontal pole (Fpz). Electromyogram (EMG) electrodes were placed on both deltoid muscles.

Quantitative EEG Analysis

Selection of Ictal EEG, Time Window, and Electrodes for the Analyses

We visually reviewed the video-EEG records, and selected ES based on the ictal EEG change of polyphasic delta or theta waves with EMG activities of rhombus or diamond shapes, coincidently occurring with clinical muscular contraction in the neck, shoulder, and/or body trunk on video recording.

Initially, the ictal record was identified visually by each muscular contraction on video and EMG recording. Then, we reviewed the ictal EEG records of polyphasic delta or theta waves, which coincided with the muscular contractions. We excluded the records that detected physiological (muscle, movement, cardiac, tongue movement, and eye movement) or non-physiological (line noise, electrode artifacts, and other equipment) artifacts.

We used the EEG data of ictal polyphasic slow waves, using the average reference (**Figure 1**). The EEG data, which were mainly preceding, coinciding with or preceding ictal muscle contractions, and presented the typical negative-positive-negative waveform were visually selected from each record. For the visual review of EEG, the sensitivity was set at 10 μV/mm with low cut and high filter of 0.5 and 70 Hz for NicoletOne or BMSI6000 and 1.6 and 60 Hz for Neurofax, respectively. We set the trigger point (0 s) for the window of EEG analysis as the start of the negative peak. Focal spasms were defined as the ES with apparently asymmetrical or asynchronous among the movements of bilateral extremities on the video, or twice or more different amplitudes of bilateral EMG.

For the computer-based analyses, we used the EEG data with monopolar montages (Fp1, Fp2, F3, F4, C3, C4, P3, P4, O1, O2, F7, F8, T3, T4, T5, and T6), using the average reference. The EEG data were calculated using MATLAB plug-in for EEGLAB. The frequency bands were classified into delta (0.5–3.9 Hz), theta (4.0–7.9 Hz), alpha (8.0–12.9 Hz), beta (13.0–29.9 Hz), and gamma (30.0–79.9 Hz) bands.

Analysis for Relative Power Spectrums

We initially analyzed the powers of each ictal EEG by individual frequency band. For the quantitative analysis, the relative power spectrum (PS) was calculated using the Welch's method with a Hamming window, for frequencies between 0.5 and 79.9 Hz. We used the EEG data with monopolar montages (Fp1, Fp2, F3, F4, C3, C4, P3, P4, O1, O2, F7, F8, T3, T4, T5, and T6), using the average as reference. The PS was calculated using MATLAB plug-in for EEGLAB. First, we analyzed and averaged PS from −0 and 500 ms on each electrode in each frequency band. The frequency bands were then classified into delta (0.5–3.9 Hz), theta (4.0–7.9 Hz), alpha (8.0–12.9 Hz), beta (13.0–29.9 Hz), and gamma (30.0–79.9 Hz) bands.

We first calculated the relative PS on each electrode during an ictal EEG. Second, the relative PSs among all electrodes were averaged for each ictal EEG (mean relative PS *per seizure*). Finally, we calculated the mean of "the mean relative PSs *per seizure*" for all ictal EEGs per patient (mean relative PS in each patient). In these analyses, we separately calculated the values by each frequency band.

Analysis for Laterality of the Ictal Relative PS (Ictal Power Laterality)

We intended to identify the differences in the EEG PS among each pair of symmetrical electrodes. We defined "ictal power laterality (IPL)" of each ictal EEG in this study using the following formula:

$$IPL = \frac{\textit{The higher relative PS value (on the right or left hemisphere)}}{\textit{The lower relative PS value (on the other electrode)}}$$

For example, if a patient had a relative PS of 0.41 dB on Fp1 and 0.64 dB on Fp2 in the delta band during an ictal EEG, the result of IPL among the pair of Fp1 and Fp2 would be 0.64/0.41 = 1.57. We first calculated the IPL of each pair of symmetrical electrodes (Fp1 vs. Fp2, F3 vs. F4, C3 vs. C4, P3 vs. P4, O1 vs. O2, F7 vs. F8, T3 vs. T4, and T5 vs. T6) during each ictal EEG. Subsequently, we calculated the mean IPL of all pairs of symmetrical electrodes during an ictal EEG (mean IPL *per seizure*) and then calculated the mean of "the mean IPLs *per seizure*" for all ictal EEGs per patient (mean IPL in each patient). In these analyses, we separately calculated these values by each frequency band.

Analysis for Cross-Power Spectrum

The cross-power spectrum (CPS) estimates the degrees of the phase lag of two discrete-time signals x and y, using the Welch's averaged and modified periodogram method of spectral estimation. We used the same data selected for the PS analysis to calculate the CPS. We calculated the CPS using MATLAB software using cross-power spectrum density. The CPS is the distribution of power per unit frequency, and is defined as:

$$Pxy(f) = \sum_{m=-\infty}^{\infty} Rxy\,(m)\, e^{-i\omega t}$$

The cross-correlation sequence is defined as:

$$Rxy\,(m) = E\left\{x_{n+m}y*_{n}\right\} = E\left\{x_{n}y_{n-m}\right\},$$

where x_n and y_n are jointly stationary random processes, $-\infty < n < \infty$, $-\infty < n < \infty$, and $E\{\cdot\}$ is the expected value operator.

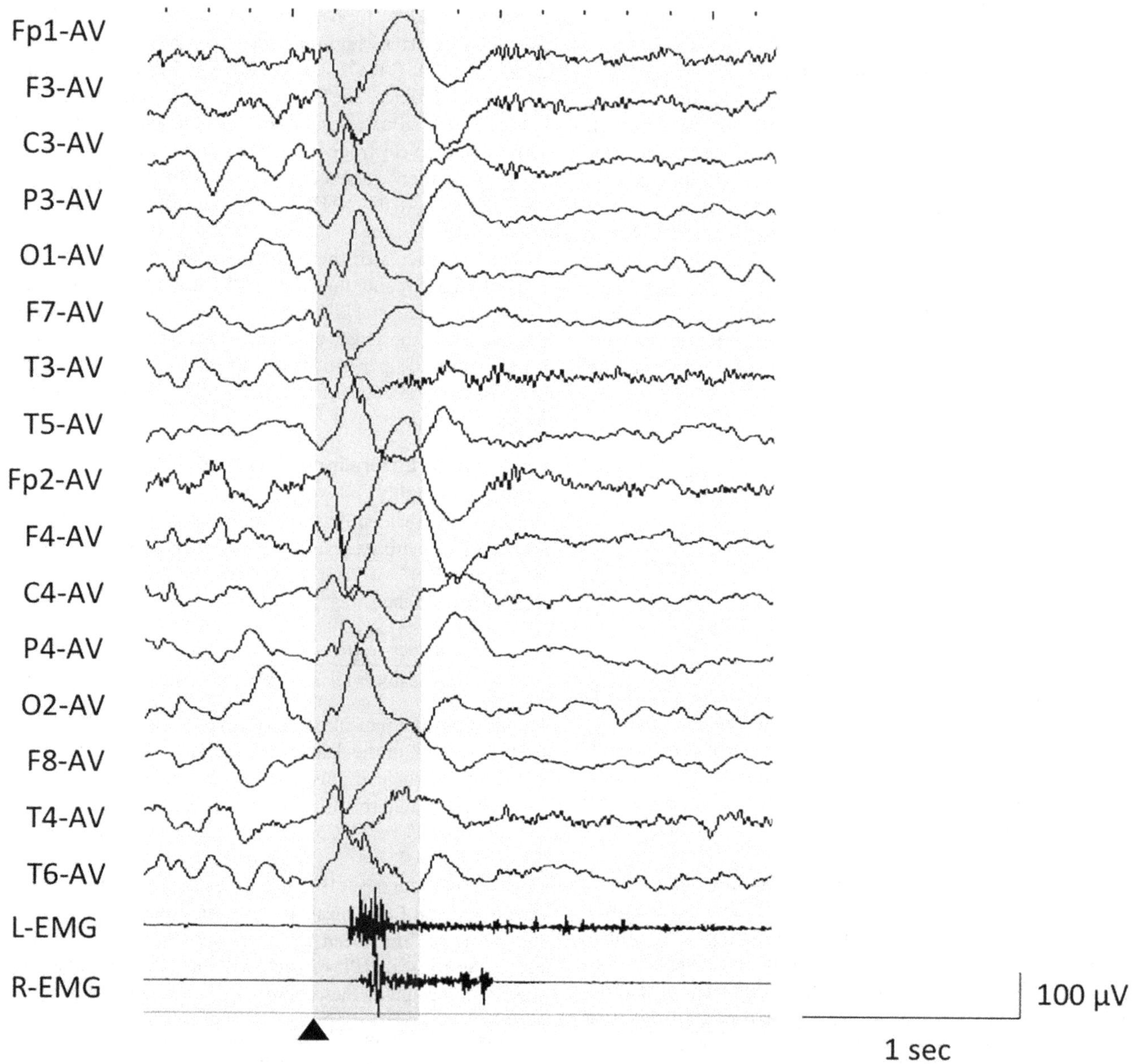

FIGURE 1 | Electroencephalography (EEG) example of epileptic spasms in monopolar montages of average reference and EEG analysis window. We used the EEG data between the trigger point (0 s, black triangle) and 500 ms (purple window) for the computer analyses.

The values of CPS represented ranged from 0 to 180 degrees on each frequency band. First, we calculated the absolute CPS of an ictal EEG at each pair of symmetrical electrodes (Fp1 vs. Fp2, F3 vs. F4, C3 vs. C4, P3 vs. P4, O1 vs. O2, F7 vs. F8, T3 vs. T4, and T5 vs. T6) in each ictal EEG. Second, we calculated the mean of the absolute CPS in all pairs of symmetrical electrodes in the ictal EEG (mean CPS *per seizure*). Finally, we calculated the mean of "the mean CPS *per seizure*" for all ictal EEGs per patient (mean CPS in each patient). In these analyses, we separately calculated these values by each frequency band.

We performed subanalysis of CPS to identify the electrode pairs from which the phase lags originated; we calculated the CPS at each electrode pair for each ictal EEG and calculated the mean of the CPS for each electrode pair during all ictal EEGs in each patient (mean CPS of each pair of symmetrical electrodes in each patient). During analysis, we also separately calculated them by each frequency band.

Statistical Analyses

All data were analyzed using GraphPad Prism 6 (GraphPad Software, La Jolla, CA, USA). For comparing the data of clinical profiles, we used the Fisher's exact probability, Welch t-, and chi-square tests, as appropriate. By removing the effect of age, we used analysis of covariance for comparing the relative PS, IPL, and CPS among the outcome groups. The mean relative PS, mean IPL, and mean CPS were individually compared between the favorable and the unfavorable outcome groups using the Welch *t*-test by each frequency band.

Multiple liner regression was used to identify significant correlations between the mean CPS of each ictal EEG in each patient and the outcomes. We calculated the optimal cut-off points of CPS values in the frequency band with statistical significance for the predictive factors of unfavorable outcome using the Youden index.

A *p*-value of < 0.05 was considered to indicate statistical significance.

RESULTS

Clinical Profiles

The details regarding the clinical information are shown in **Table 1**. The age at epilepsy onset ranged from 1 to 166 months old (mean: 23 months). The classifications of the epilepsy/epilepsy syndrome were West syndrome ($n = 10$) and combined generalized and focal epilepsy ($n = 7$). Fourteen patients developed more than two types of seizures, including tonic seizures, focal impaired awareness seizure, atonic seizures, and myoclonic seizures. The mean frequency of ES pre-operatively was 40.1 times per day (range: 5–200).

The patients' etiologies were identified in 16: tuberous sclerosis complex ($n = 5$), post-acute encephalopathy ($n = 3$), post-neonatal hypoglycemia ($n = 2$), hippocampal sclerosis (n = 1), focal cortical dysplasia ($n = 1$), chemotherapy-induced leukoencephalopathy ($n = 1$), methyl-CpG binding protein 2 (*MECP2*) duplication syndrome ($n = 1$), post-neonatal hypoxic-ischemic encephalopathy ($n = 1$), and Down syndrome ($n = 1$); one patient had both TSC and acute encephalopathy, and one patient had both *MECP2* duplication syndrome and acute encephalopathy. Three patients did not have a neurologic history prior to the onset of epilepsy.

The mean age at CC was 81.4 months (range: 17–237 months). The mean follow-up period after CC was 22.1 months (range: 8–72 months). Seven patients showed a favorable outcome (Engel classification I). Ten patients showed unfavorable outcomes (Engel II in two patients, III in four patients, and IV in four patients).

Among the outcome groups, only the age at CC was significantly higher in the favorable outcome group ($p = 0.042$) than in the unfavorable outcome group. No significant differences were seen in other factors.

TABLE 1 | Clinical profiles of patients in the favorable and unfavorable outcome groups.

	Favorable outcome group (*n* = 7)	Unfavorable outcome group (*n* = 10)	*p*-value
Sex (boys: girls)	6:1	9:1	n.s.
Types of epilepsy syndrome			n.s.
West syndrome	2	8	
Combined generalized and focal epilepsy	5	2	
Etiology			n.s.
Structural abnormality	5	6	
Genetic/chromosomal syndrome	2	1	
Unknown	0	3	
Age at epilepsy onset [months, range (mean)]	4–166 (49)	1–13 (5)	n.s.
Total number of AEDs before CC [range (mean)]	4–8 (6.6)	6–10 (7.3)	n.s.
Frequency of ES/TS			n.s.
1–20/day	5	5	
>20/day	2	5	
Artifact free ES/TS using analysis [times, range (mean)]	5–15 (9)	4–12 (8)	n.s.
Age at CC [months, range (mean)]	45–237 (125)	17–106 (51)	0.042
Procedure of CC			n.s.
Total callosotomy	6	8	
Anterior 4/5 callostomy	1	2	
Outcomes of Engel's classification			NA
I	7	–	
II	–	2	
III	–	4	
IV	–	4	
Follow-up periods [months, range (mean)]	8–36 (17)	10–72 (26)	n.s.

AEDs, antiepileptic drugs; CC, corpus callosotomy; n.s., not significant; NA, not applicable. We used Fisher's exact probability test, Welch t-test, and chi-square test, appropriately. Tuberous sclerosis complex was classified as a structural abnormality in etiology.

Selection of Ictal EEG

In total, 143 ES were visually identified in this study. The range and the median number of ES per patient were 4-15 and 9, respectively. Fifteen EEG records of ES were excluded due to non-negligible artifacts or misplacements of EEG electrodes. For the first time, SK and MS anonymously reviewed and selected ictal EEG. They discussed and excluded 15 ES due to the artifacts or misplacements of the EEG electrodes. MO performed computer analyses for the ES data. Focal spasms were seen in seven patients. All of those patients showed unfavorable outcome.

Relative PS

The mean relative PSs for each patient in the favorable and unfavorable outcome groups were 1.45 ± 2.07 (range: −0.60–49.56) (standard deviation: SD) and 2.52 (mean) ± 6.16 (range: −1.38–244.91) in the delta frequency band, 0.48 ± 1.71 (range: −2.80–38.79) and −0.55 ± 2.04 (range: −97.27–11.18) in the theta frequency band, −0.45 ± 0.41 (range: −6.28–1.63) and −1.97 ± 5.05 (range: −209.00–1.45) in the alpha frequency band, −0.42 ± 1.04 (range: −25.13–1.41) and 1.37 ± 4.61 (range:

TABLE 2 | The mean relative power spectrum of each patient in the favorable and unfavorable outcome groups.

Frequency bands	Favorable outcome group	Unfavorable outcome group	*p*-value
Delta	1.45 ± 2.07	2.52 ± 6.16	0.277
Theta	0.48 ± 1.71	−0.55 ± 2.04	0.842
Alpha	−0.45 ± 0.41	−1.97 ± 5.05	0.107
Beta	−0.42 ± 1.04	1.37 ± 4.61	0.194
Gamma	−1.00 ± 2.53	−1.35 ± 3.99	0.531

After removing age effect, we used the Welch t-test.

TABLE 3 | The mean ictal power laterality using relative power results, averaging all electrodes in each patient in the favorable and unfavorable outcome groups.

Frequency bands	Favorable outcome group	Unfavorable outcome group	*p*-value
Delta	1.51 ± 0.47	6.37 ± 11.88	0.430
Theta	1.06 ± 0.55	1.06 ± 0.89	0.176
Alpha	0.68 ± 0.28	1.14 ± 0.24	0.910
Beta	1.60 ± 1.65	11.88 ± 30.08	0.329
Gamma	1.21 ± 0.78	2.19 ± 3.50	0.885

After removing age effect, we used Welch t-test.

−8.61–192.96) in the beta frequency band, −1.00 ± 2.53 (range: −61.74–1.66) and −1.35 ± 3.99 (range: −132.61–29.65) in the gamma frequency band, respectively.

No significant differences were identified in the individual mean relative PSs in the all-frequency bands between the favorable and the unfavorable outcome groups (**Table 2**).

IPL

The mean IPLs in each patient in favorable and unfavorable outcome groups were 1.51 ± 0.47 (range: 0.73–2.21) and 6.37 ± 11.88 (range: 1.03–39.34) in the delta frequency band, 1.06 ± 0.55 (range: 0.06–1.70) and 1.06 ± 0.89 (range: 0.08–2.60) in the theta frequency band, 0.68 ± 0.28 (range: 0.20–1.01) and 1.14 ± 0.24 (range: 0.01–3.46) in the alpha frequency band, 1.60 ± 1.65 (range: 0.45–4.86) and 11.88 ± 30.08 (range: 0.13 97.09) in the beta frequency band, 1.21 ± 0.78 (range: 0.28–0.57) and 2.19 ± 3.50 (range: 0.30–11.74) in the gamma frequency band, respectively.

Although the mean IPLs in each patient tended to be higher in unfavorable outcome groups than in favorable groups, no significant differences were identified in the all-frequency bands among the groups (**Table 3**).

CPS

Figure 2 shows the bar charts of the mean CPS in each patient in the favorable and unfavorable outcome groups by each frequency bands The mean CPS in each patient in the favorable and unfavorable outcomes were 56.2 ± 9.2° (range: 0.32–179.5°) and 86.5 ± 8.4 (range: 0.19–179.7) degrees in the delta frequency band, 61.7 ± 7.8 (range: 0.53–178.4) and 85.0 ± 7.3 (range: 0.77–177.8) degrees in the theta frequency band, 76.7 ± 7.6 (range: 3.33–175.0) and 89.4 ± 5.7 (range: 2.6–171.7) degrees in the alpha frequency band, 79.3 ± 5.6 (range: 15.0–167.4) and 91.9 ± 5.3 (range: 6.6–174.3) degrees in the beta frequency band, 71.2 ± 7.4 (range: 5.0–173.1) and 90.9 ± 6.0 (range: 5.3–172.9) degrees in the theta frequency band, respectively. The numeric data are provided in **Supplementary Table 1.**

The mean CPSs in each patient in the unfavorable outcome group tended to be higher than those in the favorable outcome group in all frequency bands, and there were significant differences in the delta (p = 0.018), theta (p = 0.034), and gamma (p = 0.040) frequency bands.

The optimal cutoff values of the mean CPS in each patient for unfavorable outcome were 64.00 in the delta band (sensitivity: 100, specificity: 80%), 74.20 in the theta band (100, 80%), and 82.05 in the gamma band (100, 80%).

Subsequently, we calculated the CPS of each pair of symmetrical electrodes in each patient to identify the cortical regions that generated the differences of the mean CPS in each frequency band. Overall, 72.5% (29/40) of the pairs showed higher mean CPS values in the unfavorable than in the favorable outcome group. The CPS values were significantly higher in the unfavorable outcome group than in the favorable outcome group (p = 0.036 at F7 vs. F8 in the delta, p = 0.041 at F3 vs. F4 and p = 0.041 at F7 vs. F8 in the theta, p = 0.048 at F3 vs. F4 in the alpha, p = 0.012 at F7 vs. F8 and p = 0.010 at T3 vs. T4 in the beta, and p = 0.012 at F3 vs. F4 in the gamma frequency bands). **Figure 3** indicate the pairs of symmetrical electrodes with significant mean CPS differences among the outcomes groups. The numeric data are described in **Supplementary Table 2.**

DISCUSSION

Summary of the Results

In this study, we analyzed the relative PS, IPL, and CPS by each frequency band on the scalp ictal-EEG of ES before CC. We compared the results between the patients with favorable and unfavorable outcomes after CC. No significant differences were found in terms of the relative PS and IPL between favorable and unfavorable outcome groups. Conversely, our study revealed higher CPS values regarding the delta, theta, and gamma frequency bands; these indicated phase lags of the waves of EEG among pairs of symmetrical electrodes in patients with unfavorable outcomes, compared to those with favorable outcomes. The differences in CPS tended to be apparent in the frontal and temporal areas.

Relative PS Analyses

Previous studies on the analysis of the EEG power indicated that the emergence of gamma activity during interictal scalp EEG in patients with West syndrome positively correlated with intractableness of seizures or severity of hypsarrhythmia (17, 18). Moreover, abnormal EEGs, defined as abnormal backgrounds

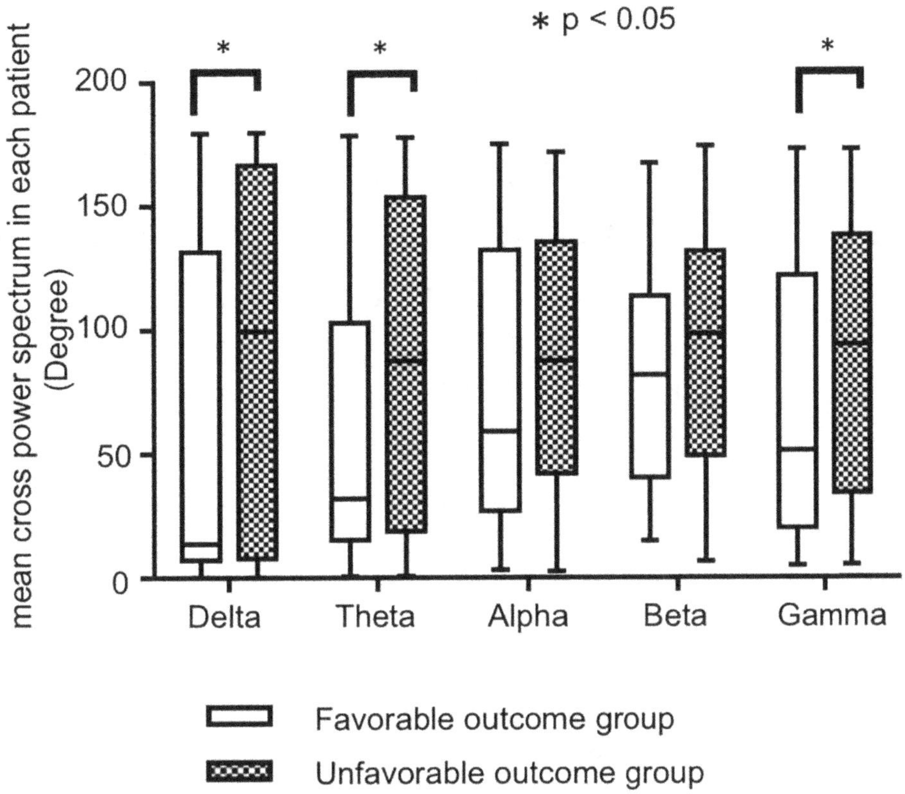

FIGURE 2 | The bar charts of the mean cross-power spectrums (CPS) in each patient by each frequency band, in favorable and unfavorable outcome groups. Although the mean CPS in each patient tended to be higher in unfavorable outcome group in all frequency bands, significant differences were seen in the delta, theta, and gamma bands.

and focal background slowing, were indicators of poor surgical outcomes in intractable epilepsy in patients with ES on inspection (19). Regarding the studies on ictal EEG of ES, Myers et al. (20) reported that less ictal slow activity was associated with better medical treatment responses in West syndrome. Using computer-based frequency analysis, Nariai et al. (21) reported that gamma and beta activities during spasms correlated with strong ictogenesis. Although we predicted that relative PS in both slow and fast activities would be higher in the unfavorable than in the favorable outcomes groups, there were no significant differences among the groups in this study. The powers of ictal activities in ES may not associate with the outcomes of CC.

IPL Analyses

We subsequently analyzed the IPL, which indicates laterality of powers of ictal EEG among bilateral hemispheres. In our previous report, we visually analyzed the ratio of the ictal peaks of the slow waves in bilateral hemispheres. The ictal slow waves were asymmetrical in patients with unfavorable outcomes after CC than in those with favorable outcomes (16). In this study, we compared the IPL, including delta to gamma frequency bands. However, this study did not show significant differences on any frequency bands, although the IPLs tended to be higher in the unfavorable than in the favorable outcome group. In our previous study on ictal slow waves, the electrodes with the most preceding seizure activity were selected for analysis (16). This study included all temporal and parasagittal electrodes for the analyses; the differences in the laterality may have been attenuated by averaging.

CPS Analyses

In our previous report using visual analysis, the peak of the negative slow wave during spasms showed more time differences among bilateral hemispheres in the unfavorable outcome group (16). Using computer-based analyses, we confirmed a larger phase lag in the unfavorable than in the favorable outcome group. Significant differences were observed in both slow activities of delta or theta bands and in gamma bands. The large phase lags in the slow frequency bands in the unfavorable group may reflect the negative peak delay in our previous report (16), and the small phase lags in the patients with favorable outcomes may reflect the approximation of epileptic excitations among bilateral hemispheres via transcallosal volleys (16, 22).

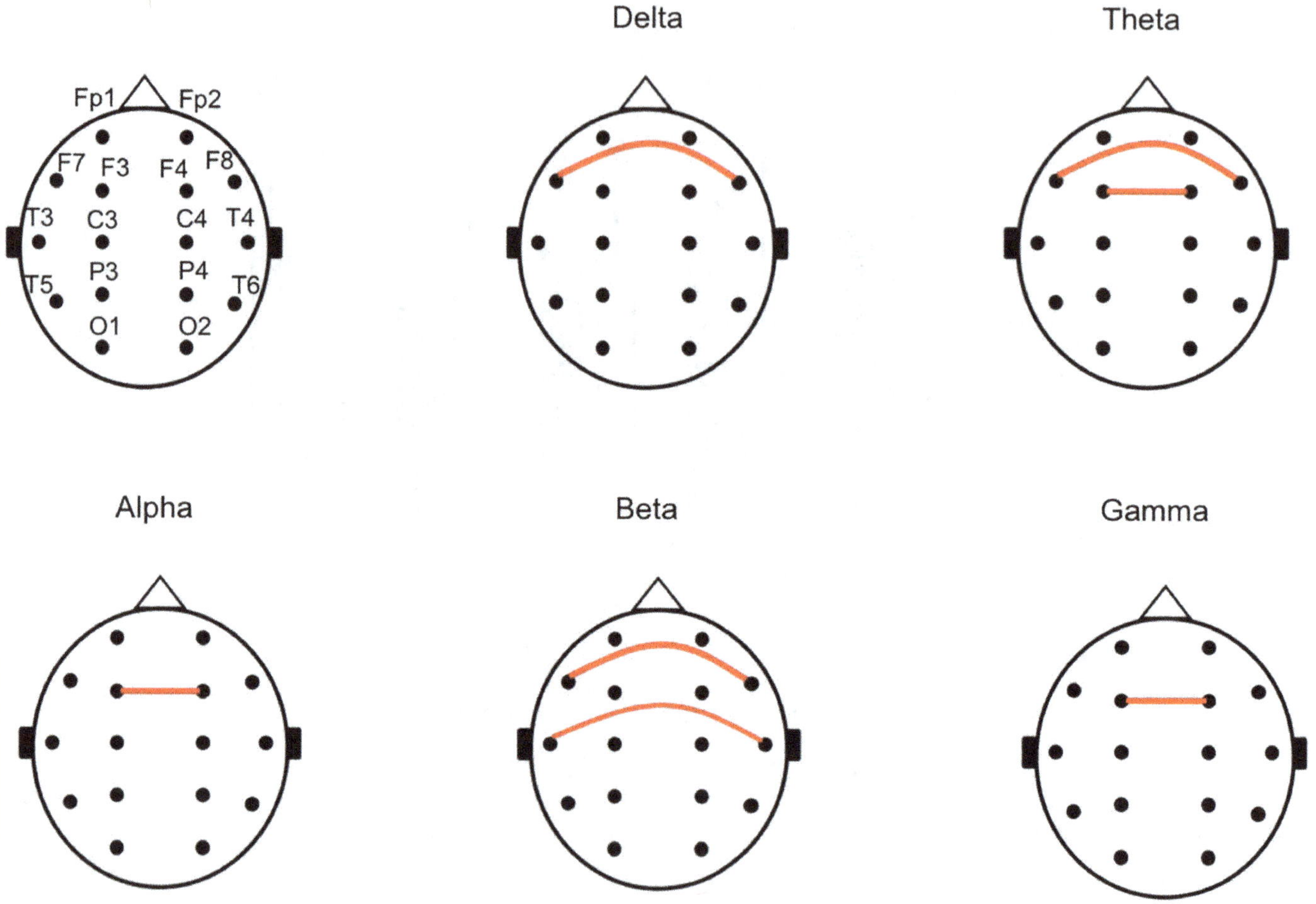

FIGURE 3 | The chart of a pair of symmetrical electrodes with large phase lags in the unfavorable outcome group. The red lines indicate the pair of symmetrical electrodes with significantly large phase lags between the unfavorable and favorable outcome groups, in the analyses for mean cross-power spectrum (CPS) of each pair of symmetrical electrodes. All of the pairs with the red line showed higher CPS in the unfavorable outcome group than in the favorable outcome group.

We additionally analyzed the mean CPS of each symmetrical pair of electrodes in each patient, to identify the origin of the phase lags. In this study, the CPS was higher among bilateral frontal and temporal regions in the unfavorable outcome group than in the favorable outcome group. The interhemispheric connection might be predominant via the anterior part of corpus callosum in the patients with favorable outcome group.

Study Limitations

Our study has some limitations. The number of the patients was not large, and the backgrounds of the patients were different. The results with statistical significances in this study became not significant after multiple comparisons. Larger samples are necessary for more definitive conclusion. Selection bias might occur, when we removed the ictal EEG data with muscle artifact. The sampling ratios (256 or 400 Hz) were lower than those in the previous studies (5, 21), and we could not analyze for more high frequency band of ripples (>80 Hz).

CONCLUSION

In conclusion, the large phase lags of delta, theta, and gamma activities among bilateral hemispheres during ES correlated with unfavorable outcomes following CC. Asynchronous activities in ES may indicate low performance of the corpus callosum in emergent seizures or severe epileptogenicity. These computed wave analyses for ictal-scalp EEG in ES may be used pre-operatively to predict outcomes of CC for ES.

ETHICS STATEMENT

The studies involving human participants were reviewed and approved by the ethical committee of Seirei Hamamatsu General Hospital. Written informed consent to participate in this study was provided by the participants' legal guardian/next of kin. Written informed consent was obtained from the minor(s)' legal guardian/next of kin for the publication of any potentially identifiable images or data included in this article.

AUTHOR CONTRIBUTIONS

MO designed the study, managed and analyzed the EEG data, performed statistical analyses, and wrote the manuscript. TO designed the study, performed statistical analyses, and revised the manuscript. SK analyzed the EEG data. MN analyzed and acquired the EEG data. SB, KO, TH, KO, and YM critically revised the manuscript. HE and AF discussed the interpretations of the data and revised the manuscript. All authors contributed to the article and approved the submitted version.

ACKNOWLEDGMENTS

We would like to sincerely thank the doctors who collaborated with us to treat the patients with intractable epilepsy.

REFERENCES

1. Fusco L, Vigevano F. Ictal clinical electroencephalographic findings of spasms in West syndrome. *Epilepsia.* (1993) 34:671–8. doi: 10.1111/j.1528-1157.1993.tb00445.x
2. Yamatogi Y, Ohtahara S. Age-dependent epileptic encephalopathy: a longitudinal study. *Folia Psychiatr Neurol Jpn.* (1981) 35:321–32. doi: 10.1111/j.1440-1819.1981.tb00233.x
3. Watanabe K, Negoro T, Okumura A. Symptomatology of infantile spasms. *Brain Dev.* (2001) 23:453–66. doi: 10.1016/S0387-7604(01)00274-1
4. Fusco L, Vigevano F. Tonic spasm seizures: a particular and previously unreported type of seizure. *Epilepsia.* (1994) 35:87.
5. Nariai H, Hussain SA, Bernardo D, Motoi H, Sonoda M, Kuroda N, et al. Scalp EEG interictal high frequency oscillations as an objective biomarker of infantile spasms. *Clin Neurophysiol.* (2020) 131:2527–36. doi: 10.1016/j.clinph.2020.08.013
6. Maehara T, Shimizu H. Surgical outcome of corpus callosotomy in patients with drop attacks. *Epilepsia.* (2001) 42:67–71. doi: 10.1046/j.1528-1157.2001.081422.x
7. Kasasbeh AS, Smyth MD, Steger-May K, Jalilian L, Bertrand M, Limbrick DD. Outcomes after anterior or complete corpus callosotomy in children. *Neurosurgery.* (2014) 74:17–28. doi: 10.1227/NEU.0000000000000197
8. Pinard JM, Delalande O, Chiron C, Soufflet C, Plouin P, Kim Y, et al. Callosotomy for epilepsy after West syndrome. *Epilepsia.* (1999) 40:1727–34. doi: 10.1111/j.1528-1157.1999.tb01590.x
9. Baba H, Toda K, Ono T, Honda R, Baba S. Surgical and developmental outcomes of corpus callosotomy for West syndrome in patients without MRI lesions. *Epilepsia.* (2018) 59:2231–9. doi: 10.1111/epi.14594
10. Itamura S, Okanishi T, Nishimura M, Kanai S, Baba S, Masuda Y, et al. Analysis for the association between corpus callosum thickness and corpus callosotomy outcomes for patients with epileptic spasms or tonic spasms. *Pediatr Neurol.* (2019) 95:79–83. doi: 10.1016/j.pediatrneurol.2019.01.012
11. Graham D, Tisdall MM, Gill D. Corpus callosotomy outcomes in pediatric patients: a systematic review. *Epilepsia.* (2016) 57:1053–68. doi: 10.1111/epi.13408
12. Sunaga S, Shimizu H, Sugano H. Long-term follow-up of seizure outcomes after corpus callosotomy. *Seizure.* (2009) 18:124–8. doi: 10.1016/j.seizure.2008.08.001
13. Iwasaki M, Uematsu M, Hino-Fukuyo N, Osawa S, Shimoda Y, Jin K, et al. Clinical profiles for seizure remission and developmental gains after total corpus callosotomy. *Brain Dev.* (2016) 38:47–53. doi: 10.1016/j.braindev.2015.04.010
14. Sorenson JM, Wheless JW, Baumgartner JE, Thomas AB, Brookshire BL, Clifton GL, et al. Corpus callosotomy for medically intractable seizures. *Pediatr Neurosurg.* (1997) 27:260–7. doi: 10.1159/000121264
15. Spencer DD, Spencer SS. Corpus callosotomy in the treatment of medically intractable secondarily generalized seizures of children. *Cleve Clin J Med.* (1989) 56:S69–78. doi: 10.3949/ccjm.56.s1.69
16. Kanai S, Oguri M, Okanishi T, Itamura S, Baba S, Nishimura M, et al. Symmetry of ictal slow waves may predict the outcomes of corpus callosotomy for epileptic spasms. *Sci Rep.* (2019) 9:19733. doi: 10.1038/s41598-019-56303-3
17. Baba S, Vakorin VA, Doesburg SM, Nagamori C, Cortez MA, Honda R, et al. EEG before and after total corpus callosotomy for pharmacoresistant infantile spasms: fast oscillations and slow-wave connectivity in hypsarrhythmia. *Epilepsia.* (2019) 60:1849–60. doi: 10.1111/epi.16295
18. Kobayashi K, Akiyama T, Oka M, Endoh F, Yoshinaga H. A storm of fast (40-150Hz) oscillations during hypsarrhythmia in West syndrome. *Ann Neurol.* (2015) 77:58–67. doi: 10.1002/ana.24299
19. Moseley BD, Nickels K, Wirrell EC. Surgical outcomes for intractable epilepsy in children with epileptic spasms. *J Child Neurol.* (2012) 27:713–20. doi: 10.1177/0883073811424463
20. Myers KA, Bello-Espinosa LE, Wei XC, Scantlebury MH. Infraslow EEG changes in infantile spasms. *J Clin Neurophysiol.* (2014) 31:600–5. doi: 10.1097/WNP.0000000000000109
21. Nariai H, Beal J, Galanopoulou AS, Mowrey WB, Bickel S, Sogawa Y, et al. Scalp EEG Ictal gamma and beta activity during infantile spasms: evidence of focality. *Epilepsia.* (2017) 58:882–92. doi: 10.1111/epi.13735
22. Ono T, Matsuo A, Baba H, Ono K. Is a cortical spike discharge "transferred" to the contralateral cortex via the corpus callosum?: an intraoperative observation of electrocorticogram and callosal compound action potentials. *Epilepsia.* (2002) 43:1536–42. doi: 10.1046/j.1528-1157.2002.13402.x

4

Cognitive and Emotional Mapping with SEEG

Daniel L. Drane[1,2,3,4*], Nigel P. Pedersen[1,2,5*], David S. Sabsevitz[6,7], Cady Block[1], Adam S. Dickey[1], Abdulrahman Alwaki[1] and Ammar Kheder[1,3]

[1] Department of Neurology, Emory University School of Medicine, Atlanta, GA, United States, [2] Emory Epilepsy Center, Atlanta, GA, United States, [3] Department of Pediatrics, Emory University School of Medicine, Atlanta, GA, United States, [4] Department of Neurology, University of Washington School of Medicine, Seattle, WA, United States, [5] Department of Biomedical Engineering, Georgia Institute of Technology and Emory University, Atlanta, GA, United States, [6] Department of Psychology and Psychiatry, Mayo Clinic, Jacksonville, FL, United States, [7] Department of Neurological Surgery, Mayo Clinic, Jacksonville, FL, United States

***Correspondence:**
Daniel L. Drane
ddrane@emory.edu
Nigel P. Pedersen
npeders@emory.edu

Mapping of cortical functions is critical for the best clinical care of patients undergoing epilepsy and tumor surgery, but also to better understand human brain function and connectivity. The purpose of this review is to explore existing and potential means of mapping higher cortical functions, including stimulation mapping, passive mapping, and connectivity analyses. We examine the history of mapping, differences between subdural and stereoelectroencephalographic approaches, and some risks and safety aspects, before examining different types of functional mapping. Much of this review explores the prospects for new mapping approaches to better understand other components of language, memory, spatial skills, executive, and socio-emotional functions. We also touch on brain-machine interfaces, philosophical aspects of aligning tasks to brain circuits, and the study of consciousness. We end by discussing multi-modal testing and virtual reality approaches to mapping higher cortical functions.

Keywords: stimulation mapping, language, passive mapping, cerebral cortex, connectivity, socioemotional, memory, SEEG

INTRODUCTION

Mapping of cortical functions in humans has provided substantial insights about the organization of the human forebrain. This review focuses on the mapping of higher cognitive functions, and will not address the mapping of primary sensory or primary motor cortices [recently covered elsewhere: (1)] nor the premotor or cingulate motor regions. We will describe the rationale for mapping in the context of its conceptual and historical development. We will then describe stimulation mapping and how it differs between subdural electrode stimulation and in the setting of stereoelectroenecephalography (SEEG). We will review language mapping and then describe broader applications of mapping to cognition and emotion and the potential for further research and technical development. Wherever relevant we will highlight controversies, key concepts, gaps in knowledge, and areas of present development.

RATIONALE AND OPPORTUNITY FOR INTRACRANIAL MONITORING FOR UNDERSTANDING SEIZURE NETWORKS AND CONDUCTING NEUROCOGNITIVE MAPPING

When seizures continue despite thoughtful medical management, epilepsy surgery is considered, often in turn resulting in invasive electrophysiology with subdural or depth electrodes. The ultimate goal of such studies is to test hypotheses about the network and location of seizure onset with a view to resective surgery, tissue ablation, or neuromodulation (2). In order to localize areas of hyperexcitability, reproduce seizures and aura, and map cortical function, electrical stimulation can also be performed while intracranial electrodes are in place, with this method arguably having afforded the greatest body of knowledge about cortical function through the last ~80 years. For much of this time in North America, this has involved a large craniotomy and placement of a subdural grid of electrodes on the surface of the brain, sometimes augmented with strip or depth electrodes. In contrast, in Europe, the approach to invasive studies has grown out of a more clinical approach with semiologic analysis, ultimately relying on less invasive depth electrodes with the overall method referred to as SEEG (3). While both methods started out as acute approaches, limited to the operating room, both rapidly developed into continuous extra-operative recording.

SEEG has been used more extensively in Europe for many years (4), but has recently become popular in North America, particularly since the use of minimally invasive procedures has increased (5). These have included the use of laser interstitial thermal therapy [LITT (6)], focused ultrasound (7), and neuromodulatory procedures [e.g., vagal nerve stimulation (VNS), responsive neurostimulation (RNS), and deep brain stimulation (DBS) of the anterior nucleus of the thalamus [DSBS-ANT (8, 9)]. With these less invasive surgical options available, patients and neurosurgeons are reluctant to use a larger procedure for evaluative purposes if the treatment is going to ultimately be more restricted and less invasive in scope. In this manuscript, we will briefly review the history of invasive EEG techniques and explore both the strengths and weaknesses of these procedures. We will discuss the use of such techniques to better understand seizure networks and brain connectivity and to study cognitive and emotional processes, then propose a research agenda that improves clinical practice and furthers our understanding of neural circuitry. The latter goal could include the standardization and dissemination of assessment techniques and the development of new cognitive and emotional testing paradigms that build upon current brain-behavior theoretical models and make use of modern technologies (e.g., augmented and virtual reality, videography, eye-tracking).

HISTORY OF SEEG AND NEUROPSYCHOLOGICAL MAPPING

Historical Antecedents of SEEG

In the late eighteenth and early nineteenth century, studies of electricity and its relationship to biology were in their infancy, with debate between Volta and Galvani about intrinsic vs. extrinsic electricity and electrical stimulation of movement (10). This debate was largely synthesized and resolved by Humboldt as Galvani's nephew first stimulated a freshly executed human cadaver in 1802, giving rise to bodily movements, inspiring the public imagination and likely contributing to the creation of the Frankenstein story. Crude localization of function was best inspired by Thomas Willis, but more fine grained cerebral localization principally occurred in the nineteenth century with clinical-pathological correlations and early motor mapping by Fritsch and Hitzig in dogs (11), and a more precise topography described by Ferrier in non-human primates (12–14). These works culminated in the "The Functions of the Brain" in 1876 (15), with later correlations to some clinical observations by Hughlings Jackson (16).

In the clinical realm, this new appreciation of the organization of the cerebral cortex developed alongside the other technical and research advances, such as stereotaxis and the string galvanometer for measuring electrical potentials. Most notably, shortly after David Ferrier's student Robert Caton recorded human brain potentials for the first time (17), Victor Horsley electrically stimulated an encephalocele then, at the behest of Hughlings Jackson, performed the first electrocorticography for epilepsy surgery (18). In 1909, Harvey Cushing reported the use of cortical stimulation in two cases of focal epilepsy (19, 20), with Emil Theodor Krause, in the same year, publishing the first map of the human motor cortex (21). This was followed by a more extensive map by Ottfreid Foerster—a major influence on Penfield's work and his approach to epilepsy surgery. In fact, the literal translation of Foerster's ideas into English and North America was so verbatim that we still use the German alternating current line frequency of 50 Hz in mapping studies till the present day—the original stimulators being simple step-down alternating current transformers.

While cerebral localization had gotten off to a somewhat pseudoscientific start, complete with racialized tropes, the phrenology of Gall and Spurzheim gave way to scientific cortical localization (22), as described above with support from the developing field of neuroanatomy, as well as to anti-localizationalist works in the early twentieth century (e.g., Karl Lashley). In clinical spheres, localization became the hallmark and unique method of neurology, growing from the prescient conjecture of Willis to an eventual clinico-pathological method of Paul Broca and, most productively, Jean Marie Charcot who essentially described the modern screening neurological examination (23). While localization in epilepsy reached a new summit in the works of Hughlings Jackson, epilepsy in the English speaking world did not keep up with the sophistication of the French fusion of Charcot's anatomical and clinical thinking that was directly mapped to the brain and its networks by Jean Talairach, the psychiatrist who pioneered, along with

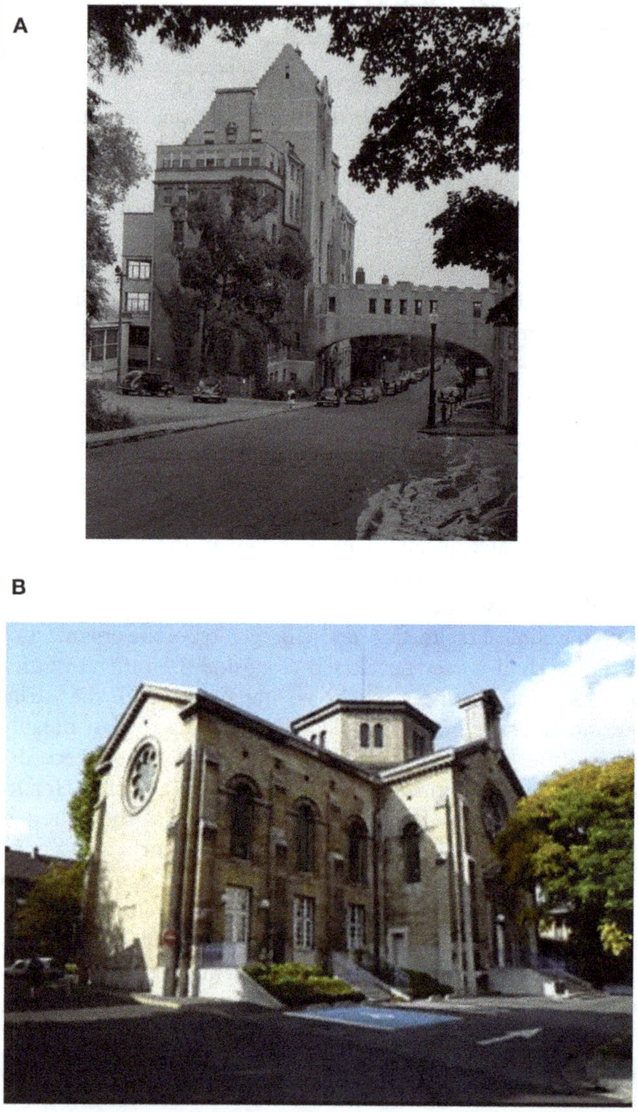

FIGURE 1 | Historical sites central to the development of cognitive mapping: **(A)** the Montreal Neurological Institute, Montreal, Canada and **(B)** St. Anne Hospital, Paris, France.

his collaborators in the 1960s, a new stereotaxic method and means of determining anatomical correlations to a standard atlas in functional neurosurgery [e.g., (24)]. While a fruitful research stereotaxic apparatus was invented by the surgeon Victor Horlsey and Robert Henry Clarke, ushering in a new era of neuroscientific discoveries, it was not used in humans until the late 1940s by the founding epileptologist Frederic Gibbs at Harvard, along with Robert Hayne, and was not accompanied by an overall anatomical and localizationalist approach to epilepsy (25). Instead, Talairach, working closely with the neurophysiologist and neurologist Jean Bancaud, developed the means to combine astute localization of seizure semiology, individualized anatomy with functional correlations, and a stereotaxic approach to hypothesis testing, culminating in the 1950s and 1960s into the method that we now know as stereoelectroencephalography (26).

While amplifiers and recording methods, along with the SEEG method were developing, it is important to note that electrical stimulation actually preceded multichannel electrophysiologic recording. Electrodes were thus crafted with stimulation in mind and this was an integral part of both intra- and extra-operative use of both subdural and SEEG-based methods. While stimulation subserves several functions, as mentioned above, we focus in this review on the application of stimulation for electrical stimulation mapping of function (ESM) which can overlap with elicitation of the seizure aura, passive mapping, and connectivity mapping.

Historical Course of Cortical Stimulation Mapping

ESM involves the application of electrical current, typically to the cerebral cortex, in an effort to determine the potential contribution of a given region to a specific cortical function (e.g., sensory, motor, cognitive, linguistic, socio-emotional). While there are a few clear objectives, mapping of function is not always separate from stimulation to elicit after discharges and seizures. For example, stimulation during language testing may be found to reproduce ictal aphasia when a run of after-discharges or focal seizure is elicited in language networks. Similarly, mapping of function may help understand both which cortex is "eloquent," but also elicit the seizure aura. Eloquence is a problematic concept and essentially equates to an observable function that is considered of high importance. However, under the right conditions and with appropriate testing, much, if not in theory all, of the cerebral cortex can be demonstrated to have a function–this is a major motivation for expanding the paradigms available for cognitive mapping. Nonetheless, eloquent cortex is conventionally considered to subserve key functions such as motor control and core components of language and speech. ESM has most frequently been employed intra- or extra-operatively in the setting of epilepsy and tumor surgery [(26–29)].

Drivers in North America

Wilder Penfield, after studying with Foerster, went on to employ direct electrical stimulation to explore the sensorimotor cortex, experiential phenomena and language functioning (30–32). Prior to that time, in clinical practice, neurosurgeons were reluctant to operate on the language dominant cerebral hemisphere for fear of creating a language disturbance (aphasia), with the exception of procedures involving the occipital lobe or anterior frontal lobe. Therefore, the introduction of ESM for language mapping opened new surgical opportunities for many patients who would have been considered at risk of harm from an open resection procedure. Penfield, along with his colleague Herbert Jasper, created what they termed the "Montreal procedure" during the 1930s, which involved testing the surgical patient while undergoing ESM in an awake state (Penfield and Jasper, 195) (33) (See **Figure 1**). Their pioneering work led to many discoveries and advancements in our knowledge of neural networks underlying language, and specifically demonstrating that such networks were much more complex and extensive than the classic language network postulated by Broca, Wernicke, Lichtheim, and others (34–37). They also showed that they could elicit both the auras of patients, which can be useful for localizing seizure networks, as well as experiential phenomena such as rich memories of events that included sensory phenomena (e.g., "I am in my grandma's house and I can smell the cookies baking"). With the advent of current regulated bipolar stimulation devices, as well as more adherence to safety limits, less electrical current is applied directly to the cortex, and rarely, if ever, are such contextually rich phenomena seen with cortical surface stimulation.

George Ojemann, one of the founding members of the regional epilepsy center at the University of Washington (UW), built upon these ESM experiences, devoting much of his research career to the use of mapping paradigms to better understand cortical function. The UW program was the second regional epilepsy center in the US, following the University of Virginia, with programs funded by a project grant from the National Institutes of Health (NIH). His seminal work in 1989 (38), which included careful language maps of 117 presurgical temporal lobe epilepsy (TLE) patients, clearly demonstrated that critical language sites are much more broadly represented across the cortex than had been conceived. Investigators heavily relied upon visual (picture) naming approaches, which were likely tapping into the widely distributed networks required for one of the more complex actions carried out by humans (i.e., to name an object requires a large swathe of cortex from the primary visual area, unimodal and polymodal association cortices including lexical access, speech monitoring, and production) [see (34, 36, 39)]. There are actually multiple stages to this process, which can be carried out for some stimuli under 1 s, while more complex material may require slightly longer (e.g., 5–8 s for some complex stimuli). The Ojemann work, which included the projects of many trainees and collaborators, led to greater knowledge of reorganization of language and normal atypical variants (e.g., extent, spatial reorganization, contributing factors) and increased knowledge of primary vs. secondary languages and their neural distribution (e.g., primary languages appear to be more focally distributed than secondary languages) (40–45). This work also delved into the study of memory and led to some provocative findings which are being given more credence with the study of focal lesions resulting from our current epoch involving the introduction of minimally invasive surgical techniques. For example, ESM memory paradigms suggested that disruption of lateral cortex could disrupt episodic memory (46, 47), and it has recently been borne out that focal lesions in such subregions can cause lasting damage to memory even when medial TL structures are spared (48). The extent to which such functions could be localized to these lateral regions remains to be determined, and it may be that both medial and lateral aspects of the TL are simply contributing TL larger, interactive networks.

Investigators at the Cleveland Clinic have also made some important contributions to our knowledge of language networks using ESM. In particular, Lüders and colleagues discovered that application of electrical stimulation of the basal temporal lobe region (fusiform gyrus) of the dominant hemisphere at a high intensity produced a significant aphasia in a subset of patients involving disruption of both comprehension and speech output (49–51). This finding sometimes seems underappreciated by the neurological community, and this region is still not routinely assessed in many clinical investigations. Of note, lower intensity stimulation of this region only resulted in naming deficits. This area was dubbed the basal temporal language area.

While Lüders and colleagues initially reported no significant language deficits resulting from resection of this region (51), subsequent studies have indeed reported impairment (52–54). The original work of Penfield also indicated that resection of this region could result in significant confrontation naming problems (32). As electrical stimulation led to comprehension deficits as well as other language symptoms, this may be additional data suggesting a more posterior location of a region that is important for single word comprehension. One group has published a couple of case studies using subdural grid mapping of epilepsy patients which suggest that the posterior basal temporal language area may be most important for relating visual images to phonological content (55). Building upon these findings, a more recent electrophysiological study, which employed cortico-cortical evoked potentials to explore regional connectivity, revealed connectivity between the basal temporal language area and a posterior language area (56). It is also possible that this reflects disruption of the ventral auditory processing pathway, perhaps when including basal temporal white matter.

Benefits and Limitations of ESM

The most obvious benefit of ESM is its potential to spare eloquent functions, which typically include language and sensorimotor function, but really should be considered more broadly to include polymodal, cognitive and emotional processing components. Limitations of ESM primarily involve limits related to the coverage that is possible through grid mapping (29) and the sparse sampling of SEEG. In general, systematic coverage is provided for a limited range of the cerebral cortex. Another key limitation is that not only is the node being stimulated affected, but it seems likely, given conveyance of evoked potentials to other regions during stimulation, that what is observed clinically could be a network effect. Other limitations include a lack of cross-center standardization, and a lack of validated, standardized tasks to cover most cognitive abilities.

Historical Course of Mapping With SEEG

European Contributions

As described above, Jean Talairach designed a robust system which allowed patient-specific mapping of cerebral anatomy to a coordinate space that included functional correlations (4). This impressive registration before the computed tomography and magnetic resonance imaging eras used ventricular position and size derived from pneumoencephalography and angiography to delimit major vessels, particularly arteries, as well as the anterior and posterior commissures. At the same time, Jean Bancaud finished his higher doctoral thesis on the correlation between neuropsychological deficits and EEG in patients with brain tumors. He saw the value of using Talairach space in defining three-dimensional representations of seizures and their propagation, and a new method was born. With the advances in technology and regulations, it became possible to move from intraoperative "acute" to intraoperative prolonged and even ambulatory "chronic" SEEG recordings in France [see (57) for a brief history of epilepsy surgery in France].

While Penfield and Jasper primarily relied on interictal spikes and cortical stimulation for his resections, Talairach and Bancaud were able to obtain ictal recordings, sometimes elicited by pro-convulsant drugs such as pentylenetetrazol, and replicated as components or as a complete sequence to understand the spatiotemporal evolution of spontaneous seizures. While paroxysmal evoked responses were also obtained by both single shock and train stimulation (4, 58, 59), this approach, in contrast to that of Penfield and Jasper, relied on the careful analysis of seizures, rather than resection based on interictal abnormalities.

There were several differences between North American and European approaches to stimulation and mapping. While North American approaches typically demarcated functional mapping from analysis of the patient's epileptic network, this was often not the case in Europe. For example, examination might occur when eliciting the seizure or components thereof, as described above. While 50 Hz stimulation was prominent in North America, the SEEG approach tended to emphasize the importance of tailoring stimulation frequency, amplitude, and train duration based on the location stimulated [e.g., (59)]. From a practical standpoint, low frequency stimulation is used for functional mapping of primary areas, for the study of functional connectivity, and of areas with a lower threshold for after-discharge and seizure (e.g., amygdala and hippocampus); high frequency stimulation, such as 50 Hz, is used for functional mapping of non-primary neocortical areas, and for triggering seizures. SEEG can be utilized to investigate and identify language networks in patients with epilepsy (60). In North America, there was a concern for "clearing" cortex that may be "eloquent" for resection, while the SEEG method tended to precede from the patient's semiology and examine function in relation to seizures. Later academic work in both arenas focused more formally on examining specific cortical functions—work that is far from exhausted today.

While SEEG can be used, unlike cortical surface mapping, to map the functions and connections of fiber bundles [e.g., (61)], much of the work of electrical mapping of the language functions of white matter has been performed intraoperatively, particularly by Duffau and colleagues. This has been achieved by mapping during tumor surgery, involving stimulation of the cortical surface and white matter tracts as they move through the surgical zone in the setting of tumor resection (62, 63). They have combined this approach in an interesting fashion with the use of neuroimaging techniques (e.g., fMRI, DTI) and neuro-dissection techniques in a multimodal manner that has contributed to more localized analyses of function and the inclusion of pathways/connections to the sometimes exclusive focus of past researchers on gray matter/cortex only (64–67). Of note, however, one criticism has been that some of this work has been based on a more crude localization using photographs of the area being stimulated, which are then matched to the available preoperative MRI scans. Therefore, there is likely much more work that can be accomplished in this area as well. These investigators have demonstrated that naming dysfunction differs by the white matter pathway that is stimulated [e.g., semantic errors tend to occur during picture naming when stimulating the inferior frontal occipital fasciculus (IFOF) while phonemic paraphasia results from stimulation of the arcuate fasciculus (67)], and that disturbance of recognition of faces and objects can occur with stimulation of the non-dominant ventral visual processing stream (68, 69). They have also published data showing that seemingly small declines in language processes (including simple speech response speed on naming) can lead to significant decline in functional status (e.g., failure to return to work relates to slowed response rate on these tasks) (70).

Benefits and Limitations of Mapping With SEEG

While the SEEG method itself affords more access to anatomically distant but functionally related areas, with superior access to sulci and deeper cortical and subcortical structures than ESM, the trade-off involves a reliance on a sparser sampling of the cortical regions of interest. A related benefit is that when a patient is implanted thoughtfully, large functional networks can be probed, rather than adjacent fragments of multiple networks as is typically the case with a subdural approach. While use of a 3D-grid approach has been described to overcome sparse sampling (71), this is largely at odds with the overall localizationalist and network thinking of the SEEG method and is generally not recommended—the large number of electrodes in one region, at the expense of covering other hypotheses or parts of the network, may increase hemorrhage risk, although electrode density as a specific risk for hemorrhage has not been studied. Furthermore, skull thickness can be a limiting factor in sampling certain areas (such as anterior temporal region). This is a major consideration in younger children. Finally, SEEG is less invasive than ESM using grids and strips, and this fits very well with the continued trend toward employing minimally invasive surgical procedures.

There are several limitations to mapping with SEEG. A major present obstacle is the learning curve in practicing the SEEG method. There is an uneven level of experience in SEEG mapping within centers which have used SEEG for decades and have well-established methods in place when compared to centers that adopted this method recently. The publication of the French guidelines on SEEG in 2018 is an effort to standardize the practice across centers and offer recommendations for those who are implementing the method (72). The interpretation of positive or negative responses during stimulation can be challenging from a functional standpoint. One of the key concepts that can impact functional mapping in SEEG is charge density given the relatively small surface area stimulated. Theoretically, the stimulation effect is local, however, a distant effect of stimulation is also likely and should be considered when interpreting stimulation results, particularly given that intercontact spacing typically means that white matter is also stimulated [human cortical thickness varies from about 1–4.5 mm, e.g., (73), and 2 mm contacts are typically not <1.5 mm apart, often more] (74, 75). Certain charge densities and frequencies may have an inhibitory effect on certain cortical areas, or may result in inhibition of downstream targets (e.g., with stimulation of the prefrontal cortex), positive clinical phenomenon, or inactivation of a network that extends beyond the area stimulated (e.g., some aphasic effects in language mapping). For all of these reasons, mapping a complex function such as language requires experience and analysis with subdural electrodes and perhaps still more with SEEG, whereas mapping primary motor or sensory function is usually straightforward despite a lower spatial resolution. Therefore, mapping must be used thoughtfully and is best tailored to individual patients and functions. Probing the presence and the effect of a focus in a large interconnected network can be accomplished with SEEG.

CURRENT STATUS OF COGNITIVE AND EMOTIONAL MAPPING WITH SEEG

Stimulation Parameters

The parameter space for stimulation can be large, but fundamental neurophysiology significantly reduces this multivariate parameter space. The variables of stimulation are intensity, montage (e.g., bipolar vs. monopolar), duration, waveform, charge balancing, frequency, and train characteristics. While not considered in this review, issues of geometry, contact size and shape, and material are also important considerations. This parameter space is made more tractable by the safety limit in charge per phase with SEEG electrodes that limits amplitude and pulse duration (with 30 $\mu C/cm^2$/phase based on animal data, electrode metal characteristics and pathological examining of human post-mortem tissue after chronic basal ganglia stimulation) (76). Waveforms have been explored to a greater extent in basal ganglia stimulation and typically a symmetrical charge balanced square wave is used in SEEG, despite other waveforms possibly providing more targeted stimulation at least in microstimulation (77)—this is yet to be studied in detail. Montage is determined by the volume of tissue that one desires to activate and there is a significant body of work pertaining to stimulation frequency for the cerebral cortex in mapping, as mentioned in a prior section [e.g., (26, 78)]. Subdural grid stimulation parameters are similar, except that a higher safety limit is typically accepted (~50 $\mu C/cm^2$/phase), perhaps given short-circuiting over the pia and through cerebrospinal fluid, based on elemental pathologic analysis of resected temporal cortical tissue after acute stimulation and subsequent temporal lobectomy (79). While these factors all serve to make the stimulation parameter space quite tractable, this should not be confused with therapeutic stimulation parameters, or higher frequency stimulation that may be inhibitory—the parameter space is under-determined, but has gradually become better explored (75).

Risks of Depth Electrode Placement

While SEEG is substantially less morbid and better tolerated than craniotomy with subdural grid placement, injury must be considered. Broadly, it is worth considering three categories of injury: Major (e.g., neurologic deficit that does not entirely resolve), minor (resolving complications), and subtle. We define the latter here as long term effects of electrode insertion in the absence of any complication. Regarding major and minor complications, the most common is hemorrhage. The largest study of complications of SEEG placement reveals a per-patient risk of hemorrhage of about 19%, and ~0.2% risk per electrode for hemorrhage, being symptomatic at a rate of about 0.05% per electrode. In this study it is noted that there is a measurable increase in hemorrhage, on a per patient basis, when the number of electrodes exceeds about 13 (80). Similar rates of symptomatic hemorrhage per electrode (0.04%) were found with a larger SEEG case series focused on broader SEEG practice (81). Overall, this is favorable to the potential harm of subdural grid placement which has a higher incidence of infection, subdural hemorrhage and cerebral edema (82).

Subtle injuries are less clear, given that studies have not yet been designed to prospectively identify these effects. Two fairly recent studies raised questions about the possibility that cognitive function, particularly memory, might be adversely affected by bilateral depth electrodes placed orthogonally through the hippocampi (83, 84). Nevertheless, both studies were retrospective in nature and limited by methodological imprecisions that could not be overcome after the fact (e.g., group differences that could not be controlled for in a retrospective clinical study). In contrast, similar studies have not been suggestive of this decline, and this has included work completed using neurostimulation devices that have been placed longitudinally along the hippocampus in both occipital and temporal lobes. Evaluations of this area have been the subject of several recent commentaries, which go into a great deal of detail, and suggest the need for prospective studies to overcome these limitations (85–87).

Promise of Cognitive Mapping With SEEG

Passive vs. Active Stimulation Mapping

Historically, as we have covered thus far in this manuscript, cognitive mapping for epilepsy presurgical candidates has involved administration of a cognitive paradigm while high frequency electrical stimulation is actively delivered. One drawback to this approach is that it requires the presence of an epileptologist to perform the stimulation and monitor the live recording for after-discharges and seizures, as well as a neuropsychologist or cognitively oriented neurologist. While 50 Hz stimulation is often appropriate for cognitive mapping, outside of the sensorimotor cortex and hippocampal formation, with both a broader range of brain structures accessed and with a greater sophistication in planning stimulation, other frequency, and train parameters can be, and perhaps ought to be chosen. With higher frequency stimulation, seizures are

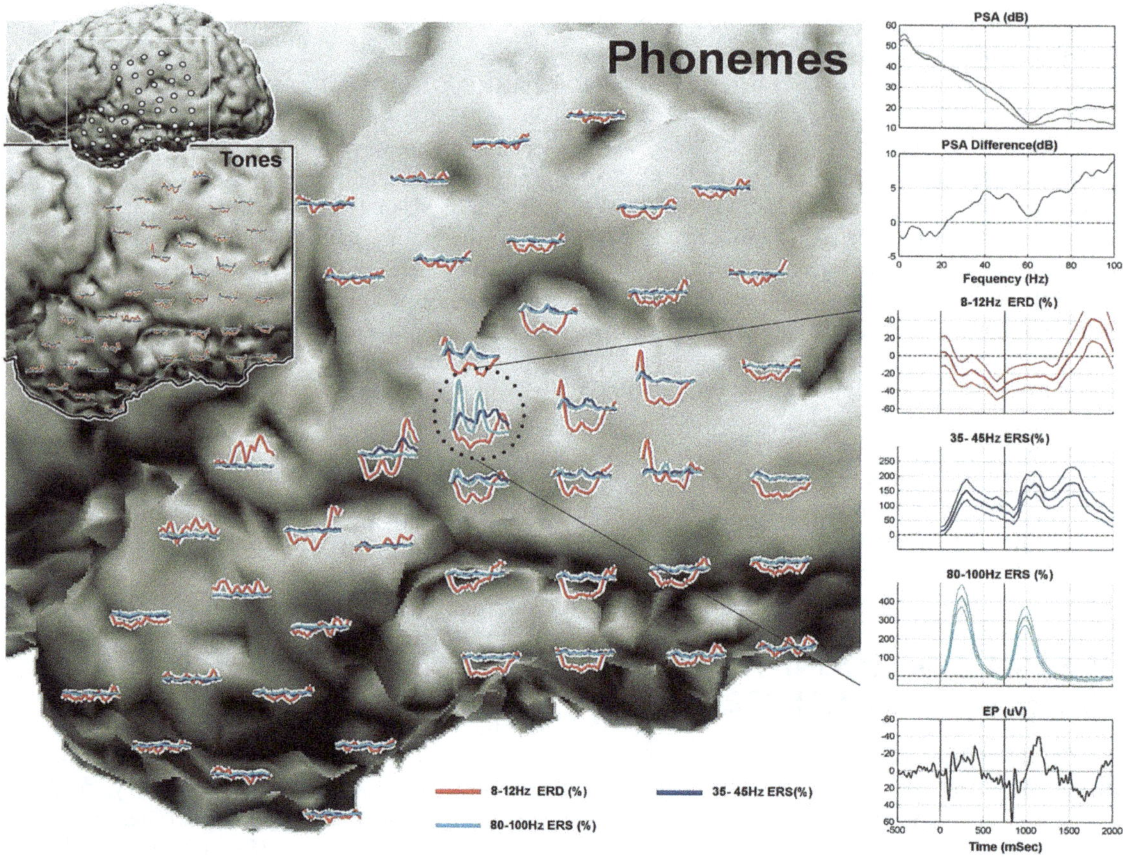

FIGURE 2 | Cortical activity during a receptive language task. From the first study of passive mapping of electrocorticographic activity during a receptive task of distinguishing tones from phonemes by Crone et al. (90). Indices during perception of tones (lower left inset with black border) vs. phonemes (expanded view of left temporal lobe). Plots of event-related power augmentation/suppression are color-coded according to frequency, and correspond to the electrode locations depicted in the upper left corner inset (white frame indicates borders of the expanded views). Detailed plots in the right column are derived from an electrode over the left superior temporal gyrus (circled). PSA, power spectral array; ESD, event related desynchronization; ERS, event related synchronization; EP, evoked potential. From Crone et al. (90).

more likely, which abort the attempt to study cognition, or contributes to after discharges which can distort assessment results by disrupting broaders network regions in more formal cognitive assessment. This cannot be entirely avoided with altered stimulation parameters, but the occurrence of focal seizures can be of some assistance in understanding the function of components of the seizure network. Nonetheless, several studies demonstrate the problem of seizures disrupting cognitive mapping. For example, in a study of 122 pediatric patients who received 50 Hz electrical stimulation mapping, sizeable percentages of patients experienced after-discharges (77%) and seizures (35%) (88). In another sample of 57 adults undergoing active mapping, seizures occurred at a similar rate (33%); in a subset of this sample who underwent language assessment, 17% experienced seizures that disrupted mapping attempts (89).

In more recent years, passive mapping of cognition has been explored (See **Figure 2**). This has been an important advance given that it is theoretically more localizing than stimulation, which can activate a network while exerting local influence, theoretically also providing cognitive evoked potentials or latency information. Conversely, brain regions related to other components of the task may be activated, arguing for a lower spatial specificity in passive mapping. Keeping both of these ideas in mind, it seems reasonable to consider this approach to mapping as complimentary, and potentially capable of acting as a second independent source of information when considering the functional organization of the cerebral cortex. From a practical standpoint, passive mapping is performed by conducting behavioral paradigms during concurrent electrocorticographic recording. In general, electrocorticographic analysis of broadband higher gamma frequencies (70–110 Hz) is typically carried out during administration of a specific cognitive or sensory task (e.g., confrontation naming, verbal fluency) (91–94). Recording of high gamma activity is best done with a sampling rate of ECOG data that is 2- to 3-times higher than the frequency of recorded activity to avoid aliasing of waveforms and a high frequency filter above 300 samples per second (S/s), fitting with most centers recording at 1 kS/s or more. After ECOG data is obtained, time-frequency analysis is performed using the bipolar montage when SEEG electrodes are used (95, 96). Bipolar montage analysis excludes common mode signals, such as muscle activity, whose high-frequency components can mimic high-gamma oscillations (97). Time-frequency analysis of event-related, high-gamma activity helps delineate the network involved in a given cognitive task (picture naming). For instance, high-gamma oscillations recorded at the onset of an auditory naming task is indicative of perceptual processing, while high-gamma activity at the end of the response represents motor processing.

Studies contrasting active and passive paradigms for language (particularly expressive) have shown reasonably equivalent results at least with respect to critical regions of common overlap [sensitivity (98, 99)]. Indeed, changes in gamma activity during passive language mapping do appear to overlap with language areas identified through electrical stimulation mapping (91, 99–102). In contrast, however, passive mapping paradigms find more regions related to task performance in general, as above, so these techniques do differ with regards to specificity, and this can lead to problems with determining core regions essential to a cognitive task. Although limited in scope, passive mapping appears efficacious when comparing mapping findings to postsurgical results; here, resection of regions that were associated with event-related gamma oscillations in passive mapping was associated with post-operative language deficits (103, 104). Much more work is required in this area, as larger studies are required that cover all behavioral paradigms of interest. Outcome validity studies are also woefully lacking for traditional active mapping paradigms as well.

Passive mapping may have some practical and accuracy advantages over active stimulation. First, passive mapping is more time efficient which lends itself well to children or adults who have difficulty completing more lengthy sessions of active cortical stimulation mapping or who cannot tolerate unpleasant sensations that can sometimes accompany stimulation mapping. It also avoids artificial perturbation of the brain, and thus reduces overall risk for after-discharges and seizures. Passive mapping is suggested to be more sensitive to localized cortical areas (e.g., as defined by language mapping: Broca's, Wernicke's, sensorimotor, basal temporal) than electrical stimulation mapping (102). In contrast, one potential limitation with passive mapping compared to active stimulation mapping, is that passive mapping, like fMRI activations, cannot determine whether regions are essential for a given cognitive task rather than simply being involved in the task (60, 105). If a region is not essential, it can still typically be included in a proposed surgical resection/ablation without harming overall function. Despite the limitations of stimulation mapping, and the potential to disrupt function more broadly than recognized or desired, it does create a "functional lesion" that may more accurately reflect the possible effect of surgical intervention. An interesting research proposition would be to use passive mapping to locate potential regions of eloquent brain tissue, and to follow this up with stimulation mapping of these areas in an attempt to better determine the potential effects of surgery.

Use of Machine Learning to Decode Passively Acquired Electrocorticography

While brain-machine interfaces are generally beyond the scope of this review, there is topical overlap with passive cognitive mapping and research directed toward the decoding of speech. Given the likely problems of under-determining activity in a single brain region from sparse sampling with SEEG, this work has relied on grids, including higher density research grids. While this represents a large body of work that shares some similarities with work on brain-machine interfaces, the most notable current achievement is the transcription of speech while recording from language-dominant frontal opercular region (106), that performs quite well with simple sentences (See **Figure 3**). This decoding of neural activity in relation to behavior is particularly suited to machine and deep learning, where a classifier can be built or trained based on neural activity and an objective measure of behavior. These approaches will provide practical and theoretical insights into the organization of cortical function, as well as potentially providing a wide-array of brain-machine interfaces.

Connectivity, Cognition, and Philosophy

While some notions of localization focus on a one to one mapping of function and brain tissue, it is obvious that functional territories cannot act in isolation. A less extreme form of localizationist thinking might hold that cortical tissue maps well to function, with it taken as implicit that subcortical structures are necessary for input and output. When considering behavior, obviously large networks, typically with multiple cortical waypoints are involved. When considering the abstractions of cognitive psychology, there can be mapping of abstract functions to some brain regions, but the agreement of neurological thinking and the functionalist concepts of cognitive psychology are imperfect (take episodic and semantic memory for examples, where these concepts do not map directly to a brain region or perhaps even a circuit). Overall, this mismatch results in a philosophical approach that grew out of medical materialism, by way of Sellars (107) and Feyerarbend (108), that has come to be known as *eliminative materialism* (109) where *folk psychological* abstractions are eliminated in favor of an ontology based around neural mechanisms [see (110), for discussion]. This is critical to mention for three reasons: Firstly, we should keep this in mind when developing new tasks that aim to test particular brain networks. Secondly, this is likely a fruitful general line of research in neuroscience, behavior, and cognitive psychology. Lastly, it marries with a vastly increased interest in neural mechanisms in philosophy and particularly in the philosophy of mind. This latter scenario is beginning to provide productive common ground for more sophisticated understandings of consciousness, cognition and brain function.

Connectivity: DTI, fMRI, CCEPs, and Limitations

As we have thus far argued, an appreciation of connectivity is critical for understanding the correspondence between cortical functions and anatomical networks. There are several ways to determine and define connectivity. It should firstly be emphasized that the gold-standard of brain connectivity remains neuroanatomical tracing. These methods are based around

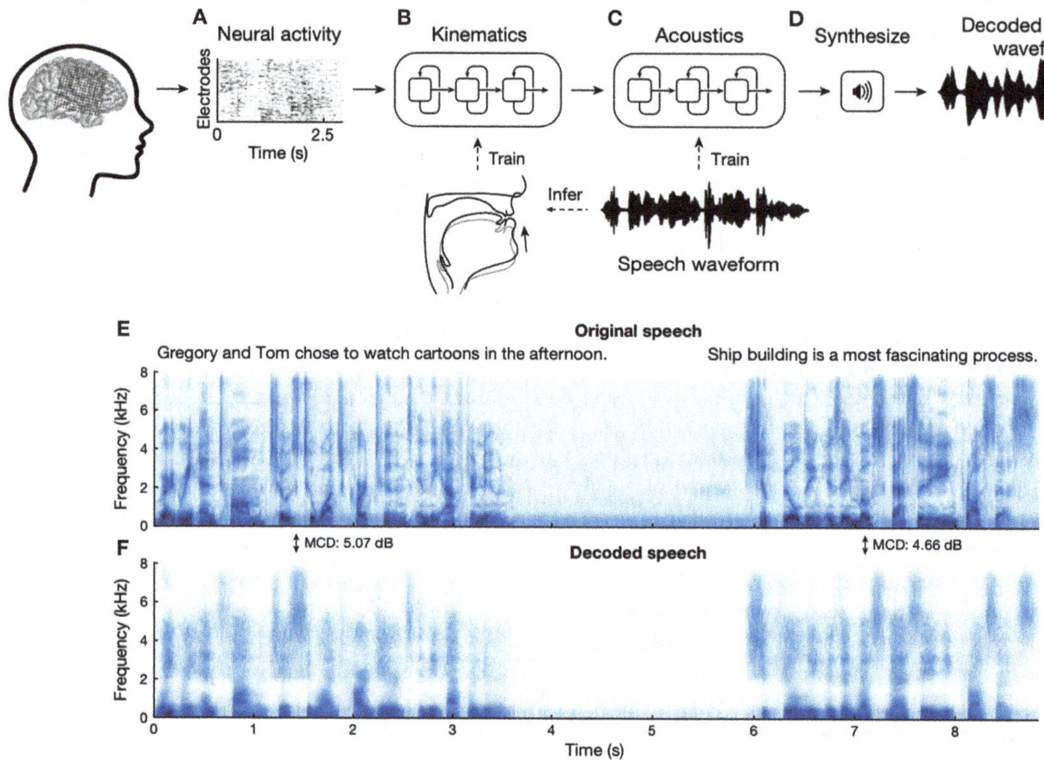

FIGURE 3 | Speech synthesis from recorded electrocorticogram during spoken sentences. **(A)** The neural decoding process begins by extracting relevant signal features from high-density cortical activity. **(B)** A neural network decodes kinematic representations of articulation from ECoG signals. **(C)** An additional algorithm decodes acoustics from the previously decoded kinematics. Acoustics are spectral features extracted from the speech waveform. **(D)** Decoded signals are then synthesized into an acoustic waveform. **(E)** Spectrogram shows the frequency content of two sentences spoken by a participant. **(F)** Spectrogram of synthesized speech from brain signals recorded simultaneously with the speech in **(E)**. From Anumanchipalli et al. (106).

the transport of stereotactically injected dyes, radiolabels or detectable proteins into the brain so that neurons projecting into the area of injection, or axons projecting from this region, can be visualized, often by autoradiography or histological methods and microscopy. Neurotropic viruses such as strains of herpes and rabies have also been used for tracing, which can be polysynaptic. More recently, viral vectors have been the principle means of determining afferent and efferent connections of a given brain region, and by using genetic methods, even of a particular cell type [see (111, 112)]. Needless to say, these methods cannot be performed in humans, meaning that our most detailed knowledge of veridical connectivity comes from non-human primates and inferences from other species. This leaves us with inference and indirect methods to determine connectivity and cortical networks essential for cognition in humans, one of which is based on and related to electrical stimulation mapping.

From the human neuroimaging literature, the indirect methods of determining human "connectivity" is often divided into *structural*, *functional*, and *effective* connectivity (113). *Structural* connectivity, not to be confused with neuroanatomical tracing, typically refers to diffusion imaging-based methods such as probabilistic and deterministic tractography. There are numerous limitations to this method, when sharp axonal branches or curves cannot be followed, the direction is not determined, nor the length of a given set of axons be determined as identical to that of the larger bundle of fibers that can be detected [see (114)]. *Functional* connectivity need not represent anatomical connectivity at all: This is where a functional assay is used, and correlated activity is determined by blood oxygen level desaturation (as in functional MRI), or perhaps by intracranial EEG. The problem is that simultaneous activation can result from two structures having a shared input. For example, activation of subcortical nuclei can result in faster activity across the cortex, but it does meaningfully represent "connectivity" between these cortical regions. *Effective* connectivity is where a connection is implied if a recording site's activity is changed by perturbation of another site. This provides causal information, but typically cannot determine if connectivity is direct or indirect. An example, pertinent to the present review of functional networks is cortico-cortical evoked potentials [CCEPs (115)], which are perhaps the closest we can get to a measure of anatomical connectivity in the human cortex (See **Figure 4**). While this technique was first described by Brazier (117), by which time it may have already been appreciated by Bancaud and Talairach, it has undergone something of a recent revival. This technique is a boon for studies of human forebrain connectivity, especially as we attempt to divide the cerebral cortex into discrete functional networks. For example, this approach to using low-frequency stimulation, longer than the time of the complete evoked potential and typically 1 Hz, and its resultant

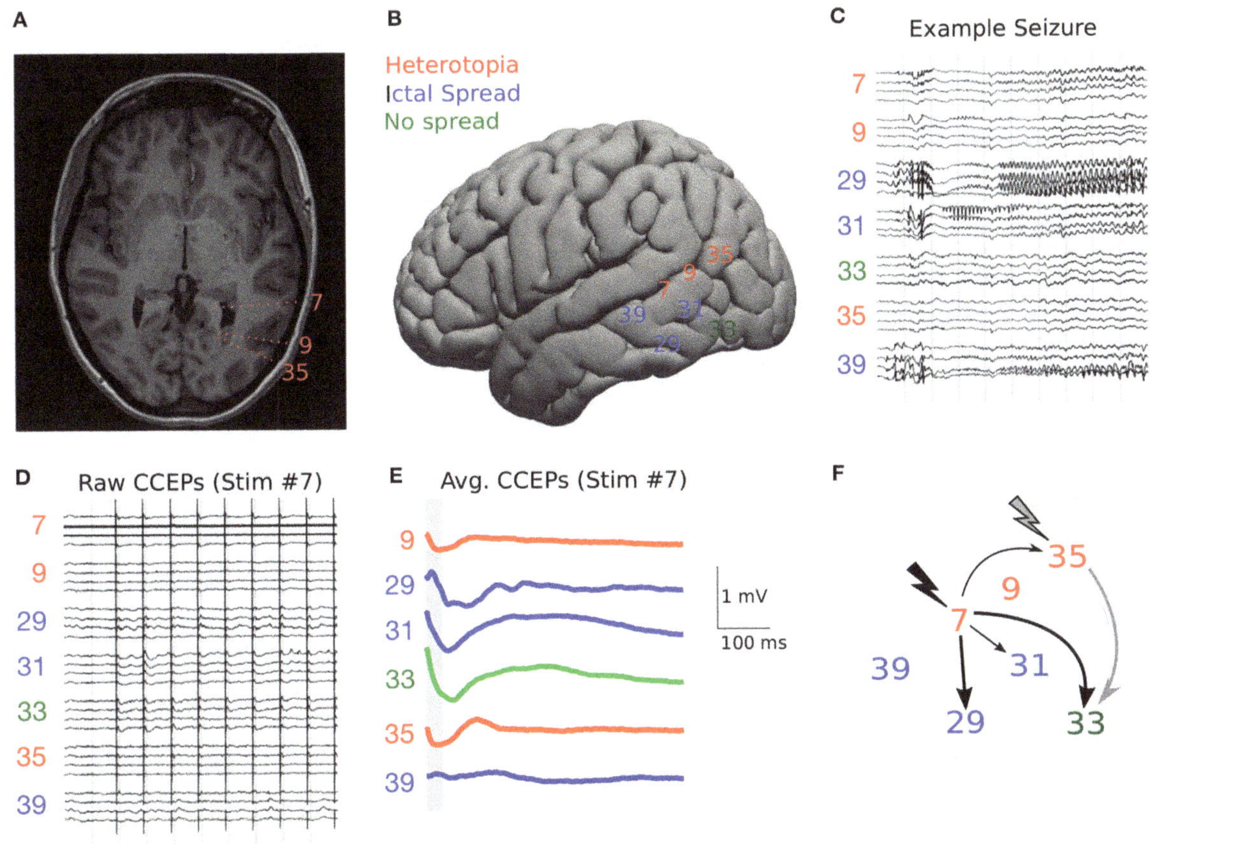

FIGURE 4 | Example of using CCEPs to study effective connectivity. **(A)** Axial MRI Brian (T1) showing two periventricular nodular heterotopias in the tirgone of the left lateral ventricle and the trajectories of electrodes 7, 9, and 35, with dashes showing the approximate location of the 10 contacts of each recording electrode. **(B)** The approximate lateral entry points of pertinent left-sided SEEG electrodes are shown as electrode numbers. **(C)** An example spontaneous left sided seizure onset is shown with gamma activity on electrode 29 contacts 1–3 (posterior hippocampus). **(D)** Raw cortico-cortical evoked potentials (CCEPS) triggered by 1 Hz bipolar stimulation anterior heterotopion (electrode 7 contacts 3–4). Evoked potentials with peak to trough amplitude >250 μV are evident on electrodes 29, 31, and 33. **(E)** Averaged CCEPs with 20–50 ms (gray bar) window of interest shown. Only the largest amplitude (root mean squared amplitude (RMSA) CCEP (taken over all 10 contacts) is shown for each electrode. **(F)** Connectivity map for stimulation to electrode 7 (black) and 35 (gray). Thick arrows represent CCEPs with RMSA >200 mV, thin arrows represent CCEPs with RMSA >100 mV. From Dickey et al. (116).

CCEPs, has been used to examine connectivity between language areas (118, 119), within the motor cortices (120). This has been of assistance in mapping and in sparing white matter intraoperatively, to preserve connectivity between the anterior and posterior language areas. For example, in one patient a 50% drop in CCEPs amplitude was associated with a long-term language deficit (61).

FUNCTIONAL MAPPING OF COGNITION AND EMOTION—ANTICIPATING FUTURE DIRECTIONS

Cognitive Function

While much progress has been made in the mapping of cognitive function, there remains considerable variability in the techniques and paradigms used (29), there are many aspects of cognition that never get assessed, and the determinations of the full networks responsible for a function is often not determined. The focus of cognitive mapping has primarily been language, and to a lesser extent, aspects of memory. This is rightfully so, as the early days of epilepsy surgery were marred by poor outcomes of cases such as Henry Molaison (121), where the severity of the resulting amnestic state overshadowed any other aspect of the case. As we have gotten better at avoiding these catastrophic outcomes, and even lessening the poor cognitive outcomes through improved testing and minimally invasive surgical options, the focus of the field can now broaden to potential deficits which were previously underappreciated and potentially overshadowed. Initial findings suggest that some of these overlooked deficits can have some profound effects on patients (70, 122). Most cognitive mapping efforts have focused on language, in particular visual object naming. Even in this well-hewn area there is little consensus on training approaches as well as best practices for clinical and research efforts. **Table 1** lists a number of cognitive and socio-emotional functions for which there is some evidence of structure-function knowledge derived primarily from cognitive mapping procedures.

TABLE 1 | Chart of positive neural stimulation sites and specific neuropsychological functions (selected sample of representative studies).

References	Function assessed	Region of stimulation	
	Language	**Left hemisphere**	**Right hemisphere**
	Visual naming		
Ojemann et al. (38)	Visual naming (general)	Cortical stimulation across language dominant temporal lobe, frontal lobe, and parietal lobe sites (with significant variability across subjects)	N/A
Hamberger et al. (123)	Visual naming (objects)	Posterior temporal lobe regions	No effects of stimulation
Duffau et al. (124)	Visual naming (objects)	Dorsal PMC and underlying white matter	N/A
Ulvin et al. (125)	Visual naming (objects)	Stimulation of VTC led to naming deficits (particularly the FG and OTS)	Stimulation of VTC led to naming deficits in a single patient with right TL language, but no other subjects
Sarubbo et al. (126)	Visual naming (general)	STG, MFG, MFG WM, AG, AG WM, MTG, ITG, STG WM, IFG WM, SMG, insula, lateral FOC, ITG, WM, MTG WM, IFG, SMG WM, lateral FOC WM, FG	AG WM, AG, MTG, WM
	Paraphasic errors during stimulation	**Left hemisphere**	**Right hemisphere**
Leclercq et al. (67)	Phonemic paraphasic errors during visual naming	AF	No disruption with stimulation
Leclercq et al. (67)	Semantic paraphasic errors during visual naming	IFOF	No disruption with stimulation
Maldonado et al. (127)	Phonemic paraphasic errors during visual naming	PostAF (WM)	No disruption with stimulation
Miozzo et al. (128)	Semantic paraphasic errors during visual naming	Mid-middle temporal gyrus	No disruption with stimulation
Miozzo et al. (128)	Phonemic paraphasic errors during visual naming	Middle and posterior STG	No disruption with stimulation
	Auditory naming (naming to description)	**Left hemisphere**	**Right hemisphere**
Hamberger et al. (123)	Naming to verbal description (definitions) presented orally	Anterior temporal lobe	No disruption with stimulation
	Transmodal naming	**Left hemisphere**	**Right hemisphere**
Abel et al. (129)	Visual and Auditory Naming of Same Semantic Concept (e.g., famous person)	Anterior temporal lobe	No disruption with stimulation
	Proper noun naming	**Left hemisphere**	**Right hemisphere**
Abel et al. (129)	Famous person naming	Anterior temporal lobe/temporal pole	No disruption with stimulation
	Language comprehension	**Left hemisphere**	**Right hemisphere**
Sarubbo et al. (126)	Comprehension	SPL, STG, insula, SPL WM, SMG WM, MFG WM, STG WM	MFG WM, STG, hippocampus, MFG, STG WM, AG WM, MTG WM, AG, insula, ITG WM, ITG, PostCG, SMFG, MTG
	Semantic processing	**Left hemisphere**	**Right hemisphere**
Ulvin et al. (125)	Picture matching (semantically related)	No disruption from stimulation of VTC	No disruption from stimulation of VTC
Sarubbo et al. (126)	Semantic processing	MTG WM, insula, MTG, STG, hippocampus, MG WM, ITG, FG, ITG WM, STG WM, MFG, IFG, IFG WM, putamen, lateral FOC, FG WM, SFG, WM	No disruption
	Reading	**Left hemisphere**	**Right hemisphere**
Roux et al. (130)	Oral reading	Inferior aspect of pre- and Post CG, SMG, AG, and posterior STG, IFG, MFG, posterior MTG	Inferior aspect of pre- and Post CG, IFG
Roux et al. (130)	Articulation errors in oral reading	Inferior aspect of Pre- and Post CG	Inferior aspect of Pre- and Post CG
Roux et al. (130)	Ocular-induced reading errors	IFG	IFG
Sarubbo et al. (126)	Reading	ITG, FG, MTG, IOG, ITG WM, MTG WM, FG WM, IOG WM	ITG, ITG WM
Sabsevitz et al. (131)	Reading	Lateral fusiform gyrus (VWFA)	N/A

(Continued)

TABLE 1 | Continued

References	Function assessed	Region of stimulation	
	Language	**Left hemisphere**	**Right hemisphere**
	Acoustic responses/disruption	**Left hemisphere**	**Right hemisphere**
Sarubbo et al. (126)	Acoustic responses	STG, STG WM, MTG	STG, MTG, STG WM, MTG WM
Sarubbo et al. (126)	Phonological	ITG, MTG, MTG WM, FG, IFG WM, STG, SPL WM, ITG WM, IFG, MFG, STG WM, AG WM, MFG WM, PostCG WM, SS, PreCG WM, AG, PostCG, SPL, SMG WM, PreCG, SMG, insula	No disruption
Duffau et al. (124)	Speech production	Ventral PMC and underlying WM	N/A
Sarubbo et al. (126)	Speech production	IFG, IFG WM, PreCG, PreCG WM, MFG, STG, insula, MFG WM, STG WM	PreCG WM, PreCG, MFG, IFG, insula, MFG WM, IFG WM, putamen
Sarubbo et al. (126)	Speech articulation	SMG WM, SMG, PostCG, PreCG WM, PostCG WM, PreCG, IFG, MFG, IFG WM, MFG WM, STG, AG WM, AG, insula, SFG WM	SMG, SMG WM, IFG, MFG SFG WM, MFG WM
	Somatosensory	**Left hemisphere**	**Right hemisphere**
Maldonado et al. (127)	Somatosensory	PostCG	PostCG
Sarubbo et al. (126)	Somatosensory	SPL WM, SPL, PostCG WM, precuneus, PostCG, PreCG, PreCG WM	SPL, PostCG WM, PostCG, SPL WM, SMG, AG, SMG, insula, pre-cuneus, STG, AG WM, PreCG
	Motor function	**Left hemisphere**	**Right hemisphere**
Blanke et al. (132)	Eye movements	Posterior portion of MFG, SFG; no response from IFG or precentral gyrus	Posterior portion of MFG, SFG; no response from IFG or precentral gyrus
Sarubbo et al. (126)	Eye movement control	MFG, MFG WM, SFG WM, PreCG, PreCG WM, SFG	MFG, MFG WM, SFG, SFG WM
Maldonado et al. (127)	Speech initiation/articulation	PO, horizontal portion of the lateral segment of the SLF III.	N/A
Sarubbo et al. (126)	Language initiation and motor planning	CN, SFG WM, SFG, MFG WM, insula, IFG, lateral FOC WM, IFG WM, MFG, putamen, lateral FOC	CN
Sarubbo et al. (126)	Motor	PreCG WM, SFG, PreCG, SFG WM, putamen, insula, MFG	preCG WM, SFG, putamen, SFG WM, PreCG, insular, MFG, MFG WM, PostCG, SLF, Post CG WM, IFG, IFG WM
Sarubbo et al. (126)	Motor control	SFG WM, SFG, MFG WM, MFG, CG, PostCG WM, PostCG, PreCG	SFG, SFG WM, MFG, CG, IFG, IFG WM, insula, MFG WM, putamen, precuneus
	Consciousness/mental phenomenology	**Left hemisphere**	**Right hemisphere**
Halgren et al. (133)	Déjà vu/"dreamy state"	Hippocampus and Amygdala	Hippocampus and Amygdala
Gloor (134)	Déjà vu	Lateral TL with spread to medial TL region	Lateral TL with spread to medial TL region
Bartolomei et al. (135)	Déjà vu	Entorhinal cortex, Perirhinal cortex hippocampus, amygdala (while this sensation could occur after stimulation of any of these structures it was much more common after entorhinal stimulation)	Entorhinal cortex, Perirhinal cortex hippocampus, amygdala (while this sensation could occur after stimulation of any of these structures it was much more common after entorhinal stimulation)
Bartolomei et al. (135)	Reminiscence of scenes	Perirhinal cortex	Perirhinal cortex
Sarubbo et al. (126)	"Mentalizing"	No disruption	MFG WM, IFG, MFG, SFG, IFG WM, SFG WM, CG, CN, insula
	Emotional responses	**Left hemisphere**	**Right hemisphere**
Lanteaume et al. (136)	Experience of negative emotions	Amygdala	Amygdala
Lanteaume et al. (136)	Experience of positive emotions	Amygdala	No effect elicited in right hemisphere
	Visual processing	**Left hemisphere**	**Right hemisphere**
Sarubbo et al. (126)	Visual	FG, IOG WM, FG WM, MOG WM, IOG	AG WM, AG, IOG, MTG WM, MOG WM, hippocampus, FG, IOG WM, SPL WM, SOG WM, MOG, MTG, ITG, FG WM, STG WM, SMG WM

(Continued)

TABLE 1 | Continued

References	Function assessed	Region of stimulation	
	Language	**Left hemisphere**	**Right hemisphere**
	Visuo-perceptual/visual-spatial	**Left hemisphere**	**Right hemisphere**
Vignal et al. (137)	Facial hallucinations	No effect of stimulation	Ventrolateral prefrontal cortex
Barbeau et al. (138)	Famous face recognition	Passive mapping with intracerebral recordings demonstrates early involvement of the FG simultaneously with the IFG, then multiple regions of the ventral visual WM stream, and finally involvement of the hippocampus (much more pronounced in right hemisphere than left)	Passive mapping with intracerebral recordings demonstrates early involvement of the FG simultaneously with the IFG, then multiple regions of the ventral visual WM stream, and finally involvement of the hippocampus (much more pronounced in right hemisphere than left)
Fernandez Coello et al. (68)	Recognition of faces and select objects	N/A	Stimulation of ventral visual processing stream (IFOF and ILF)
Roux et al. (139)	Spatial neglect	N/A	Posterior part of the right STG and MTG, IPL, and inferior post CG and IFG. SLF II and SOFF
Bush et al. (140)	Spatial navigation	Increases in low and high frequency theta power are observed at the onset of movement in the hippocampus and lateral temporal lobe regions	Increases in low and high frequency theta power are observed at the onset of movement in the hippocampus and lateral temporal lobe regions
Maidenbaum et al. (141)	Spatial navigation	Entorhinal theta band activity is related to task performance	Entorhinal theta band activity is related to task performance
Sarubbo et al. (126)	Spatial perception	AG WM, AG	SMG, SMG WM, AG, AG WM, STG, SPL WM STG WM, MFG WM, PostCG WM, SPL, CG, MTG, PreCG WM, MFG
	Arithmetic skills	**Left hemisphere**	**Right hemisphere**
Duffau et al. (142)	Multiplication/subtraction	AG	N/A
Yu et al. (143)	Subtraction—but not multiplication disrupted at right hemisphere sites	N/A	IPL and AG
	Memory functions		
Haglund et al. (144) and Ojemann et al. (46)	Verbal episodic memory	Disrupted by stimulation of lateral TL cortex	No evidence of disruption from right TL stimulation
Coleshill et al. (145)	Verbal episodic memory	Disrupted by stimulation of amygdala and hippocampus	N/A
Ezzyat et al. (146)	Verbal episodic memory	Memory was enhanced at some frequencies by stimulation of lateral TL cortex in setting of SEEG	N/A
	Executive functions		
Bonini et al. (147)	Metacognitive evaluation of accuracy estimates	SMA	SMA
Puglisi et al. (148)	response inhibition	No disruption with stimulation	Non-dominant FL

AF, arcuate fasciculus; AG, angular gyrus; CG, cingulate gyrus; FL, frontal lobe; FG, fusiform gyrus; FOC, fronts-orbital cortex; IFG, inferior frontal gyrus; IFOF, inferior frontal occipital fasciculus; ILF, inferior longitudinal fasciculus; IOG, inferior occipital gyrus; IPL, inferior parietal lobule; ITG, inferior temporal gyrus; MFG, middle frontal gyrus; MOG, middle occipital gyrus; MTGG, middle temporal gyrus; N/A, no assessment was completed; OTS, occipital temporal sulcus; PMC, pre-motor cortex; PO, parietal operculum; PostAF, posterior arcuate fasciculus; PostCG, postcentral gyrus; PreCG, precentral gyrus; SFG, superior frontal gyrus; SLF II/SLF III, superior longitudinal fasciculus; SMA, supplementary motor area; SMG, supra marginal gyrus; SOFF, superior occipital frontal fasciculus; SOG, superior occipital gyrus; SPL, superior parietal lobule; STG, superior temporal gyrus; TL, temporal lobe; VTC, ventral temporal cortex; VWFA, visual word form area; WM, white matter.

Language

Language mapping often involves administration of relatively simple tasks to test basic, automatic speech functions, such as counting or reciting overlearned phrases. Object naming is considered the "gold standard" for mapping language and allows for a broad sampling of the language network; however, more targeted, multitask testing may be needed to increase sensitivity as naming alone has been shown to miss 31% of temporoparietal and 43% of frontal language sites (149). It is widely accepted that language involves a more distributed network than Broca's and Wernicke's area and that anatomically dissociable regions exist that are specialized for specific linguistic subroutines which interactively support the construct of language (34, 39, 150, 151). Regions spanning the ventral temporal and occipital lobes and fusiform area appear to contribute heavily to recognition (primarily right hemisphere, but some left) of visual objects and faces, while coexisting areas on the left are important for naming (152–156). Naming itself is a complex

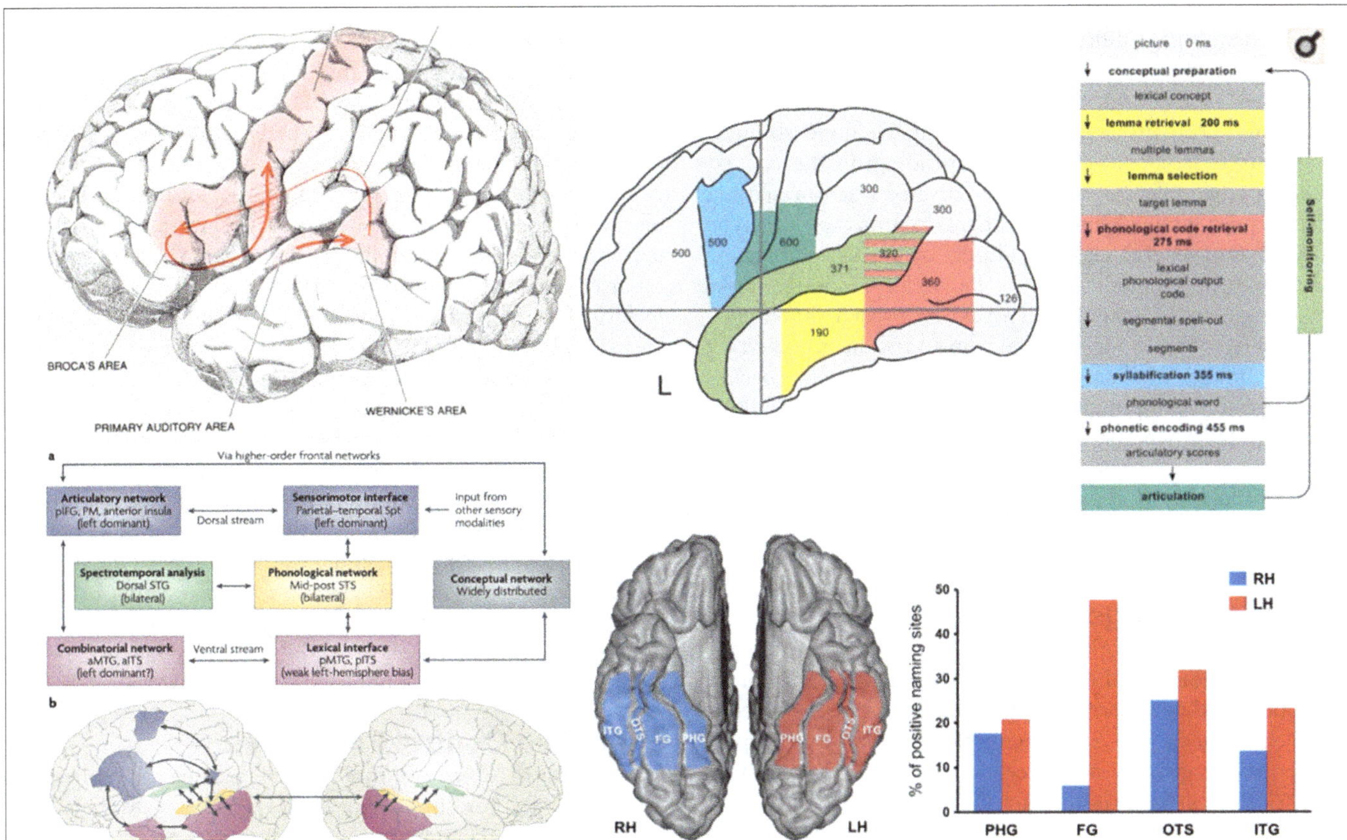

FIGURE 5 | Models and Anatomy of Language Networks reveal the large area of the cerebral cortical involved in language. Top left: Geschwind's (169) illustration of the Broca-Wernicke model of language. Top right: Indefrey's (170) model of cortical activity (showing evoked potential latencies by region in milliseconds) during a confrontation naming task, demonstrating some of the cortical extent of language processing. Bottom left: Hickok and Poeppel (39) dual stream model of the cortical anatomy of auditory language comprehension and response where auditory processing is bilateral and involves bilateral superior temporal sulci and unimodal auditory cortex from which activity is conveyed to either a dorsal stream for, motor and articulatory analysis and phonological representation, vs. a ventral stream for lexical and conceptual representation (aITS, anterior inferior temporal sulcus; aMTG, anterior middle temporal gyrus; pIFG, posterior inferior frontal gyrus; PM, premotor cortex). Bottom right: From Ulvin et al. (125), showing the regions in which stimulation can result in specific naming deficits ("positive naming sites"), identifying the crucial role of the dominant fusiform basal temporal region in naming (ITG, inferior temporal gyrus; FG, fusiform gyrus; OTS, occipitotemporal sulcus; PHG, parahippocampal gyrus).

construct, which can differ by modality of stimulus presentation [e.g., naming sounds vs. naming pictures (157)], object type [i.e., different object types map to different brain region (158, 159)], and level of classification [e.g., proper nouns have been more associated with the temporal pole while common nouns seem more broadly distributed (160)]. Naming can also vary by task parameters such as having a patient name objects/persons based on verbal descriptions (e.g., "the current President of the US") rather than based on a sensory representation [e.g., naming a washing machine based on the sound it makes or its visual image (161)]. The latter tasks require the subject to determine the semantic content before applying the name, and are therefore slightly more complex. Orthographic or written letter content seems to be managed by a posterior temporal component of this stream [e.g., visual word form area (131, 162, 163)]. Aspects of the mid superior temporal gyrus and sulcus are dedicated to processing phonology or speech sounds, consistent with adjacency to unimodal auditory association cortex, while more posterior areas of the superior temporal gyrus and inferior parietal lobule involved in phonological access and retrieval, and areas in lateral middle and inferior temporal lobe, posterior inferior parietal lobe (angular gyrus) and dorsolateral frontal cortex that are involved in processing semantics [i.e., the meaning of pictures, words, phrases, etc. (29, 150, 164, 165)]. And this is of course all contingent on patient-specific factors like intelligence (44), gender (166), and handedness (167, 168) to name but a few.

Given the complexity and multidimensional nature of language, there is a need to develop and use tasks that differentially engage or drive these linguistic processes so mapping can be better tailored to the functional anatomy of the area being mapped (See **Figure 5**). For example, (171) have put forward the idea that language networks consist of functionally specialized "cores" and domain general "periphery." Interactions between language nodes and with other brain networks are thought to subserve different language functions which may differ depending on task parameters. For example, the word "nail" has different meanings depending on the context of use, and will likely engage different subnetworks when presented as body part, an object, or as an action. This conceptualization of language is consistent with fMRI findings, such as those of Tyler et al. (172), which have shown that the same stimulus can activate different brain regions depending on the context of the task (e.g., different regions are activated when presenting a given object and asking the patient to think of the type of object, the general class of object, or the specific name of the object). It could therefore be useful to design tasks with a single set of stimuli that could be used to potentially activate different brain regions depending upon the broader task demands. On the other hand, cognitive psychological approaches to language are often function- and theory-based. Both cognitive theory and underlying brain mechanisms and understanding of the functional organization of the cerebral cortex will be key, related to the idea of *eliminative materialism*, above. In other words, preceding from neurologically plausible concepts of the organization of language is also critical.

Beyond Language

To date, much less work has been done on mapping non-language functions—and the notion of non-eloquence in brain areas outside of dominant hemisphere language regions needs to be challenged. The right hemisphere is known to play an important role in visual perception and spatial processing (173, 174), object/face recognition (155, 158, 175–178), socio-emotional processing (7), navigation and learning in a spatial context (179), and attention/neglect (180), and there is great need to develop tasks to assess these functions for the purposes of stimulation mapping.

Visual-Spatial Processing, Construction, Navigation

Some work exists in the area of spatial processing and navigation with regards to ESM/SEEG, but most represent "one-off" case studies and an occasional targeted experiment rather than a planned effort to study these functions with these technologies. However, deficits in many of these functions can lead to varying degrees of disability for the patient. One example is unilateral spatial neglect, which involves an inability to attend to one side of space (most often the left side with right sided lesions). Line bisection and cancellation tasks are commonly used to assess spatial neglect and discrimination behaviorally, and this function has in turn been mapped to the posterior parietal cortex—more specifically the inferior and superior parietal lobules but also portions of the posterior temporal lobe (139). Mental rotation tasks, where the patient has to determine whether two objects are the same or different by mentally rotating them, can also be used to test the non-dominant parietal lobe (181, 182). Functional MRI studies have implicated bilateral superior parietal, frontal, and inferotemporal cortices during mental rotation with greater non-dominant, right parietal activation often seen (183). Facial perception and line orientation have likewise been tied to the non-dominant parietal lobe (specifically the parietal-occipital junction) as well as the non-dominant posteroinferior frontal lobe (184). Impairment on these tasks tend to contribute to social dysfunction and can impair work performance as well, although this is an area that has never been well-studied.

Navigation has also been studied in humans, but the tasks, physiology and circuits have some dissimilarities with the large knowledge from rodent studies. Firstly, studies of neocortical theta are likely irrelevant to the navigation-related activity that is extensively characterized in rodents. Attention has focused on lower frequency components of the intracranial medial temporal lobe EEG, but while non-hippocampal theta has been reported, in relation to virtual maze tasks up to 8 Hz (185), including in relation to possible grid cells of the entorhinal area (141, 186), hippocampal task-related candidate theta activity has been described at 1–4 Hz and around 8 Hz (140, 187–190) also see (191). Furthermore, periods of enriched theta are very brief (188) and are not coordinated along the human septo-hippocampal axis (192). Given the large number of diverse cortical inputs to the hippocampal formation inferred in humans, spatial tasks may only influence as-yet unidentified subregions of the hippocampus. Similarly, rodent work has called attention to the hippocampal formation, given a role in learning of spatial tasks, but spatial learning and perception obviously involves multiple regions of both neo- and allocortex, again ripe for dissection with task development.

Executive Control Processes

Monitoring of executive functions is particularly important during frontal resections, but it is important to note that executive functions involve more distributed cortico-cortico and cortico-subcortical networks, and deficits in this domain can develop with damage outside the frontal lobes (193). Executive functions include processes such as planning, shifting from one mental set to another, updating and monitoring of information, problem solving, metacognition, abstract reasoning, and inhibitory control (194). While little work has been done in this area when it comes to cognitive mapping, tasks to consider could include inhibitory control (e.g., Stroop/color-word interference tests, Go/No Go tests), working memory (e.g., reverse digit sequencing), verbal generative fluency (e.g., saying as many words starting with a particular letter within a short period of time) and mental flexibility (e.g., Oral Trail Making Test requiring alternating recitation of ascending numbers and letters). As an example, researchers used SEEG to demonstrate that the supplementary motor area has a role in evaluating the accuracy of actions (147). Similarly, Puglisi et al. (148) used a simplified Stroop paradigm in a ESM setting, and reported that sparing the identified subcortical sites in the non-dominant frontal lobe region led to preserved executive functions as compared to patients who did not previously receive this mapping.

Learning and Memory

Clinical memory evaluation using ESM and SEEG paradigms has also been minimally explored and is rarely used in clinical practice, although changes in memory comprise some of the worst potential deficits of epilepsy surgical procedures. Estimates of memory decline, which are limited by greater variations in test usage, nevertheless range from 40 to 60% in temporal lobe cases (195–198). These numbers are more modest with minimally invasive surgical procedures but still occur (48, 199). Moreover, we have argued that the current clinical tests of memory are woefully inadequate to fully capture the complexity of memory. Almost all clinically available tasks require the patient to learn solely auditory/verbal or visual content, which they must learn and recall for a very brief period of time. In actuality, human memory is a much more complex construct in which such recall has to be integrated into existing memories (semantic and autobiographical knowledge) and is typically learned in a multimodal fashion (i.e., requires the integration of multisensory and motor input, linguistic/semantic interpretation, etc.) with coding of temporal, spatial, and emotional context. It is possible that we are only testing the most basic of memory subsystems in the process of learning and consolidating information required for effective adaptation to life. Therefore, we need to develop much more advanced measures and test paradigms to allow us to explore these broader aspects of memory. Some of these paradigms can be as simple as combining modalities of learning (e.g., putting a name with a face) and other aspects have only become possible with the advent of technological advances (e.g., virtual reality). Ideally, an array of tasks varying in complexity with dissociable sub-components will allow for the "mental chronometric" process of determining the neural substrates of the basic components (e.g., networks underlying simple encoding of different stimulus modalities) and the broader systems level interactions (e.g., integrating encoded percepts across stimulus modalities, integrating these new memories with existing semantic and autobiographical knowledge bases, processing modulatory feedback from emotional and linguistic systems), which obviously form multiple "scaleable" levels of integrated complexity.

The use of memory paradigms combined with properly designed electrophysiological study (e.g., CCEPs, single unit recordings) could powerfully increase our knowledge of this critical brain function. Recent work with human and non-human primates, for example, is exploring the relationship between the electrophysiology of sleep (e.g., occurrence of sleep spindles) to memory consolidation processes (200–202). Of note, standard clinical neuropsychological batteries only assess patients after time spans under 1 h and never assess patients after periods of sleep (203). This type of work could be carried out in the EMU with intracranially implanted patients, although not without its own set of confounds (e.g., accounting for potential changes in memory related to recent seizure occurrence, changes in antiseizure medications, and a disruptive hospital environment and sleep schedule). Nevertheless, SEEG paradigms with the use of CCEPs is potentially a powerful tool to explore the sub-circuitry of memory processes. George Ojemann carried out a number of memory studies using ESM over the years, and some of his research suggested that the memory system was more complicated than suggested by theoretical models [e.g., episodic memory was disrupted by stimulation of the lateral temporal cortex: (44, 144)]. These findings have more recently been supported by more recent stimulation work through DARPA [i.e., stimulation of lateral TL cortex enhanced memory at some frequencies (146)], and by some initial clinical data involving minimalistic approaches to surgery [lateral TL ablations led to significant verbal memory dysfunction despite preservation of medial TL structures (48)].

Extraoperative single unit recordings can be made when intracranial electrodes are implanted for clinical reasons in patients with refractory epilepsy [see (204)]. While they have provided important insights into memory and cognition, there are a number of limitations. Particularly, it is difficult to continue to record from the same unit for long periods, cell types can be inferred, but not exquisitely defined, and the few neurons that can be recorded, as well as the inability to cover all areas involved in every function (205).

Finally, the possibility of an "*electric Wada*" seems surprisingly absent from the epilepsy surgery landscape. At least, in the case of patients undergoing invasive monitoring with hippocampal electrodes, it is possible to carry out Wada memory paradigms while disrupting subregions and interconnections of the hippocampus and amygdala or even broader structures (145). This seems particularly relevant in this era of minimally invasive surgical procedures as compared to prior surgical epochs where essentially all patients were undergoing procedures that resected multiple regions of the temporal lobe (including much of the temporal pole, anterior inferior and middle temporal gyrus, fusiform, basal temporal lobe, entorhinal/perirhinal cortex, etc.). The Wada is a blunt test in its own right, with many studies suggesting variability in which brain regions are being affected by the delivery of drug [e.g., sodium amobarbital, brevital (206)]. This was less of a problem with open resective surgery but the Wada test may not adequately reflect the potential outcome of a stereotactic laser amygdalophippocampotomy, which primarily affects the amgdalohippocampal complex. Creating an electric Wada appears to be an area where SEEG will be well-suited, but disruptive stimulation will need to be thoughtfully deployed with very low current intensities and careful tailoring based on the stimulation site: Most patients that would be candidates will have medial temporal onset zones—higher frequency stimulation readily causes seizures when applied to the hippocampus and is often avoided (72).

Social-Emotional Functions

There is increasing recognition of the importance of brain functions beyond cognitive processing, as the preservation of social cognition, emotional processing, and empathy may be equally important in determining quality of life (207), and often represent some of core areas of dysfunction in disorders such as autism and schizophrenia (208, 209). Over the years, socio-emotional tasks (e.g., recognizing emotional state from facial expressions, emotional prosody, self-other distinction, empathy, embodied rotation, and theory of mind tasks) have been shown to depend heavily on the limbic system with significant contributions from the amygdalohippocampal complex, the insula, the cingulate cortex, the anterior temporal lobe (e.g., superior temporal pole), select regions of the broader temporal lobe (e.g., the right temporo-parietal junction), the right dorso-medial prefrontal cortex, the bilateral inferior parietal lobules, and more recently the "default mode network (DMN)" (210–215). The latter is a proposed network derived from functional neuroimaging research that appears to activate whenever an individual is not actively engaged in a task in their environment, and which has been linked to a wide range of cognitive [e.g., forming self-relevant mental constructs, planning for future (216)] and social functions in its own right [e.g., social understanding of others, morality (211, 214)]. These findings relating socio-emotional functions to neural underpinnings were originally formulated from naturally occurring lesion studies in humans and ablation studies in non-human primates (217–221), and have been augmented over the years by data derived from functional neuroimaging studies and to a lesser extent electrophysiological investigation (222, 223). Catani et al. (224) provide a thorough review of the contributors over the past century and a half to these developments, and offer an updated model for the neural substrates underlying emotion, memory, and behavior. These authors reviewed the pioneering work of Papez (225), Yakolev (226), and MacLean (227, 228) among notable contributors, and incorporated the DMN into these earlier models, noting that this network shares neuroanatomical overlap with Papez's circuit. More specifically, the medial aspects of the DMN correspond to the most dorsal aspects of the Papez circuit and are interconnected through the dorsal cingulum. While this is an interesting model, it is worth noting that Papez's circuit was proposed as a mechanism of emotion (225) before the idea of the hippocampus in memory took hold (121), after which Papez's circuit was then recast as a mechanism for memory. Similarly, while ontogeny has some vague relation to the work of MacLean (227), this is a model that has insufficient detail to have explanatory traction in functional localization. Nevertheless, the use of cortical and subcortical mapping paradigms, rarely performed in the thalamus and hypothalamic hamartoma, have not been fully realized as the valuable opportunities that they represent, particularly through the merging of technological advances to create real-life emotional processing situations (e.g., using virtual and augmented reality techniques) that can be coupled with novel data collection methods (e.g., CCEPs, machine learning). In many regards, despite these regions or connections to them being disrupted in many epilepsy surgeries and tumor cases, there has been little clinical attention focused on this likely critical area of function for all of the reasons previously cited.

Theory of mind in particular has emerged as an important facet of social cognition and is one of the few areas that has received some degree of attention in the surgical setting. Critical to this ability—which involves the inference of others' mental/affective states and prediction of behavior(s)—are the posterior inferior frontal gyrus, dorsolateral prefrontal cortex, posterior superior temporal gyrus, and right temporo-parietal junction (207, 229, 230). One such measure that has been adapted to the neurosurgical setting is the *Reading the Mind in the Eyes task* (229), which was developed for use in the autistic population. This task consists of patients matching one of four affective states to 36 serially presented photographs depicting only the eye region of human faces. Use of this novel task has facilitated mapping of theory of mind, and research has shown that patients do not completely recover this ability following pars opercularis resection (231, 232). Additionally, however, we recently had a teenager decline drastically on this task (normal to impaired) who underwent a left stereotactic laser amygdalohippocampotomy only, and whose dysfunction has persisted over time (233). This highlights the need for further study of the regions critical for such functions as well as individual variability that may occur across patients. Finally, mapping of the insular cortex has also led to some interesting disruptions of potential socio-emotional functions, as well as internal perceptions or *interoception*, including pain sensation, interoceptive awareness, emotions, self-recognition, empathy, motivation, craving, alterations in breathing, and time perception (234).

Consciousness

An ontology of consciousness is developing, with a key and important example of the necessity of a clear ontology in Antti Revonsuo's *Inner Presence* (235). This has helped neuroscience move away from imprecise and all-encompassing notions of consciousness, as well as behavioral approaches to consciousness from clinical neurology, where the level of arousal is a major interest. While important recent work has taken this latter approach to study minimally conscious states, often in the setting of diffuse or at least non-focal brain injury [e.g., (236)], other work has brought us close to examining subject-reported inner experience. Of particular note is the extension of Baars "Global Workspace Theory" from the 1980s [see (237)] to neural substrates and cognitive theory. This approach has informed both cognitive and psychological ideas regarding *phenomenal consciousness* (see Revonsuo) or subjective awareness—a core component of consciousness—such as in the work of Dehaene [e.g., (238)], or in the sphere of SEEG studies, where this has been developed by Naccache et al. (239–246). This work argues, with empirical evidence, that association cortices are fundamental to phenomenal consciousness. Disfunction of these regions in turn leads to a loss of awareness. It is important to note that while phenomenal consciousness may represent a core component of consciousness perhaps its *sine qua non*, there are other elements that are necessary to normal conscious experience that call for mechanistic explanations, such as metacognition, reflection, selfhood, embodiment, autobiographical narrative, introspection, etc. While all of these seem amenable to well-designed studies that might take advantage of the spatial and temporal resolution of SEEG, sparse sampling needs to be overcome, perhaps by combination with functional imaging methods. When rejecting the behaviorist notion that subjective report is not scientific, and accepting that within certain wide bounds, subjectivity is a core and valid type of data [see, for example (238)]. With a better framework for considering the important constituents of consciousness (e.g., wakefulness, perception, attention, multi-modal representation, mnemonic processing, meta-cognitive processes), the time seems right to begin exploring aspects of these mechanisms. To achieve this, new tasks and experimental paradigms are needed.

Modernization and Standardization of Testing Paradigms and Techniques

It is important to take a highly individualized and functional anatomically informed approach to task selection to optimize mapping/monitoring for any given patient. In addition to greater focus on task development, there is a need to develop effective and innovative methods for administering cognitive testing during ESM more considerate to efficiency and portability of both stimuli and capture methods. Laptop-based systems are widely utilized to display stimuli to patients (e.g., Powerpoint presentations) and allow for extensive stimuli to be stored and displayed electronically but the transition to computers alone does not address the often unstructured and highly variable testing methods used across institutions. Increased consensus in this regard would be valuable in allowing for more comprehensive research endeavors with larger samples across collaborating institutions and further identification of best practices. It would also allow for sharing of common test stimuli, making it possible for more groups to consider more sophisticated mapping paradigms that often take a great deal of preparation time to create. Consensus is becoming increasingly possible through development of specific surgical brain mapping software packages/applications that can be used in a standardized fashion across institutions. One such open-source testing platform is NeuroMapper, which was developed by one of the authors of this manuscript (DSS) (See **Figure 6**). It is utilized to administer a variety of cognitive paradigms to patients in a highly customized and flexible manner *via* dual iPads, allowing for highly individualized mapping by using baseline performance to select stimulus sets for mapping. This then allows examiners to quickly and easily code patient responses (e.g., correct/incorrect, types of errors made) and monitor changes in task accuracy and reaction times in real time, as well as to obtain video records of patients responses for later review. Another useful feature of NeuroMapper is its portability, given the relatively reduced size and weight of the iPad vs. more traditional laptop/computer setups.

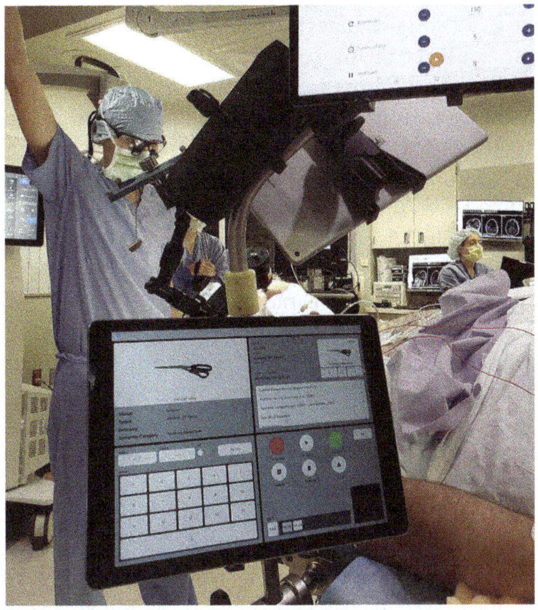

FIGURE 6 | Intraoperative use of the iPad-based Neuromapper tool. Written informed consent was obtained from the individual for the publication of any potentially identifiable images.

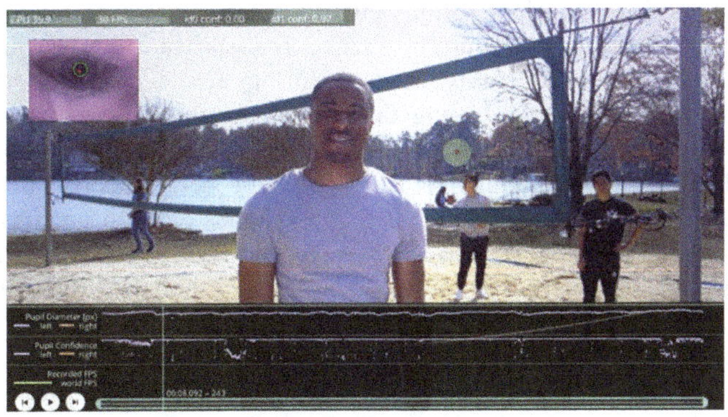

FIGURE 7 | Emory Multimodal Memory Test. A new multimodal tool that is under development for the assessment of multiple domains of cognition and their integration, along with simultaneous recorded eye position and pupil diameter data. Written informed consent was obtained from the individual for the publication of any potentially identifiable images.

We have already suggested many areas of additional test development (e.g., expanded testing of language, adaptation, and creation of tasks of socio-emotional function), but would also like to encourage the exploration of virtual reality and augmented reality techniques to expand the depth and range of constructs that are being examined. These technologies allow for an immersive experience which can be tightly controlled, observed, measured, and manipulated in a manner that allows us to move beyond simple measurement of function yet provides control of the environment while altering task components in a systematic manner. Given the construct of memory, for example, we can continue to test simple episodic recall of a list of words, a story, an object, or a visual scene, but we can also more easily add greater context to the learning, which can pull from semantic (factual information) and autobiographical information (the subject's own personal experiences) and can include both established and novel experiences and information as well. With eye-tracking, motion capture technologies, video-recording, and simultaneous electrophysiological measurement, we can study the patient thoroughly and in a precision manner not previously possible with paper and pencil or even computer-administered tasks. Our own group has created a series of video-vignettes (See **Figure 7**) with professional actors, which require the patient to learn the content of a brief episodic occurrence in the life of one or more individuals, while learning to recognize those individuals (including face, voice, etc.), the settings in which each event takes place, incidental occurrences in the background, and the interactions between these factors (e.g., "Which person was seen in a given context?" and "What other individuals and objects were present?"). We have created extensive foils that include altering subtle characteristics of each scene and its content to test the limits of recall, including potentially the stylistic manner of information retrieval (e.g., subtasks that can potentially tease out the reliance upon familiarity or recognition or a failure of pattern-separation vs. a failure of language, semantics, or other factors). With current technology and artistic capabilities scenes can be subtly manipulated to allow for the ultimate alternate test forms (e.g., making changes in objects or persons while leaving every other aspect of the scene exactly the same) or to apply eye-tracking mechanisms to determine if changes in repetitive scenes were even noticed based on existing literature on the visual fixation differences for novel vs. old information in patients and controls [a finding observed in human and non-human primates (247, 248)]. These sorts of complex tasks would be ideally suited to a situation in which passive mapping is being used, yet a simplified version (e.g., face-name learning) can be completed using an active stimulation paradigm.

Some examples of the use of virtual reality and electrophysiological studies together already exist both with human, rodents, and non-human primates. Several studies have used virtual reality systems combined with implanted electrodes, for example, to study processes such as spatial navigation in rodents and non-human primates (249, 250). These studies have provided a number of interesting findings, facilitating insight into the neural substrates of allocentric (i.e., a more general, global directional sense) and egocentric navigation (a more local system, based on familiar landmarks and their spatial relationships), and other factors that facilitate or hinder navigation. It appears that the hippocampal formation is critical for allocentric navigation (along with parahippocampal and retrosplenial cortex), but that egocentric processes activate neural systems outside of the medial TL (including medial and posterior parietal lobe regions and caudate nucleus).

In humans, a group in France has started piloting the use of a virtual reality headset during awake surgeries in the operating room, using this system to test language but also to explore the ability to understand social gestures (251). There were limitations to what could be accomplished, but they are working on solutions to these issues through ongoing research. Over the last 2 years, virtual tasks have exploded, with ecologically realistic or episodic memory in a shop environment (252, 253), spatial orientation (254), attention (255), and large-scale spatial learning (256). Similarly, standard objects to use in creating these environments (257), and free programming tools (e.g., Unity by Unity Technologies) are making this easier and more standardized (See **Figure 8**). Combining these rich tasks with intracranial electrophysiology will be difficult, given the complex and unfolding nature of tasks, but much may also be learned. Overall, virtual and augmented reality paradigms will increase our ability to study complex phenomena in a highly controlled manner, and should lead to further insights into the neural substrates of complex behavior of all sorts, which will be helpful for better understanding disease states, navigating neurosurgical procedures to provide optimal benefit with the greatest sparing of function, enhancing our ability to use neuromodulation procedures to treat disease (e.g., seizures, depression) and potentially enhance/restore neurological function, and create the opportunity to develop brain-machine interfaces (259), such as those that have allowed the creation of a bionic prosthetic limb. Of note, all of these "futuristic" advances also call for the need for close collaboration with neuroethicists, discussion between cognitive psychologists and neuroscientists, and potentially input from neurophilosophy, to determine the best path forward in these new frontiers [e.g., (260)].

CONCLUSIONS

Cognitive and emotional mapping with SEEG holds great promise both as a clinical tool and research paradigm for significantly improving our understanding of brain structure-function networks. As laid out in this paper, by augmenting a rich history cortical stimulation mapping and SEEG mapping with advances in neuroimaging (e.g., connectivity metrics; precision volumetrics), neuropsychology/neurophilosophy (e.g., updating old models with advances in brain modeling and theory; adding new measures that tap the rich, complexity of thought and memory), technology (e.g., virtual/augmented reality for humans and non-human primates alike), electrophysiological processing and computational modeling (e.g., CCEPs, machine learning algorithms), the field is poised to make rapid advances. Such potential gains could not only improve the care of patients with brain tumors and epilepsy, but potentially allow us to better understand other neurological diseases (e.g., semantic dementia vs. Alzheimer's disease) while developing more targeted, novel treatments. For example, by understanding the neural circuitry of cognition and emotion and their dysfunction, we may be able to develop more specific drug treatments, better position neuromodulatory devices, or even learn to "relink" damaged pathways and circuits. There is still much exciting "building block" work to be done in each of these subfields, and those of us working with these tools and paradigms should be establishing consortiums to share ideas, resources, and data to enable exponential growth in this field over the next couple of decades.

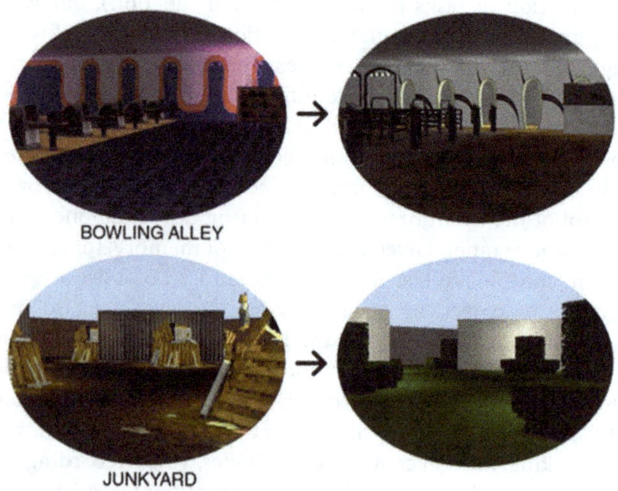

FIGURE 8 | Examining meta-memory with a spatial task. In this virtual reality task from the Cleary Lab (258), subjects can rate feelings of familiarity and deja vu after flying through spatially similar scenes. This is presently being used in the setting of SEEG to examine the anatomy and network activity associated with familiarity. It is also under development with contemporary virtual reality hardware and software.

AUTHOR'S NOTE

This manuscript reflects a review of the relevant published research related to cognitive and behavioral mapping using passive and active stimulation electrophysiological paradigms. It has not been published in any other source and is the original work of the cited authors. DD and NP created an outline for the article, wrote major components, and invited and supervised co-authors with specific expertise in relevant areas to write subsections of the paper. All authors were given an opportunity to edit the manuscript prior to submission for publication.

AUTHOR CONTRIBUTIONS

DD and NP planned the paper, created an outline, recruited co-authors to assist with writing specific subsections, wrote several subsections of the paper, and provide editorial oversight. DS, CB, AD, AA, and AK were assigned subsections to write based on their specific expertise, carried out systematic literature searches, and prepared a draft of their assigned section. All co-authors contributed to the editorial process. All authors contributed to the article and approved the submitted version.

FUNDING

DD's efforts on this paper were supported in part by funding received from the National Institutes of Health/National Institute of Neurological Disorders and Stroke (NIH/NINDS, R01NS088748). He also receives funding from additional grants from the NIH (R01MH118514; R01NS110347), as well as Medtronic, Inc. (A1321808). NPP was supported in part by funding received from the NIH/NINDS (K08NS105929) and CURE Epilepsy.

ACKNOWLEDGMENTS

We would like to thank our undergraduate students, Noah Okado and Rogelio Cortez-Cuevas, with their assistance in the preparations of **Figures 7**, **8**, and our neurophilosophy collaborators, Drs. Anne Cleary and Joseph Neisser for contributing ideas related to our use of a deja vu assessment task.

REFERENCES

1. Arya R, Ervin B, Holloway T, Dudley J, Horn PS, Buroker J, et al. Electrical stimulation sensorimotor mapping with stereo-EEG. *Clin Neurophysiol.* (2020) 131:1691–701. doi: 10.1016/j.clinph.2020.04.159
2. Chauvel P, Gonzalez-Martinez J, Bulacio J. Presurgical intracranial investigation in epilepsy surgery. *Handb Clin Neurol.* (2019) 161:45–71. doi: 10.1016/B978-0-444-64142-7.00040-0
3. Cardinale F, Casaceli G, Raneri F, Miller J, Lo Russo G. Implantation of stereoelectroencephalography electrodes: a systematic review. *J Clin Neurophysiol.* (2016) 33:490–502. doi: 10.1097/WNP.00000000000 00249
4. Talairach J, Bancaud J, Bonis A, Szikla G, Tournoux P. Functional stereotactic exploration of epilepsy. *Confin Neurol.* (1962) 22:328–31. doi: 10.1159/000104378
5. Katz JS, Abel TJ. Stereoelectroencephalography versus subdural electrodes for localization of the epileptogenic zone: what is the evidence? *Neurotherapeutics.* (2019) 16:59–66. doi: 10.1007/s13311-018-0 0703-2
6. Willie JT, Laxpati NG, Drane DL, Gowda A, Appin A, Hao C, et al. Real-time magnetic resonance-guided amygdalohippocampotomy for mesial temporal lobe epilepsy. *Neurosurgery.* (2014) 74:569–84. doi: 10.1227/NEU.0000000000000343
7. Martin AK, Huang J, Hunold A, Meinzer M. Dissociable roles within the social brain for self-other processing: a HD-tDCS study. *Cereb Cortex.* (2019) 29:3642–54. doi: 10.1093/cercor/bhy238
8. Lee DJ, Lozano CS, Dallapiazza RF, Lozano AM. Current and future directions of deep brain stimulation for neurological and psychiatric disorders. *J Neurosurg.* (2019) 131:333–42. doi: 10.3171/2019.4.JNS181761
9. Skarpaas TL, Jarosiewicz B, Morrell MJ. Brain-responsive neurostimulation for epilepsy (RNS® System). *Epilepsy Res.* (2019) 153:68–70. doi: 10.1016/j.eplepsyres.2019.02.003
10. Piccolino M, Bresadola M. *Shocking Frogs: Galvani, Volta, and the Electric Origins of Neuroscience.* Oxford University Press, Oxford Scholarship Online (2013).
11. Fritsch G, Hitzig E. Über die elektrische erregbarkeit des grosshirns. *Arch Anat Physiol Wissen.* (1870) 37:300–32.
12. Engelhardt E. Cerebral localization of higher functions: the period between Thomas Willis and Paul Broca. *Dementia and Neuropsychologia.* (2019) 13:238–43. doi: 10.1590/1980-57642018dn13-020014
13. Ferrier S. Experimental researches in cerebral physiology and pathology. *West Riding Lunatic Asylum Med Rep.* (1873) 3:30–96. doi: 10.1136/bmj.1.643.457
14. Willis T. *De anima brutorum, quae hominis vitalis ac sensitiua est, exercitationes duae.* Leyden, IL: Joannis Antonii Huguetan and Soc (1676).
15. Lewes G. The functions of the brain. *Nature.* (1876) 15:73–4. doi: 10.1038/015073a0
16. Hughlings Jackson J. *Selected Writings of John Hughlings Jackson* (Taylor J, editor). New York, NY: Basic Books (1958).
17. Caton R. The electric currents of the brain. *Br Med J.* (1875) 2:278.
18. Horsley V, Clarke RH. The structure and functions of the cerebellum examined by a new method. *Brain.* (1908) 31:45–124. doi: 10.1093/brain/31.1.45
19. Cushing H. A note upon the faradic stimulation of the postcentral gyrus in conscious patients. *Brain.* (1909) 32:44–53. doi: 10.1093/brain/32.1.44
20. Isitan C, Yan Q, Spencer DD, Alkawadri R. Brief history of electrical cortical stimulation: a journey in time from Volta to Penfield. *Epilepsy Res.* (2020) 166:106363. doi: 10.1016/j.eplepsyres.2020.106363
21. Krause F. Die operative behandlung der epilepsie. *Med Klin Berlin.* (1909) 5:1418–22.
22. Greenblatt SH. Phrenology in the science and culture of the 19th century. *Neurosurgery.* (1995) 37:790–804. doi: 10.1227/00006123-199510000-00025
23. Charcot JM. *Lectures on the diseases of the nervous system*, Vol 3. London: New Sydenham Society (1889)
24. Talairach J, Szikla G. *Atlas d'anatomie stereotaxique du telencephale.* Paris: Masson & Cie (1967).
25. Jensen RL, Stone JL, Hayne RA. Introduction of the human Horsley-Clarke stereotactic frame. *Neurosurgery.* (1996) 38:563–567. doi: 10.1097/00006123-199603000-00029
26. Bancaud J, Talairach J, Bonis A. *La Stéréoencéphalographie dans l'épilepsie.* Paris: Masson & Cie (1965).
27. Bancaud J, Talairach J. Méthodologie de l'exploration SEEG et de l'intervention chirurgicale dans l'épilepsie [Methodology of stereo EEG exploration and surgical intervention in epilepsy]. *Rev Otoneuroophtalmol.* (1973) 45:315–28.
28. Haglund MM, Berger MS, Shamseldin M, Lettich E, Ojemann GA. Cortical localization of temporal lobe language sites in patients with gliomas. *Neurosurgery.* (1994) 34:567–76. doi: 10.1227/00006123-199404000-00001
29. Hamberger MJ. Cortical language mapping *in* epilepsy: a critical review. *Neuropsychol Rev.* (2007) 17:477–89. doi: 10.1007/s11065-007-9046-6

30. Foerster O, Altenburger H. Elektrobiologische Vorgänge an der menschlichen Hirnrinde. *Dtsch Z Nervenheilkd.* (1935) 135:277–88. doi: 10.1007/BF01732786
31. Penfield W, Jasper H. *Epilepsy and the Functional Anatomy of the Human Brain.* Boston, MA: Little, Brown and Co (1954). doi: 10.1097/00007611-195407000-00024
32. Penfield W, Roberts L. *Speech and Brain-Mechanisms.* Princeton, NJ: Princeton University Press (1959).
33. Snyder PJ, Whitaker HA. Neurologic heuristics and artistic whimsy: the cerebral cartography of Wilder Penfield. *J Hist Neurosci.* (2013) 22:277–91. doi: 10.1080/0964704X.2012.757965
34. Drane DL, Pedersen NP. Knowledge of language function and underlying neural networks gained from complex partial seizures and epilepsy surgery. *Brain Lang.* (2019) 189:20–33. doi: 10.1016/j.bandl.2018.12.007
35. Dronkers N, Baldo JV. Language: aphasia. In: Squire LR, editor *Encyclopedia of Neuroscience.* Cambridge, MA: Elsevier Ltd. (2009). p. 343–8.
36. Duffau H, Moritz-Gasser S, Mandonnet E. A re-examination of neural basis of language processing: proposal of a dynamic hodotopical model from data provided by brain stimulation mapping during picture naming. *Brain Lang.* (2014) 131:1–10. doi: 10.1016/j.bandl.2013.05.011
37. Lichtheim L. On aphasia. *Brain.* (1885) 433–84. doi: 10.1093/brain/7.4.433
38. Ojemann G, Ojemann J, Lettich E, Berger M. Cortical language localization in left, dominant hemisphere. An electrical stimulation mapping investigation in 117 patients. *J Neurosurg.* (1989) 71:316–26. doi: 10.3171/jns.1989.71.3.0316
39. Hickok G, Poeppel D. The cortical organization of speech processing. *Nat Rev Neurosci.* (2007) 8:393–402. doi: 10.1038/nrn2113
40. Corina DP, Loudermik BC, Detwiler L, Martin RF, Brinkley JF, Ojemann G. Analysis of naming errors during cortical stimulation mapping: implications for models of language representation. *Brain Lang.* (2010) 115:101–12. doi: 10.1016/j.bandl.2010.04.001
41. Ojemann GA. Individual variability in cortical localization of language. *J Neurosurg.* (1979) 50:164–9. doi: 10.3171/jns.1979.50.2.0164
42. Ojemann SG, Berger MS, Lettich E, Ojemann GA. Localization of language function in children: results of electrical stimulation mapping. *J Neurosurg.* (2003) 98:465–70. doi: 10.3171/jns.2003.98.3.0465
43. Drane DL, Roraback-Carson J, Hebb AO, Hersonskey T, Lucas T, Ojemann GA, et al. Cortical stimulation mapping and Wada results demonstrate a normal variant of right hemisphere language organization. *Epilepsia.* (2012) 53:1790–8. doi: 10.1111/j.1528-1167.2012.03573.x
44. Ojemann GA, Whitaker HA. The bilingual brain. *Arch Neurol.* (1978) 35:409–12. doi: 10.1001/archneur.1978.00500310011002
45. Ojemann GA, Whitaker H. Language localization and variability. *Brain Lang.* (1978) 6:239–60. doi: 10.1016/0093-934X(78)90061-5
46. Ojemann GA, Creutzfeldt O, Lettich E, Haglund MM. Neuronal activity in human lateral temporal cortex related to short-term verbal memory, naming and reading. *Brain.* (1988) 111(Pt 6):1383–403. doi: 10.1093/brain/111.6.1383
47. Ojemann G, Mateer C. Human language cortex: localization of memory, syntax, and sequential motor-phoneme identification systems. *Science.* (1979) 205:1401–3. doi: 10.1126/science.472757
48. Drane DL. MRI-guided stereotactic laser ablation for epilepsy surgery: promising preliminary results for cognitive outcome. *Epilepsy Res.* (2018) 142:170–5. doi: 10.1016/j.eplepsyres.2017.09.016
49. Lüders H, Hahn J, Lesser RP, Dinner DS, Morris HH 3rd, Wyllie E, et al. Basal temporal subdural electrodes in the evaluation of patients with intractable epilepsy. *Epilepsia.* (1989) 30:131–42. doi: 10.1111/j.1528-1157.1989.tb05445.x
50. Lüders H, Lesser RP, Dinner DS, Morris HH, Hahn J. Language disturbances produced by electrical stimulation of the basal temporal region. *Ann Neurol.* (1985) 18:151.
51. Lüders J, Lesser RP, Hahn J, Dinner DS, Morris HH, Wyllie E, et al. Basal temporal language area. *Brain.* (1991) 114:743–54. doi: 10.1093/brain/114.2.743
52. Bartha L, Benke T, Bauer G, Trinka E. Interictal language functions in temporal lobe epilepsy. *J Neurol Neurosurg Psychiatry.* (2005) 76:808–14. doi: 10.1136/jnnp.2004.045385
53. Bartha L, Trinka E, Ortler M, Donnemiller E, Felber S, Bauer G, et al. Linguistic deficits following left selective amygdalohippocampectomy: a prospective study. *Epilepsy Behav.* (2004) 5:348–57. doi: 10.1016/j.yebeh.2004.02.004
54. Pouratian N, Bookheimer SY, Rubino G, Martin NA, Toga AW. Category-specific naming deficit identified by intraoperative stimulation mapping and postoperative neuropsychological testing. *Case Rep J Neurosurg.* (2003) 99:170–6. doi: 10.3171/jns.2003.99.1.0170
55. Usui K, Ikeda A, Takayama M, Matsuhashi M, Yamamoto J-I, Satoh T, et al. Conversion of semantic information into phonological representation: a function in left posterior basal temporal area. *Brain.* (2003) 126:632–41. doi: 10.1093/brain/awg057
56. Araki K, Terada K, Usui K, Usui N, Araki Y, Baba K, et al. Bidirectional neural connectivity between basal temporal and posterior language areas in humans. *Clin Neurophysiol.* (2015) 126:682–8. doi: 10.1016/j.clinph.2014.07.020
57. Kahane P, Arzimanoglou A, Benabid A-L, Chauvel P. Epilepsy surgery in France. In: Luders HO, editor. *Textbook of Epilepsy Surgery.* London: Informa Healthcare (2008). p. 46–53.
58. Bancaud J. Apport de l'exploration fonctionnelle par voie stéréotaxique à la chirurgie de l'épilepsie. *Neurochirurgie.* (1959) 5:55–112.
59. Talairach J, Bancaud J. Stereotaxic approach to epilepsy. Methodology of anatomo- functional stereotaxic investigations. *Progr Neurol Surg.* (1973) 5:297–354. doi: 10.1159/000394343
60. Trébuchon A, Liégeois-Chauvel C, Gonzalez-Martinez JA, Alario F-X. Contributions of electrophysiology for identifying cortical language systems in patients with epilepsy. *Epilepsy Behav.* (2020) 112:1525–5050. doi: 10.1016/j.yebeh.2020.107407
61. Yamao Y, Suzuki K, Kunieda T, Matsumoto R, Arakawa Y, Nakae T, et al. Clinical impact of intraoperative CCEP monitoring in evaluating the dorsal language white matter pathway. *Hum Brain Mapp.* (2017) 38:1977–91. doi: 10.1002/hbm.23498
62. Duffau H, Peggy Gatignol ST, Mandonnet E, Capelle L, Taillandier L. Intraoperative subcortical stimulation mapping of language pathways in a consecutive series of 115 patients with Grade II glioma in the left dominant hemisphere. *J Neurosurg.* (2008) 109:461–71. doi: 10.3171/JNS/2008/109/9/0461
63. Duffau H. Stimulation mapping of white matter tracts to study brain functional connectivity. *Nat Rev Neurol.* (2015) 11:255–65. doi: 10.1038/nrneurol.2015.51
64. Herbet G, Moritz-Gasser S, Boiseau M, Duvaux S, Cochereau J, Duffau H. Converging evidence for a cortico-subcortical network mediating lexical retrieval. *Brain.* (2016) 139:3007–21. doi: 10.1093/brain/aww220
65. Martino J, Brogna C, Robles SG, Vergani F, Duffau H. Anatomic dissection of the inferior fronto-occipital fasciculus revisited in the lights of brain stimulation data. *Cortex.* (2010) 46:691–9. doi: 10.1016/j.cortex.2009.07.015
66. Yordanova YN, Cochereau J, Duffau H, Herbet G. Combining resting state functional MRI with intraoperative cortical stimulation to map the mentalizing network. *NeuroImage.* (2019) 186:628–36. doi: 10.1016/j.neuroimage.2018.11.046
67. Leclercq D, Duffau H, Delmaire C, Capelle L, Gatignol P, Ducros M, et al. Comparison of diffusion tensor imaging tractography of language tracts and intraoperative subcortical stimulations. *J Neurosurg.* (2010) 112:503–11. doi: 10.3171/2009.8.JNS09558
68. Fernandez Coello A, Duvaux S, De Benedictis A, Matsuda R, Duffau H. Involvement of the right inferior longitudinal fascicle in visual hemiagnosia: a brain stimulation mapping study. *J Neurosurg.* (2013) 118:202–5. doi: 10.3171/2012.10.JNS12527
69. Gil-Robles S, Carvallo A, Jimenez M, Gomez Caicoya A, Martinez R, Ruiz-Ocaña C, et al. Double dissociation between visual recognition and picture naming: a study of the visual language connectivity using tractography and brain stimulation. *Neurosurgery.* (2013) 72:678–86. doi: 10.1227/NEU.0b013e318282a361
70. Moritz-Gasser S, Herbet G, Maldonado IL, Duffau H. Lexical access speed is significantly correlated with the return to professional activities after awake surgery for low-grade gliomas. *J Neuro Oncol.* (2012) 107:633–41. doi: 10.1007/s11060-011-0789-9

71. Munyon C, Sweet J, Luders H, Lhatoo S, Miller J. The 3-dimensional grid: a novel approach to stereoelectroencephalography. *Neurosurgery.* (2015) 11:127–34. doi: 10.1227/NEU.0000000000000649
72. Isnard J, Taussig D, Bartolomei F, Bourdillon P, Catenoix H, Chassoux F, et al. French guidelines on stereoelectroencephalography (SEEG). *Clin Neurophysiol.* (2018) 48:5–13. doi: 10.1016/j.neucli.2017.11.005
73. von Economo C. *The Cytoarchitectonics of the Human Cerebral Cortex.* London: Oxford University Press (1929).
74. Borchers S, Himmelbach M, Logothetis N, Karnath HO. Direct electrical stimulation of human cortex - the gold standard for mapping brain functions? *Nat Rev Neurosci.* (2011) 13:63–70. doi: 10.1038/nrn3140
75. Mohan UR, Watrous AJ, Miller JF, Lega BC, Sperling MR, Worrell GA, et al. The effects of direct brain stimulation in humans depend on frequency, amplitude, white-matter proximity. *Brain Stimul.* (2020) 13:1183–95. doi: 10.1016/j.brs.2020.05.009
76. Cogan SF, Ludwig KA, Welle CG, Takmakov P. Tissue damage thresholds during therapeutic electrical stimulation. *J Neural Eng.* (2016) 13:021001. doi: 10.1088/1741-2560/13/2/021001
77. Bari BA, Ollerenshaw DR, Millard DC, Wang Q, Stanley GB. Behavioral and electrophysiological effects of cortical microstimulation parameters. *PLoS ONE.* (2013) 8:e82170. doi: 10.1371/journal.pone.0082170
78. Bancaud J, Talairach J. Organisation fonctionnelle de l'aire motrice supplémentaire. Enseignements apportés par la stéréo-E.E.G [Functional organization of the supplementary motor area. Data obtained by stereo-E.E.G]. *Neurochirurgie.* (1967) 13:343-56. French.
79. McCreery DB, Agnew WF, Yuen TG, Bullara L. Charge density and charge per phase as cofactors in neural injury induced by electrical stimulation. *IEEE Trans Bio Med Eng.* (1990) 37:996–1001. doi: 10.1109/10.102812
80. Jones JC, Alomar S, McGovern RA, Firl D, Fitzgerald Z, Gale J, Gonzalez-Martinez JA. Techniques for placement of stereotactic electroencephalographic depth electrodes: Comparison of implantation and tracking accuracies in a cadaveric human study. *Epilepsia.* (2018) 59:1667–1675. doi: 10.1111/epi.14538
81. Cardinale F, Rizzi M, Vignati E, Cossu M, Castana L, d'Orio P, et al. Stereoelectroencephalography: retrospective analysis of 742 procedures in a single centre. *Brain.* (2019) 142:2688–704. doi: 10.1093/brain/awz196
82. Arya R, Mangano FT, Horn PS, Holland KD, Rose DF, Glauser TA. Adverse events related to extraoperative invasive EEG monitoring with subdural grid electrodes: a systematic review and meta-analysis. *Epilepsia.* (2013) 54:828–39. doi: 10.1111/epi.12073
83. Helmstaedter C, Gielen GH, Witt JA. The immediate and short-term effects of bilateral intrahippocampal depth electrodes on verbal memory. *Epilepsia.* (2018) 59:e78–84. doi: 10.1111/epi.14019
84. Ljung H, Nordlund A, Strandberg M, Bengzon J, Källén K. Verbal memory decline from hippocampal depth electrodes in temporal lobe surgery for epilepsy. *Epilepsia.* (2017) 58:2143–52. doi: 10.1111/epi.13931
85. Drane DL, Gross RE. Hippocampal depth electrodes in epilepsy surgery: diagnostic or damaging? *Epilepsy Curr.* (2018) 18:104–6. doi: 10.5698/1535-7597.18.2.104
86. Drane DL, Pedersen NP, Hewitt KC, Jordan T. Promise and perils of SEEG for cognition and emotion in the epilepsy surgery setting. In: S. U. Schuele, editor. *A Practical Approach to Stereo EEG*, New York, NY: Springer (2021) 431–438.
87. Meador KJ, Halpern CH, Hermann BP. Cognitive safety of intracranial electrodes for epilepsy. *Epilepsia.* (2018) 59:1132–7. doi: 10.1111/epi.14197
88. Aungaroon G, Vera AZ, Horn PS, Byars AW, Greiner HM, Tenney JR, et al. After-discharges and seizures during pediatric extra-operative electrical cortical stimulation functional brain mapping: incidence, thresholds, and determinants. *Clin Neurophysiol.* (2017) 128:2078–86. doi: 10.1016/j.clinph.2017.06.259
89. Bank AM, Schevon CA, Hamberger MJ. Characteristics and clinical impact of stimulation-evoked seizures during extraoperative cortical mapping. *Epilepsy Behav.* (2014) 34:6–8. doi: 10.1016/j.yebeh.2014.03.004
90. Crone NE, Boatman D, Gordon B, Hao L. Induced electrocorticographic gamma activity during auditory perception. Brazier Award-winning article. *Clin Neurophysiol.* (2001) 112:565–82. doi: 10.1016/S1388-2457(00)00545-9
91. Babajani-Feremi A, Wheless JW, Papanicolaou JW, Wang Y, Fifer MS, Flinker A, et al. Spatial-temporal functional mapping of language at the bedside with electrocorticography. *Neurology.* (2016) 87:2604. doi: 10.1212/01.wnl.0000511287.40052.8d
92. Miller KJ, Schalk G, Hermes D, Ojemann JG, Rao RP. Spontaneous decoding of the timing and content of human object perception from cortical surface recordings reveals complementary information in the event-related potential and broadband spectral change. *PLoS Comput Biol.* (2016) 12:e1004660. doi: 10.1371/journal.pcbi.1004660
93. Su DK, Ojemann JG. Electrocorticographic sensorimotor mapping. *Clin Neurophysiol.* (2013) 124:1044–8. doi: 10.1016/j.clinph.2013.02.114
94. Van Poppel M, Wheless JW, Clarke DF, McGregor A, McManis MH, Perkins FF, et al. Passive language mapping with magnetoencephalography in pediatric patients with epilepsy. *J Neurosurg Pediatrics.* (2012) 10:96–102. doi: 10.3171/2012.4.PEDS11301
95. Bagshaw AP, Jacobs J, LeVan P, Dubeau F, Gotman J. Effect of sleep stage on interictal high-frequency oscillations recorded from depth macroelectrodes in patients with focal epilepsy. *Epilepsia.* (2009) 50:617–28. doi: 10.1111/j.1528-1167.2008.01784.x
96. Burke JF, Sharan AD, Sperling MR, Ramayya AG, Evans JJ, Healey MK, et al. Theta and high-frequency activity mark spontaneous recall of episodic memories. *J Neurosci.* (2014) 34:11355–65. doi: 10.1523/JNEUROSCI.2654-13.2014
97. Jerbi K, Freyermuth S, Dalal S, Kahane P, Bertrand O, Berthoz A, et al. Saccade related gamma-band activity in intracerebral EEG: dissociating neural from ocular muscle activity. *Brain Topogr.* (2009) 22:18–23. doi: 10.1007/s10548-009-0078-5
98. Korostenskaja M, Wilson AJ, Rose DF, Brunner P, Schalk G, Leach J, et al. Real-time functional mapping with electrocorticography in pediatric epilepsy: comparison with fMRI and ESM findings. *Clin EEG Neurosci.* (2014) 45:205–11. doi: 10.1177/1550059413492960
99. Swift JR, Coon WG, Guger C, Brunner P, Bunch M, Lynch T, et al. Passive functional mapping of receptive language areas using electrocorticographic signals. *Clin Neurophysiol.* (2018) 129:2517–24. doi: 10.1016/j.clinph.2018.09.007
100. Arya R, Wilson JA, Vannest J, Byars AW, Greiner HM, Buroker J, et al. Electrocorticographic language mapping in children by high-gamma synchronization during spontaneous conversation: comparison with conventional electrical cortical stimulation. *Epilepsy Res.* (2015) 110:78–87. doi: 10.1016/j.eplepsyres.2014.11.013
101. Arya R, Wilson JA, Fujiwara H, Rozhkov L, Leach JL, Byars AW, et al. Presurgical language localization with visual naming associated ECoG high-gamma modulation in pediatric drug-resistant epilepsy. *Epilepsia.* (2017) 58:663–73. doi: 10.1111/epi.13708
102. Wang Y, Fifer MS, Flinker A, Korzeniewska A, Cervenka MC, Anderson WS, et al. Spatial-temporal functional mapping of language at the bedside with electrocorticography. *Neurology.* (2016) 86:1181–9. doi: 10.1212/WNL.0000000000002525
103. Cervenka MC, Corines J, Boatman-Reich DF, Eloyan A, Sheng X, Franaszczuk PJ, et al. Electrocorticographic functional mapping identifies human cortex critical for auditory and visual naming. *NeuroImage.* (2013) 69:267–76. doi: 10.1016/j.neuroimage.2012.12.037
104. Kojima K, Brown EC, Matsuzaki N, Rothermel R, Fuerst D, Shah A, et al. Gamma activity modulated by picture and auditory naming tasks: intracranial recording in patients with focal epilepsy. *Clin Neurophysiol.* (2013) 124:1737–44. doi: 10.1016/j.clinph.2013.01.030
105. Cuisenier P, Testud B, Minotti L, El Bouzaïdi Tiali S, Martineau L, Job A-S. Relationship between direct cortical stimulation and induced high-frequency activity for language mapping during SEEG recording. *J Neurosurg.* (2020) 2020:1–11. doi: 10.3171/2020.2.JNS192751
106. Anumanchipalli GK, Chartier J, Chang EF. Speech synthesis from neural decoding of spoken sentences. *Nature.* (2019) 568:493–8. doi: 10.1038/s41586-019-1119-1
107. Sellars W. Empiricism and the philosophy of mind. In: Feigl H, Scriven M, editor. *The Foundations of Science and the Concepts of Psychology and Psychoanalysis: Minnesota Studies in the Philosophy*

of Science, Vol. 1. Minneapolis, MN: University of Minnesota Press (1956). p. 253–329.

108. Feyerabend P. Mental events and the brain. *J Philos.* (1963) 40:295–6. doi: 10.2307/2023030
109. Cornman J. On the elimination of 'sensations' and sensations. *Rev Metaphys.* (1968) XXII:15–35.
110. Churchland PM. *Matter and Consciousness.* Cambridge, MA: MIT Press (1984).
111. Zaborszky L, Wouterlood FG, Lanciego JL, editors. *Neuroanatomical Tract Tracing 3: Molecules, Neurons, and Systems.* 3rd ed. New York, NY: Springer (2006).
112. Lanciego JL, Wouterlood FG. Neuroanatomical tract-tracing techniques that did go viral. *Brain Struct Function.* (2020) 225:1193–224. doi: 10.1007/s00429-020-02041-6
113. Park HJ, Friston K. Structural and functional brain networks: from connections to cognition. *Science.* (2013) 342:1238411. doi: 10.1126/science.1238411
114. Mortazavi F, Oblak AL, Morrison WZ, Schmahmann JD, Stanley HE, Wedeen VJ, Rosene DL. Geometric Navigation of Axons in a Cerebral Pathway: Comparing dMRI with Tract Tracing and Immunohistochemistry. *Cereb Cortex.* (2018) 28:1219–1232. doi: 10.1093/cercor/bhx034
115. Matsumoto R, Kunieda T, Nair D. Single pulse electrical stimulation to probe functional and pathological connectivity in epilepsy. *Seizure.* (2017) 44:27–36. doi: 10.1016/j.seizure.2016.11.003
116. Dickey AS, Isbaine F, Fasano RE, Cabaniss BT, Gross RE, Willie JT, et al. Single-pulse electrical stimulation mapping of the connectivity of malformations of cortical development. *Presented at the annual meeting of the American Epilepsy Society (AES).* Washington, DC (2017).
117. Brazier MA. Evoked responses recorded from the depths of the human brain. *Ann NY Acad Sci.* (1964) 112:33–59. doi: 10.1111/j.1749-6632.1964.tb26741.x
118. Matsumoto R, Nair DR, LaPresto E, Najm I, Bingaman W, Shibasaki H, Lüders HO. Functional connectivity in the human language system: a cortico-cortical evoked potential study. *Brain.* (2004) 127:2316–30. doi: 10.1093/brain/awh246
119. Yamao Y, Matsumoto R, Kikuchi T, Yoshida K, Kunieda T, Miyamoto S. Intraoperative Brain Mapping by Cortico-Cortical Evoked Potential. *Front Hum Neurosci.* (2021) 15:635453. doi: 10.3389/fnhum.2021.635453
120. Matsumoto R, Nair DR, LaPresto E, Bingaman W, Shibasaki H, Lüders HO. Functional connectivity in human cortical motor system: a cortico-cortical evoked potential study. *Brain.* (2007) 130:181–97. doi: 10.1093/brain/awl257
121. Scoville WB, Milner B. Loss of recent memory after bilateral hippocampal lesions. *J Neurol Neurosurg Psychiatr.* (1957) 296:1–22. doi: 10.1136/jnnp.20.1.11
122. Rossi M, Nibali MC, Torregrossa F, Bello L, Grasso G. Innovation in neurosurgery: the concept of cognitive mapping. *World Neurosurg.* (2019) 131:364–70. doi: 10.1016/j.wneu.2019.06.177
123. Hamberger MJ, Goodman RR, Perrine K, Tamny T. Anatomic dissociation of auditory and visual naming in the lateral temporal cortex. *Neurology.* (2001) 56:56–61. doi: 10.1212/wnl.56.1.56
124. Duffau H, Capelle L, Denvil D, Gatignol P, Sichez N, Lopes M, et al. The role of dominant premotor cortex in language: a study using intraoperative functional mapping in awake patients. *Neuroimage.* (2003) 20:1903–14. doi: 10.1016/S1053-8119(03)00203-9
125. Ulvin LB, Jonas J, Brissart H, Colnat-Coulbois S, Thiriaux A, Vignal JP, et al. Intracerebral stimulation of left and right ventral temporal cortex during object naming. *Brain Lang.* (2017) 175:71–6. doi: 10.1016/j.bandl.2017.09.003
126. Sarubbo S, Tate M, De Benedictis A, Merler S, Moritz-Gasser S, Herbet G, et al. A normalized dataset of 1821 cortical and subcortical functional responses collected during direct electrical stimulation in patients undergoing awake brain surgery. *Neuroimage.* (2020) 28:104892. doi: 10.1016/j.dib.2019.104892
127. Maldonado IL, Moritz-Gasser S, de Champfleur NM, Bertram L, Moulinié G, Duffau H. Surgery for gliomas involving the left inferior parietal lobule: new insights into the functional anatomy provided by stimulation mapping in awake patients. *J Neurosurg.* (2011) 115:770–9. doi: 10.3171/2011.5.JNS112
128. Miozzo M, Williams AC, McKhann GM 2nd, Hamberger MJ. Topographical gradients of semantics and phonology revealed by temporal lobe stimulation. *Hum Brain Mapp.* (2017) 38:688–703. doi: 10.1002/hbm.23409
129. Abel TJ, Rhone AE, Nourski KV, Kawasaki H, Oya H, Griffiths TD, et al. Direct physiologic evidence of a heteromodal convergence region for proper naming in human left anterior temporal lobe. *J Neurosci.* (2015) 35:1513–20. doi: 10.1523/JNEUROSCI.3387-14.2015
130. Roux FE, Lubrano V, Lauwers-Cances V, Trémoulet M, Mascott CR, Démonet JF. Intra-operative mapping of cortical areas involved in reading in mono- and bilingual patients. *Brain.* (2004) 127(Pt 8):1796–810. doi: 10.1093/brain/awh204
131. Sabsevitz DS, Middlebrooks EH, Tatum W, Grewal SS, Wharen R, Ritaccio AL. Examining the function of the visual word form area with stereo EEG electrical stimulation: a case report of pure alexia. *Cortex.* (2020) 129:112–8. doi: 10.1016/j.cortex.2020.04.012
132. Blanke O, Spinelli L, Thut G, Michel C, Perrig S, Landis T, et al. Location of the human frontal eye field as defined by electrical cortical stimulation: anatomical, functional and electrophysiological characteristics. *Neuroreport.* (2000) 11:1907–13. doi: 10.1097/00001756-200006260-00021
133. Halgren E, Walter RD, Cherlow DG, Crandall PH. Mental phenomena evoked by electrical stimulation of the human hippocampal formation and amygdala. *Brain.* (1978) 101:83–117. doi: 10.1093/brain/101.1.83
134. Gloor P. Experiential phenomena of temporal lobe epilepsy. Facts and hypotheses. *Brain.* (1990) 113 (Pt 6):1673–94. doi: 10.1093/brain/113.6.1673
135. Bartolomei F, Barbeau E, Gavaret M, Guye M, McGonigal A, Régis J, et al. Cortical stimulation study of the role of rhinal cortex in déjà vu and reminiscence of memories. *Neurology.* (2004) 63:858–64. doi: 10.1212/01.WNL.0000137037.56916.3F
136. Lanteaume L, Khalfa S, Régis J, Marquis P, Chauvel P, Bartolomei F. Emotion induction after direct intracerebral stimulations of human amygdala. *Cereb Cortex.* (2007) 17:1307–13. doi: 10.1093/cercor/bhl041
137. Vignal JP, Chauvel P, Halgren E. Localised face processing by the human prefrontal cortex: stimulation-evoked hallucinations of faces. *Cogn Neuropsychol.* (2000) 17:281–91. doi: 10.1080/026432900380616
138. Barbeau EJ, Taylor MJ, Regis J, Marquis P, Chauvel P, Liégeois-Chauvel C. Spatio temporal dynamics of face recognition. *Cerebral Cortex.* (2008) 18:997–1009. doi: 10.1093/cercor/bhm140
139. Roux FE, Dufor O, Lauwers-Cances V, Boukhatem L, Brauge D, Draper L, et al. Electrostimulation mapping of spatial neglect. *Neurosurgery.* (2011) 69:1218–31. doi: 10.1227/NEU.0b013e31822aefd2
140. Bush D, Bisby JA, Bird CM, Gollwitzer S, Rodionov R, Diehl B, et al. Human hippocampal theta power indicates movement onset and distance travelled. *Proc Natl Acad Sci USA.* (2017) 114:12297–302. doi: 10.1073/pnas.1708716114
141. Maidenbaum S, Miller J, Stein JM, Jacobs J. Grid-like hexadirectional modulation of human entorhinal theta oscillations. *Proc Natl Acad Sci USA.* (2018) 115:10798–803. doi: 10.1073/pnas.1805007115
142. Duffau H, Denvil D, Lopes M, Gasparini F, Cohen L, Capelle L, et al. Intraoperative mapping of the cortical areas involved in multiplication and subtraction: an electrostimulation study in a patient with a left parietal glioma. *J Neurol Neurosurg Psychiatry.* (2002) 73:733–8. doi: 10.1136/jnnp.73.6.733
143. Yu X, Chen C, Pu S, Wu C, Li Y, Jiang T, et al. Dissociation of subtraction and multiplication in the right parietal cortex: evidence from intraoperative cortical electrostimulation. *Neuropsychologia.* (2011) 49:2889–95. doi: 10.1016/j.neuropsychologia.2011.06.015
144. Haglund MM, Ojemann GA, Schwartz TW, Lettich E. Neuronal activity in human lateral temporal cortex during serial retrieval from short-term memory. *J Neurosci.* (1994) 14:1507–15. doi: 10.1523/JNEUROSCI.14-03-01507.1994
145. Coleshill SG, Binnie CD, Morris RG, Alarcón G, van Emde Boas W, Velis DN, et al. Material-specific recognition memory deficits elicited by unilateral hippocampal electrical stimulation. *J Neurosci.* (2004) 24:1612–6. doi: 10.1523/JNEUROSCI.4352-03.2004

146. Ezzyat Y, Wanda PA, Levy DF, Kadel A, Aka A, Pedisich I, et al. Closed-loop stimulation of temporal cortex rescues functional networks and improves memory. *Nat Commun*. (2018) 9:365. doi: 10.1038/s41467-017-02753-0
147. Bonini F, Burle B, Liégeois-Chauvel C, Régis J, Chauvel P, Vidal F. Action monitoring and medial frontal cortex: leading role of supplementary motor area. *Science*. (2014) 343:888–91. doi: 10.1126/science.1247412
148. Puglisi G, Sciortino T, Rossi M, Leonetti A, Fornia L, Conti Nibali M, et al. Preserving executive functions in nondominant frontal lobe glioma surgery: an intraoperative tool. *J Neurosurg*. (2018) 131:474–80. doi: 10.3171/2018.4.JNS18393
149. Wellmer J, Weber C, Mende M, von der Groeben F, Urbach H, Clusmann H, et al. Multitask electrical stimulation for cortical language mapping: hints for necessity and economic mode of application. *Epilepsia*. (2009) 50:2267–75. doi: 10.1111/j.1528-1167.2009.02192.x
150. Binder JR, Desai RH, Graves WW, Conant LL. Where is the semantic system? A critical review and meta-analysis of 120 functional neuroimaging studies. *Cereb Cortex*. (2009) 19:2767–96. doi: 10.1093/cercor/bhp055
151. Hickok G, Poeppel D. Towards a new functional anatomy of language. *Cognition*. (2004) 92:1–12. doi: 10.1016/j.cognition.2003.11.001
152. Binder JR, Tong JQ, Pillay SB, Conant LL, Humphries CJ, Raghavan M, et al. Anterior temporal lobe regions essential for picture naming: a voxel-level correlation analysis in left language dominant temporal lobe epilepsy surgery. *Epilepsia*. (2020) 61:1939–48. doi: 10.1111/epi.16643
153. Damasio AR. Time-locked multiregional retroactivation: a systems-level proposal for the neural substrates of recall and recognition. *Cognition*. (1989) 33:25–62. doi: 10.1016/0010-0277(89)90005-X
154. Damasio H, Grabowski TJ, Tranel D, Hichwa RD, Damasio A. A neural basis for lexical retrieval. *Nature*. (1996) 380:499–505. doi: 10.1038/380499a0
155. Drane DL, Ojemann JG, Phatak V, Loring DW, Gross RE, Hebb AO, et al. Famous face identification in temporal lobe epilepsy: Support for a multimodal integration model of semantic memory. *Cortex*. (2013) 49:1648–67. doi: 10.1016/j.cortex.2012.08.009
156. Hickok G, Poeppel D. Dorsal and ventral streams: a framework for understanding the functional neuroanatomy of language. *Cognition*. (2004) 92:67–99. doi: 10.1016/j.cognition.2003.10.011
157. Tranel D, Damasio H, Eichhorn GR, Grabowski T, Ponto LL, Hichwa RD. Neural correlates of naming animals from their characteristic sounds. *Neuropsychologia*. (2003) 41:847–54. doi: 10.1016/S0028-3932(02)00223-3
158. Drane DL, Ojemann GA, Aylward EH, Ojemann JG, Johnson LC, Silbergeld DL, et al. Category-specific naming and recognition deficits in temporal lobe epilepsy surgical patients. *Neuropsychologia*. (2008) 46:1242–55. doi: 10.1016/j.neuropsychologia.2007.11.034
159. Gomez J, Pestilli F, Witthoft N, Golarai G, Liberman A, Poltoratski S, et al. Functionally defined white matter reveals segregated pathways in human ventral temporal cortex associated with category-specific processing. *Neuron*. (2015) 85:216–27. doi: 10.1016/j.neuron.2014.12.027
160. Tranel D. The left temporal pole is important for retrieving words for unique concrete entities. *Aphasiology*. (2009) 23:867. doi: 10.1080/02687030802586498
161. Hamberger MJ, Miozzo M, Schevon CA, Morrison C, Carlson C, Mehta AD, et al. Functional differences among stimulation-identified cortical naming sites in the temporal region. *Epilepsy Behav*. (2016) 60:124–9. doi: 10.1016/j.yebeh.2016.04.021
162. Cohen L, Dehaene S, Naccache L, Lehéricy S, Dehaene-Lambertz G, Hénaff MA, et al. The visual word form area: spatial and temporal characterization of an initial stage of reading in normal subjects and posterior split-brain patients. *Brain*. (2000) 123(Pt 2):291–307. doi: 10.1093/brain/123.2.291
163. Henry C, Gaillard R, Volle E, Chiras J, Ferrieux S, Dehaene S, et al. Brain activations during letter-by-letter reading: a follow-up study. *Neuropsychologia*. (2005) 43:1983–9. doi: 10.1016/j.neuropsychologia.2005.04.007
164. Binder JR. Current controversies on Wernicke's area and its role in language. *Curr Neurol Neurosci Rep*. (2017) 17:58. doi: 10.1007/s11910-017-0764-8
165. Perrine K. Future directions for functional mapping. *Epilepsia*. (1994) 35:S90–102. doi: 10.1111/j.1528-1157.1994.tb05991.x
166. Mateer C, Polen S, Ojemann GA. Sexual variation in cortical localization of naming as determined by stimulation mapping. Commentary on McGlone 1980. *Behav Brain Sci*. (1982) 5:310–1. doi: 10.1017/S0140525X00012188
167. Devinsky O, Perrine K, Hirsch J, McMullen W, Pacia S, Doyle W. Relation of cortical language distribution and cognitive function in surgical epilepsy patients. *Epilepsia*. (2000) 41:400–4. doi: 10.1111/j.1528-1157.2000.tb00180.x
168. Schwartz TH, Devinsky O, Doyle W, Perrine K. Preoperative predictors of anterior temporal language areas. *J Neurosurg*. (1998) 89:962–70. doi: 10.3171/jns.1998.89.6.0962
169. Geschwind N. The organization of language. *Science*. (1979) 170:940–4. doi: 10.1126/science.170.3961.940
170. Indefrey P. The spatial and temporal signatures of word production components: a critical update. *Front Psychol*. (2011) 2:255. doi: 10.3389/fpsyg.2011.00255
171. Fedorenko E, Thompson-Schill SL. Reworking the language network. *Trends Cogn Sci*. (2014) 18:120–6. doi: 10.1016/j.tics.2013.12.006
172. Tyler LK, Stamatakis EA, Bright P, Acres K, Abdallah S, Rodd JM, et al. Processing objects at different levels of specificity. *J Cogn Neurosci*. (2004) 16:351–62. doi: 10.1162/089892904322926692
173. Roth EC, Hellige JB. Spatial processing and hemispheric asymmetry. Contributions of the transient/magnocellular visual system. *J Cogn Neurosci*. (1998) 10:472–84. doi: 10.1162/089892998562889
174. Takamiya N, Maekawa T, Yamasaki T, Ogata K, Yamada E, Tanaka M, et al. Different hemispheric specialization for face/word recognition: a high-density ERP study with hemifield visual stimulation. *Brain Behav*. (2020) 10:e01649. doi: 10.1002/brb3.1649
175. Levine SC, Banich MT, Koch-Weser MP. Face recognition: a general or specific right hemisphere capacity? *Brain Cogn*. (1988) 8:303–25. doi: 10.1016/0278-2626(88)90057-7
176. Jonas J, Descoins M, Koessler L, Colnat-Coulbois S, Sauvée M, Guye M, et al. Focal electrical intracerebral stimulation of a face-sensitive area causes transient prosopagnosia. *Neuroscience*. (2012) 222:281–8 doi: 10.1016/j.neuroscience.2012.07.021
177. Jonas J, Rossion B, Krieg J, Koessler L, Colnat-Coulbois S, Vespignani H, et al. Intracerebral electrical stimulation of a face-selective area in the right inferior occipital cortex impairs individual face discrimination. *Neuroimage*. (2014) 99:487–97. doi: 10.1016/j.neuroimage.2014.06.017
178. Jonas J, Jacques C, Liu-Shuang J, Brissart H, Colnat-Coulbois S, Maillard L, et al. A face-selective ventral occipito-temporal map of the human brain with intracerebral potentials. *Proc Natl Acad Sci USA*. (2016) 113:E4088–97. doi: 10.1073/pnas.1522033113
179. Burgess N, Maguire EA, O'Keefe J. The human hippocampus and spatial and episodic memory. *Neuron*. (2002) 35:625–41. doi: 10.1016/S0896-6273(02)00830-9
180. Karnath H-O, Rorden C. The anatomy of spatial neglect. *Neuropsychologia*. (2012) 50:1010–7. doi: 10.1016/j.neuropsychologia.2011.06.027
181. Corballis MC. Mental rotation and the right hemisphere. *Brain Lang*. (1997) 57:100–21. doi: 10.1006/brln.1997.1835
182. Parsons TD, Larson P, Kratz K, Thiebaux M, Bluestein B, Buckwalter JG, et al. Sex differences in mental rotation and spatial rotation in a virtual environment. *Neuropsychologia*. (2004) 42:555–62. doi: 10.1016/j.neuropsychologia.2003.08.014
183. Hawes Z, Sokolowski HM, Ononye CB, Ansari D. Neural underpinnings of numerical and spatial cognition: an fMRI meta-analysis of brain regions associated with symbolic number, arithmetic, mental rotation. *Neurosci Biobehav Rev*. (2019) 103:316–36. doi: 10.1016/j.neubiorev.2019.05.007
184. Fried I, Mateer C, Ojemann GA, Wohns R, Fedio P. Organization of visuospatial functions in human cortex: evidence from electrical stimulation. *Brain*. (1982) 105:349–71. doi: 10.1093/brain/105.2.349
185. Kahana MJ, Sekuler R, Caplan JB, Kirschen M, Madsen JR. Human theta oscillations exhibit task dependence during virtual maze navigation. *Nature*. (1999) 399:781–4. doi: 10.1038/21645
186. Chen D, Kunz L, Wang W, Zhang H, Wang W-X, Schulze-Bonhage A, et al. Hexadirectional modulation of theta power in human entorhinal cortex during spatial navigation. *Curr Biol*. (2018) 28:3310–4. doi: 10.1016/j.cub.2018.08.029
187. Ekstrom AD, Caplan JB, Ho E, Shattuck K, Fried I, Kahana MJ. Human hippocampal theta activity during virtual navigation. *Hippocampus*. (2005) 15:881–9. doi: 10.1002/hipo.20109

188. Aghajan Z, Schuette P, Fields TA, Tran ME, Siddiqui SM, Hasulak NR, et al. Theta oscillations in the human medial temporal lobe during real-world ambulatory movement. *Curr Biol.* (2017) 27:3743–51.e3. doi: 10.1016/j.cub.2017.10.062
189. Miller J, Watrous AJ, Tsitsiklis M, Lee SA, Sheth SA, Schevon CA, et al. Lateralized hippocampal oscillations underlie distinct aspects of human spatial memory and navigation. *Nat Commun.* (2018) 9:2423. doi: 10.1038/s41467-018-04847-9
190. Goyal A, Miller J, Qasim SE, Watrous AJ, Zhang H, Stein JM, et al. Functionally distinct high and low theta oscillations in the human hippocampus. *Nat Commun.* (2020) 11:2469. doi: 10.1038/s41467-020-15670-6
191. Jacobs J. Hippocampal theta oscillations are slower in humans than in rodents: implications for models of spatial navigation and memory. *Philos Trans R Soc B Biol Sci.* (2014) 369:20130304. doi: 10.1098/rstb.2013.0304
192. Mormann F, Osterhage H, Andrzejak RG, Weber B, Fernández G, Fell J, et al. Independent delta/theta rhythms in the human hippocampus and entorhinal cortex. *Front Hum Neurosci.* (2008) 2:3. doi: 10.3389/neuro.09.003.2008
193. Koziol LF, Budding DE, editors. *Subcortical Structures and Cognition: Implications for Neuropsychological Assessment.* Newark, NJ: Springer (2009).
194. Henri-Bhargava A, Stuss DT, Freedman M. Clinical assessment of prefrontal lobe functions. *Continuum.* (2018) 24:704–26. doi: 10.1212/CON.0000000000000609
195. Baxendale S, Thompson PJ, Sander JW. Neuropsychological outcomes in epilepsy surgery patients with unilateral hippocampal sclerosis and good preoperative memory function. *Epilepsia.* (2013) 54:e131–4. doi: 10.1111/epi.12319
196. Gleissner U, Helmstaedter C, Schramm J, Elger CE. Memory outcome after selective amygdalohippocampectomy in patients with temporal lobe epilepsy: one-year follow-up. *Epilepsia.* (2004) 45:960–2. doi: 10.1111/j.0013-9580.2004.42203.x
197. Helmstaedter C, Petzold I, Bien CG. The cognitive consequence of resecting nonlesional tissues in epilepsy surgery–results from MRI- and histopathology-negative patients with temporal lobe epilepsy. *Epilepsia.* (2011) 52:1402–8. doi: 10.1111/j.1528-1167.2011.03157.x
198. Seidenberg M, Hermann B, Wyler AR, Davies K, Dohan FC Jr, Leveroni C. Neuropsychological outcome following anterior temporal lobectomy in patients with and without the syndrome of mesial temporal lobe epilepsy. *Neuropsychology.* (1998) 12:303–16. doi: 10.1037/0894-4105.12.2.303
199. Gross RE, Stern MA, Willie JT, Fasano RE, Saindane AM, Soares BP, et al. Stereotactic laser amygdalohippocampotomy for mesial temporal lobe epilepsy. *Ann Neurol.* (2018) 83:575–87. doi: 10.1002/ana.25180
200. Cairney SA, Guttesen A, El Marj N, Staresina BP. Memory consolidation is linked to spindle-mediated information processing during sleep. *Curr Biol.* (2018) 28:948–54. doi: 10.1016/j.cub.2018.01.087
201. Jiang X, Gonzalez-Martinez J, Halgren E. Coordination of human hippocampal sharpwave ripples during NREM sleep with cortical theta bursts, spindles, downstates, and upstates. *J Neurosci.* (2019) 39:8744–61. doi: 10.1523/JNEUROSCI.2857-18.2019
202. Lambert I, Tramoni-Negre E, Lagarde S, Roehri N, Giusiano B, Trebuchon-Da Fonseca A, et al. Hippocampal interictal spikes during sleep impact long-term memory consolidation. *Ann Neurol.* (2020) 87:976–87. doi: 10.1002/ana.25744
203. Drane DL. Neuropsychological evaluation of the epilepsy surgical candidate. In: Barr WB, Morrison C, editors. *Handbook on the Neuropsychology of Epilepsy.* New York, NY: Springer (2015) 87–121.
204. Chari A, Thornton RC, Tisdall MM, Scott RC. Microelectrode recordings in human epilepsy: a case for clinical translation. *Brain Commun.* (2020) 2:fcaa082. doi: 10.1093/braincomms/fcaa082
205. Quian Quiroga R. Plugging in to human memory: advantages, challenges, and insights from human single-neuron recordings. *Cell.* (2019) 179:1015–32. doi: 10.1016/j.cell.2019.10.016
206. Coubes P, Baldy-Moulinier M, Zanca M, Boire JY, Child R, Bourbotte G, et al. Monitoring sodium methohexital distribution with [99mTc]HMPAO with single photon emission computed tomography during Wada test. *Epilepsia.* (1995) 36:1041–9. doi: 10.1111/j.1528-1157.1995.tb00964.x
207. Herbet G, Moritz-Gasser S. Beyond language: mapping cognition and emotion. *Neurosurg Clin.* (2019) 30:75–83. doi: 10.1016/j.nec.2018.08.004
208. Ameis SH, Catani M. Altered white matter connectivity as a neural substrate for social impairment in Autism Spectrum Disorder. *Cortex.* (2015) 62:158–81. doi: 10.1016/j.cortex.2014.10.014
209. Savla GN, Vella L, Armstrong CC, Penn DL, Twamley EW. Deficits in domains of social cognition in schizophrenia: a meta-analysis of the empirical evidence. *Schizophrenia Bull.* (2013) 39:979–92. doi: 10.1093/schbul/sbs080
210. Blair RJ. The amygdala and ventromedial prefrontal cortex in morality and psychopathy. *Trends Cogn Sci.* (2007) 11:387–92. doi: 10.1016/j.tics.2007.07.003
211. Li W, Mai X, Liu C. The default mode network and social understanding of others: what do brain connectivity studies tell us. *Front Hum Neurosci.* (2014) 8:74. doi: 10.3389/fnhum.2014.00074
212. Raichle ME, MacLeod AM, Snyder AZ, Powers WJ, Gusnard DA, Shulman GL. A default mode of brain function. *Proc Natl Acad Sci USA.* (2001) 98:676–82. doi: 10.1073/pnas.98.2.676
213. Raichle ME, Snyder AZ. A default mode of brain function: a brief history of an evolving idea. *NeuroImage.* (2007) 37:1083–99. doi: 10.1016/j.neuroimage.2007.02.041
214. Schilbach L, Eickhoff SB, Rotarska-Jagiela A, Fink GR, Vogeley K. Minds at rest? Social cognition as the default mode of cognizing and its putative relationship to the "default system" of the brain. *Consciou Cogn.* (2008) 17:457–67. doi: 10.1016/j.concog.2008.03.013
215. Martin E, Jeanmonod D, Morel A, Zadicario E, Werner B. High-intensity focused ultrasound for noninvasive functional neurosurgery. *Ann Neurol.* (2009) 66:858–61. doi: 10.1002/ana.21801
216. Buckner RL, Andrews-Hanna JR, Schacter DL. The brain's default network: anatomy, function, and relevance to disease. *Ann NY Acad Sci.* (2008) 1124:1–38. doi: 10.1196/annals.1440.011
217. Aggleton JP, Passingham RE. Syndrome produced by lesions of the amygdala in monkeys (Macacamulatta). *J Comp Physiol Psychol.* (1981) 95:961–77. doi: 10.1037/h0077848
218. Brown S, Schäfer EA. An investigation into the functions of the occipital and temporal lobes of the monkey's brain. *Philos Trans R Soc Lond.* (1888) 179B:303–27. doi: 10.1098/rstb.1888.0011
219. Klüver H, Bucy PC. "Psychic blindness" and other symptoms following bilateral temporal lobectomy in Rhesus monkeys. *Am J Physiol.* (1937) 119:352–3.
220. Klüver H, Bucy PC. Preliminary analysis of functions of the temporal lobes in monkeys. *Arch Neurol Psychiatry.* (1939) 42:979–1000. doi: 10.1001/archneurpsyc.1939.02270240017001
221. Marlowe WB, Mancall EL, Thomas JJ. Complete Klüver-Bucy syndrome in man. *Cortex.* (1975) 11:53–9. doi: 10.1016/S0010-9452(75)80020-7
222. Cox CL, Uddin LQ, Di Martino A, Castellanos FX, Milham MP, Kelly C. The balance between feeling and knowing: affective and cognitive empathy are reflected in the brain's intrinsic functional dynamics. *Soc Cogn Affect Neurosci.* (2012) 7:727–37. doi: 10.1093/scan/nsr051
223. Molnar-Szakacs I, Uddin LQ. Self-processing and the default mode networks: interactions with the mirror neuron system. *Front Human Neurosci.* (2013) 7:571. doi: 10.3389/fnhum.2013.00571
224. Catani M, Dell'acqua F, Thiebaut de Schotten M. A revised limbic system model for memory, emotion and behaviour. *Neurosci Biobehav Rev.* (2013) 37:1724–37. doi: 10.1016/j.neubiorev.2013.07.001
225. Papez JW. A proposed mechanism of emotion. *Arch Neurol Psychiatry.* (1937) 38:725–43. doi: 10.1001/archneurpsyc.1937.02260220069003
226. Yakovlev PJ. Motility, behavior and the brain; stereodynamic organization and neural coordinates of behavior. *J Nervous Mental Dis.* (1948) 107:313–35. doi: 10.1097/00005053-194810740-00001
227. MacLean PD. Psychosomatic disease and the 'visceral brain': recent developments bearing on the Papez theory of emotion. *Psychosom Med.* (1949) 11:338–53. doi: 10.1097/00006842-194911000-00003
228. MacLean PD. Some psychiatric implications of physiological studies on frontotemporal portion of limbic system (visceral brain). *Electroencephalogr Clin Neurophysiol.* (1952) 4:407–18. doi: 10.1016/0013-4694(52)90073-4
229. Baron-Cohen S, Wheelwright S, Hill J, Raste Y, Plumb I. The "Reading the Mind in the Eyes" Test revised version: a study with normal adults, and adults with Asperger syndrome or high-functioning autism. *J Child*

Psychol Psychiatry Allied Discipl. (2001) 42:241–51. doi: 10.1111/1469-7610.00715
230. Döhnel K, Schuwerk T, Meinhardt J, Sodian B, Hajak G, Sommer M. Functional activity of the right temporo-parietal junction and of the medial prefrontal cortex associated with true and false belief reasoning. *NeuroImage.* (2012) 60:1652-61. doi: 10.1016/j.neuroimage.2012.01.073
231. Herbet G, Lafargue G, Bonnetblanc F, Moritz-Gasser S, Duffau H. Is the right frontal cortex really crucial in the mentalizing network? A longitudinal study in patients with a slow-growing lesion. *Cortex.* (2013) 49:2711–27. doi: 10.1016/j.cortex.2013.08.003
232. Herbet G, Lafargue G, Bonnetblanc F, Moritz-Gasser S, Menjot de Champfleur N, Duffau H. Inferring a dual-stream model of mentalizing from associative white matter fibres disconnection. *Brain.* (2014) 137:944–59. doi: 10.1093/brain/awt370
233. Ono KE, Bearden DJ, Adams E, Doescher J, Koh S, Eksioglu Y, et al. Cognitive and behavioral outcome of stereotactic laser amydalohippocampotomy in a pediatric setting. *Epilepsy Behav Rep.* (2020) 14:100370. doi: 10.1016/j.ebr.2020.100370
234. Hofman MA, Falk D, editors. *Progress in Brain Research*, Vol. 195. Amsterdam: Elsevier (2012). p. 123–63.
235. Revonsuo A. *Inner Presence: Consciousness as Biological Phenomenon.* Cambridge, MA: MIT Press (2006).
236. Giacino JT, Fins JJ, Laureys S, Schiff ND. Disorders of consciousness after acquired brain injury: the state of the science. *Nat Rev Neurol.* (2014) 10:99–114. doi: 10.1038/nrneurol.2013.279
237. Baars BJ. *On Consciousness.* Oxford: Nautilus Press (2019).
238. Dehaene S. *Consciousness and the Brain.* New York, NY: Viking (2014).
239. Arthuis M, Valton L, Regis J, Chauvel P, Wendling F, Naccache L, et al. Impaired consciousness during temporal lobe seizures is related to increased long-distance cortical-subcortical synchronization. *Brain.* (2009) 132:2091–101. doi: 10.1093/brain/awp086
240. Gaillard R, Dehaene S, Adam C, Clemenceau S, Hasboun D, Baulac M, et al. Converging intracranial markers of conscious access. *PLoS Biol.* (2009) 7:e61. doi: 10.1371/journal.pbio.1000061
241. Naccache L, Marti S, Sitt JD, Trübutschek D, Berkovitch L. Why the P3b is still a plausible correlate of conscious access? A commentary on Silverstein et al., 2015. *Cortex.* (2016) 85:126–8. doi: 10.1016/j.cortex.2016.04.003
242. Naccache L. Why and how access consciousness can account for phenomenal consciousness. *Philos Trans R Soc Lond B Biol Sci.* (2018) 373:20170357 doi: 10.1098/rstb/2017.0357
243. Bartolomei F, Naccache L. The global workspace (GW) theory of consciousness and epilepsy. *Behav Neurol.* (2011) 24:67–74. doi: 10.3233/BEN-2011-0313
244. Bartolomei F, McGonigal A, Naccache L. Alteration of global workspace in focal epilepsy: the global workspace alteration theory. *Epilepsy Behav.* (2014) 30:17–23. doi: 10.1016/j.yebeh.2013.09.012
245. Bonini F, Lambert I, Wendling F, McGonigal A, Bartolomei F. Altered synchrony and loss of consciousness during frontal lobe seizures. *Clin Neurophysiol.* (2016) 127:1170–5. doi: 10.1016/j.clinph.2015.04.050
246. Lambert I, Arthius M, McGonigal A, Wendling F, Bartolomei F. Alteration of global workspace during loss of consciousness: a study of parietal seizures. *Epilepsia.* (2012) 53:2014–110. doi: 10.1111/j.1528-1167.2012.03690.x
247. Lagun D, Manzanares C, Zola SM, Buffalo EA, Agichtein E. Detecting cognitive impairment by eye movement analysis using automatic classification algorithms. *J Neurosci Methods.* (2011) 201:196–203. doi: 10.1016/j.jneumeth.2011.06.027
248. Zola SM, Manzanares CM, Clopton P, Lah JJ, Levey AI. A behavioral task predicts conversion to mild cognitive impairment and Alzheimer's disease. *Am J Alzheimer's Dis Other Dement.* (2013) 28:179–84. doi: 10.1177/1533317512470484
249. Aronov D, Tank DW. Engagement of neural circuits underlying 2D spatial navigation in a rodent virtual reality system. *Neuron.* (2014) 84:442–56. doi: 10.1016/j.neuron.2014.08.042
250. Lester AW, Moffat SD, Wiener JM, Barnes CA, Wolbers T. The aging navigational system. *Neuron.* (2017) 95:1019–35. doi: 10.1016/j.neuron.2017.06.037
251. Bernard F, Lemée JM, Aubin G, Ter Minassian A, Menei P. Using a virtual reality social network during awake craniotomy to map social cognition: prospective trial. *J Med Internet Res.* (2018) 20:e10332. doi: 10.2196/10332
252. Corriveau Lecavalier N, Ouellet É, Boller B, Belleville S. Use of immersive virtual reality to assess episodic memory: a validation study in older adults. *Neuropsychol Rehabil.* (2020) 30:462–80. doi: 10.1080/09602011.2018.1477684
253. Ouellet É, Boller B, Corriveau-Lecavalier N, Cloutier S, Belleville S. The virtual shop: a new immersive virtual reality environment and scenario for the assessment of everyday memory. *J Neurosci Methods.* (2018) 303:126–35. doi: 10.1016/j.jneumeth.2018.03.010
254. da Costa R, Pompeu JE, de Mello DD, Moretto E, Rodrigues FZ, Dos Santos MD, et al. Two new virtual reality tasks for the assessment of spatial orientation: preliminary results of tolerability, sense of presence and usability. *Dement Neuropsychol.* (2018) 12:196–204. doi: 10.1590/1980-57642018dn12-020013
255. Climent G, Rodríguez C, García T, Areces D, Mejías M, Aierbe A, et al. New virtual reality tool (Nesplora Aquarium) for assessing attention and working memory in adults: a normative study. *Appl Neuropsychol Adult.* (2019) 1–13. doi: 10.1080/23279095.2019.1646745
256. König SU, Clay V, Nolte D, Duesberg L, Kuske N, König P. Learning of spatial properties of a large-scale virtual city with an interactive map. *Front Hum Neurosci.* (2019) 13:240. doi: 10.3389/fnhum.2019.00240
257. Peeters D. A standardized set of 3-D objects for virtual reality research and applications. *Behav Res Methods.* (2018) 50:1047–54. doi: 10.3758/s13428-017-0925-3
258. Cleary AM, Brown AS, Sawyer BD, Nomi JS, Ajoku AC, Ryals AJ. Familiarity from the configuration of objects in 3-dimensional space and its relation to déjà vu: a virtual reality investigation. *Conscious Cogn.* (2012) 21:969–75. doi: 10.1016/j.concog.2011.12.010
259. Caldwell DJ, Ojemann JG, Rao R. Direct electrical stimulation in electrocorticographic brain-computer interfaces: enabling technologies for input to cortex. *Front Neurosci.* (2019) 13:804. doi: 10.3389/fnins.2019.00804
260. Zuk P, Torgerson L, Sierra-Mercado D, Lázaro-Muñoz G. Neuroethics of neuromodulation: an update. *Curr Opin Biomed Eng.* (2018) 8:45–50. doi: 10.1016/j.cobme.2018.10.003

5

Distinguishing Dependent-Stage Secondary Epileptogenesis in a Complex Case of Giant Hypothalamic Hamartoma with Assistance of a Computational Method

Zhao Liu[1,2], *Guoming Luan*[1,2,3*], *Chuanzuo Yang*[4], *Yuguang Guan*[1], *Changqing Liu*[1], *Jing Wang*[5], *Mengyang Wang*[5] *and Qingyun Wang*[4]

[1] Department of Functional Neurosurgery, Sanbo Brain Hospital, Capital Medical University, Beijing, China, [2] Beijing Key Laboratory of Epilepsy, Epilepsy Center, Sanbo Brain Hospital, Capital Medical University, Beijing, China, [3] Beijing Institute for Brain Disorders, Beijing, China, [4] Department of Dynamics and Control, Beihang University, Beijing, China, [5] Department of Neurology, Sanbo Brain Hospital, Capital Medical University, Beijing, China

***Correspondence:**
Guoming Luan
luangm3@163.com

Besides gelastic seizures, hypothalamic hamartoma (HH) is also noted for its susceptibility to remote secondary epileptogenesis. Although clinical observations have demonstrated its existence, and a three-stage theory has been proposed, how to determine whether a remote symptom is spontaneous or dependent on epileptic activities of HH is difficult in some cases. Herein, we report a case of new non-gelastic seizures in a 9-year-old female associated with a postoperatively remaining HH. Electrophysiological examinations and stereo-electroencephalography (SEEG) demonstrated seizure onsets with slow-wave and fast activities on the outside of the HH. By using computational methodologies to calculate the network dynamic effective connectivities, the importance of HH in the epileptic network was revealed. After SEEG-guided thermal coagulation of the remaining HH, the patient finally was seizure-free at the 2-year follow-up. This case showed the ability of computational methods to reveal information underlying complex SEEG signals, and further demonstrated the dependent-stage secondary epileptogenesis, which has been rarely reported.

Keywords: stereo-electroencephalography, refractory focal epilepsy, epileptogenic zone localization, coupled neuronal population model, epileptogenic networks, hypothalamic hamartoma

INTRODUCTION

As a rare congenital malformation disease, hypothalamic hamartoma (HH) has four major impacts on patients, especially in the pediatric populations: precocious puberty (PP) (1), seizures that are mainly gelastic seizures (GS) (2), cognitive and behavioral impairments (3), and developmental delays (4). Among the symptoms, GS is a hallmark, mostly drug resistant and is verified by stereo-electroencephalography (SEEG) as originating from HH (5, 6). However, due to the observation of multiple other seizure types associated with extra-lesion areas, a hypothesis of secondary epileptogenesis, that persistent seizure activities from HH could induce seizure activities in various neocortical areas, has been suggested (5, 7). According to Morell's postulation, secondary epileptogenesis develops in three stages (i.e., dependent, intermediate, and independent) (8, 9).

Previous clinical observations have demonstrated the existence of the independent stage, but methods to distinguish this stage once the secondary epileptogenesis emerges have rarely been described (7). Since the 1990s, computational methods based on various theoretical models have been developed and used to solve problems that were too complex for manual interpretations (10–14).

In this paper, we report a giant (diameter > 5 cm) HH case, whose epilepsy control did not merely fail after a secondary-stage surgery approach, but secondary epileptogenesis also developed. Despite the difficulty of diagnosing the stage of secondary epileptogenesis with information from magnetic resonance imaging (MRI) scans, scalp video electroencephalograms EEGs, and SEEG, use of a novel computational method based on SEEG data suggested the possibility of a dependent stage, and the patient's seizure control finally succeeded with SEEG-guided thermal coagulation.

CASE PRESENTATION

A 9-year-old female was admitted to our epilepsy center because of an almost 8.5-year history of compulsive bursts of giggles, which probably started since 8 months of age. At that time, giggles were not confirmed because the sounds merely sounded like a peculiar noise. A giant HH, which was approximately 35 × 32 × 25 mm had grown to the interpeduncular cistern as revealed by an MRI scan (**Figure 1A**). GS were diagnosed at 2 years of age, and two resective operations had been conducted separately at 6 months and 1.5 years later. Both operations were via the same trans-right-frontal-basal approach and about 50% of the lesion had been removed (**Figure 1B**), and pathological examinations verified the diagnosis of HH. After the first operation, carbamazepine therapy of 100 mg per day was given. Unfortunately, the two operations and medical therapy did not improve the compulsive giggles. Later, since 7 years of age, carbamazepine had been ceased by her mother without medical consultation. The patient had no antiepileptic drugs and her GS had not changed until her admission to our center due to a recent aggravation with two times of a new seizure type. These two seizures started with a loss of consciousness and then developed to her eyes turning to the left and then tonic-clonic seizure of the four limbs. This lasted for about 2–3 min. The patient had medium-level academic achievement, and her mother reported no obvious behavioral deterioration. Nevertheless, the patient was described as short-tempered and hard to communicate with.

Her physical and neurological examinations were normal. The Wechsler Intelligence Scale for Children—Chinese Revised showed that her full intelligence quotient was at an average level with a score of 97. All routine blood, blood coagulation, and biochemical tests, as well as infection immunoassay results, urinalysis, electrocardiogram, and chest radiography showed normal results.

For epilepsy evaluation, both scalp video-EEG (VEEG) and MRI scans were conducted. Structural imaging showed that the remaining HH was connected to the hypothalamus (**Figure 1B**).

VEEG were recorded with a Nicolet video-EEG monitoring system (Thermo Fisher Scientific, Waltham, MA, USA) and digitized at the rate of 1,024 Hz with the international standard 10–10 electrode montage. The online band-pass filter was set to 1.6–150 Hz. The monitor recorded for 7 days and video observations demonstrated two types of clinical seizures. The first was the bursts of giggles, which persisted for about 5 s, and the second one was the loss of consciousness followed by head-turning to the left, which lasted about 20 s. No obvious giggles were observed during the second procedure, and associated auras were denied.

In the inter-ictal period, intermittent poly-spikes and slow-wave activities were recorded in the right frontal area (F8, Fp2, F4) and the right temporal area (M2, T4). In the peri-ictal period, the EEG onset zone was located in the right hemisphere and was obvious in the anterior area (Fp2, F4, C4, M2, F8, T8) with low-voltage fast activities. Two seconds later, the clinical symptoms started. **Figure 2A** shows the VEEG waveforms of 6 s pre-ictal and 11 s early-ictal period of the second seizure type. The GS showed similar VEEG performances.

From these data, three hypotheses for the secondary partial seizures emerged; these shared the same mechanisms with GS induced either by HH or some region in the neocortex. Likewise, it might independently oscillate similar to VEEG performances with GS induced by HH.

To accurately explore the seizure onset zone, five intracranial electrodes were stereotaxically implanted with a robot-assisted stereotaxic operation system (ROSA). The SEEG depth electrodes (16 contacts, length: 2 mm, diameter: 0.8 mm; 1.5 mm apart) were manufactured by ALICS Co Ltd., Besancon, France. The diameter of the depth electrode was 0.8 mm. The electrodes were placed into the remaining HH via the right anterior temporal lobe (electrodes A–D) or right anterior frontal lobe (electrode E). The SEEGs were recorded using a common reference electrode (Nicolet^{TM} system; 128 channels; sampling rate, 1024 Hz). The impedance of all the recording electrode nodes was kept below 50 kΩ; otherwise, the nodes would be excluded from analyses. Bipolar derivation was chosen to avoid possible bias deriving either from a not completely inactive common reference or from interference due to a volume conduction effect. To verify the correct placement of the electrodes, a postimplantation (DynaCT; Siemens, Malvern, PA, USA) scan was performed and reconstructed images were digitally fused with the presurgical MRI dataset using the fusion system within ROSA.

Finally, electrodes A–D were implanted as planned while the tip of electrode E was placed into the hippocampus. As a result, electrode nodes A1–5, B1–5, C1–3, and D1–4 were located within the remaining HH; nodes A8–11, B7–9, D7–10, and E4–5 were located within the hippocampus; nodes A14–15, B12–17, C14–17, and D15–17 were located within the right superficial temporal lobe; nodes E16–17 were located within the right superficial frontal lobe; and the other nodes were located within the white matter. **Figure 3A** shows all nodes within the remaining HH. SEEGs were monitored for 3 days after implantation, and a total of four seizures in two types were captured.

Figure 2B shows that SEEGs for all the inter-ictal discharges were located within the temporal lobe (A8–11, B6–7, B11–12,

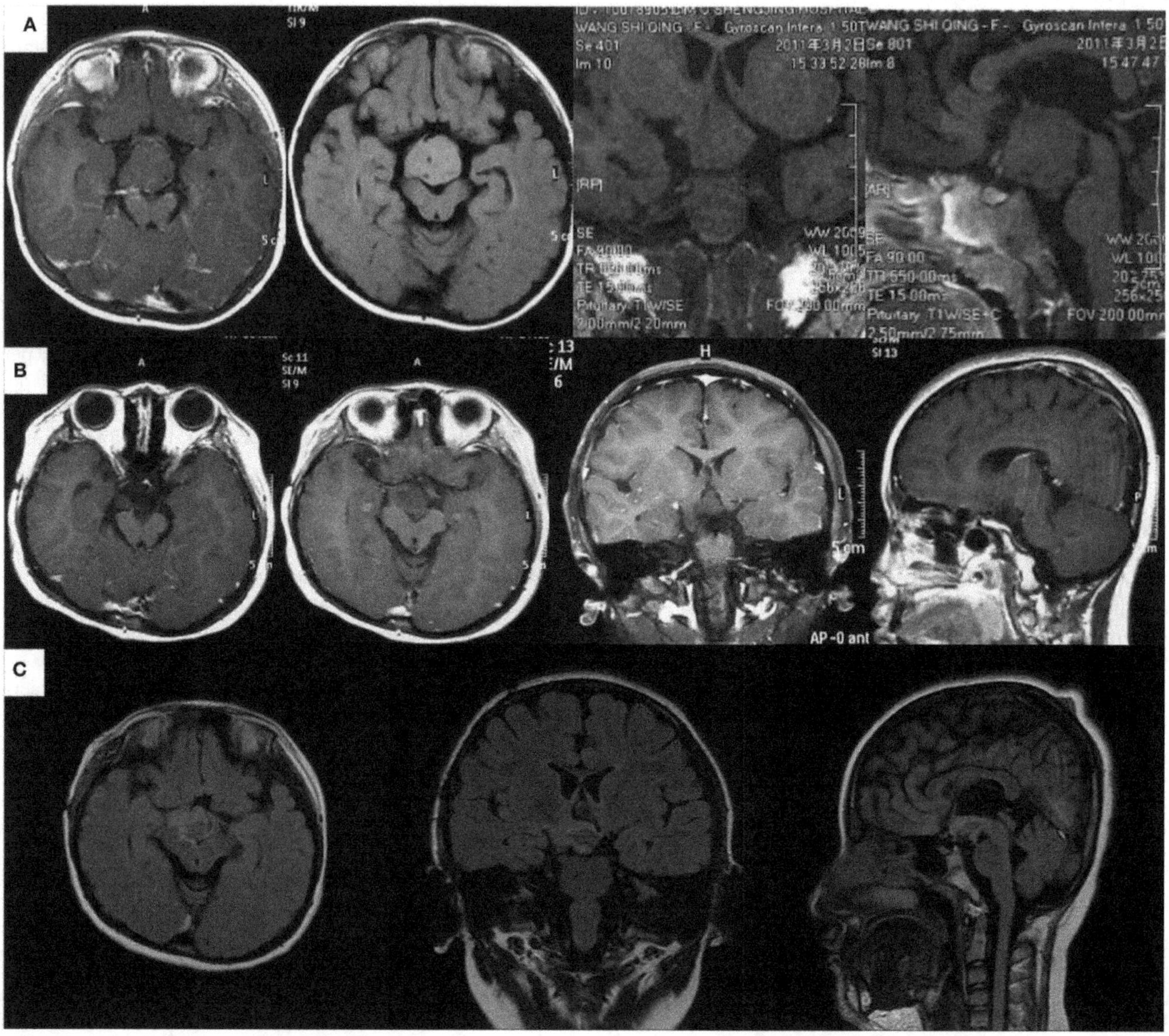

FIGURE 1 | Magnetic resonance imaging scans of the patient at different ages. **(A)** Images at 2.5 years of age before the first resective operation the giant HH (about 35 × 32 × 25 mm, images from left to right are the axial contrasted T1 image, axial T2 FLAIRE image, coronal T1 image, and sagittal T1 image). **(B)** Images at 3.5 years of age after the second resective operation demonstrated about 25% of the lesion had remained (images from left to right are two axial contrasted T1 images in different slices, contrasted coronal T1 image, and contrasted sagittal T1 image). **(C)** Images 7 days after the ablation showed that almost all the par connection between the HH and the hypothalamus has been coagulated. (Images from left to right are axial, sagittal, and coronal T2 FLAIRE images).

D7–9, and E4–5). Unexpectedly, seizure onsets of the two types, even the GS, originated from the hippocampus (E4–5 and D7–9) with spike-waves in fast activities as shown in **Figure 2C**. The time intervals between onset activities and clinical symptoms (giggles or head-turning) were about 14 s.

Because this diverged from clinical experiences, that GS were mostly induced by electrical/physiological activities of HH, the SEEG data were further analyzed by a hemi-manual computational method, which was previously introduced (10; in Matlab 2017). This computational method calculated the SEEG dataset in all bands. Using the adaptive direct transfer function, the SEEG data were integrated into a frequency domain. We then essentially used the Granger causality technique (15) and a time-variant autoregressive model to evaluate the statistical interdependence of multiple simultaneous time series, considering the Kalman filtering algorithm (16). Each node stood for its adjacent neural population. Finally, the instant out-degree of each node in a network was drawn, which stood for the impact of the node on other neural ensembles in the production of synchronous discharges. **Figure 3B** shows the analyzing process; more details have been described in our previous study (10). For this case, two time periods, which were

TABLE 1 | Parameters of SEEG-guided radiofrequency coagulation.

Ablation nodes	Power rate (W)	Impedance pre-abl. (Ω)	Impedance post-abl. (Ω)	Ablation time(s)
A (1,2)	3.5	840	750	120
A (2,3)	3.5	800	760	120
A (3,4)	3.5	870	750	120
A (4,5)	3.0	923	800	30
B (1,2)	3.5	615	470	60
B (2,3)	3.5	590	440	60
B (3,4)	3.5	>1000	610	60
B (3,4)	3.0	690	485	30
C (1,2)	3.0	950	900	60
C (2,3)	3.0	960	900	60
A2–B1	3.5	707	670	60
A3–B1	3.5	750	600	60
A4–B2	3.5	890	-	Termination*
B1–C2	3.5	850	800	60

*The ablation times and power rate were set according to location of the nodes. When the nodes were close to hypothalamus, a lower rate (3.0 W) with lower time (30 s or 60 s) would be chosen. *The ablation of A4–B2 was terminated because of the intolerance headache.*

5 min before (pre-ictal) and 90 s after (early-ictal) seizure onset, were analyzed, as these datasets could reflect neural network evolution during seizure activities. Thereafter, prominent out-degrees within HH (B1–2, C1–3, and D2–4) were demonstrated in the pre-ictal period (**Figure 3C**), although the hippocampus (E4–5) persistently showed dominant out-degrees.

From these data, our hypothesis was that the patient showed a dependent-stage elevated secondary epileptogenesis, and therefore, radiofrequency ablation therapy targeting the remaining HH was designed. The parameters are listed in **Table 1**.

Of note, when seizures ceased right after the ablation, post-ablation SEEG monitoring recorded an abrupt decrease of inter-ictal discharges. In addition, the patient had a curative feeling, and the parent described a personality change in the patient as becoming gentler and easier to communicate with. Post-ablation MRI showed a satisfying ablation of the par connection between the HH and the hypothalamus (**Figure 1C**). After the ablation, an oxcarbazepine therapy of 600 mg per day was given as the postoperative antiepileptic drug. At the 2-year follow-up, there was no sign of relapse and VEEGs (four times for 16 h) showed continued "running down" of inter-ictal discharges. The oxcarbazepine was gradually withdrawn to 300 mg per day. No intelligence decline and behavioral deterioration was observed and the change of personality seemed to be permanent.

DISCUSSION

In this case, the existence of the dependent stage of secondary epileptogenesis was first suggested. Secondary epileptogenesis was defined by Morell as the involvement of a previously normal neural network by an interconnected actively discharging an epileptogenic area (9), which might be related to the kindling procedure (17). Three stages were postulated: the dependent stage, the intermediate stage, and the independent stage (8). When driven by the primary focus, epileptic activities could be ceased after exclusion of the primary focus in the dependent stage. After temporary persistence, secondary epileptic activities would finally cease after the removal of the primary focus. However, in the dependent stage, in spite of removal of the primary focus, secondary epileptogenesis epileptic activities may persist. A kindling phenomenon, which was described by Goddard (17), was believed to be the cause. Repetition of kindling-like seizure activities may recruit uninvolved neural populations into epileptic networks and the rate of kindling-like activities may decide the secondary-epileptogenesis stage. However, because of the controversy regarding the definition, and the imperfect fit of animal models to the human epileptic syndrome, "secondary epileptogenesis" remained controversial except in the HHs.

Kindling-like activities have been revealed in human HH tissues. In a series of pathological researches, it was recognized that clusters of 80–90% HH neurons, which have an interneuron-like phenotype, work as a pacemaker and the other HH neurons, which are large cells with pleomorphic soma and dendrites, function as a neurotransmitter (18–21). These activities could propagate to the temporal lobe through the left fornix (22) or to the frontal lobe through the mammillary-thalamo-cingulate pathway (23). Scholly et al. have reported HH cases consistent with the independent stage (5, 7). Parvizi et al. suggested that the development of non-GS types in GS with HHs correlates with older age and longer duration of epilepsy (24), while GS related to frontal, parietal lobe epilepsy or hippocampal sclerosis has also been reported (25). Several reports suggested that seizure types besides GS in HHs were related to neocortical seizure activities (5, 26).

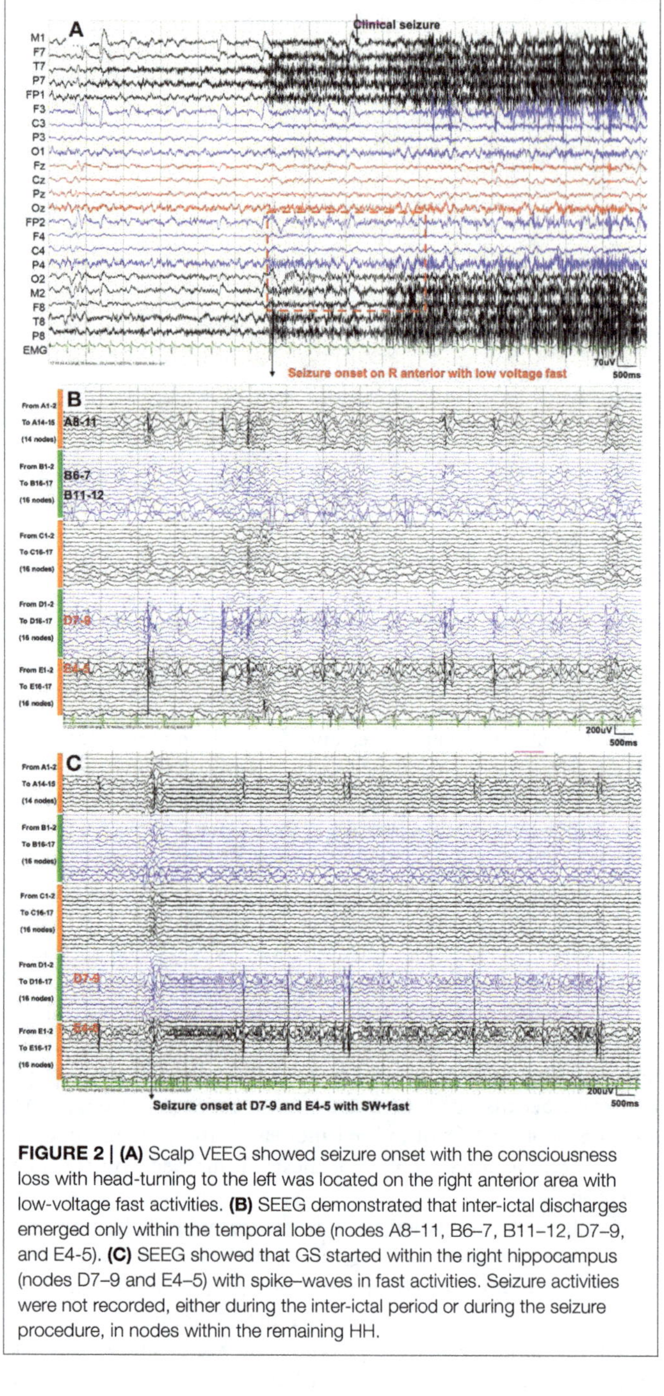

FIGURE 2 | (A) Scalp VEEG showed seizure onset with the consciousness loss with head-turning to the left was located on the right anterior area with low-voltage fast activities. **(B)** SEEG demonstrated that inter-ictal discharges emerged only within the temporal lobe (nodes A8–11, B6–7, B11–12, D7–9, and E4-5). **(C)** SEEG showed that GS started within the right hippocampus (nodes D7–9 and E4–5) with spike-waves in fast activities. Seizure activities were not recorded, either during the inter-ictal period or during the seizure procedure, in nodes within the remaining HH.

In the current case study, the cessation of the seizures, especially non-gelastic seizures after thermal coagulation of par connection and no relapse in the 2-year follow-up, strongly suggested that these seizure activities correlated with the remaining HH. Although electrophysiological examination, especially SEEG, could not directly confirm this correlation, and the SEEG directly indicated seizure onset in the right hippocampus (E4–5, D7–9) (**Figure 2C**), it might be induced by a lack of HH tissues and the insufficient sensitivity of the SEEG equipment. As previously mentioned, the seizure activities of the HHs were generated by the intrinsic pacemaker neurons (18–21). In this case, the majority of the HH was excluded. The remaining volume of the HH may not generate potentials that could be recorded. The maximum frequency of our SEEG equipment was 1,024 Hz, and it was therefore probable that high-frequency neural oscillations could not be recognized. There was also a window period for anti-epileptic drug treatment, and oxcarbazepine was added after the thermocoagulation. The medication therapy was not believed to play a dominant role, because carbamazepine was not reported to work on seizure control. Considering all these factors, there was a high probability that the patient was in the dependent stage of secondary epileptogenesis, which has seldom been reported.

In similar clinical processes, recognizing the correlation between dependent-stage secondary epileptogenesis and HH preoperatively is crucial to prevent damages from surgical interventions. Computational methods might provide perspectives beyond the manual interpretation of SEEG data.

In recent years, different computational methods have been widely applied to epilepsy clinical studies. Sinha et al. have developed a simulated resection method for neurosurgical outcome prediction based on calculating the escape time, which indicates the possibility of a normal neural population generating abnormal behavior (27). Bartolomei et al. have developed the epileptogenicity index calculation (EI) method, which considers the intensity and frequency of unit neural ensemble activity, to determine the epileptogenic zone (13) Using this method, Scholly et al. analyzed SEEG data of a HH patient (5). The method applied in this study considered the interactive influence of neural populations, which was indicated by the out-degrees of each node, and the dynamical alteration of a seizure network. This was the main strength of this approach. In our previous research (10), the accuracy of our computational method for epileptogenic zone location was 82.86%, and the detection rate was 85.29%.

The calculated results demonstrated that nodes in the hippocampus dominated either in the pre-ictal or in the early-ictal period and nodes within the HH showed prominent results in the pre-ictal at 5 min (**Figures 3C,D**). We interpreted these results as an indication of hippocampal involvement and as a functional state of the remaining HH in the seizure network. The calculated out-degrees indicated the influenced range of a single neural population. This included populations within the remaining HH that would process less out-degrees for the outputs of the HH and were fewer than those of the hippocampus. Whether this method overcame the relatively low potential induced by the exclusion of the majority of the lesion needs to be further studied. One future problem to solve is how to reduce the interference from the signal *per se*. In addition, the pre-ictal appearance of the prominent HH out-degree and dominant hippocampus out-degree could be interpreted as the hippocampus having become the main functional unit, and the HH might work as a pacemaker. A recent *in vivo* study showed that the loss of neuronal network

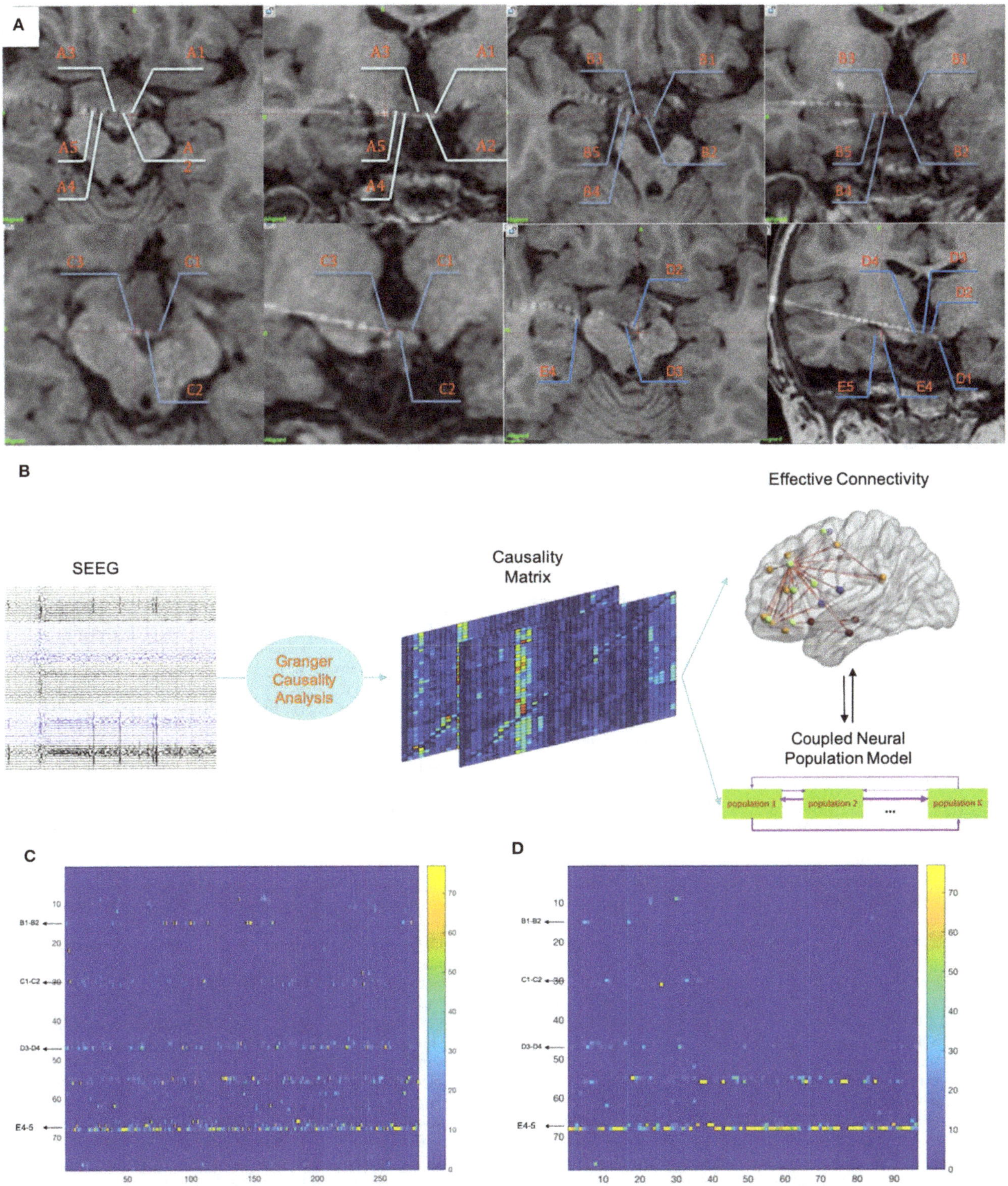

FIGURE 3 | (A) Fusion images of CT and T1 images demonstrated locations of the electrode nodes. Nodes A1–5, B1–5, C1–3, and D1–4 were located within the remaining HH. E4–5 were located in the right hippocampus that occurred during implantation. **(B)** The whole procedure of the computational method. More details have been described in a previous study (10). **(C)** The results of calculations of the 5 min SEEG data before seizure onset demonstrated that nodes within the remaining HH (nodes B1–2, C1–2, and D3–4) also contained prominent out-degrees, while nodes within the hippocampus (nodes E4–5) contained dominant out-degrees. **(D)** The results of calculations of the 90 s ictal data showed dominant out-degrees within the hippocampus (nodes E4–5). Numbers in the vertical axis correspond to nodes of the electrodes: 1:14 = A1–2:A14–15; 15:29 = B1–2:B15–16; 30:45 = C1–2:C16–17; 46:61 = D1–2:D16–17; 62:77 = E1–2:E16–17.

resilience in the inter- and pre-ictal period might precede seizures (28), which indicated the importance of inter- and pre-ictal periods. Furthermore, the nodes within the white matter were not excluded. Theoretically, electrical activities of white matter are secondary to those of the neural populations, and the involvement of the white matter does not change the results generated by the whole network.

There were some limitations to the study, which could not be resolved by the present techniques. Besides the previously mentioned signal bias, the low coverage rate of SEEGs might omit important neural populations only by non-detection, and the method still has to be explored in larger clinical studies.

In conclusion, the importance of this case was that not only the existence of the dependent stage of secondary epileptogenesis was verified, but also the ability of computational methods to reveal information that could not be manually interpreted was demonstrated. In clinical processes, secondary epileptogenesis needs to be considered, and in the future, computational methods might suggest novel diagnoses and treatment of epilepsy.

AUTHOR CONTRIBUTIONS

ZL collected the patient information, conceptualized and designed the study, performed the SEEG-guided thermocoagulation, and drafted the manuscript. CY and QW conducted the computational calculations. MW and JW performed the clinical data analyses. GL, YG, and CL conducted the electrode implantations.

ACKNOWLEDGMENTS

This work was supported by the National Natural Science Foundation of China (81790650, 81790654, and 11932003) and the Beijing Municipal Science & Technology Commission (Z161100002616016).

REFERENCES

1. Ramos CO, Latronico AC, Cukier P, Macedo DB, Bessa DS, Cunha-Silva M, et al. Long-term outcomes of patients with central precocious puberty due to hypothalamic hamartoma after GnRHa treatment: anthropometric, metabolic, and reproductive aspects. *Neuroendocrinology.* (2018) 106:203–10. doi: 10.1159/000477584
2. Striano S, Santulli L, Ianniciello M, Ferretti M, Romanelli P, Striano P. The gelastic seizures-hypothalamic hamartoma syndrome: facts, hypotheses, and perspectives. *Epilepsy Behav.* (2012) 24:7–13. doi: 10.1016/j.yebeh.2012.02.013
3. Wagner K, Wethe JV, Schulze-Bonhage A, Trippel M, Rekate H, Prigatano GP, et al. Cognition in epilepsy patients with hypothalamic hamartomas. *Epilepsia.* (2017) 58 Suppl 2:85–93. doi: 10.1111/epi.13759
4. Berkovic SF, Arzimanoglou A, Kuzniecky R, Harvey AS, Palmini A, Andermann F. Hypothalamic hamartoma and seizures: a treatable epileptic encephalopathy. *Epilepsia.* (2003) 44:969–73. doi: 10.1046/j.1528-1157.2003.59102.x
5. Scholly J, Staack AM, Kahane P, Scavarda D, Regis J, Hirsch E, et al. Hypothalamic hamartoma: epileptogenesis beyond the lesion? *Epilepsia.* (2017) 58 Suppl 2:32–40. doi: 10.1111/epi.13755
6. Marashly A, Lew S, Koop J. Successful surgical management of New Onset Refractory Status Epilepticus (NORSE) presenting with gelastic seizures in a 3 year old girl. *Epilepsy Behav Case Rep.* (2017) 8:18–26. doi: 10.1016/j.ebcr.2017.05.002
7. Scholly J, Valenti MP, Staack AM, Strobl K, Bast T, Kehrli P, et al. Hypothalamic hamartoma: is the epileptogenic zone always hypothalamic? Arguments for independent (third stage) secondary epileptogenesis. *Epilepsia.* (2013) 54 Suppl 9:123–8. doi: 10.1111/epi.12456
8. Morrell F, deToledo-Morrell L. From mirror focus to secondary epileptogenesis in man: an historical review. *Adv Neurol.* (1999) 81:11–23. doi: 10.1016/B978-012422150-5/50043-3
9. Morrell F. Secondary epileptogenesis in man. *Arch Neurol.* (1985) 42:318–35. doi: 10.1001/archneur.1985.04060040028009
10. Yang C, Luan G, Wang Q, Liu Z, Zhai F, Wang Q. Localization of epileptogenic zone with the correction of pathological networks. *Front Neurol.* (2018) 9:143. doi: 10.3389/fneur.2018.00143
11. Aupy J, Wendling F, Taylor K, Bulacio J, Gonzalez-Martinez J, Chauvel P. Cortico-striatal synchronization in human focal seizures. *Brain.* (2019) 142:1282–95. doi: 10.1093/brain/awz062
12. Schmeiser B, Wagner K, Schulze-Bonhage A, Mader I, Wendling AS, Steinhoff BJ, et al. Surgical treatment of mesiotemporal lobe epilepsy: which approach is favorable? *Neurosurgery.* (2017) 81:992–1004. doi: 10.1093/neuros/nyx138
13. Bartolomei F, Chauvel P, Wendling F. Epileptogenicity of brain structures in human temporal lobe epilepsy: a quantified study from intracerebral EEG. *Brain.* (2008) 131(Pt 7):1818–30. doi: 10.1093/brain/awn111
14. Wendling F, Bartolomei F, Bellanger JJ, Chauvel P. Epileptic fast activity can be explained by a model of impaired GABAergic dendritic inhibition. *Eur J Neurosci.* (2002) 15:1499–508. doi: 10.1046/j.1460-9568.2002.01985.x
15. Granger CWJ. Investigating causal relations by econometric models and cross-spectral methods. *Econometrica.* (1969) 37:424–38. doi: 10.2307/1912791
16. Arnold M, Milner XHR, Witte H, Bauer R, Braun C. Adaptive AR modeling of nonstationary time series by means of Kalman filtering. *IEEE Trans Biomed Eng.* (1998) 45:553–62. doi: 10.1109/10.668741
17. Goddard GV. Development of epileptic seizures through brain stimulation at low intensity. *Nature.* (1967) 214:1020–1. doi: 10.1038/2141020a0
18. Wu J, Xu L, Kim DY, Rho JM, St John PA, Lue LF, et al. Electrophysiological properties of human hypothalamic hamartomas. *Ann Neurol.* (2005) 58:371–82. doi: 10.1002/ana.20580
19. Fenoglio KA, Wu J, Kim DY, Simeone TA, Coons SW, Rekate H, et al. Hypothalamic hamartoma: basic mechanisms of intrinsic epileptogenesis. *Semin Pediatr Neurol.* (2007) 14:51–9. doi: 10.1016/j.spen.2007.03.002
20. Wu J, Gao M, Shen JX, Qiu SF, Kerrigan JF. Mechanisms of intrinsic epileptogenesis in human gelastic seizures with hypothalamic hamartoma. *CNS Neurosci Ther.* (2015) 21:104–11. doi: 10.1111/cns.12348
21. Kerrigan JF, Parsons A, Tsang C, Simeone K, Coons S, Wu J. Hypothalamic hamartoma: neuropathology and epileptogenesis. *Epilepsia.* (2017) 58 Suppl 2:22–31. doi: 10.1111/epi.13752
22. Leal AJ, Moreira A, Robalo C, Ribeiro C. Different electroclinical manifestations of the epilepsy associated with hamartomas connecting to the middle or posterior hypothalamus. *Epilepsia.* (2003) 44:1191–5. doi: 10.1046/j.1528-1157.2003.66902.x
23. Kahane P, Ryvlin P, Hoffmann D, Minotti L, Benabid AL. From hypothalamic hamartoma to cortex: what can be learnt from depth recordings and stimulation? *Epileptic Disord.* (2003) 5:205–17.
24. Parvizi J, Le S, Foster BL, Bourgeois B, Riviello JJ, Prenger E, et al. Gelastic epilepsy and hypothalamic hamartomas: neuroanatomical analysis of brain lesions in 100 patients. *Brain.* (2011) 134(Pt 10):2960–8. doi: 10.1093/brain/awr235
25. Kovac S, Diehl B, Wehner T, Fois C, Toms N, Walker MC, et al. Gelastic seizures: incidence, clinical and EEG features in adult patients undergoing video-EEG telemetry. *Epilepsia.* (2015) 56:e1–5. doi: 10.1111/epi.12868
26. Valentin A, Lazaro M, Mullatti N, Cervantes S, Malik I, Selway RP, et al. Cingulate epileptogenesis in hypothalamic hamartoma. *Epilepsia.* (2011) 52:e35–9. doi: 10.1111/j.1528-1167.2011.03060.x
27. Sinha N, Dauwels J, Kaiser M, Cash SS, Brandon Westover M, Wang Y, et al. Predicting neurosurgical outcomes in focal epilepsy patients using computational modelling. *Brain.* (2017) 140:319–32. doi: 10.1093/brain/aww299
28. Chang WC, Kudlacek J, Hlinka J, Chvojka J, Hadrava M, Kumpost V, et al. Loss of neuronal network resilience precedes seizures and determines the ictogenic nature of interictal synaptic perturbations. *Nat Neurosci.* (2018) 21:1742–52. doi: 10.1038/s41593-018-0278-y

6

Robot Assisted MRI-Guided LITT of the Anterior, Lateral and Medial Temporal Lobe for Temporal Lobe Epilepsy

Kunal Gupta[1,2]*, Adam S. Dickey*[3]*, Ranliang Hu*[4]*, Edward Faught*[3] *and Jon T. Willie*[1,5*]

[1] Department of Neurosurgery, Emory University Hospital, Atlanta, GA, United States, [2] Department of Neurosurgery, Indiana University Health, Indianapolis, IN, United States, [3] Department of Neurology, Emory University Hospital, Atlanta, GA, United States, [4] Department of Radiology, Emory University Hospital, Atlanta, GA, United States, [5] Department of Neurological Surgery, Washington University School of Medicine, Washington, DC, United States

***Correspondence:**
Jon T. Willie
jontwillie@wustl.edu

Robotic systems have fundamentally altered the landscape of functional neurosurgery. These allow automated stereotaxy with high accuracy and reliability, and are rapidly becoming a mainstay in stereotactic surgeries such as deep brain stimulation (DBS), stereoelectroencephalography (SEEG), and stereotactic laser ablation/MRI guided laser interstitial thermal therapy (MRgLITT). Robotic systems have been effectively applied to create a minimally invasive approach for diagnostics and therapeutics in the treatment of epilepsy, utilizing robots for expeditious and accurate stereotaxy for SEEG and MRgLITT. MRgLITT has been shown to approach open surgical techniques in efficacy of seizure control while minimizing collateral injury. We describe the use of robot assisted MRgLITT for a minimally invasive laser anterior temporal lobotomy, describing the approach and potential pitfalls. Goals of MRgLITT are complete ablation of the epileptogenic zone and avoiding injury to uninvolved structures. In the middle fossa these include structures such as cranial nerves in the skull base and cavernous sinus and the thalamus. These can be mitigated with careful trajectory planning and control of laser ablation intensity.

Keywords: temporal lobe epilepsy, LITT (laser interstitial thermal therapy), ROSA (robotized stereotactic assistant), temporal lobectomy, SEEG (stereoelectroencephalography)

INTRODUCTION

Advancements in robotic and laser technology have dramatically altered the landscape of functional neurosurgery. The principal application of robotics in functional neurosurgery has been automated stereotaxy, providing a potentially expeditious workflow for cases involving multiple sequential and unrelated trajectories, as exemplified by stereoelectroencephalography (SEEG). A number of robotic stereotactic devices are currently available in North America, including the Neuromate robotic system (Renishaw), ROSA ONE Brain robotic platform (Zimmer Biomet), and Stealth Autoguide cranial robotic guidance platform (Medtronic). Robots are rapidly becoming a mainstay in surgical stereotaxy and studies have demonstrated that the accuracy of robotic guidance systems can approach that of gold-standard stereotactic frames (1–4).

Likewise, the modern surgical application of laser technology combines a number of advancements, narrow-caliber cooled-fibers for laser interstitial thermal therapy and magnetic resonance thermography for non-invasive real-time imaging of tissue temperature, into a minimally invasive therapeutic strategy. Two commercial platforms utilizing this technology are currently available for central nervous system application in North America, NeuroBlate (Monteris) and Visualase (Medtronic). Robotic stereotaxy and laser technology can be combined as a minimally invasive therapy, providing surgeons a method to ablate tissue across a number of subspecialties including epilepsy and neuro-oncology.

Laser ablation of the temporal lobe is especially challenging due to its complex shape and volume. MRgLITT has been successfully applied to ablation of the mesial temporal lobe for laser amygdalohippocampotomy, with up to 53% freedom from focal seizures impairing awareness reported after 12 months (5, 6), with variable outcomes likely resulting from important differences in patient selection and technical execution. In particular, temporal lobe epileptogenic zones may extend outside the entorhinal cortex, amygdala, and hippocampus. However, previous case series of MRgLITT for temporal lobe epilepsy describe approaches intended to deliver a minimally invasive analog to an open selective amygdalohippocampectomy. In cases where a wider epileptogenic zone is identified by SEEG or other approaches, a more extensive resection or ablation may be indicated. Complete laser ablation of the mesial, anterior and lateral structures requires a combination of multiple lateral and posterior approaches, which could be difficult to achieve expeditiously with a stereotactic frame set up in a single configuration. Advances in robotic stereotactic targeting allows the placement of multiple LITT bolts and laser cannulae expeditiously and accurately, with potentially fewer restrictions upon available trajectories (7, 8). Here, we present the use of robotic assisted MRgLITT for ablation of the anterior temporal lobe using multiple stereotactic trajectories to create a temporal lobe ablation volume analogous to open anterior temporal lobotomy.

CASE REPORT

A 32-year-old right handed female presented with a 2-year history of medically refractory right temporal lobe epilepsy. Her seizures comprised 2 semiologies; the first consisted of focal seizures with déjà vu, out of body sensation and dream-like state, shortness of breath, nausea, diaphoresis, and bilateral hand paresthesia. These sometimes progress to behavioral arrest and loss of awareness. She reported post-ictal tiredness, fear and confusion. These initially occurred 2–20 times per day, however the frequency reduced to 1–3 times per month with lacosamide treatment, and followed a catamenial pattern. Her second seizure semiology consisted of generalized tonic seizures, characterized by arm extension and stiffening, lasting a few minutes, with 2 h of post-ictal confusion. These were infrequent, having occurred twice since the onset of her seizures. She has an existing diagnosis of depression and took citalopram for this. She denied specific risk factors, precipitating events, or other psychiatric comorbidities. She reported, however, that she was hospitalized with fever of unknown origin at age 19-years-old and again at 20-years-old (10–11 years prior to seizure onset). Her other medical history was unremarkable and she had not had prior epilepsy surgery or evaluation. She had failed trials of levetiracetam, oxcarbazepine, and lamotrigine. Cerebrospinal fluid and blood serology were negative for auto-antibodies. She was neurologically non-focal on examination.

Long-term video scalp electroencephalography (LTvEEG) captured 10 events. Two events were characterized by whole body tremors and pelvic thrusting without electrographic correlate (and were deemed non-epileptic events). For two events she reported a dreamlike state that often occurred prior to her seizures, however these had no electrographic change. Six typical events were captured, during which she described her typical semiology of a rushing feeling, bilateral hand paresthesia and nausea; she did not exhibit behavioral arrest. During these typical events, right frontal temporal polymorphic delta and theta activity were noted, maximal in F8/T2. She underwent neuropsychological testing, which demonstrated average to above average function with mild dysfunction in both verbal and non-verbal domains. While there was a slight split favoring non-verbal performance, other areas conflicted this, including better visual naming vs. auditory naming. Therefore, her neuropsychological testing was felt to be non-lateralizing.

Her brain MRI showed no structural abnormalities (**Figures 1A,B**). Volumetric quantification of her hippocampi (NeuroQuant) demonstrated that her combined hippocampal volume was in the 95th percentile (9.41cc). Functional MRI demonstrated bilateral language lateralization (left > right Broca's area representation, left Wernicke's area, and right supplementary motor area activation) as well as bilateral parahippocampal gyrus activation with memory tasks. Positron emission tomography (PET) was performed; an area in the right Rolandic operculum demonstrated hypometabolism ($z = -2.78$) however this was felt to be discordant with her semiology and therefore of low clinical relevance during epilepsy multi-disciplinary team discussion. Ictal single-photon emission computerized tomography (SPECT) was attempted but injection of isotope was unable to be timed appropriately with a seizure. Results were therefore reported as interictal SPECT, which showed an area of hypometabolism in right inferior temporal lobe. Magnetoencephalography (MEG) demonstrated a single interictal spike in right medial basal temporal lobe. Her case was discussed in an epilepsy multi-disciplinary team meeting; given her semiology and LTvEEG findings it was reasoned that the most likely location for seizure onset was her right mesial temporal lobe. As she did not have mesial temporal sclerosis (and therefore did not meet criteria to skip invasive monitoring), it was recommended that she undergo stereoelectroencephalography (SEEG). Given mixed language dominance and potentially discordant neuropsychological memory results, she also underwent Wada testing, which unambiguously confirmed left sided support of memory and language.

Stereoelectroencephalography (SEEG) was performed targeting the right temporal lobe and related networks. Sampled locations included mesial structures (entorhinal cortex, parahippocampal gyrus, amygdala, hippocampus), basal structures (fusiform gyrus), lateral structures (superior,

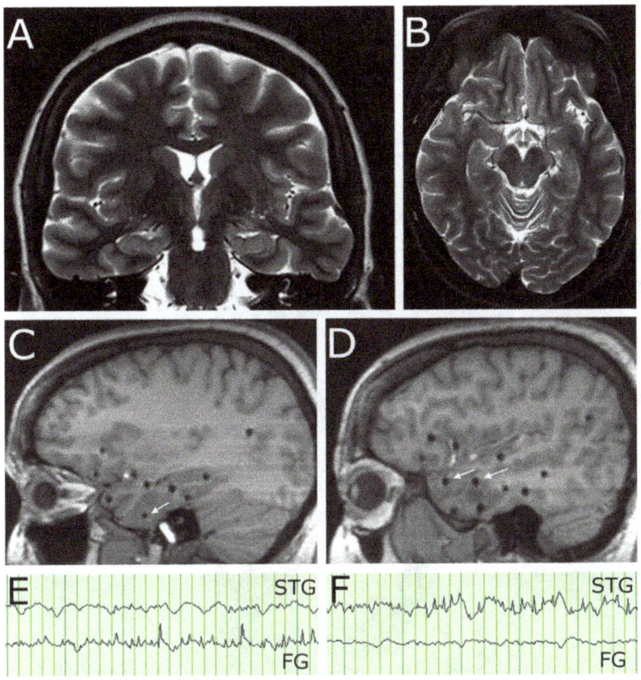

FIGURE 1 | Pre-operative imaging demonstrates no abnormality on MRI and location of SEEG electrode contacts involved in the seizure network. **(A)** Coronal T2 MRI and **(B)** axial T2 MRI show normal appearance of the temporal lobes bilaterally. **(C)** Sagittal T1 MRI at the level of the mesial temporal lobe. White arrow indicates SEEG electrode contact in the fusiform gyrus with spread pattern electrographic activity during a captured seizure. **(D)** Sagittal T1 MRI at level of the lateral temporal neocortex. White arrows indicate SEEG electrode contacts in the superior temporal gyrus (anterior arrow) and middle temporal gyrus (posterior arrow) involved in spread patterns during subclinical seizures. **(E)** A clinical seizure (characterized by behavioral arrest and oral automatism) had EEG onset with rhythmic theta spiking, maximal on a contact in fusiform gyrus (FG) near the basal temporal pole, which evolved in frequency and morphology and then spread to other contacts in the neocortex of the superior, middle, and inferior temporal gyrus. Note that at onset of this clinical seizure, a contact in the superior temporal gyrus (STG) was not involved. **(F)** A subclinical seizure recorded on the same day had an onset of rhythmic theta spiking, maximal on a contact in the superior temporal gyrus (STG) which evolved in frequency and morphology and also spread to other contacts in the neocortex of the superior, middle, and inferior temporal gyrus. Note that at the onset of this subclinical seizures a contact in the fusiform gyrus (FG) implicated as the clinical seizure onset was not involved.

middle, and inferior temporal gyrus), and limbic lobe associated structures (insula, frontal and temporal opercula, orbitofrontal cortex, retrosplenial cingulate cortex). Twelve electrode arrays were placed in total, utilizing robotic assisted stereotaxy (ROSA robot), and the patient was monitored for 4-weeks. She had one typical clinical seizure (characterized by behavioral arrest and oral automatism noticed by patient's spouse) which was first detected in the contacts located in the fusiform gyrus (**Figures 1C,E**) with spread to the superior, middle, and inferior temporal gyrus. She also had subclinical seizures with a similar onset, as well as two independent seizure onset zones in the lateral superior temporal gyrus or the lateral inferior temporal gyrus (**Figures 1D,F**). In each of these three locations, however, low voltage fast activity was not detected, suggesting that the true epileptogenic zone had not been captured. Given the widespread and multi-focal right temporal involvement for the electrographic seizures, it was determined that the patient would benefit from anterior temporal lobectomy. Options of surgical therapy by conventional open anterior lobectomy vs. MRI-guided laser interstitial thermal therapy (MRgLITT) were presented, and she ultimately expressed a preference for a minimally invasive approach.

MRgLITT was performed utilizing the ROSA stereotactic robot, at 6 trajectories encompassing the right temporal lobe. The patient's head was secured within a stereotactic frame base ring (CRW, Integra) and then affixed to the ROSA robot. Stereotactic registration was performed and the robotic articulated arm was navigated to each trajectory. In each location a twist-drill hole was made and laser bolts (Visualase, Medtronic) were placed. Once the bolts had been placed, alignment stylets were inserted to target (**Figure 2A**) and an O-arm (Medtronic) 3-dimensional image was obtained to ensure that the trajectories were accurate (**Figure 2B**). The distance to target from the top of each bolt was recorded for laser fiber insertion. The alignment stylets were removed and the bolts and surrounding scalp were covered with a sterile impermeable adhesive barrier (Ioban) (**Figure 2C**). The patient was transferred to the interventional MRI suite, positioned supine on the MRI table with the right shoulder bumped and the head turned laterally. A head coil was positioned to allow access to all the bolts and the adhesive barrier was prepped with betadine (**Figure 2D**). The area was then draped with sterile towels (**Figure 2E**) and the Ioban was removed for each trajectory, exposing the underlying sterile field. For each trajectory, and the laser fiber was inserted to the appropriate depth (**Figure 2F**), using the distance from the bolt to the target that had been recorded earlier.

A 980 nm/15 w diode laser (Visualase, Medtronic) was used to ablate all six trajectories, with the intention of confluent ablation of the medial temporal structures (extending posteriorly to the landmark of the lateral mesencephalic sulcus), as well as temporal pole, basal temporal lobe, and lateral temporal lobe extending 5 cm from the temporal tip. **Figure 3** demonstrates orthogonal images for each laser fiber and the resultant Visualase ablation volumes for each trajectory. Two trajectories began in the parietal-occipital region to cannulate the long axes of the hippocampus/uncus (**Figures 3A,B**) and the rhinal cortices and medial temporal pole (**Figures 3C,D**), two oblique lateral trajectories began in the posterolateral temporal region and terminated in the superior (**Figures 3E,F**) and inferior (**Figures 3G,H**) lateral temporal pole, and two lateral trajectories completed the lateral neocortical ablation at the level of the uncus (**Figures 3I,J**) and the hippocampal body (**Figures 3K,L**). A final volumetric MRI confirmed the extent of the ablation (**Figure 4B**), and demonstrates the complete ablation of the targeted structures. The final ablation volume was 49.9 cm^3 [itksnap.org (9)]. At the end of the case, the bolts were removed and a single interrupted suture was placed at each bolt site (**Figure 2G**).

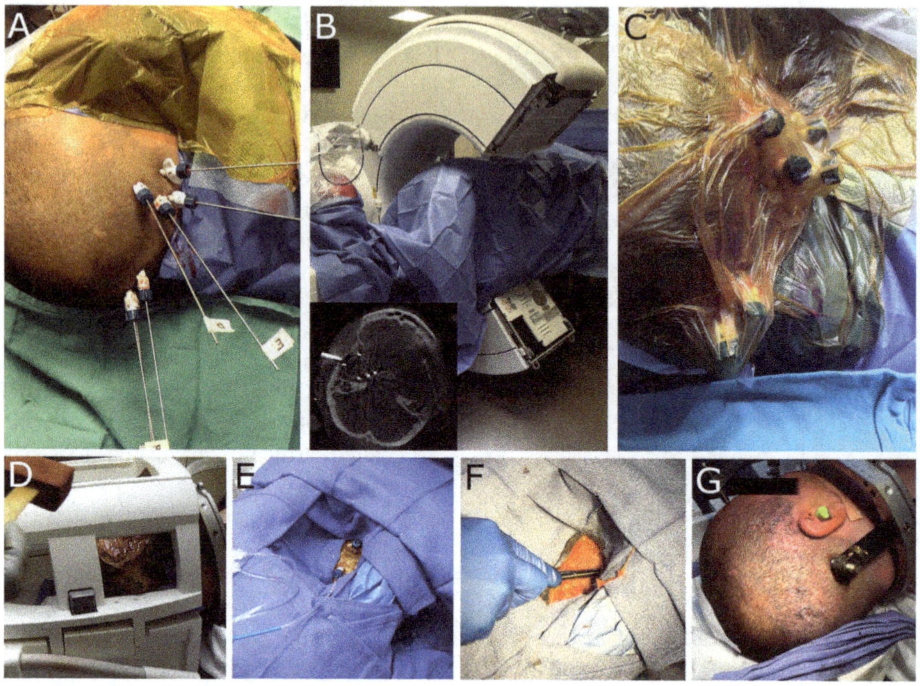

FIGURE 2 | Intra-operative images demonstrating robotic workflow for implantation of laser bolts and subsequent MRgLITT in an interventional MRI suite. **(A)** Visualase bolts have been implanted and alignment stylets have been passed to target. **(B)** The patient is draped and the O-arm (Medtronic) is used to visualize each trajectory; inset demonstrates representative axial image and alignment stylets. **(C)** A sterile adhesive barrier (Ioban) is placed over the bolts prior to patient transfer to iMRI. **(D)** The head coil is placed and the area prepped with betadine. **(E)** Sterile towels are used to drape the head coil and allow access to the laser bolts; laser fibers are inserted through each bolt for laser ablation. **(F)** At the end of the case the bolts are removed and a single suture placed at each insertion site. **(G)** The end cosmetic result from multiple small incisions. Minimal hair removal is possible, however, in this case the patient shaved her own head prior to surgery.

Total anesthesia time was 9.8 h, and total operative time was 8.85 h.

Immediately after surgery the patient had no gross neurological deficits. By post-operative day 1, however, she was noted to have the onset of right facial weakness. This gradually progressed by post-operative day 3 to an inability to close her right eye (House Brackman grade 4). Direct thermal injury during the ablation was considered unlikely to have occurred as the laser fiber was intentionally placed 8 mm away from the middle fossa skull base, and deficit took time to develop. She underwent repeat CT that demonstrated stable post-ablation changes (**Figure 4A**). She remained admitted for 3 days to ensure that radiographic imaging and clinical symptoms were stable prior to discharge. She was advised to tape the right eye closed to prevent exposure keratopathy. She was evaluated by ophthalmology as an out-patient: a left superior quadrantanopsia was noted on formal Goldman visual field testing; 3rd, 4th and 6th cranial nerves were functioning normally; and she was advised on continued eye-care to prevent exposure keratopathy. She and her husband reported cluster of 11 focal impaired-awareness seizures immediately after discharge however no further seizures by 6-weeks after surgery. At 6-weeks post-op she was noted to have worsening hemifacial weakness (now House Brackman grade 5). A brain MRI was obtained as an out-patient to evaluate her ablation (**Figure 4C**) and determine an etiology for her symptoms. Immediately after surgery there was evidence of mild enhancement of the distal canalicular, labyrinthine, geniculate and tympanic segments of the facial nerve (**Figure 5B**) compared to pre-operative imaging (**Figure 5A**). At 3-month follow-up there was intense perineural enhancement of the greater-superficial petrosal nerve, geniculate ganglion and tympanic segment of facial nerve (**Figure 5C**).

At 6-months after surgery, her hemifacial weakness had improved considerably to House Brackman grade 2, not visible at rest and she was able to close her right eye completely, and some residual reduced acuity of hearing with the right ear. She reported subjective headaches and insomnia but she did not find these symptoms bothersome enough to warrant further investigation. Her husband also reported multiple episodes of brief staring and unresponsiveness, and the patient denied recollection of these events, and given history of non-epileptic events, the episodes remained unconfirmed. These events occurred several times per week, without conversion to generalized seizure. Given the history of non-epileptic events, these episodes could not be discriminated from possible focal impaired awareness seizures, and lacosamide dosing was increased by her treating neurologist.

At 12-months after surgery, she reported complete resolution of her hemifacial weakness, however she acknowledged subjectively reduced acuity of right-sided hearing. She was

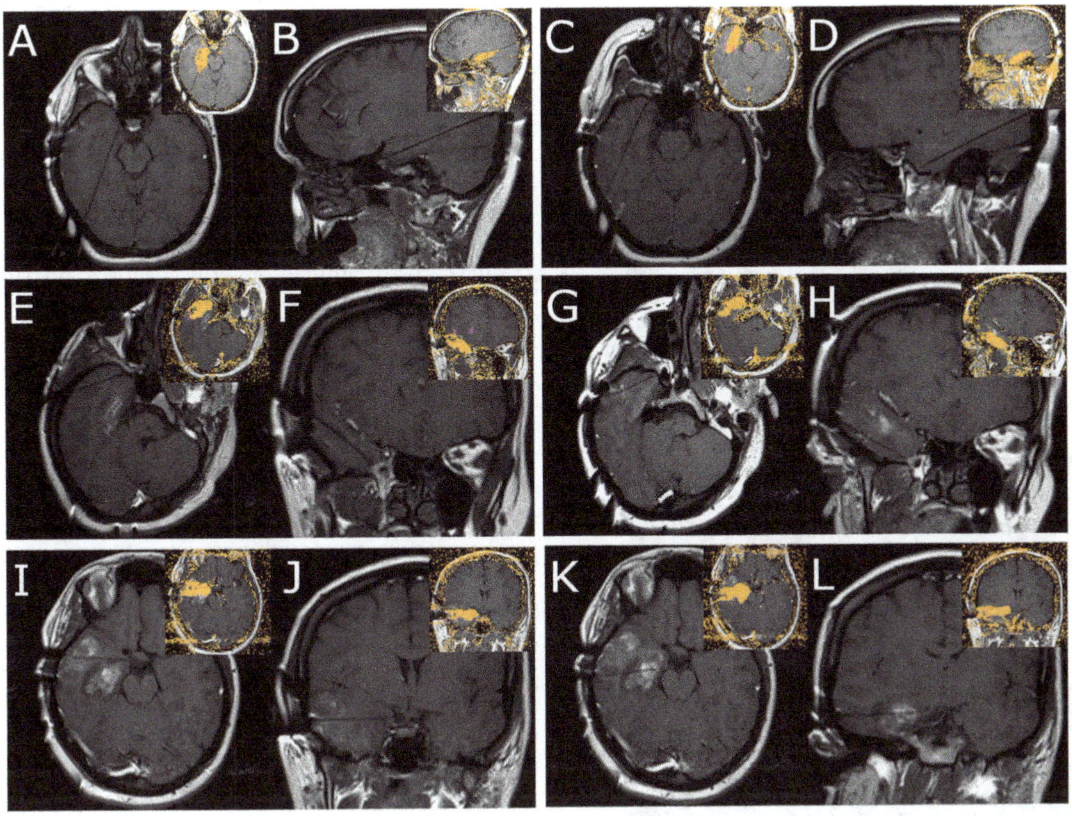

FIGURE 3 | Panel demonstrates MRI images obtained during MRgLITT ablation of the right temporal lobe. Each panel demonstrates two orthogonal views along the laser fiber; inset images demonstrate the resultant ablation volume as determined by the Visualase system for each trajectory (Medtronic). **(A,B)** Panel demonstrates mesial hippocampal laser fiber trajectory. **(C,D)** Panel demonstrates medial temporal pole laser fiber trajectory. **(E,F)** Panel demonstrates superior lateral temporal pole laser fiber trajectory. **(G,H)** Panel demonstrates inferior lateral temporal pole laser fiber trajectory. **(I,J)** Panel demonstrates lateral approach to uncus laser fiber trajectory. **(K,L)** Panel demonstrates lateral approach to hippocampal body laser fiber trajectory.

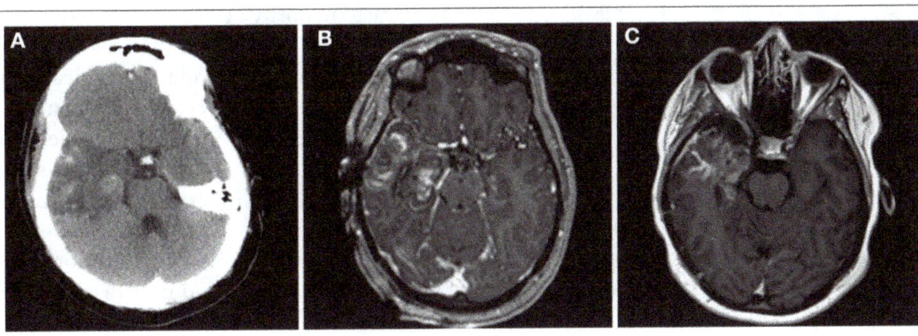

FIGURE 4 | Panel demonstrates intra-operative and peri-operative patient imaging. **(A)** Axial CT obtained on post-operative day 2 demonstrates cerebral edema at the ablation site. **(B)** Post-ablation contrast-enhanced T1 axial MRI that demonstrates ablation of temporal lobe from the temporal pole to the level of the lateral mesencephalic sulcus and collicular plate at the time of surgery. **(C)** Contrast-enhanced (fluid dark) T1 axial MRI demonstrates the ablation 3 months after surgery.

referred to otorhinolaryngology, but chose not to pursue this. She denied new memory complaints and did not submit to post-operative neuropsychological assessment. Notably, follow up history and physical examinations did not detect visual defects or complaints, although we did not pursue formal ophthalmological evaluations. She and her husband denied any further episodes of impaired awareness since the increase in lacosamide dosing and no generalized seizures since surgery.

DISCUSSION

Robot-assisted MRI-guided laser interstitial thermal therapy provides a novel tool in the neurosurgeon's armamentarium

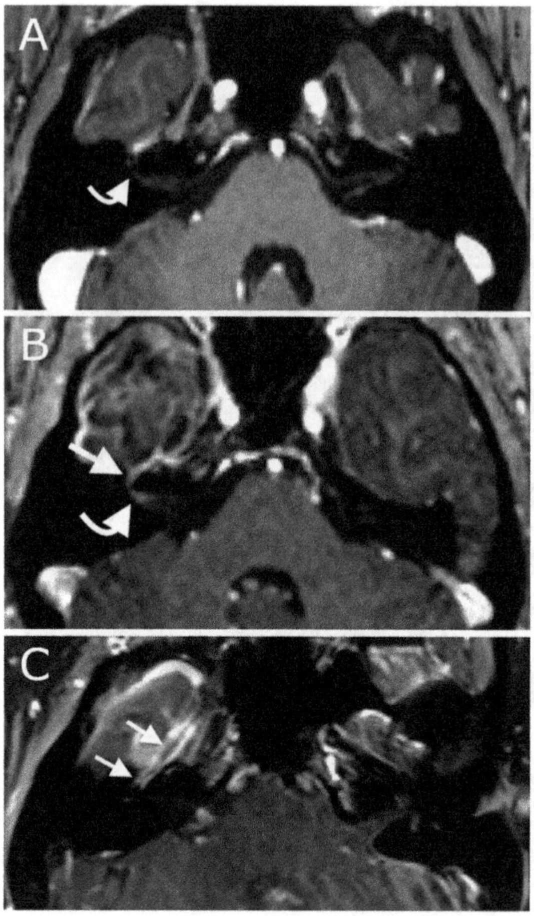

FIGURE 5 | Panel demonstrates MRI scans of the internal acoustic meatus and facial nerve ipsilateral to the ablation. **(A)** Axial contrast-enhanced T1 pre-operative MRI demonstrates normal appearance of the facial nerve without abnormal enhancement. **(B)** Axial contrast-enhanced T1 intra-operative MRI demonstrates mild enhancement of the distal canalicular, labyrinthine and geniculate segments of the facial nerve at the time of surgery. **(C)** Coronal contrast-enhanced T1 MRI demonstrates intense enhancement of the facial nerve 3-months after surgery.

for the treatment of epilepsy (and other subspecialties such as neuro-oncology and movement disorders). In particular, the surgical techniques that we describe combine novel robotic stereotaxy with laser technology to provide a minimally invasive approach for laser temporal lobotomy. A surgical strategy that utilizes robot-assisted stereoencephalography (SEEG) and MRgLITT is particularly powerful as it combines minimally invasive intracranial diagnostics with minimally invasive therapy. LITT ablation of the mesial temporal lobe has now been reported from multiple epilepsy surgery centers in North America, and such ablations have often utilized robotic and SEEG techniques (6). Nonetheless, a similarly large experience describing the potential indications, outcomes, and adversities of temporal lobe ablations that are large, complex, atypical, and/or extra-mesial remains to be established. This report stands out as an illustration of bringing multiple technologies to bear on a particularly atypical case and raises issues needing to be addressed in larger future series.

For patients diagnosed with MTLE, larger temporal lobe resections are associated with a greater chance of seizure freedom, presumably by eliminating occult epileptogenic tissues. The highly selective laser technique that is typically reported targets the amygdala, hippocampus, subiculum, and part of the entorhinal cortex. By contrast, open anterior temporal lobectomy generally also includes resection of the temporal pole, all of the rhinal cortices within the anterior fusiform and parahippocampal gyri, as well as anterior portions of the lateral temporal lobe, all of which may harbor occult epileptogenic tissues. Middle ground is represented by open "selective" amygdalohippocampectomy techniques which typically include much of the rhinal cortices. Thus, it comes as no surprise that despite efforts to select patients ideal for each of these procedures, overall seizure freedom rates have been reported as ~68–78% achieved by anterior temporal lobectomy in lesional cases (10, 11) vs. ~64% achieved by open selective amygdalohippocampectomy (12) vs. 53% seizure freedom with SLAH (5, 6). Complication rates attributed to open temporal lobectomy are also reduced with SLAH, including reduced incidence of visual field deficits (13, 14) and reduced neuropsychological deficits in naming and object recognition (15), as well as reduced hospitalization times and an improved patient experience. Nevertheless, the uniqueness of the case we report herein precludes any direct comparison to more extensive published results regarding open anterior temporal lobectomy or SLAH.

Improved patient experience with MRgLITT may also expand access to epilepsy surgery for patients fearful of open surgery. When patients are asked their opinions about epilepsy surgery beforehand, a majority (74%) expressed "anxiety of the unknown" prior to surgery, even though after surgery the vast majority (94%) reported surgery increased their independence and only a minority (19%) complained of wide-ranging psychological and neurological long-term adverse effects such as fatigue, memory, and concentration impairment (16). These anxieties don't necessarily reflect the complication rates attributable to open surgery; in the seminal study by Wiebe et al. 10% (4/40) incurred an unexpected adverse event (1 thalamic infarct causing sensory changes, 1 wound infection, and 2 declines in verbal memory interfering with occupation) and 55% (22/40) had expected non-disabling visual quadrantanopsia (17). Nevertheless, in our experience, a non-trivial fraction of patients will refuse a standard open anterior temporal lobectomy but will consider the less invasive laser ablation, even if the volume of tissue targeted for destruction is the same.

We have previously described outcomes of LITT to target lesion boundaries and networks explored by SEEG (18). In our case example, we used robotic MRgLITT to achieve an ablation comparable to anterior temporal lobectomy. An extensive treatment area was recommended based upon SEEG results which generally suggested multifocal mesial-lateral temporal lobe epilepsy. Failure to identify a particular region of rhythmic spiking and/or low voltage fast activity precluded the use of LITT to target only a small area (e.g., mesial temporal) for ablation and puts our patient at greater risk of not achieving or maintaining seizure freedom (19). Thus, our team offered extensive right temporal lobectomy, but the patient expressed an interest in avoiding a typical surgical incision and a likely visual field defect. She likewise expressed understanding that despite potential feasibility, ablation might not achieve as predictable an outcome as open surgery. The complex shape of the temporal lobe and mesial temporal structures in particular must be considered due to the limitations imposed by linear stereotactic trajectories. The curvature of the hippocampus and uncus limits the anterior medial extent of the ablation and a more lateral entry must be utilized to place the laser fiber in the uncus (20). Due to the medial curvature of the posterior hippocampal formation at the region of the lateral mesencephalic sulcus, however, the posterior body of the hippocampus could be missed. For this reason, we used two occipital trajectories to ablate the parahippocampal gyrus and rhinal cortices, the amygdala and uncus, and the head and body of the hippocampus. The remaining planum polare and inferior temporal pole and lateral temporal neocortex (including the superior temporal sulcus) were ablated using four lateral trajectories. Additional lateral trajectories were included in this particular case to assure a confluent ablation of the lateral temporal cortices, because the SEEG results implicated a widespread medial-lateral temporal epileptogenic zone. Fewer trajectories might be required to target the combination of the temporopolar and medial temporal structures alone. The combination of posterior and lateral approach trajectories is easily accommodated within a robotic workflow.

For trajectory planning, deliberate considerations must be made to (i) target the appropriate tissue for ablation and (ii) avoid key structures to minimize the risk of complications from off-target injury. In particular for the mesial temporal lobe, cranial nerves within the cavernous sinus, along the tentorium, and within the skull base are vulnerable to thermal injury, as well as the optic tracts and lateral geniculate nucleus (LGN) of the thalamus which overly the body of the hippocampus. This patient did incur an ipsilateral facial nerve injury, which resolved with conservative management by 6-months after surgery. Proximity to the skull base was considered during surgical planning, and the trajectory in this location was planned 8 mm away from the skull base to account for the expected diameter of the ablation. As the patient seemed to have no facial nerve palsy immediately after surgery but developed hemifacial weakness progressively over the first 3 days after surgery, this suggests that direct thermal injury during the ablation was not the cause. Given prior reports of prolonged blood brain barrier disruption following laser ablation including a published case of delayed optic neuritis (21), it is possible that thermal ablation may rarely precipitate autoimmune central nervous system inflammatory conditions, as in this case resembling typical Bell's palsy. Supporting this hypothesis, the facial nerve itself showed minimal changes on immediate post-operative imaging, and was found to avidly contrast-enhance on imaging obtained 3-months after surgery. Despite our attention to the location and course of the facial nerve in the skull base when ablating the basal temporal lobe, the observed nerve injury testifies to the sensitivity of this nerve to direct thermal and/or indirect inflammatory injury. We urge even greater respect for proximity to this nerve with regard to laser trajectory proximity and relative power settings. Inherent constraints of gradient echo-weighted imaging-based thermometry near bone remain a limitation of commercially available MRgLITT systems and highlight a need for further technological developments.

CONCLUSION

We described the application of robotic stereotaxy and MR-guided laser interstitial thermal therapy in a combined minimally invasive surgical workflow for anterior temporal lobotomy. Robot guided MRgLITT provides a number of benefits, including those associated with minimally invasive techniques such as smaller incisions and reduced length of stay, with comparable surgical efficacy. Complications remain possible with minimally invasive techniques, and must be considered and mitigated with prior knowledge and experience. Minimally invasive techniques such as MRgLITT will not entirely replace open surgical techniques, however complement existing treatments and offer alternate therapeutic strategies in selected patients. MRgLITT may also expand access to epilepsy surgery for patients who refuse open surgery.

AUTHOR CONTRIBUTIONS

KG and JW conceptualized the manuscript. KG, AD, and JW wrote the manuscript. RH and EF provided data. All authors approved the final manuscript.

REFERENCES

1. Bradac O, Steklacova A, Nebrenska K, Vrana J, De Lacy P, Benes V. Accuracy of varioguide frameless stereotactic system against frame-based stereotaxy: prospective, randomized, single-center study. *World Neurosurg.* (2017) 104:831–40. doi: 10.1016/j.wneu.2017.04.104
2. Vakharia VN, Sparks R, O'keeffe AG, Rodionov R, Miserocchi A, Mcevoy A, et al. Accuracy of intracranial electrode placement for stereoencephalography: a systematic review and meta-analysis. *Epilepsia.* (2017) 58:921–32. doi: 10.1111/epi.13713
3. Neudorfer C, Hunsche S, Hellmich M, El Majdoub F, Maarouf M. Comparative study of robot-assisted versus conventional frame-based deep brain stimulation stereotactic neurosurgery. *Stereotact Funct Neurosurg.* (2018) 96:327–34. doi: 10.1159/000494736
4. Mirzadeh Z, Chen T, Chapple KM, Lambert M, Karis JP, Dhall R, et al. Procedural variables influencing stereotactic accuracy and efficiency in deep brain stimulation surgery. *Oper Neurosurg.* (2019) 17:70–8. doi: 10.1093/ons/opy291
5. Gross RE, Stern MA, Willie JT, Fasano RE, Saindane AM, Soares BP, et al. Stereotactic laser amygdalohippocampotomy for mesial temporal lobe epilepsy. *Ann Neurol.* (2018) 83:575–87. doi: 10.1002/ana.25180
6. Wu C, Jermakowicz WJ, Chakravorti S, Cajigas I, Sharan AD, Jagid JR, et al. Effects of surgical targeting in laser interstitial thermal therapy for mesial temporal lobe epilepsy: a multicenter study of 234 patients. *Epilepsia.* (2019) 60:1171–83. doi: 10.1111/epi.15565
7. Chan AY, Tran DK, Gill AS, Hsu FP, Vadera S. Stereotactic robot-assisted MRI-guided laser thermal ablation of radiation necrosis in the posterior cranial fossa: technical note. *Neurosurg Focus.* (2016) 41:E5. doi: 10.3171/2016.4.FOCUS1622

8. Miller BA, Salehi A, Limbrick DD Jr, Smyth MD. Applications of a robotic stereotactic arm for pediatric epilepsy and neurooncology surgery. *J Neurosurg Pediatr.* (2017) 20:364–70. doi: 10.3171/2017.5.PEDS1782
9. Yushkevich PA, Piven J, Hazlett HC, Smith RG, Ho S, Gee JC, et al. User-guided 3D active contour segmentation of anatomical structures: significantly improved efficiency and reliability. *Neuroimage.* (2006) 31:1116–28. doi: 10.1016/j.neuroimage.2006.01.015
10. Mcintosh AM, Kalnins RM, Mitchell LA, Fabinyi GC, Briellmann RS, Berkovic SF. Temporal lobectomy: long-term seizure outcome, late recurrence and risks for seizure recurrence. *Brain.* (2004) 127:2018–30. doi: 10.1093/brain/awh221
11. Josephson CB, Dykeman J, Fiest KM, Liu X, Sadler RM, Jette N, et al. Systematic review and meta-analysis of standard vs selective temporal lobe epilepsy surgery. *Neurology.* (2013) 80:1669–76. doi: 10.1212/WNL.0b013e3182904f82
12. Tanriverdi T, Olivier A, Poulin N, Andermann F, Dubeau F. Long-term seizure outcome after mesial temporal lobe epilepsy surgery: corticalamygdalohippocampectomy versus selective amygdalohippocampectomy. *J Neurosurg.* (2008) 108:517–24. doi: 10.3171/JNS/2008/108/3/0517
13. Jermakowicz WJ, Wu C, Neal E, Cajigas I, D'haese PF, Donahue DJ, et al. Clinically significant visual deficits after laser interstitial thermal therapy for mesiotemporal epilepsy. *Stereotact Funct Neurosurg.* (2019) 97:347–55. doi: 10.1159/000504856
14. Voets NL, Alvarez I, Qiu D, Leatherday C, Willie JT, Sotiropoulos S, et al. Mechanisms and risk factors contributing to visual field deficits following stereotactic laser amygdalohippocampotomy. *Stereotact Funct Neurosurg.* (2019) 97:255–65. doi: 10.1159/000502701
15. Drane DL, Loring DW, Voets NL, Price M, Ojemann JG, Willie JT, et al. Better object recognition and naming outcome with MRI-guided stereotactic laser amygdalohippocampotomy for temporal lobe epilepsy. *Epilepsia.* (2015) 56:101–13. doi: 10.1111/epi.12860
16. Ozanne A, Graneheim UH, Ekstedt G, Malmgren K. Patients' expectations and experiences of epilepsy surgery–a population-based long-term qualitative study. *Epilepsia.* (2016) 57:605–11. doi: 10.1111/epi.13333
17. Wiebe S, Blume WT, Girvin JP, Eliasziw M, Effectiveness and Efficiency of Surgery for Temporal Lobe Epilepsy Study G. A randomized, controlled trial of surgery for temporal-lobe epilepsy. *N Engl J Med.* (2001) 345:311–8. doi: 10.1056/NEJM200108023450501
18. Gupta K, Cabaniss B, Kheder A, Gedela S, Koch P, Hewitt KC, et al. Stereotactic MRI-guided laser interstitial thermal therapy for extratemporal lobe epilepsy. *Epilepsia* (2020). 61:1723–34. doi: 10.1111/epi.16614
19. Grinenko O, Li J, Mosher JC, Wang IZ, Bulacio JC, Gonzalez-Martinez J, et al. A fingerprint of the epileptogenic zone in human epilepsies. *Brain.* (2018) 141:117–31. doi: 10.1093/brain/awx306
20. Gross RE, Boulis NM. *Neurosurgical Operative Atlas Functional Neurosurgery.* New York, NY; Stuttgart: Thieme Publishers (2018).
21. Morris SA, Rollo M, Rollo P, Johnson J, Grant GA, Friedman E, et al. Prolonged blood-brain barrier disruption following laser interstitial ablation in epilepsy: a case series with a case report of postablation optic neuritis. *World Neurosurg.* (2017) 104:467–75. doi: 10.1016/j.wneu.2017.05.009

7

Large-Scale Desynchronization During Interictal Epileptic Discharges Recorded with Intracranial EEG

Elie Bou Assi [1,2*†], *Younes Zerouali* [1,3†], *Manon Robert* [1], *Frederic Lesage* [3,4], *Philippe Pouliot* [3,4] *and Dang K. Nguyen* [1,2]

[1] *University of Montreal Hospital Research Center (CRCHUM), University of Montreal, Montreal, QC, Canada,* [2] *Department of Neuroscience, University of Montreal, Montreal, QC, Canada,* [3] *Institute of Biomedical Engineering, Polytechnique Montreal, Montreal, QC, Canada,* [4] *Montreal Heart Institute, Montreal, QC, Canada*

Correspondence:
Elie Bou Assi
elie.bou.assi.chum@ssss.gouv.qc.ca

It is increasingly recognized that deep understanding of epileptic seizures requires both localizing and characterizing the functional network of the region where they are initiated, i. e., the epileptic focus. Previous investigations of the epileptogenic focus' functional connectivity have yielded contrasting results, reporting both pathological increases and decreases during resting periods and seizures. In this study, we shifted paradigm to investigate the time course of connectivity in relation to interictal epileptiform discharges. We recruited 35 epileptic patients undergoing intracranial EEG (iEEG) investigation as part of their presurgical evaluation. For each patient, 50 interictal epileptic discharges (IEDs) were marked and iEEG signals were epoched around those markers. Signals were narrow-band filtered and time resolved phase-locking values were computed to track the dynamics of functional connectivity during IEDs. Results show that IEDs are associated with a transient decrease in global functional connectivity, time-locked to the peak of the discharge and specific to the high range of the gamma frequency band. Disruption of the long-range connectivity between the epileptic focus and other brain areas might be an important process for the generation of epileptic activity. Transient desynchronization could be a potential biomarker of the epileptogenic focus since 1) the functional connectivity involving the focus decreases significantly more than the connectivity outside the focus and 2) patients with good surgical outcome appear to have a significantly more disconnected focus than patients with bad outcomes.

Keywords: intracranial electroencephalography, epileptiform discharges, epileptic focus, epilepsy surgery, surgical outcome, functional connectivity

INTRODUCTION

Networks at Work

It has long been recognized that most anatomical subdivisions of the brain exhibit some degree of functional specialization (1, 2), and localization of the neural substrate of brain function has constituted the workhorse of neuroscientists for decades. More recently, it was shown that a deeper understanding of brain functions could be gained by investigating functional specialization at the scale of brain networks. Functional networks emerge as sets of brain regions that exchange information in a spontaneous and transient fashion through synchronization of their activity (3, 4), a process commonly referred to as "functional connectivity." Importantly, healthy functioning of brain networks relies on precise levels of connectivity among its constituting structures, and alterations of functional connectivity were shown to be involved in various neurological diseases (5).

Epilepsy as a Network Disease

In epilepsy, it is increasingly recognized that deep understanding of seizures requires both localizing and characterizing the functional network of the region where they are initiated, which is usually referred to as the epileptic focus. As was originally postulated by Spencer, seizures arise when an epileptic focus disrupts the balance of functional connectivity within a network, thereby driving its constituting regions into aberrant discharges (6). This theoretical framework is supported empirically by a number of studies showing permanent alterations in brain connectivity in epilepsy. Indeed, resting-state brain functional connectivity in epileptic patients is significantly different from control subjects (7–9). Interestingly, abnormal increases in functional connectivity seem to be closely associated with evolution of the disease (10) and local hypersynchrony/ hyposynchrony were found to be potential electrophysiological/hemodynamic biomarkers for localizing the epileptic focus (11–15). This clinical perspective was further investigated during epileptiform discharges (16) and seizures (17–19), during which regions with elevated connectivity spatially overlapped with the clinically defined epileptic focus. However, it is still unclear whether functional connectivity increases or decreases at seizure onset, as both findings are reported in the literature. Those contrasting findings cannot be attributed to different recording modalities since contradictions arise both from magnetoencephalography (MEG) (20, 21) and intracranial electroencephalography (iEEG) (22–28) studies. In addition, although those studies evaluate functional connectivity using different metrics, most of them use broad-band cross-correlation and mean phase coherence, which were shown to perform relatively similarly on simulations (29) and *in vitro* (30) studies. At least three possible explanations could explain these discrepancies: (1) the definition of the electrical onset of seizures can vary among epileptologists; (2) the changes in connectivity that culminate in seizures might begin before visually identified electrical onset, and (3) different frequency bands could act as distinct information transfer channels during seizures, which has been seldom investigated.

Ictal vs. Interictal Networks

In addition to seizures, epilepsy is characterized by brief asymptomatic electrical discharges called interictal epileptiform discharges (IEDs). Given their sharp shape on electroencephalographic recordings and the large spatial overlap of their generators with the epileptic focus (31), IEDs might be an easier proxy than seizures to study the alterations of functional connectivity in epilepsy. Indeed, it was found that functional connectivity during IEDs might be informative for identifying the epileptic focus as they co-localize with the site of seizure onset (32–36). However, all of those studies evaluated functional connectivity in a relatively large window, which mixes the changes specific to IEDs with those preceding and following IEDs.

In the present study, we hypothesized that functional connectivity exhibits significant variations in the amplitude of synchronization time-locked to the appearance of IEDs, as recorded by intracranial macroelectrodes. In addition, we hypothesized that the epileptic focus displays smaller high-frequency synchrony during IEDs than other brain regions.

METHODS

Patients

For this study, we retrospectively collected data from patients with pharmacoresistant epilepsy who were admitted at the epilepsy monitoring unit of the University of Montreal Hospital Center. Thirty-five consecutive patients undergoing iEEG recordings as part of their pre-surgical evaluation were recruited for this study. In case patients had more than one epilepsy surgery, only the first invasive investigation was considered in this study. The research project was approved by the University of Montreal hospital research center ethics committee (approval reference number: 18.016).

Recordings

All iEEG recordings were acquired from a combination of subdural strip, grid (10 mm spacing, 2.3 mm diameter of exposed area per contact, AD-TECH, WI, USA) and depth electrodes (5 mm spacing, 1.6 mm contact per contact, AD-TECH, WI). iEEG signals were sampled at 2 kHz and digitized (eAMP 64 channel EEG amplifier, Stellate now Natus medical, CA). Electrode contacts were labeled according to timing of the epileptic activity they display during seizures into 3 classes: focus (F—involved at onset), propagation (P—involved after seizure spread), and silent (S—not involved). An expert epileptologist (D.K.N.) reviewed seizure traces and assigned class labels to each electrode contact.

Data Processing

For each patient, we randomly selected a subset of IEDs among continuous recordings and extracted a three-second epoch around the positive peak of IEDs, as marked by an expert epileptologist (-2 to 1 s). To avoid sleep cycles' effect on IEDs, these were selected from awake state day recordings. An average of 51 IEDs were randomly selected per patient to provide a global picture of their interictal epileptiform activity. Data epochs were mirror band-pass filtered in consecutive frequency bands (theta-θ: 4-7Hz, alpha-α: 8-12Hz, beta-β: 12-30Hz, gamma1-$\gamma 1$: 30-60Hz, and gamma2-$\gamma 2$: 60-120Hz) with a finite impulse response (FIR) filter defined using a Kaiser window, as implemented in Brainstorm (37). The backward and forward filtering technique was used to keep the phase of signals intact. In order to avoid edge effects, only the $[-1, 0.5]$ s window was considered for analysis. We then evaluated pairwise connectivity among iEEG electrode contacts within a frequency-adapted sliding window. We set the sliding window to two periods of the middle frequency per band (θ: 363 ms; α: 200 ms; β: 95 ms; $\gamma 1$: 44 ms; $\gamma 2$: 22 ms) and computed in each window the phase-locking value (PLV) (38), which is a measure of synchrony bounded between 0 (asynchrony) and 1 (synchrony). We thus obtained one N_e x

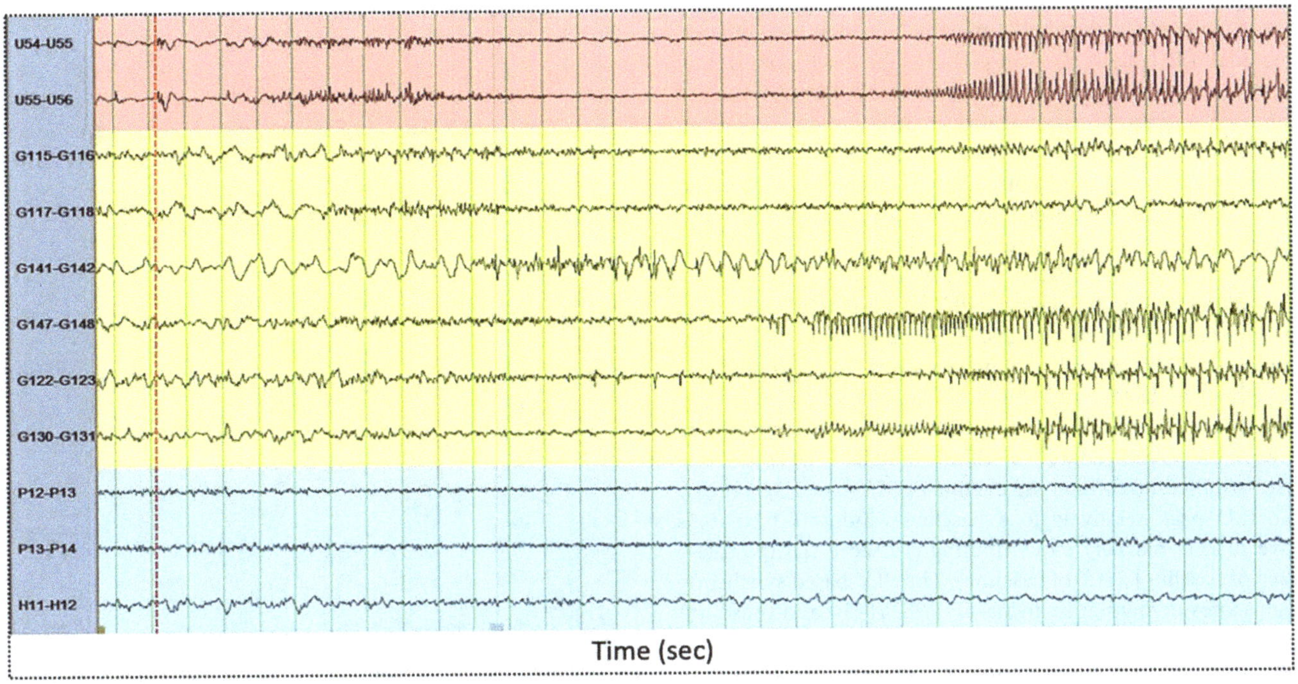

FIGURE 1 | Illustrative examples of intracranial EEG ictal signals recorded by electrodes within the focus area (red), propagation area (yellow) and silent area (blue). The x-axis displays time (in seconds). Green vertical lines are spaced one second each. The red dashed vertical line displays electrical seizure onset.

N_e PLV-based synchrony matrix for each time window and frequency band, where N_e is the number of electrode contacts. For details regarding the mathematical basis of PLV, readers are referred to (38). In brief, PLV is a measure of synchrony which computes a degree of phase-locking between the components the components of 2 time series at each latency. The PLV at each time instant t is then computed as the average value:

$$PLV_t = \frac{1}{N}\left|\sum_{n=1}^{N} exp\left(j\theta\left(t,n\right)\right)\right|$$

where $\theta\ (t,n)$ is the difference between phases of the 2 given signals at time t and trial n, and N is the number of trials.

We recall that the size of the sliding window used for analysis of the time course of connectivity was frequency adaptive. Since phase locking of Hilbert-transformed signals assesses coupling among oscillators, the analysis window was selected in terms of cycles of oscillation. In this work, we chose 2 cycles of oscillation to balance the need for sufficient temporal resolution and signal-to-noise ratio.

Dynamics of Global PLV-Based Synchrony

PLV-based synchrony values were averaged within each matrix to obtain a single time course for each IED and frequency band, representing the dynamics of global PLV-based synchrony. Since those matrices are symmetrical, only upper off-diagonal values were averaged. Time courses of PLV-based synchrony were then averaged over IEDs for each frequency band to reveal band-specific dynamics. In order to identify the time windows during which the global PLV-based synchrony level departs significantly from chance level, we designed a band-specific non-parametric statistical procedure. First, electrode signals were randomly shuffled across IEDs, such that electrode signal $X_{i,k}$ from electrode i and IED k is replaced by the signal $X_{i,l}$, where l is a IED index and $k \neq l$. This procedure disrupts the connectivity structure among sensors while preserving the IED shape (39). Dynamics of global connectivity is then computed using the procedure described in the previous section. The shuffling operation is iterated 1,000 times to produce confidence intervals (99% percentile, corresponding to $p<=0.01$) on the global level of PLV-based synchrony at each time window.

To further ensure that observed dynamic changes of PLV-based synchrony are specific to IEDs, we repeated the described analysis on randomly selected epochs. For each patient, 50 markers were set randomly on the DC component of iEEG signals to avoid any bias toward epileptic activity. Epochs [-2, 1] s were then exported and analyzed.

IED-Locked PLV-Based Synchrony Changes

We then computed the dynamics of PLV-based synchrony according to the connectivity types: the links among electrodes in the focus (F-F), among electrodes in the propagation area (P-P), among electrodes in silent areas (S-S) and across areas (F-P, F-S, P-S) were averaged separately within each connectivity matrix. The focus area (or seizure onset zone), the propagation zone, and silent electrodes were determined by an expert epileptologist based on visual interpretation of seizure recordings. The focus area was defined as the one displaying the first unequivocal intracranial EEG sign of change from the background that leads to a clear sustained rhythmic discharge, without return to background activity. The propagation zone is composed of other electrodes (areas) showing ictal activity but with a delay with regard to the onset zone. **Figure 1** shows illustrative examples of iEEG ictal signals recorded by electrodes within the focus area (red), propagation area (yellow) and silent area (blue) This electrode classification (based on ictal recordings) was then used to compute the dynamics of PLV-based synchrony during interictal epileptiform discharges. **Figure 2** displays illustrative examples of IEDs as recorded in the focus area (red), propagation area (yellow), and silent area (blue).

The dynamics of PLV-based synchrony of each connectivity type were then averaged across IEDs to obtain an average time course. We then quantified the change in PLV-based synchrony at the IED peak relatively to a baseline window (-1 to−0.5s relative to IED marker) by computing a z-score ([IED peak—average of baseline] / std. of baseline). The PLV-based synchrony change scores involving the focus—F-F/F-P/F-S—and those not involving the focus—P-P/P-S/S-S—were analyzed separately.

We then assessed the relationship between the changes in PLV-based synchrony of each connectivity type and the surgical outcome of patients. We categorized patients as having either good (Engel I and II post-surgical outcome scores) or bad (Engel III or IV) and assessed the effect of surgical outcome and frequency bands on PLV-based synchrony changes. Since data patients with good and bad outcomes had unequal variances, we conducted non-parametric *t*-tests: for each frequency band, we computed the t-statistic to measure the difference of average PLV-based synchrony change between patients with good and bad outcomes. This statistic was compared against 100 000 surrogate t-statistic generated by randomly shuffling patients across groups. Differences between patients with respect to surgical outcome were considered significant if the t-statistic exceeded 500 random t-statistics, which corresponds to a Bonferroni-corrected 5% significance level.

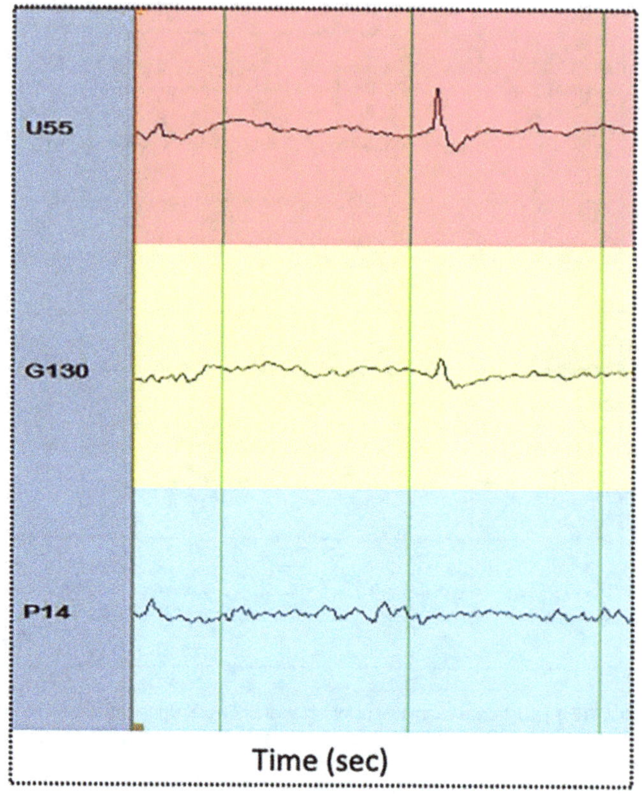

FIGURE 2 | Illustrative examples of IEDs as recorded in the focus area (red), propagation area (yellow), and silent area (blue). The x axis displays time (in seconds). Green vertical lines are spaced one second each.

RESULTS

Patients

In total, 35 patients (15 female, age 34.0 ± 10.8 years—demographic and clinical data are provided in **Table 1**) were recruited and an average of 51 IEDs (average 51.5±8.0) were selected for each patient. Twenty-one and ten patients were categorized as having good and bad surgical outcomes, respectively. Follow-up was not available for four subjects and were thus excluded from the surgical outcome association analysis.

Dynamics of Global PLV-Based Synchrony

As can be seen from **Figure 3**, the global level of PLV-based synchrony changes in a frequency-dependent manner. Low frequency bands (θ, α, β) display an increase in PLV-based synchrony time-locked to the appearance of the IEDs while high frequency bands display a decrease in PLV-based synchrony. However, those changes exceed the confidence interval only for the γ2 band. PLV-based synchrony changes for low-frequency bands were not statistically significant. Interestingly, such changes were absent from global PLV-based synchrony during randomly selected epochs, for any frequency band (**Figure 4**).

We found no significant interplay between low and high frequency bands. By correlating the average relative changes in functional connectivity across low and high frequency bands (theta/alpha/beta X gamma1/gamma2) across patients, we found no statistically significant linear associations.

IED Changes of PLV-Based Synchrony According to Connectivity Type

We compared changes of PLV-based synchrony at the IED peak relative to a preceding baseline period separately for connectivity involving the focus and connectivity not involving the focus:

When analyzing PLV-based synchrony involving the focus (**Figure 5**, left), non-parametric pairwise *t*-tests revealed that IED-locked high-frequency (γ1: $p = 0.0088$; γ2: $p = 0.0183$) PLV-based synchrony is significantly different between patients with good and bad outcomes. However, those differences did not survive Bonferroni correction (γ1: $p = 0.088$; γ2: $p = 0.18$). No significant differences in low-frequency IED-locked PLV-based synchrony were found between patients with good and bad outcomes (θ: $p = 0.95$, α: $p = 0.26$, β: $p = 0.31$). We then averaged IED-locked PLV-based synchrony changes within low

TABLE 1 | Demographic and clinical characteristics of patients.

ID	Age Range	Gender	Ep. Dur.	Total contacts (Depth)	Contacts localization	Resection	Engel	F.-U.
1	[40-49]	M	19	84 (30)	Ins L, Temp L,	mTemp L	IA	4
2	[40-49]	M	4	128 (60)	mTemp L, mTemp R, Ins L, Ins R,Fr L, Fr R, Par L, Par R	mTemp L	IB	6
3	[40-49]	F	13	69 (15)	Ins R, mTemp R	Op-Ins R	IIIA	4
4	[50-59]	M	33	128 (8)	Fr R, Par R, Oc R, mTemp R, Fr L	Par R	IA	2.5
5	[40-49]	F	33	62 (10)	Op-Ins L, Temp L, Fr L	Op-Ins L	IA	1
6	[40-49]	M	24	114 (36)	mTemp L, Ins L, Temp L,	mTemp L	IIIA	3
7	[30-39]	F	21	48	Fr R, Fr L	Fr R	IID	2
8	[50-59]	M	43	134	Fr R, Fr L, Temp R,	Fr R	IA	5.5
9	[50-59]	M	50	108 (8)	Par L, Ins L, Temp L, Fr L, Fr R	Insula L	IB	7
10	[30-39]	F	32	118 (28)	Temp L, mTemp L,Ins R,Temp R, mTemp R	Insula R	IA	3.5
11	[50-59]	F	9	28 (20)	Ins L, Temp L	mTemp L	IA	4
12	[20-29]	M	17	130	Fr R, Fr L	Fr L	IA	6
13	[50-59]	M	16	106 (8)	mTemp L, Ins L, Fr L,	Fr L	IA	4
14	[70-79]	F	40	100 (4)	Temp R, ParR, Occ R, Op-Ins R, Fr R, Par R, mTemp R	mTemp R	IC	3
15	[30-39]	M	30	106 (12)	mTemp L, mTemp R, Ins R, Ins L, Par R, Par L, Fr L, Fr R, Temp R, Temp L,	Temp R	-	-
16	[30-39]	M	41	82 (16)	mTemp R, Ins R, Fr R, Temp R, Par R	Ins R	IV	0.3 **
17	[30-39]	F	13	58	Occ L, Occ R, Temp R, Par R,	Occ R + Temp R + Par R	IA	2.5
18	[30-39]	M	23	118 (44)	Fr L, Temp L, OP-Ins L,	Fr R	IIIB	3
19	[20-29]	F	20	152 (8)	Par L, Occ L, Temp L, Fr L, Fr R	Occ L	IA	5
20	[20-29]	F	20	98 (5)	Fr R, Temp R, Ins R, mTemp R,	mTemp R	-	-
21	[40-49]	F	7	102 (24)	Op-Ins L, Temp L, Occ L, Par L, mTemp L.	Op-Ins L	IIIA	4
22	[20-29]	F	16	104	Fr R, Fr L	Fr L	IIIB	3
23	[50-59]	M	44	140	Fr R, Fr L, Par L, Temp L,	Fr L	IA	5
24	[30-39]	M	23	140	Fr R, Par R, Fr L	Premotor R	IV	4
25	[20-29]	F	8	92	Fr R, Fr L	Fr R	IA	4.5
26	[50-59]	M	34	108 (4)	Fr L, Par L	Fr L	IA	5.5
27	[30-39]	F	19	124 (8)	Fr R, Op-Ins R, Temp R,	Fr R + Ins R	IA	3
28	[20-29]	M	12	116 (8)	Ins L, Fr L, Temp L,	Fr L + Temp L	-	-
29	[30-39]	M	5	112 (8)	Fr L, Ins L, Temp L,	Fr + Ins R	IIIA	2
30	[40-49]	M	35	100 (12)	Fr R, Temp R, Par R, Ins R	Fr-Op R + Ins R	IA	3
31	[30-39]	M	26	126 (32)	Ins L, Fr L, Temp L, Par L, mTemp L	-	-	-
32	[20-29]	F	12	74	Fr L, Par L, Temp L	inf-Rol L	IA	2
33	[50-59]	F	47	106 (14)	Ins L, Op-Ins L, Temp L, Par, Fr L	mTemp L	IIIA	2
34	[50-59]	M	31	96 (28)	Ins L, OP-Ins L, Temp L, Par L, mTemp L	Op-Ins L	IA	2
35	[20-29]	M	20	108 (16)	Fr R, Temp R, Par R, Occ R, Ins R	Fr R	IVA	2

*Reported age corresponds to age at surgery (mTemp: mesio-temporal; Op-Ins: operculo-insular; biTemp: bitemporal; Fr: frontal; Ins: insular; Occ: occipital; Par: Parietal R: right; L: left; Fr-Op: frontal operculum; inf-Rol: inferior rolandic; **: case of SUDEP; F.-U.: follow-up in number of years).*

($\theta + \alpha + \beta$) and high ($\gamma1+\gamma2$) frequencies and repeated the non-parametric test. We found that IED-locked high-frequency PLV-based synchrony was significantly lower in patients with good than in patients with bad outcome ($p = 0.023$, corrected) while no difference was found for low-frequency PLV-based synchrony ($p = 0.59$, uncorrected).

When analyzing PLV-based synchrony not involving the focus (**Figure 5**, right), we found that neither high ($\gamma1$: $p = 0.43$; $\gamma2$: $p = 0.48$—corrected) nor low (θ: $p = 0.93$, α: $p = 0.67$, β: $p = 0.46$—uncorrected) frequency IED-locked PLV-based synchrony differed between patients with good and bad outcomes. After averaging PLV-based synchrony changes within bands, differences between patients with good and bad outcomes were not significant (low freq.: $p = 0.92$; high freq.: $p = 0.092$—corrected).

Illustrative Cases

Patient 1 is a 35 year-old male with persistent nocturnal seizures (2–3 per day) despite eight antiepileptic drug trials. A presurgical evaluation revealed on surface EEG left fronto-temporal IEDs while ictal single-photon emission computed tomography (SPECT) and interictal positron emission tomography

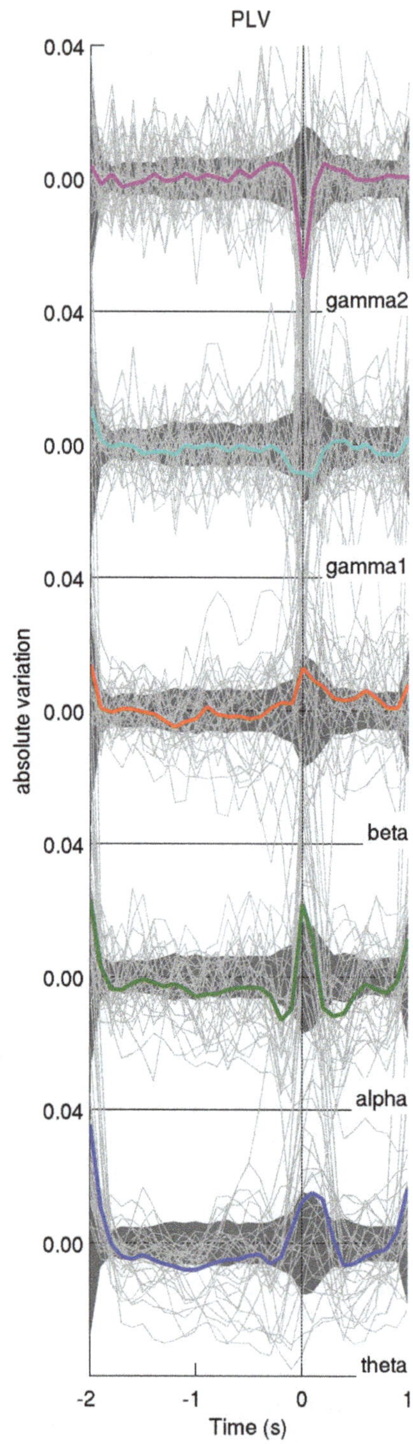

FIGURE 3 | Average time course of the iEEG functional connectivity. The average PLV across pairs of iEEG contacts for each patient is represented with a light solid line and the average across patients is displayed in thick colored lines. Confidence intervals for the average across patients are displayed as a dark shaded area. The time axis is centered on the peak of IEDs (time 0). In general, the average functional connectivity, as measured with the phase-locking value (PLV), increases at IED peak for lower frequency bands (<30 Hz) and decreases for higher frequency bands (>30 Hz). The y-axis displays absolute variation in terms of z-score.

(PET) imaging showed, respectively hyperperfusion and hypometabolism over the left inferior frontal gyrus and anterior insula. MEG dipole imaging of IEDs showed a dense cluster of dipoles over the left superior temporal gyrus, anterior insula and left inferior frontal gyrus. IEEG recordings showed frequent interictal spiking activity in the anterior insula and broad onset of seizures, including the insula, the inferior frontal gyrus, the orbito-frontal gyrus and the superior temporal gyrus. The patient subsequently underwent an insulectomy (see **Figure 6**, top) that rendered him seizure-free for 6 months prior to recurrence. Interestingly, the resection site does not overlap with the site of maximal decrease of functional connectivity in the gamma2 band at the peak of IEDs (**Figure 6**, top), which was rather located in the lateral inferior frontal gyrus. Importantly, a second surgery targeting the lateral inferior frontal gyrus and orbitofrontal cortex subsequently rendered the patient seizure-free (follow-up of 2 years).

Patient 2 is a 23-year-old female with pharmacoresistant non-lesional right occipital lobe epilepsy. Scalp EEG revealed frequent spiking over bilateral temporo-occipital regions with right predominance. Seizures started with low-voltage fast activity over the right occipito-temporal regions. Interictal PET and ictal SPECT imaging revealed, respectively hypometabolism and hyperperfusion over the same regions. MEG dipole imaging revealed a dense cluster over the right occipito-temporal region. Those observations were confirmed with iEEG recordings that showed frequent spiking over occipital and posterior temporal contacts. Surgical resection of the occipito-temporal junction (**Figure 6**, bottom), which overlapped with two "hot spots" showing maximal decrease of functional connectivity at IED peak, rendered the patient seizure-free (follow-up of 2 years).

DISCUSSION

In this work, we investigated the role of PLV-based synchrony during the generation of IEDs at the macroscopic scale of brain networks using a relatively large cohort of patients ($N = 35$) with an average of 51 IEDs per patient. In addition, we explored the link between changes in levels of PLV-based synchrony at the IED peak and the surgical outcome of patients.

Network Desynchronization in Epilepsy

We found that the high frequency ($\gamma1 + \gamma2$) component of iEEG signals during interictal epileptiform discharges is associated with a statistically significant transient decrease in functional connectivity, time locked to the peak of the IEDs. Our results are in line with observations made during seizures; Mormann et al. found that seizures are consistently preceded by a state of hyposynchronization involving both the epileptic focus and distant brain areas (24). Burns et al. demonstrated a specific association between decreased synchronization at seizure onset and the epileptic focus, as surgical resection of the regions that display desynchronization at seizure onset correlated with good outcome in patients with refractory epilepsy (40). Our results are concordant with that study, as we showed significant relationship between the degree of desynchronization of the

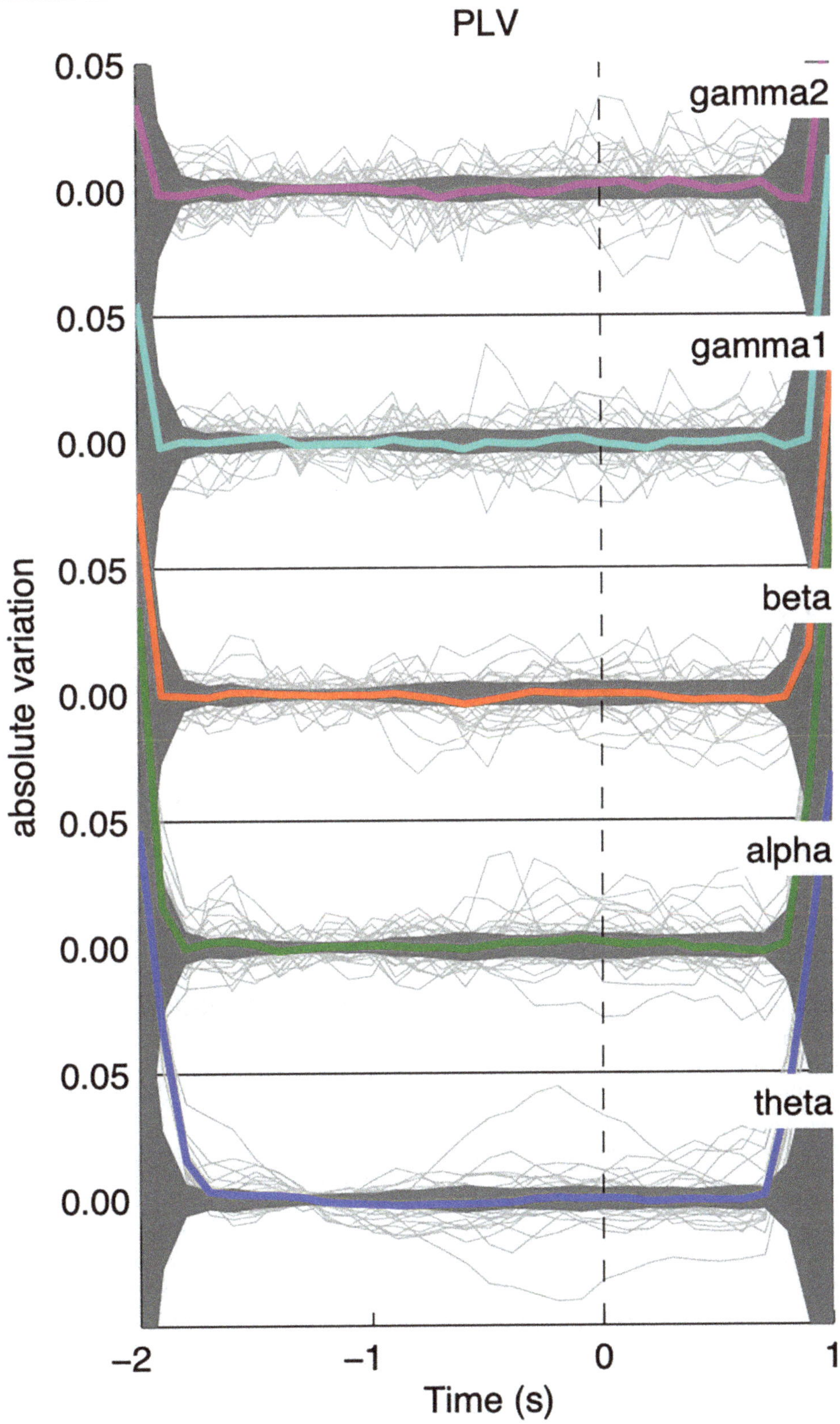

FIGURE 4 | Average time course of the shuffled iEEG functional connectivity; results were only flat noise and no change in connectivity was observed for all frequency bands.

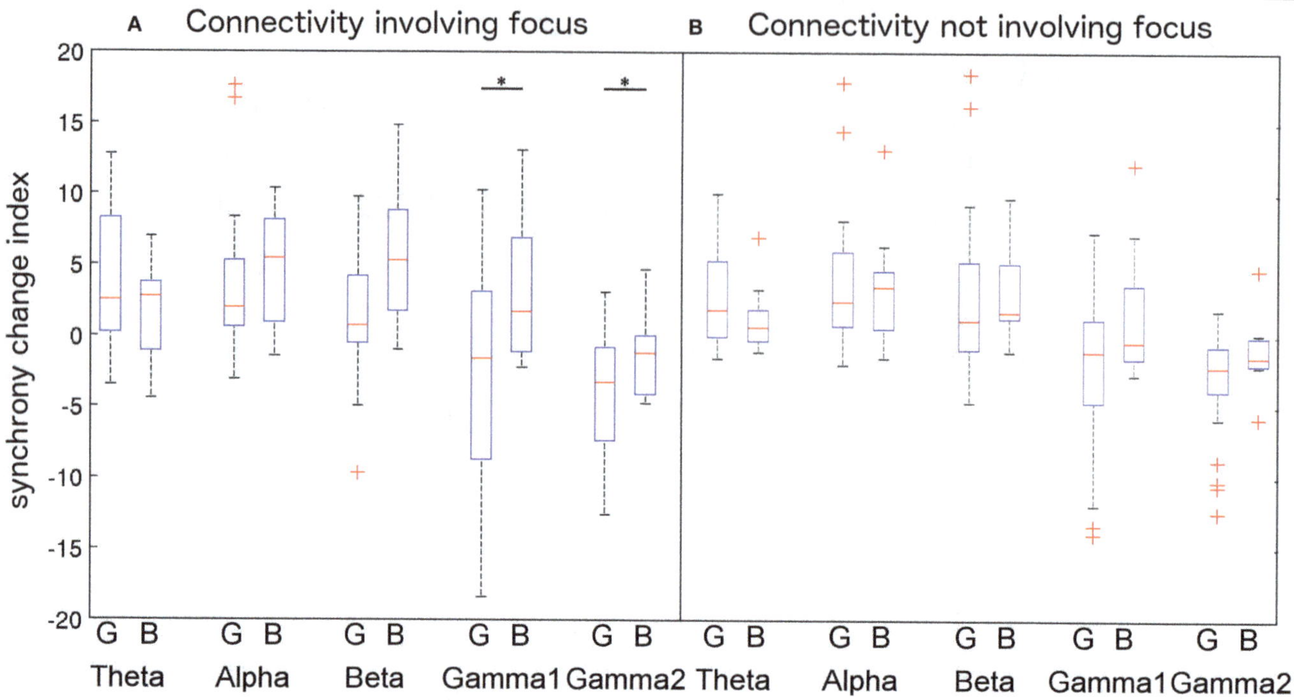

FIGURE 5 | Comparison of PLV variations among the (good outcome—G vs. bad outcome—B) patients groups for each frequency band using a 2-way ANOVA. Connectivity involving the epileptic focus (F-F, F-P, and F-S connections, **A**) increases in lower frequency bands and decrease in higher frequency bands. Differences between patients groups reach significance at the 5% level for gamma1 and gamma2 bands. Connectivity not involving the focus (P-P, P-S, and S-S, **B**) shows similar trends but differences were not significant. Outliers are represented with a "+" symbol. Significant differences are represented with a "*" symbol.

resected region with the surgical outcome of patients. Taken together with previous studies on long-range synchronization in epilepsy, our results suggest that transient desynchronization is observed during interictal epileptiform discharges.

Importantly, our study showed that decreases in PLV-based synchrony during IEDs were restricted to the gamma 1 and gamma 2 frequency bands. By recording simultaneously unit activity in pairs of neurons and the local field potential in slice preparations of rats hippocampus, Netoff and Schiff observed that seizure initiation is marked by a decrease of synchrony both between pairs of neurons and between individual neurons and the local field potential (30). This transient decrease in synchrony was specific to seizure initiation since epileptic bursts were associated with increased synchrony both between individual neurons and between neurons and the local field potential. In humans, simultaneous recordings of multiunit activity using microelectrode arrays and local field potentials revealed that microscopic seizures are initiated in very focal regions while the majority of the clinically defined seizure onset zone is silent. Transition to macroscopic seizures is thought to result from the coalescence of small seizing territories into a synchronized neural mass. At this stage, synchrony between the seizing cortex and the silent regions of the brain drops below baseline levels (41). Our results and those from studies showing transient desynchronization (40, 42, 43) at seizure onset are in line with this explanation.

The emergence of a hypersynchronous state, i.e., seizures, in weakly coupled networks has also been studied using numerical simulations. Nishikawa and Motter showed that any network under quantized total interactions could reach hypersynchronous states (44). In their simulations, they showed that weakly coupled networks can reach hypersynchrony after a phase of relative disconnection during which some specific links are removed (44), which supports the hypothesis that functional decoupling is a possible mechanism for seizure initiation.

Functional Isolation Through Desynchronization

More than fifty years ago, Cannon proposed the "Law of denervation" to account for increased neuronal sensitivity following deprivation of the nervous connections from which they routinely receive inputs (45). In a series of observations on neurons in the spinal cord (46) and the cortex (47, 48) it was demonstrated that isolation of a patch of neurons after incision of its lateral connections increases its sensitivity to both chemical agents and electrical stimulation, thereby lowering the threshold for eliciting epileptiform activity. Can desynchronization transiently mimic functional isolation in human cortex such as to promote epileptiform activity?

Warren et al. used iEEG to compare the resting-state functional connectivity of the epileptic focus in epileptic patients to that of homologous regions in control patients suffering from facial pain injury and implanted with depth electrodes (43). They found that connectivity of the epileptic focus with surrounding regions was significantly reduced as compared

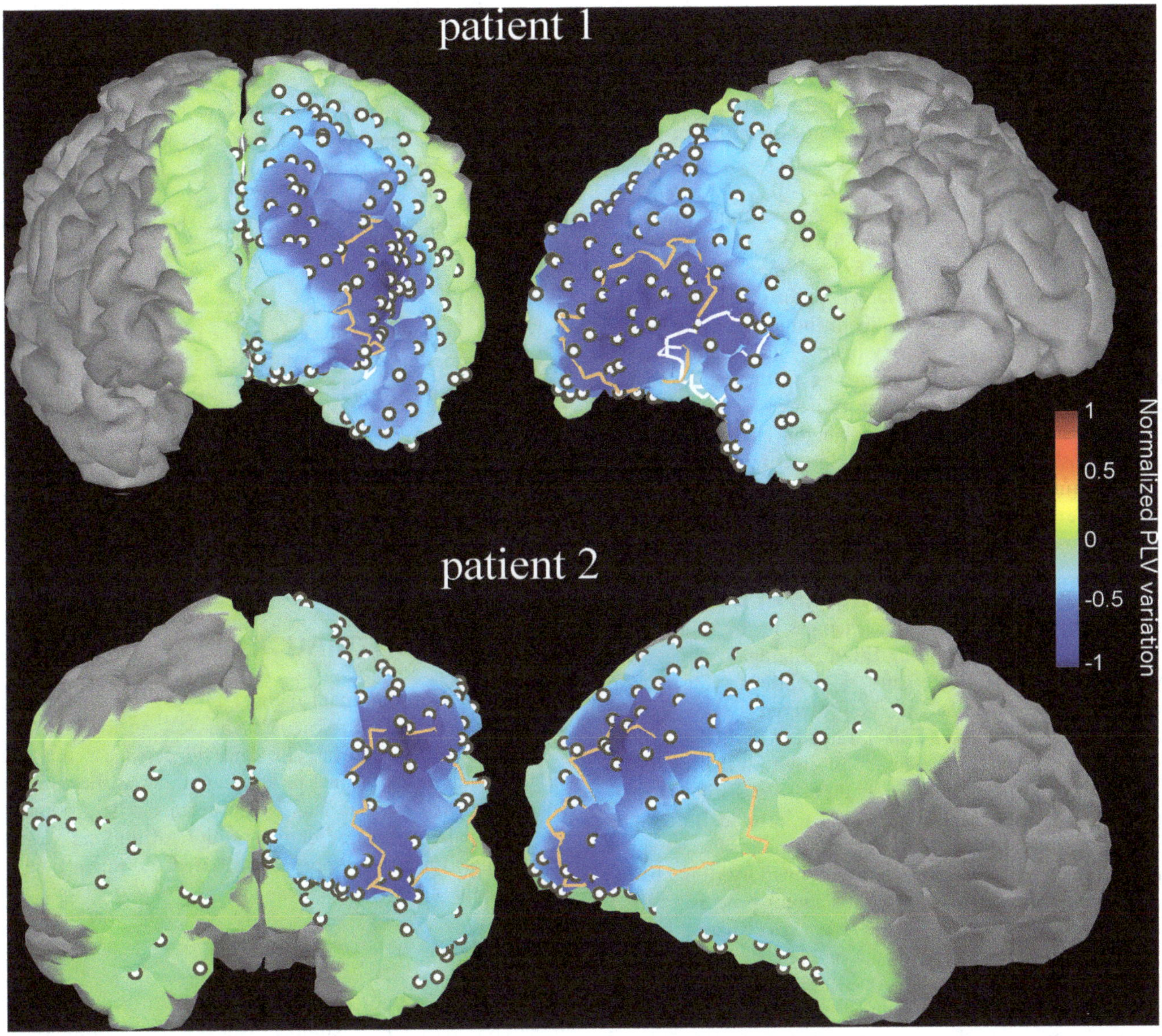

FIGURE 6 | Variation of functional connectivity in the high gamma band (60–120 Hz) as measured with PLV index at the IED peak with respect to baseline (-1 to−0.5 s) for two illustrative patients. The variation index was computed for each electrode contact then interpolated over the underlying cortical surface using an in-house algorithm. The resection site targeted by a later surgery is overlaid as a thick contour. The first patient (upper row) had 2 surgeries; the first one targeted mainly the anterior insula (white contour line) while the maximal decrease of PLV was found in the lateral inferior frontal gyrus. The second surgery (orange contour line) targeted left orbitofrontal and frontal lateral regions, which was concordant with the sites of maximal PLV variation. For the second patient, the resected site (orange contour line) overlaps with the two sites with maximal PLV variation. The PLV projection onto the modeled cortex was threshold; only points on the projection of the cortex which account for 95% of the variance were kept.

to both intra-focus connections and homologous connections in control patients (43). They concluded that the epileptic focus was "functionally disconnected" from the rest of the brain in epilepsy. Recently, Burns et al. supported this view by analyzing seizures in human patients. They found that seizures can be robustly described with a finite set of states including an "isolated focus" state during which the focus exhibits decreased connectivity with the rest of the brain (40). Interestingly, patients who display the isolated focus state in early stages of seizures are those with good postsurgical outcomes while patients who do not display such a state have bad outcomes.

In line with that study, we found in our work that IED-locked high frequency ($\gamma1+\gamma2$) PLV-based synchrony was significantly lower in patients with good outcome than in patients with bad outcome. In other words, patients with good postsurgical outcome have a significantly more disconnected focus during IEDs than patients with bad outcome. We speculate that the epileptic focus is under the influence of resting-state networks during interictal periods and transient desynchronization is necessary to achieve transition toward the spiking and ictal states. More specifically, we found that IED-locked gamma-band PLV-based synchrony was significantly lower in patients with good outcome than in patients with bad outcome when analyzing connectivity within the focus ($p < 0.05$, corrected). We were not able to reveal differences in discriminative power (among patients with good vs. bad outcomes) between $\gamma 1$ and $\gamma 2$ frequency bands.

Clearly, we must remain prudent before translating this work into clinical practice since findings are based on group analyses using retrospective data from a modest number of patients. Further studies with larger cohorts of patients are required to better characterize the contribution of gamma (and subdivisions of gamma) frequency bands. Furthermore, in this work, electrodes were labeled according to the timing of the epileptic activity they displayed during seizures as classified by an expert epileptologist. Exploring how changing electrode class can impact the observed results could be an interesting future avenue. Given the sample size of our study, we could not investigate the effect of antiseizure medications on functional connectivity patterns or postoperative seizure control.

Frequency-Specific Networks in Epilepsy

Our findings suggest band-specific changes in the time course of functional connectivity during IEDs. Although changes were only significant for the $\gamma 2$ band, a preliminary distinction between frequency bands can be observed by comparing higher (>30 Hz) and lower (<30 Hz) bands, which respectively displayed decrease and increase in connectivity at the IED peak. This distinction is expected since they have distinct neural correlates and physiological roles in the healthy brain. Indeed, the low frequency range of the local field potentials reflects mainly synaptic activity and was associated with memory (theta band) (49, 50), arousal (alpha band) (51) and motor processing (beta band) (52), while higher frequencies reflect partly neural spiking activity (53) and were associated with higher cognitive functions such as visual (54) and auditory (55) perception. In epilepsy, the spectral power of high frequencies (>50 Hz) was shown to increase prior to seizure initiation in both humans (56–58) and animal models (59).

Relative contributions of synchronized neural activity within specific frequency bands to epileptiform activity are yet poorly understood. Most of the previous studies investigating epilepsy-related changes in functional connectivity using EEG (either intracranial or scalp) assessed coupling in the broad band signal, which is mainly dominated by lower frequencies given the well-described 1/f shape of the power density spectrum on electrophysiological signals. In addition, we found a distinction between high (>60 Hz) and low (<60 Hz) gamma bands to connectivity changes. This distinction is in line with changes in the power spectrum density of EEG prior to seizures, which shows a bimodal distribution with two statistically independent peaks in the (low: 30–60 Hz, high: 60–120 Hz) gamma range (57).

CONCLUSION

This study suggests that the emergence of interictal epileptiform activity is time-locked with a decrease in functional connectivity in the $\gamma 2$ frequency range. Moreover, IED-locked gamma band PLV-based synchrony was significantly lower in patients with good than in patients with bad outcome recalling to a network configuration in which the epileptogenic focus is functionally isolated from the rest of the brain. While further studies with a larger cohort of patients are required, our results show promise for the design of quantitative methods capable of quantitatively localizing the epileptic focus.

AUTHOR CONTRIBUTIONS

EB and YZ wrote the main manuscript text. EB formatted the manuscript and submitted it. YZ and MR retrieved the data. YZ performed the analysis. FL and PP acted as consultants for the study design, signal processing, and statistical analysis. DKN annotated the interictal epileptiform discharges and was the principal investigator of this study. All authors reviewed the manuscript. All authors contributed to the article and approved the submitted version.

FUNDING

This work was supported by the Canadian Institutes of Health Research (CIHR, Grant Number: 390044), the Institute for Data Valorization (IVADO, Grant Number: PD-2018b-AP-03), the Canada Research Chair in Epilepsy and Functional Anatomy of Human Brain (Grant Number: 232075), and the Natural Sciences and Engineering Research Council of Canada (NSERC, Discovery Grant Number: 289987).

REFERENCES

1. Desmond JE, Sum JM, Wagner AD, Demb JB, Shear PK, Glover GH, et al. Functional MRI measurement of language lateralization in Wada-tested patients. *Brain.* (1995) 118:1411–9. doi: 10.1093/brain/118.6.1411
2. Geschwind N. Anatomical and functional specialization of the cerebral hemispheres in the human. *Bull Mem Acad R Med Belg.* (1979) 134:286–97.
3. Roelfsema PR, Engel AK, Konig P, Singer W. The role of neuronal synchronization in response selection: a biologically plausible theory of structured representations in the visual cortex. *J Cogn Neurosci.* (1996) 8:603–25. doi: 10.1162/jocn.1996.8.6.603
4. Varela F, Lachaux JP, Rodriguez E, Martinerie J. The brainweb: phase synchronization and large-scale integration. *Nat Rev Neurosci.* (2001) 2:229–39. doi: 10.1038/35067550
5. He BJ, Shulman GL, Snyder AZ, Corbetta M. The role of impaired neuronal communication in neurological disorders. *Curr Opin Neurol.* (2007) 20:655–60. doi: 10.1097/WCO.0b013e3282f1c720
6. Spencer SS. Neural networks in human epilepsy: evidence of and implications for treatment. *Epilepsia.* (2002) 43:219–27. doi: 10.1046/j.1528-1157.2002.26901.x
7. Clemens B, Puskas S, Besenyei M, Spisak T, Opposits G, Hollody K, et al. Neurophysiology of juvenile myoclonic epilepsy: EEG-based network and graph analysis of the interictal and immediate preictal states. *Epilepsy Res.* (2013) 106:357–69. doi: 10.1016/j.eplepsyres.2013.06.017
8. Elshahabi A, Klamer S, Sahib AK, Lerche H, Braun C, Focke NK. Magnetoencephalography reveals a widespread increase in network connectivity in idiopathic/genetic generalized epilepsy. *PLoS ONE.* (2015) 10:e0138119. doi: 10.1371/journal.pone.0138119

9. Maccotta L, He BJ, Snyder AZ, Eisenman LN, Benzinger TL, Ances BM, et al. Impaired and facilitated functional networks in temporal lobe epilepsy. *Neuroimage Clin.* (2013) 2:862–72. doi: 10.1016/j.nicl.2013.06.011
10. Morgan VL, Rogers BP, Sonmezturk HH, Gore JC, Abou-Khalil B. Cross hippocampal influence in mesial temporal lobe epilepsy measured with high temporal resolution functional magnetic resonance imaging. *Epilepsia.* (2011) 52:1741–9. doi: 10.1111/j.1528-1167.2011.03196.x
11. Antony AR, Alexopoulos AV, González-Martínez JA, Mosher JC, Jehi L, Burgess RC, et al. Functional connectivity estimated from intracranial EEG predicts surgical outcome in intractable temporal lobe epilepsy. *PLoS ONE.* (2013) 8:e77916. doi: 10.1371/journal.pone.0077916
12. Bettus G, Bartolomei F, Confort-Gouny S, Guedj E, Chauvel P, Cozzone PJ, et al. Role of resting state functional connectivity MRI in presurgical investigation of mesial temporal lobe epilepsy. *J Neurol Neurosurg Psychiatry.* (2010) 81:1147–54. doi: 10.1136/jnnp.2009.191460
13. Bettus G, Wendling F, Guye M, Valton L, Regis J, Chauvel P, et al. Enhanced EEG functional connectivity in mesial temporal lobe epilepsy. *Epilepsy Res.* (2008) 81:58–68. doi: 10.1016/j.eplepsyres.2008.04.020
14. Pittau F, Grova C, Moeller F, Dubeau F, Gotman J. Patterns of altered functional connectivity in mesial temporal lobe epilepsy. *Epilepsia.* (2012) 53:1013–23. doi: 10.1111/j.1528-1167.2012.03464.x
15. Schevon CA, Cappell J, Emerson R, Isler J, Grieve P, Goodman R, et al. Cortical abnormalities in epilepsy revealed by local EEG synchrony. *Neuroimage.* (2007) 35:140–8. doi: 10.1016/j.neuroimage.2006.11.009
16. Dai Y, Zhang W, Dickens DL, He B. Source connectivity analysis from MEG and its application to epilepsy source localization. *Brain Topogr.* (2012) 25:157–66. doi: 10.1007/s10548-011-0211-0
17. Bou Assi E, Rihana S, Nguyen DK, Sawan M. Effective connectivity analysis of iEEG and accurate localization of the epileptogenic focus at the onset of operculo-insular seizures. *Epilepsy Res.* (2019) 152:42–51. doi: 10.1016/j.eplepsyres.2019.02.006
18. Elshoff L, Muthuraman M, Anwar AR, Deuschl G, Stephani U, Raethjen J, et al. Dynamic imaging of coherent sources reveals different network connectivity underlying the generation and perpetuation of epileptic seizures. *PLoS ONE.* (2013) 8:e78422. doi: 10.1371/journal.pone.0078422
19. van Mierlo P, Carrette E, Hallez H, Raedt R, Meurs A, Vandenberghe S, et al. Ictal-onset localization through connectivity analysis of intracranial EEG signals in patients with refractory epilepsy. *Epilepsia.* (2013) 54:1409–18. doi: 10.1111/epi.12206
20. Amor F, Baillet S, Navarro V, Adam C, Martinerie J, Quyen Mle. V. Cortical local and long-range synchronization interplay in human absence seizure initiation. *Neuroimage.* (2009) 45:950–62. doi: 10.1016/j.neuroimage.2008.12.011
21. Parra J, Kalitzin SN, Iriarte J, Blanes W, Velis DN, Lopes da Silva FH. Gamma-band phase clustering and photosensitivity: is there an underlying mechanism common to photosensitive epilepsy and visual perception? *Brain.* (2003) 126:1164–72. doi: 10.1093/brain/awg109
22. Bartolomei F, Wendling F, Bellanger JJ, Regis J, Chauvel P. Neural networks involving the medial temporal structures in temporal lobe epilepsy. *Clin Neurophysiol.* (2001) 112:1746–60. doi: 10.1016/S1388-2457(01)00591-0
23. Kramer MA, Eden UT, Kolaczyk ED, Zepeda R, Eskandar EN, Cash SS. Coalescence and fragmentation of cortical networks during focal seizures. *J Neurosci.* (2010) 30:10076–85. doi: 10.1523/JNEUROSCI.6309-09.2010
24. Mormann F, Andrzejak RG, Kreuz T, Rieke C, David P, Elger CE, et al. Automated detection of a preseizure state based on a decrease in synchronization in intracranial electroencephalogram recordings from epilepsy patients. *Phys Rev E Stat Nonlin Soft Matter Phys.* (2003) 67:021912. doi: 10.1103/PhysRevE.67.021912
25. Mormann F, Lehnertz K, David PE, Elger C. Mean phase coherence as a measure for phase synchronization and its application to the EEG of epilepsy patients. *Physica D.* (2000) 144:358–69. doi: 10.1016/S0167-2789(00)00087-7
26. Schindler K, Elger CE, Lehnertz K. Increasing synchronization may promote seizure termination: evidence from status epilepticus. *Clin Neurophysiol.* (2007) 118:1955–68. doi: 10.1016/j.clinph.2007.06.006
27. Schindler KA, Bialonski S, Horstmann MT, Elger CE, Lehnertz K. Evolving functional network properties and synchronizability during human epileptic seizures. *Chaos.* (2008) 18:33119. doi: 10.1063/1.2966112
28. Varotto G, Tassi L, Franceschetti S, Spreafico R, Panzica F. Epileptogenic networks of type II focal cortical dysplasia: a stereo-EEG study. *Neuroimage.* (2012) 61:591–8. doi: 10.1016/j.neuroimage.2012.03.090
29. Wendling F, Ansari-Asl K, Bartolomei F, Senhadji L. From EEG signals to brain connectivity: a model-based evaluation of interdependence measures. *J Neurosci Methods.* (2009) 183:9–18. doi: 10.1016/j.jneumeth.2009.04.021
30. Netoff TI, Schiff SJ. Decreased neuronal synchronization during experimental seizures. *J Neurosci.* (2002) 22:7297–307. doi: 10.1523/JNEUROSCI.22-16-07297.2002
31. Hufnagel A, Dumpelmann M, Zentner J, Schijns O, Elger CE. Clinical relevance of quantified intracranial interictal spike activity in presurgical evaluation of epilepsy. *Epilepsia.* (2000) 41:467–78. doi: 10.1111/j.1528-1157.2000.tb00191.x
32. Englot DJ, Rolston JD, Wang DD, Kirsch HE, Nagarajan SS, Chang EF. 206 spikes, slowing, and functional connectivity: multimodal magnetoencephalography in epilepsy surgery. *Neurosurgery.* (2016) 63:181. doi: 10.1227/01.neu.0000489775.61051.9c
33. Iannotti GR, Grouiller F, Centeno M, Carmichael DW, Abela E, Wiest R, et al. Epileptic networks are strongly connected with and without the effects of interictal discharges. *Epilepsia.* (2016) 57:1086–96. doi: 10.1111/epi.13400
34. Jmail N, Gavaret M, Bartolomei F, Chauvel P, Badier JM, Benar CG. Comparison of brain networks during interictal oscillations and spikes on magnetoencephalography and intracerebral EEG. *Brain Topogr.* (2016) 29:752–65. doi: 10.1007/s10548-016-0501-7
35. Luo C, An D, Yao D, Gotman J. Patient-specific connectivity pattern of epileptic network in frontal lobe epilepsy. *NeuroImage.* (2014) 4:668–75. doi: 10.1016/j.nicl.2014.04.006
36. Malinowska U, Badier JM, Gavaret M, Bartolomei F, Chauvel P, Benar CG. Interictal networks in magnetoencephalography. *Hum Brain Mapp.* (2014) 35:2789–805. doi: 10.1002/hbm.22367
37. Tadel F, Baillet S, Mosher JC, Pantazis D, Leahy RM. Brainstorm: a user-friendly application for MEG/EEG analysis. *Comp Intell Neurosci.* (2011) 2011:13. doi: 10.1155/2011/879716
38. Lachaux JP, Rodriguez E, Martinerie J, Varela FJ. Measuring phase synchrony in brain signals. *Hum Brain Mapp.* (1999) 8:194–208. doi: 10.1002/(SICI)1097-0193(1999)8:4<194::AID-HBM4>3.0.CO;2-C
39. Zerouali Y, Pouliot P, Robert M, Mohamed I, Bouthillier A, Lesage F, et al. Magnetoencephalographic signatures of insular epileptic spikes based on functional connectivity. *Hum Brain Mapp.* (2016) 37:3250–61. doi: 10.1002/hbm.23238
40. Burns SP, Santaniello S, Yaffe RB, Jouny CC, Crone NE, Bergey GK, et al. Network dynamics of the brain and influence of the epileptic seizure onset zone. *Proc Natl Acad Sci.* (2014) 111:E5321. doi: 10.1073/pnas.1401752111
41. Schevon CA, Weiss SA, McKhann, G. Jr., Goodman RR, Yuste R, et al. Evidence of an inhibitory restraint of seizure activity in humans. *Nat Commun.* (2012) 3:1060. doi: 10.1038/ncomms2056
42. Khambhati AN, Davis KA, Oommen BS, Chen SH, Lucas TH, Litt B, et al. Dynamic network drivers of seizure generation, propagation and termination in human neocortical epilepsy. *PLOS Comp Biol.* (2015) 11:e1004608. doi: 10.1371/journal.pcbi.1004608
43. Warren CP, Hu S, Stead M, Brinkmann BH, Bower MR, Worrell GA. Synchrony in normal and focal epileptic brain: the seizure onset zone is functionally disconnected. *J Neurophysiol.* (2010) 104:3530–9. doi: 10.1152/jn.00368.2010
44. Nishikawa T, Motter AE. Network synchronization landscape reveals compensatory structures, quantization, and the positive effect of negative interactions. *Proceed Natl Acad Sci USA.* (2010) 107:10342. doi: 10.1073/pnas.0912444107
45. Cannon WB. A law of denervation. *Am J Med Sci.* (1939) 1:198. doi: 10.1097/00000441-193912000-00001
46. Cannon WB, Haimovici H. The sensitization of motoneurones by partial "Denervation". *Am J Physiol.* (1939) 126:731–40. doi: 10.1152/ajplegacy.1939.126.3.731
47. Echlin FA. The supersensitivity of chronically "isolated" cerebral cortex as a mechanism in focal epilepsy. *Electroencephalogr Clin Neurophysiol.* (1959) 11:697–722. doi: 10.1016/0013-4694(59)90110-5

48. Echlin FA, Battista A. Epileptiform seizures from chronic isolated cortex. *Arch Neurol.* (1963) 9:154–70. doi: 10.1001/archneur.1963.00460080064009
49. Axmacher N, Henseler MM, Jensen O, Weinreich I, Elger CE, Fell J. Cross-frequency coupling supports multi-item working memory in the human hippocampus. *Proc Natl Acad Sci USA.* (2010) 107:3228. doi: 10.1073/pnas.0911531107
50. Kaplan R, Bush D, Bonnefond M, Bandettini PA, Barnes GR, Doeller CF, et al. Medial prefrontal theta phase coupling during spatial memory retrieval. *Hippocampus.* (2014) 24:656–65. doi: 10.1002/hipo.22255
51. Bollimunta A, Mo J, Schroeder CE, Ding M. Neuronal mechanisms and attentional modulation of corticothalamic alpha oscillations. *J Neurosci.* (2011) 31:4935–43. doi: 10.1523/JNEUROSCI.5580-10.2011
52. Khanna P, Carmena JM. Neural oscillations: beta band activity across motor networks. *Curr Opin Neurobiol.* (2015) 32:60–7. doi: 10.1016/j.conb.2014.11.010
53. Buzsáki G, Anastassiou CA, Koch C. The origin of extracellular fields and currents - EEG. ECoG, LFP and spikes. *Nat Rev Neurosci.* (2012) 13:407. doi: 10.1038/nrn3241
54. Rodriguez E, George N, Lachaux JP, Martinerie J, Renault B, Varela FJ. Perception's shadow: long-distance synchronization of human brain activity. *Nature.* (1999) 397:430–33. doi: 10.1038/17120
55. Steinmann S, Leicht G, Ertl M, Andreou C, Polomac N, Westerhausen R, et al. Conscious auditory perception related to long-range synchrony of gamma oscillations. *Neuroimage.* (2014) 100:435–43. doi: 10.1016/j.neuroimage.2014.06.012
56. Allen PJ, Fish DR, Smith SJ. Very high-frequency rhythmic activity during SEEG suppression in frontal lobe epilepsy. *Electroencephalogr Clin Neurophysiol.* (1992) 82:155–9. doi: 10.1016/0013-4694(92)90160-J
57. Fisher RS, Webber WR, Lesser RP, Arroyo S, Uematsu S. High-frequency EEG activity at the start of seizures. *J Clin Neurophysiol.* (1992) 9:441–8. doi: 10.1097/00004691-199207010-00012
58. Lee SA, Spencer DD, Spencer SS. Intracranial EEG seizure-onset patterns in neocortical epilepsy. *Epilepsia.* (2000) 41:297–307. doi: 10.1111/j.1528-1157.2000.tb00159.x
59. Grenier F, Timofeev I, Steriade M. Neocortical very fast oscillations (ripples, 80-200 Hz) during seizures: intracellular correlates. *J Neurophysiol.* (2003) 89:841–52. doi: 10.1152/jn.00420.2002

8

Combination of Matching Responsive Stimulations of Hippocampus and Subiculum for Effective Seizure Suppression in Temporal Lobe Epilepsy

Fang Zhang[1,2,3], *Yufang Yang*[1,2,3], *Yongte Zheng*[1,2,3], *Junming Zhu*[3,4], *Ping Wang*[2] *and Kedi Xu*[1,2,3*]

[1] *Qiushi Academy for Advanced Studies, Zhejiang University, Hangzhou, China,* [2] *Key Laboratory of Biomedical Engineering of Education Ministry, Department of Biomedical Engineering Zhejiang University, Hangzhou, China,* [3] *Zhejiang Provincial Key Laboratory of Cardio-Cerebral Vascular Detection Technology and Medicinal Effectiveness Appraisal, Zhejiang University, Hangzhou, China,* [4] *Department of Neurosurgery, Second Affiliated Hospital of Zhejiang University, Hangzhou, China*

***Correspondence:**
Kedi Xu
xukd@zju.edu.cn

Responsive neural stimulation (RNS) is considered a promising neural modulation therapy for refractory epilepsy. Combined stimulation on different targets may hold great promise for improving the efficacy of seizure control since neural activity changed dynamically within associated brain targets in the epileptic network. Three major issues need to be further explored to achieve better efficacy of combined stimulation: (1) which nodes within the epileptogenic network should be chosen as stimulation targets? (2) What stimulus frequency should be delivered to different targets? and (3) Could the efficacy of RNS for seizure control be optimized by combined different stimulation targets together? In our current study, Granger causality (GC) method was applied to analyze epileptogenic networks for finding key targets of RNS. Single target stimulation (100 μA amplitude, 300 μs pulse width, 5s duration, biphasic, charge-balanced) with high frequency (130 Hz, HFS) or low frequency (5 Hz, LFS) was firstly delivered by our lab designed RNS systems to CA3, CA1, subiculum (SUB) of hippocampi, and anterior nucleus of thalamus (ANT). The efficacy of combined stimulation with different groups of frequencies was finally assessed to find out better combined key targets with optimal stimulus frequency. Our results showed that stimulation individually delivered to SUB and CA1 could shorten the average duration of seizures. Different stimulation frequencies impacted the efficacy of seizure control, as HFS delivered to CA1 and LFS delivered to SUB, respectively, were more effective for shortening the average duration of electrographic seizure in Sprague-Dawley rats ($n = 3$). Moreover, the synchronous stimulation of HFS in CA1 combined with LFS in SUB reduced the duration of discharge significantly in rats ($n = 6$). The combination of responsive stimulation at different targets may be an inspiration to optimize stimulation therapy for epilepsy.

Keywords: combined stimulation, granger causality, responsive neural stimulation, temporal lobe epilepsy, rat

INTRODUCTION

Neural modulation is gradually accepted by those patients with medicine-refractory epilepsy who are not candidates for surgery resection (1, 2). Compared with Vagus nerve stimulation (VNS) and deep brain stimulation, which deliver scheduled stimulation on open-loop mode, responsive neural stimulation (RNS) delivers electrical stimulation in response to the neural activity of the target tissue and is emerging as one of the most promising approaches for refractory epilepsy treatment (3). Several clinical multi-center outcome studies demonstrated a median reduction in seizure frequency of 53% at 2 years and 72% at 6 years with the treatment of RNS (4, 5). However, the efficacy of RNS is still far from optimal due to the various stimulation parameters, complex stimulation targets for seizure control, and limited understanding of neural modulation mechanism (6). Stimulation targets and parameters of RNS are intimately related to the efficacy of seizure control. Understanding the knowledge of seizure initiation and propagation is crucial for looking for ideal stimulation targets. It has been demonstrated that limbic structures, primarily the hippocampus, amygdala, subiculum, and entorhinal cortex, are the sites of seizure initiation in temporal lobe epilepsy (TLE), moreover, the initiation and propagation varies between subjects (7). The targets for RNS are typically seizure onset zones in clinical studies. To optimize the efficacy, extensive studies were performed to look for more effective stimulation brain targets in recent studies (8–10). Most of the explored potential targets were those directly involved in seizure generation, propagation, or served as a hub to control an epileptic network (3). Specifically, besides the classical epileptic foci of CA3 and CA1 in hippocampi, other targets, such as subiculum (SUB) and anterior nucleus of thalamus (ANT) which have a tight connection with the mesial temporal lobe structure, were also proven to be potential stimulation targets of seizure suppression (11). Except for the stimulation targets, optimal stimulation parameters for aborting seizure activity are still unclear (12). Among the complex stimulus parameter space, stimulation frequency is a vital parameter and has distinct effects on different brain targets (13). In general, stimulation with a high frequency range (>70 Hz) is deemed to be effective for seizure control, since it may demonstrate the acute suppressive effects on neuronal synchrony by preferential activation of GABA-ergic inhibitory neurons and alter extracellular potassium concentrations (14). Nevertheless, stimulation with low frequency (<10 Hz) delivered to white matter tracts evokes a large, coordinated population burst which then leads to a period of reduced population firing mediated by slow after-hyperpolarization and GABA-B currents (15, 16), and attenuates seizure severity in multiple rodent models and non-human primate models (17, 18). Both high frequency and low frequency stimulations applied in animal and clinical studies were proven to be effective for seizure control (19–22). However, to the best of our knowledge, whether high frequency or low frequency stimulation applied at each different target has different efficacy for seizure control in the same animal model of temporal lobe epilepsy has not been well-explored. Overall, the identification of new targets and approaches for brain stimulation in epilepsy control is particularly compelling.

As the research progressed, epilepsy came to be understood as a disorder of the large neural network, the activity of which depends on the dysfunction of widespread regions in the brain rather than a single epileptic focus (23). Right now, the main approach of neural modulation for seizure control is delivered to a single target region alone, which may not sufficiently alter the dynamics of networks during seizures and may underline the suboptimal efficacy of RNS for seizure control (24). Therefore, it might be more effective to alter the dynamics of brain networks during seizures if responsive stimulation could be delivered to multi-targeted brain regions. Hence, simultaneously combined stimulations on different targets hold great feasibility for improving the efficacy of seizure control. Only a few studies were performed to evaluate this hypothesis. One of the most intriguing works was simultaneously activating inhibitory luminopsins on dentate gyrus and ANT of the rat brain, which was proven to be more effective than inhibition of each single individual structure (25). Overall, three major issues are worthy of further exploration to optimize the efficacy of RNS for seizure suppression: How to find key targets of combined stimulations in the epileptic network? How to choose the stimulus frequency of combined stimulation? And whether the efficacy could be optimized by combined stimulation matched with the ideal stimulus frequency of each different key target?

To answer the questions above, epileptic activity should be assessed in terms of functional connectivity and dynamics of neuronal networks (23). Among the many methods of functional connectivity, Granger causality (GC) is a reliable tool to estimate the interactions from time-series data during seizure onset and propagation (26, 27) and has the potential to help localize the ictal network (28, 29). In addition, if multiple neuronal groups have been recorded simultaneously, the conditional GC can distinguish the interaction relationship between direct vs. indirect interactions (30). In this work, epileptic activity was assessed in terms of functional connectivity and dynamics of neuronal GC method to find out key targets for brain stimulation. We then applied high frequency or low frequency responsive stimulation with our own designed RNS system for seizure control on a TLE rat model to evaluate the effect of single brain target stimulation on different potential targets for seizure control. Finally, combined stimulations with different groups of frequencies were delivered to key targets simultaneously to explore whether the combined stimulation with matching frequency could abort seizures efficiently.

MATERIALS AND METHODS

Subject and Surgery

Sprague-Dawley rats weighing 250–300 g were used for induction of the chronic TLE model. The process of rats treated with lithium and pilocarpine for seizure induction was based on our prior work (31). In brief, a dose of lithium chloride (12.7 mg/100 g) was pre-administered to the rats intraperitoneally. One day later, atropine sulfate was injected into pretreated rats to reduce saliva secretion (1 ml, i.p., 30 min before pilocarpine injection). Rats were then treated with 32 mg/kg pilocarpine dissolved in saline and supplemented every 30 min by a repeated

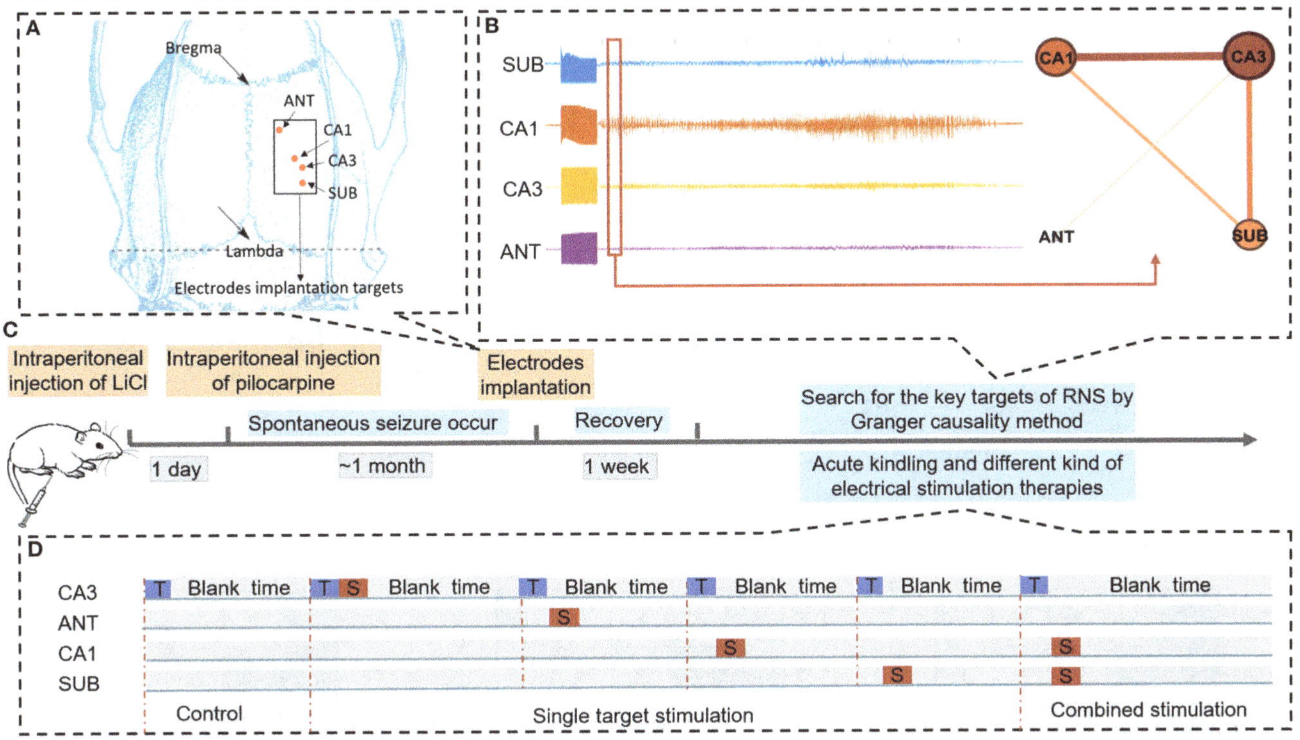

FIGURE 1 | Schematic of experiments. **(A)** Schematic diagram of brain targets for electrode implantation. **(B)** Searching for key nodes of RNS during acute seizure onset within the epileptogenic network by Granger causality method. **(C)** Time flow chart of the experiment. **(D)** Three different conditions to evaluate the efficacy of different neural stimulation protocols for alleviating seizure severity. "T" in the blue rectangle represents trigger stimulation induced to R-CA3 to produce the acute seizure. "S" in the red rectangle represents therapeutic stimulation. In the control condition, there is only trigger stimulation delivered to CA3. In the single target stimulation condition, therapeutic stimulation was delivered to each of the four nodes. In combined stimulation, different therapeutic stimulation was delivered to both CA1 and SUB.

dose (16 mg/kg) until a sequence of animal behaviors of status epilepticus (SE) were observed. Once rats had SE lasting over 90 min, a dose of diazepam (20 mg/kg) was given to terminate the continuous convulsive seizure. After completing the whole process, rats were taken back to home cages and spontaneous seizures were monitored by video cameras. Approximately 1 month later, once spontaneous recurrent seizures were observed, rats were operated under propofol anesthesia and chronically implanted with tripolar electrodes for local field potentials' (LFPs) recording and neural stimulation. The tripolar electrode was made of 65 μm diameter teflo-coated microfilament electrodes, and their tips were spaced 500 μm from each other. One of the three electrodes was used for signal recording, and the other two strands (0.5 mm tip exposed) twisted together were paired for neural stimulation. Each rat was implanted with four tripolar electrodes for recording and stimulation, which were implanted into the ANT (−1.5 mm AP, +1.5 mm ML, −5.6 mmDV), CA1 (−3.6 mm AP, +2.0 mm ML, −3.0 DV) as shown in **Figure 1A**, CA3 (−4.2 mm AP, +3.0 mm ML, −3.7 mm DV), and subiculum (SUB, −6.0 mm AP, +3.0 mm ML, −3.0 mm DV) regions in the right hemisphere. In addition, a ground sliver electrode was implanted over the posterior fontanelle and a reference electrode was epidurally inserted on the region far from other record electrodes. After implantation, the electrodes were connected to a miniature receptacle. The whole assembly was finally fixed to the skull by dental cement.

The whole process of our experiment was shown in **Figure 1C**. All experimental procedures were performed in accordance with the Animal Care and Use Committee of Zhejiang University and achieved ethical approval (Zhejiang University 15896).

Acute Seizure Induction and Electroencephalography Acquisition and Analysis

Rats' behaviors were monitored by cameras and LFPs were recorded by our custom-made responsive neural stimulator; the detailed designs were described in our previous work (32–34) and depicted in **Supplementary Figure 1**. Specifically, an interface programmed on the computer was used in an online pattern, which contains neural signal recording function, real-time neural signal display interface, auto seizure detection function based on Ostu's algorithm (35), and real-time neural stimulation function to satisfy all needs of experiments in this work. The LFPs signals were recorded and digitized at 1,000 Hz, bandpass filtered from 0.1 to 500 Hz, notch filtered 50 Hz signal to reduce power frequency interference, and then shown in the display interface for seizure detection and stored for offline analysis.

The acute seizure induction experiment was performed 1 week after surgery. The process was similar to Tiwalade's prior work (36). Trigger stimulation, a sequence of biphasic square pulses with 200 μA amplitude, 1 ms pulse width, and 60 Hz frequency

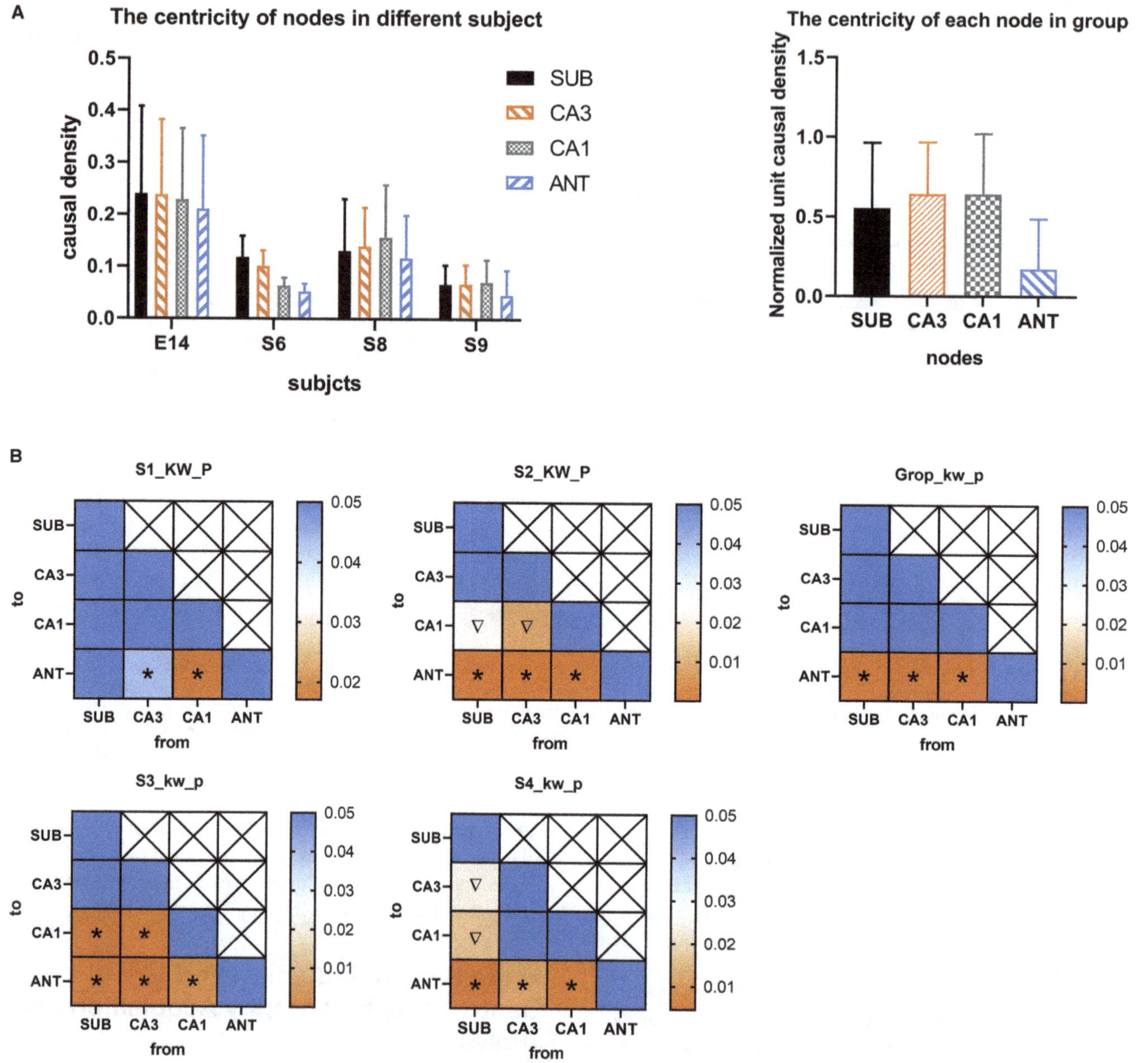

FIGURE 2 | (A) The normalized weighted causality density (wcd_u) of each node during seizure onset activity in different four rats. **(B)** Color-coded significance value matrices were obtained from the pairwise computation of wcd_u between each different node. The square with icon represents significant differences between two corresponding nodes. colors indicate the magnitude of the *p*-value. To outline the *p*-value small than 0.05, only *p*-value range from 0 to 0.05 were presented by colors. The symbol "*" represents wcd_u in the abscissa node is significantly larger than that in the ordinate node, while the symbol "∇" represents wcd_u in the abscissa node is significantly less than that in the ordinate node.

lasting for 5 s, was manually delivered to CA3 in the hippocampus to evoke acute seizures. The acute seizure onset was identified when the value of time-domain features including line-length (LL), average amplitude (AMP), and slope (SLP) all exceeded the threshold which was calculated by OSTU algorithm in all detected channels (34). Each acute seizure induction stimulation was performed with an interval longer than 10 min. Only those rats with six successive successful induction seizures were used as the subjects in the subsequent experiments.

Key Targets Identification for Responsive Stimulation by Granger Causality Analysis

GC analysis was adopted to identify directed interaction between pairs of signals in multichannel signals. The main idea of GC is based on autoregressive (AR) modeling, in which a signal Y "Granger-causal" another signal X if the future of X can be predicted by the past Y and X. Moreover, the prediction error of X can be decreased with past Y as compared to only being predicted by the past values of X itself (37). For example, assuming two

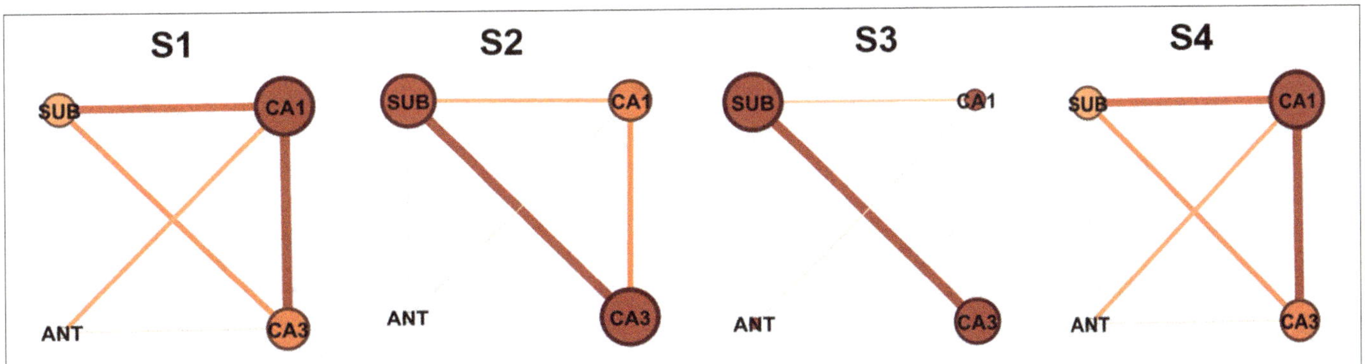

FIGURE 3 | Network characteristics of the nodes in different four rats. The size of the node and the darkness of color are in direct proportion to the G-causality value between different nodes. The width of the line represents the interaction strength between pairs of nodes. In each network illustration, the line thickness of weighted edges is proportional to the GC values, when significantly. Node size and color are proportional to the Ncd_u value for each node.

TABLE 1 | The performance of seizure detection algorithm in the acute seizures.

Subjects	Detected seizures	Detected duration(min)	Time Delay(s)	False alarm (/hr)	Detection rate
#S1	17	85	0.035	8	100%
#S2	15	75	1.088	10	100%
#S3	17	85	0.113	2	100%
#S4	18	90	0.807	2	100%
#S5	15	75	0.048	4	100%
#S6	18	90	0.173	13	100%
Total	100	500	0.377	6.5	100%

signals X(t) and Y(t) are covariance stationarity:

$$X(t) = \sum_{j=1}^{p} A_X X(t-j) + \varepsilon_1(t) \quad (1)$$

$$X(t) = \sum_{j=1}^{p} B_{XX} X(t-j) + \sum_{j=1}^{p} B_{XY} Y(t-j) + \varepsilon_2(t) \quad (2)$$

A univariate AR model of signal X is made by using past X values to predict future X values, as shown in (1). A bivariate AR model is calculated in (2), which combined the past X and Y to predict the future values of X. Here, p past values are included to predict the current value (p is the optimal AR model order), A_X, B_{XX}, *and* B_{XY} are the coefficients of AR models, and ε_1, $and \varepsilon_2$ are the prediction errors of signal X, respectively. As shown in (3), $F_{Y\to X}$ is the interaction magnitude of GC (from Y to X), calculated by the log ratio of the prediction error variances for AR model. When Y reduces the prediction error of X, the log ratio is positive and Y "Granger-cause" X. Instead, the opposite interaction can be assessed by reversing the positions of two signals.

$$F_{Y\to X} = In \frac{var(\varepsilon_1(t))}{var(\varepsilon_2(t))} \quad (3)$$

In this study, LFP data recorded from each of the four electrodes were analyzed for G-causality in the time domain using the Multivariate Granger Causality (MVGC) toolbox (38). GC was calculated in the first 5 s of seizure onset using the following parameters: window size of 2,000 samples, 50% window overlap, the number of surrogates 10 to determine the statistically significant connectivity between electrodes, and the AR model order was estimated using Bayesian Information Criterion (BIC) to a maximum of 30 lags, subsequently, pairwise GC values were calculated by MVGC routines (tsdata_to_var). then, unit causal density, $cd_u(i)$, which is the summed causal interactions involving node i, normalized by the number of nodes were measured for inferring the centricity of each electrode targeted in ANT, CA1, CA3, and SUB. Nodes with high values of cd_u can be considered to be causal hubs within the circuit (39). while unit causal density varied in order of magnitude from seizure to seizure and weighted cdu(i) [wcdu(i)] were calculated by cdu(i) dividing causal density [the sum of cdu(i)] to raise the comparability of data in different seizure event. The formula is depicted as follows, where n denotes the number of nodes.

$$cd_u(i) = \frac{1}{n} \sum_{i \neq j} F_{X_i \to X_j} \quad (4)$$

$$wcd(i) = \frac{cd_u(i)}{\sum_1^n cd_u(i)} \quad (5)$$

In order to illustrate the network by graphs clearly, networks were visualized by simple graphical depictions (**Figure 1B**); in this network, nodes represent targets of recording channels and edges represent G-causality between two nodes.

Generally speaking, cdu or wcdu of each node was a useful description of dynamic complexity, which reflected the total degree of inflow and outflow causal information. As is known, during the propagation of epileptic activity, transient information flow occurs among extensive brain networks. The brain regions with high cd_u or wcd_u values may indicate that they take an active part in the information interactions within the network. Therefore, these brain regions are considered to be causal hubs and are more likely targets than others for neuromodulation. Moreover, these nodes were likely to be key targets of RNS for seizure control.

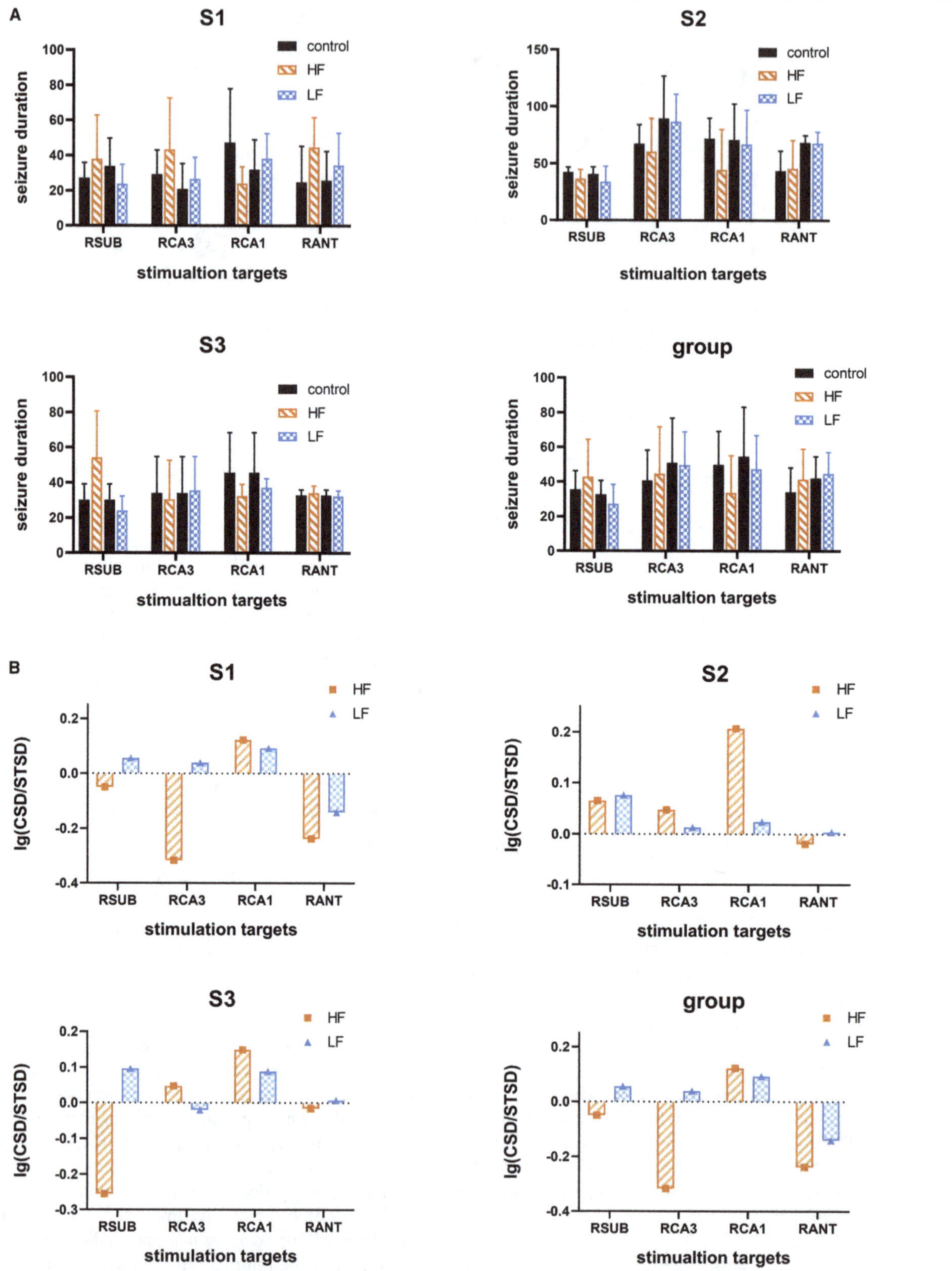

FIGURE 4 | The therapeutic effect of single target stimulation for seizure suppression. **(A)** The seizure duration under control condition and single target stimulation condition with high frequency (HF, 130 Hz) or low frequency (LF, 5 Hz). Data are represented as mean ± standard error (M ± SEM). **(B)** Logarithm (to the base 10) of the average seizure duration's ratio. The ratio of average seizure duration in the control condition without therapeutic stimulation to that in single target therapeutic

(Continued)

FIGURE 4 | stimulation with high frequency (130 Hz) or with low frequency (5 Hz). The bar value higher than zeros represents it was effective for seizure suppression, the higher the better. "CSD" represent the average seizure duration under control condition which without therapeutic stimulation. "STSD" represents the average seizure duration under single target therapeutic stimulation.

Single Target Stimulation on Key Targets

To evaluate the efficacy of seizure suppression in key targets which were found by GC, biphasic and charge-balanced therapeutic stimulation (100 μA amplitude, 300 μs pulse width, 5 s duration) with high frequency (130 Hz) or low frequency (5 Hz) was delivered to each of the four selected targets, namely SUB, CA3, CA1, and ANT, in three subjects after evoked seizures. As shown in **Figure 1D**, each rat will receive a single target stimulation condition and sham control condition, respectively, after acute seizure induction. The sham control condition received a fake stimulation without current after an evoked seizure was detected. While in the single target stimulation condition, therapeutic stimulation was delivered to one of the selected targets once acute seizure was detected. Each sham control condition trial was interleaved with one single target stimulation trial to access the efficacy of seizure control with different therapeutic protocols (high frequency or low frequency). To ensure the background of each trial is consistent, a 10-min interval was set between evoked stimulation delivery. Different stimulus types were randomly organized. For further statistical analyses, at least six trials were included in each different condition with different therapeutic stimulation protocols in the same test subject.

Combined Stimulations of Key Targets

To explore whether the combined stimulations of key targets would improve the efficacy of seizure control, combined therapeutic stimulations were delivered to potential therapeutic targets evaluated by the single target stimulation experiment. The process of the combined stimulation experiment was similar to the single target stimulation experiment. The combined stimulation condition would deliver the different combinations of high and low frequency stimulations to different targets simultaneously.

The Indicator of Seizure Severity

The duration of evoked seizures was counted as the indicator of seizure severity in this study since it was related to essential improvements in GABA functions (40). Teager energy (TE), which was found to be a reliable indicator for providing temporal markers for seizure onset and offset, was calculated in CA3 for counting seizure duration (41, 42). The LFP recorded in CA3 with 90 s before evoked stimulation was used as baseline. The criteria to select valid seizure activities was identified with a threshold of the mean of TE plus five times the standard deviation calculated by the baseline. Two typical examples of seizure duration counting were shown in **Supplementary Figure 2**.

Statistics Methods

Two different statistical analysis methods were used in this work. Kruskal-Wallis was applied to assess the significance of wcd_u between each different node. Student's t-test (t-test) was used to evaluate the significance of electrographic seizure duration changes between the control condition and stimulation condition under different therapeutic stimulation protocols. A $p < 0.05$ was identified as statistically significant.

RESULTS

Performance of Seizure Detection

The performance of the seizure detection algorithm was evaluated in six subjects before it was applied to our custom-made neural stimulator. As shown in **Table 1**, the seizure detection rate was 100% with an average 0.377 second time delay on account of a tiny step of the time window (120 ms) which was used for feature construction. However, a high false alarm rate was also reached in the meantime for the same reason. To reduce the impact of the false alarm, the function of auto seizure detection was disenabled until trigger stimulation for evoking acute seizure was delivered. Besides, once seizure onset was detected by the algorithm, the function of seizure detection was disenabled to ensure only one sequence of therapeutic stimulation was delivered for the corresponding evoked seizure treatment.

Key Targets Identification in The Temporal Lobe Epilepsy Model

According to the GC analysis results, nodes with a high value of wcd_u were considered as key targets of RNS for aborting seizures at the seizure onset network. As shown in **Figure 2**, four rats with successful induction of seizures were used in this analysis. A total of 76 seizures, excluding those with motion artifacts, S1 (n = 18), S2 (n = 19), S3 (n = 20), and S4 (n = 19), were randomly selected from four subjects and used for G-causality analysis. The wcd_u depicted by **Figure 2A** indicated the importance of each corresponding node. Based on this result, the significance value of wcd_u between each two different nodes was calculated by Kruskal-Wallis to demonstrate the significant difference of importance degree (**Figure 2B**). The results indicated that the target with the highest value wcd_u was varied among different subjects, however, the target with the lowest value was ANT which is uniform among the four subjects.

To visualize the interactions between nodes, graphical networks of acute seizure onset were shown in **Figure 3**. The nodes represent different electrode targets and the width of the line represents the mean value of G-causality calculated above. The node with a larger size and a darker color is more likely to be the key target. In each rat individually, the key nodes found by graphical networks and interaction characteristics had a strong similarity between the results depicted by wcd_u in **Figure 2** to some extent.

Above all, ANT should be excluded from key targets because it had the least influence among all stimulation targets. The target

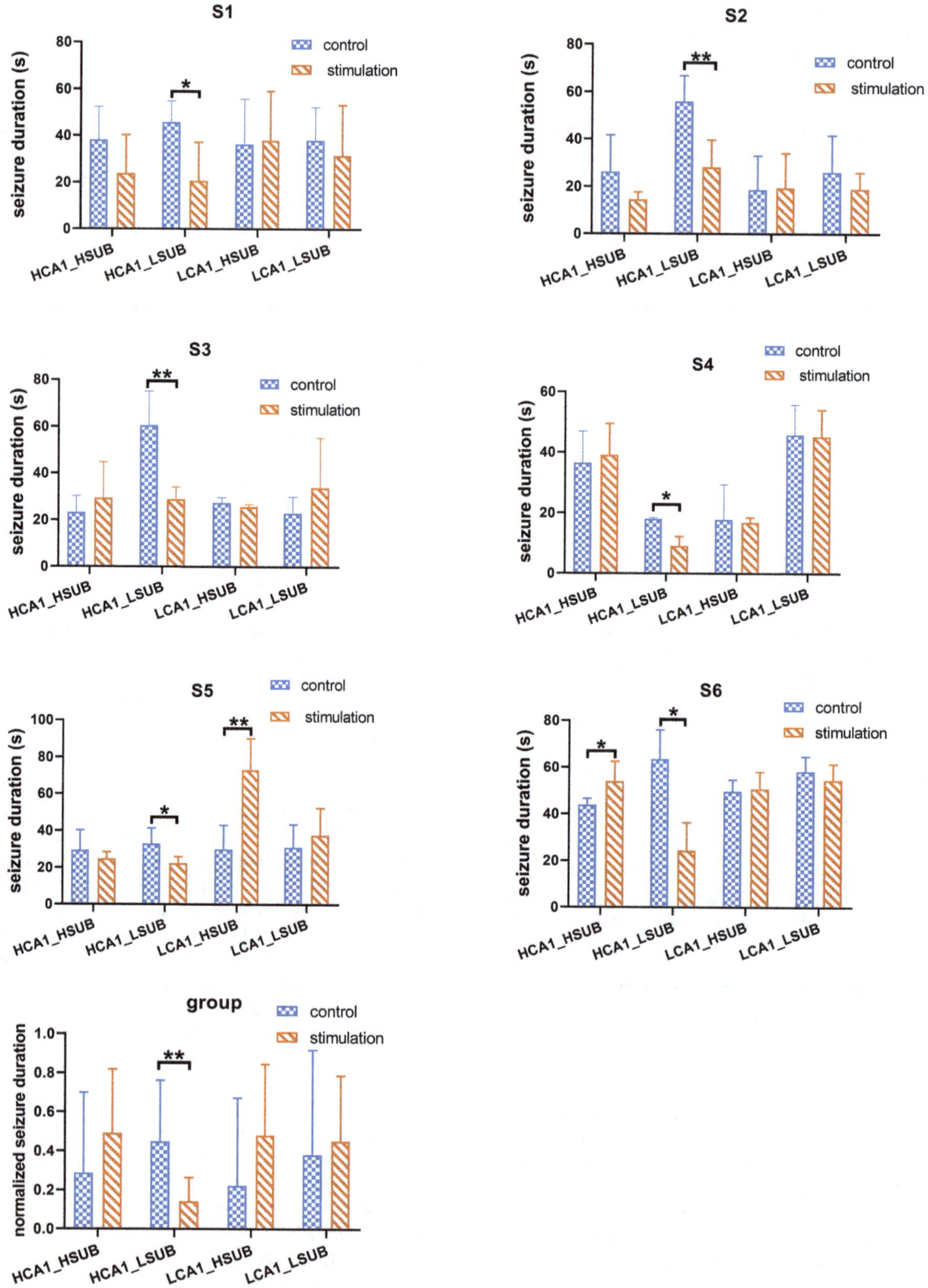

FIGURE 5 | The efficacy of combined stimulation under different stimulation protocols. HF_HF represents that both CA1 and SUB received HFS simultaneously. HF_LF represents that CA1 received HFS while SUB received LFS. LF_HF represents that LFS delivered to CA1 while HFS delivered to SUB. LF_LF represents LFS delivered to both CA1 and SUB in the same time. "*" represents $p < 0.05$. "**" represents $p < 0.01$.

of CA1, CA3, and SUB played more important roles in acute seizures of our TLE rat model, which were identified as two key targets in the following study.

Seizure Depression With Single Target Stimulation

To further evaluate the electrical stimulation efficacy on selected targets, high frequency stimulation (HFS, 130 Hz, 300 μs, 100 μA, 5 s) or low frequency stimulation (LFS, 5 Hz, 300 μs, 100 μA, 5 s) was delivered to one of four selected targets, namely SUB, CA3, CA1, and ANT, in three subjects. A total of 256 evoked seizures were statistically analyzed for evaluating the efficacy of single target stimulation. As shown in **Figure 4A**, there was no significant decrease (t-test, $p > 0.05$) of electrographic seizure duration between control condition and single target stimulation condition. The single target stimulation in all targets referred above was unable to shorten the electrographic seizure duration in this acute TLE model statistically. However, compared with other stimulation protocols, the result that LFS in SUB and HFS in CA1 reduced the average electrographic seizure duration was seen in all three rats (without a statistical difference). To further explore whether the HFS and LFS had different efficacy of seizure suppression, logarithm (to the base 10) of the ratio between average electrographic seizure duration in the control condition and that in stimulation condition was calculated. The average electrographic seizure duration in the control condition is longer than that in the stimulation condition when the logarithm value is bigger than zero. As displayed in **Figure 4B**, the results were consistent among three subjects that the logarithm value of LFS delivered to SUB is higher than HFS, while the logarithm value is larger when HFS was induced to CA1. Further, it also showed the stimulation protocol could shorten electrographic seizure duration. The larger value it has, the more effective it is. Therefore, it was suggested that SUB and CA1 may have a different response to LFS and HFS, while neither HFS and LFS could shorten the average seizure duration when delivered to ANT. In general, each different key node may have a distinct optimal stimulus frequency for seizure control. In this experiment SUB and CA1 may play a more important part than ANT for seizure control.

Seizure Depression With Combined Stimulations

Since the single target stimulation approach may underline the suboptimal efficacy of seizure control, it is important to consider whether the efficacy could be improved by combined stimulation. We further tested the combined stimulation on SUB and CA1 with different stimulation frequencies. Another three subjects were included in the combination stimulation experiment, as shown in **Figure 5**, the duration of 288 evoked seizures under combined stimulation in total six different subjects were statistically analyzed. The results illustrated only the combination of HFS in CA1 and LFS in SUB could significantly decrease the electrographic seizure duration of evoked seizures in all six tested subjects (t-test, $p < 0.05$). This result matched with the above single target stimulation result, that combined stimulations were able to shorten electrographic seizure duration efficiently when the stimulation frequency matched with optimal frequency in each target. It is particularly important to point out stimulation with unmatched frequency might even enhance the seizure activity, which may worsen the treatment of epilepsy. As shown in **Figure 5**, combined HFS in SUB with LFS in CA1 significantly increased the electrographic seizure duration in rat S5. Similarly, the seizure severity also deteriorated when both CA1 and SUB received HFS in rat S6.

DISCUSSION

The purpose of this research was to investigate whether the efficacy of brain stimulation for seizure control could be improved by combined stimulations of key targets with matched frequency. Three main findings could be noted as follows: (1) Key targets were proven more effective in seizure control tested by single target stimulation experiment, which was in line with the targets found by GC method; (2) The stimulus frequency played an important role in the stimulation approach for seizure control. Each different key node may have a prior stimulus frequency between 130 and 5 Hz for seizure control since LFS delivered to SUB and HFS delivered to CA1 could shorten the average electrographic seizure duration; and (3) Combined stimulation with matched frequency could significantly decrease the duration of evoked electrographic seizures, which was more effective than single target stimulation.

Epilepsy is a network disorder with potential aberrance in nodes and/or pathways (43). A deeper understanding of the dynamics of epileptogenic networks may control and regulate seizure activity more effectively. As a way to measure the dynamic of epileptogenic networks, GC estimates of connectivity in the network have been shown to have some reference value. It has shown similar results to dynamic causal modeling, which has plausible estimates of human seizure propagation pathway and is in line with pathways demonstrated with DTI as well (44). However, the mathematical protocol for epileptogenic network analysis like GC does not merely help in understanding those progresses but also has a guiding value for establishing the RNS treatment strategies for epilepsy. Such techniques are practical and have potential to be used in clinical treatment. In this work, GC was used to find the key targets which have tight interconnections with other nodes during seizure onset, and it has the potential to aid therapeutic intervention like RNS. The single target stimulation for evaluating the efficacy of seizure suppression in each different node showed that the mean electrographic seizure duration could be shortened when key targets found by GC received matched therapeutic stimulation, while others are not. It suggested that GC could provide valuable insights into looking for potential targets for RNS in the specific epileptogenic network, though much more work should be carried out to support this conclusion.

The current neuromodulation technique is considered as a complementary rather than alternative treatment option to those patients who cannot benefit from conventional treatment (3). The approach of single target stimulation may underline the limited efficacy, since lots of regions involved in epileptic activity may occupy a vital position in seizure onset (45, 46). Therefore, the stimulation delivered to a single region alone might not abort seizure activity sufficiently (25, 46), which was also supported by a single target stimulation experiment in this study. To sum up, it is worthwhile to investigate the combined stimulation method (47). However, to our knowledge, only a few studies were performed on this aspect. Li et.al concentrated on a novel electrical stimulation approach involving distributed multielectrode microstimulation at the epileptic focus, which proved that distributed stimulation delivered together may be more effective to seizure control (48). Bertram et.al mainly focused on the circuits that support the different stages of seizures developed from a system's view of epilepsy. But this study was at the theoretical stage and no animal experiment was performed to evaluate the relationship between the epileptogenic network and stimulation pattern (46). Tung et.al introduced how precise multi-focal control of pathological circuits with optogenetic stimulation can be advantageous for the treatment of epilepsy (25). Nevertheless, whether a similar answer would be achieved on RNS, a more clinically achievable method has not been explored. In the current research, we only chose key targets that were found by GC method and evaluated by single target stimulation as our targets for combined stimulations. It is interesting to note that the key targets found by GC method are not exactly the most effective node for decreasing the average electrographic seizure duration in our acute TLE model. CA3 was proven to be a key node in seizure onset by GC but stimulation of CA3 was unable to shorten electrographic seizure duration in the single target stimulation experiment, which is not consistent with the previous studies (49). One possible explanation for the ineffective CA3 stimulation is that the trigger stimulation was also located in CA3 shortly before (3s in average) therapeutic stimulation. More studies of single or combined target brain stimulation could be performed on the chronic TLE model which may mimic clinical situations better.

In addition to the location of stimulation, the frequency of stimulation is another crucial factor of brain stimulation that inhibits seizure activity. Both HFS and LFS were studied for seizure control. HFS has been proven to be effective in many clinical and animal studies and LFS of a white matter tract reduced epileptiform discharges and seizures in patients (13). Similar to our result, HFS was more effective than LFS in CA1, which is in accord with a prior work that focused on comparing the efficacy between HFS and LFS delivered to the hippocampus in epileptic rats (50). Not all of our results were consistent with other studies. Both HFS and LFS delivered to SUB were demonstrated to be effective in seizure control (22, 51). However, LFS was superior to HFS in SUB in our current study. Moreover, the combined stimulation with matched frequencies in SUB and CA1 illustrated more effectiveness in seizure control. The effectiveness of combined stimulation may partly be on account of the stimulation energy since the combined stimulation will deliver twice as much electricity into the brain compared with single target stimulation. On the other hand, the matched optimal stimulation frequency is the most important factor for effective seizure control, for combined stimulation with unmatched frequency increased seizure duration conversely. These findings indicated that the efficacy of combined stimulation may be achieved by accumulating the effect of single target stimulation.

The evoked stimulation only induced to those pilocarpine model with spontaneous seizure; it demonstrated many pathophysiological mechanisms associated with epileptogenesis already exist before induced stimulation, including mossy fiber sprouting and interneuron loss ad granule cell dispersion in the dentate gyrus (52). It increased sensitivity for induced seizures to the kindling model in this pilocarpine-pretreated model. In our study, every induced electrographic seizure combined with behavior, however, it is a pity that not all behavior combined with electrographic seizure was collected and analyzed in this study. There was an essential difference between a spontaneous seizure and induced seizure since the stimulation targets located in CA3 may the reason CA1 and SUB have a higher GC value than ANT, although this model still provided a platform for us to study effective RNS protocols to reduce the severity of seizures. Effective RNS remains a choke point for long-term spontaneous seizure detection.

Our findings in this work provide valuable insights into the combined brain stimulation approach to improve the efficacy of seizure control. We do not deny the existence of other effective protocols of combined stimulation. However, it is difficult to evaluate the most effective one for seizure control by going through all the combined stimulation protocols, due to the existence of sophisticated conditions in this work. Besides, the stimulation frequencies selected in this current work were according to previous works and mainly depended on trial and error. Moreover, the acute TLE model was used in this study because of the limitation of the seizure detection algorithm, which has a very unified seizure type among different trials and subjects similar to kainic acid model (53). This is also different from various seizure onset types that existed in the clinical and chronic TLE animal model. If the different combinations of key targets did exist in different seizure onset types, it is still important to consider how to alter the approach of brain stimulation to improve the efficacy of seizure control. Combining all key targets found in different types of seizures together or a adaptive stimulation will be needed in such a situation. Therefore, more focus is needed on the intrinsic relationship between the epileptogenic network and stimulus parameters, and more methods are required to find out the most appropriate brain modulation method for refectory epilepsy in the future.

AUTHOR CONTRIBUTIONS

FZ, YZ, and KX designed this study. FZ organized the data. FZ and YY performed the data analysis and drafted the manuscript. JZ, PW, and KX revised the manuscript. All authors approved the final manuscript.

FUNDING

This work was supported by the grant from National

Key R&D Program of China (2018YFA0701400), the National Natural Science Foundation of China (31627802, 81873911), the Public Projects of Zhejiang Province (2019C03033), and the Fundamental Research Funds for the Central Universities (2019XZZX001-01-01, 2020FZZX001-05 and 2021KYY600403-0001).

REFERENCES

1. Mogul DJ, van Drongelen W. Electrical control of epilepsy. *Annu Rev Biomed Eng.* (2014) 16:483–504. doi: 10.1146/annurev-bioeng-071813-104720
2. Kwan P, Brodie MJ. Early identification of refractory epilepsy. *N Engl J Med.* (2000) 342:314–19. doi: 10.1056/NEJM200002033420503
3. Schulze-Bonhage A. Brain stimulation as a neuromodulatory epilepsy therapy. *Seizure.* (2017) 44:169–75. doi: 10.1016/j.seizure.2016.10.026
4. Jobst BC, Kapur R, Barkley GL, Bazil CW, Berg MJ, Bergey GK, et al. Brain-responsive neurostimulation in patients with medically intractable seizures arising from eloquent and other neocortical areas. *Epilepsia.* (2017) 58:1005–14. doi: 10.1111/epi.13844
5. Geller EB, Skarpaas TL, Gross RE, Goodman RR, Barkley GL, Bazil CW, et al. Brain-responsive neurostimulation in patients with medically intractable mesial temporal lobe epilepsy. *Epilepsia.* (2017) 58:994–1004. doi: 10.1111/epi.13740
6. Sisterson ND, Wozny TA, Kokkinos V, Constantino A, Richardson RM. Closed-loop brain stimulation for drug-resistant epilepsy: towards an evidence-based approach to personalized medicine. *Neurotherapeutics.* (2019) 16:119–27. doi: 10.1007/s13311-018-00682-4
7. Toyoda I, Bower MR, Leyva F, Buckmaster PS. Early activation of ventral hippocampus and subiculum during spontaneous seizures in a rat model of temporal lobe epilepsy. *J Neurosci.* (2013) 33:11100–15. doi: 10.1523/JNEUROSCI.0472-13.2013
8. Huang L. Search for new targets of deep brain stimulation for epilepsy treatment. *J Neurol Res Therapy.* (2016) 1:23–33. doi: 10.14302/issn.2470-5020.jnrt-15-800
9. Wang Y, Liang J, Xu C, Wang Y, Kuang Y, Xu Z, et al. Low-frequency stimulation in anterior nucleus of thalamus alleviates kainate-induced chronic epilepsy and modulates the hippocampal Eeg rhythm. *Exp Neurol.* (2016) 276:22–30. doi: 10.1016/j.expneurol.2015.11.014
10. Bayat A, Skopin MD, Joshi S, Siddu M, Mukharesh L, Jahan S, et al. Effects of low-frequency electrical stimulation of the anterior piriform cortex on kainate-induced seizures in rats. *Epilepsy Behav.* (2017) 72:1–7. doi: 10.1016/j.yebeh.2017.04.002
11. D'Arcangelo G, Panuccio G, Tancredi V, Avoli M. Repetitive low-frequency stimulation reduces epileptiform synchronization in limbic neuronal networks. *Neurobiol Dis.* (2005) 19:119–s28. doi: 10.1016/j.nbd.2004.11.012
12. S, Fisher R. Neurostimulation for epilepsy: do we know the best stimulation parameters. *Epilepsy Curr.* (2011) 11:203–4. doi: 10.5698/1535-7511-11.6.203
13. Rajdev P, Ward M, Irazoqui P. Effect of stimulus parameters in the treatment of seizures by electrical stimulation in the Kainate animal model. *Int J Neural Syst.* (2011) 21:51–62. doi: 10.1142/S0129065711002730
14. Schiller Y, Bankirer Y. Cellular mechanisms underlying antiepileptic effects of low- and high-frequency electrical stimulation in acute epilepsy in neocortical brain slices *in vitro*. *J Neurophysiol.* (2007) 97:1887–902. doi: 10.1152/jn.00514.2006
15. Toprani S, Durand DM. Fiber tract stimulation can reduce epileptiform activity in an *in-vitro* bilateral hippocampal slice preparation. *Experi Neurol.* (2013) 240:28–43. doi: 10.1016/j.expneurol.2012.10.022
16. Toprani S, Durand DM. Long-lasting hyperpolarization underlies seizure reduction by low frequency deep brain electrical stimulation. *J Physiol.* (2013) 591:5765–90. doi: 10.1113/jphysiol.2013.253757
17. Han CL, Hu W, Stead M, Zhang T, Zhang JG, Worrell GA, et al. Electrical stimulation of hippocampus for the treatment of refractory temporal lobe epilepsy. *Brain Res Bull.* (2014) 109:13–21. doi: 10.1016/j.brainresbull.2014.08.007
18. Wozny TA, Lipski WJ, Alhourani A, Kondylis ED, Antony A, Richardson RM. Effects of hippocampal low-frequency stimulation in idiopathic non-human primate epilepsy assessed via a remote-sensing-enabled neurostimulator. *Exp Neurol.* (2017) 294:68–77. doi: 10.1016/j.expneurol.2017.05.003
19. Rashid S, Pho G, Czigler M, Werz MA, Durand DM. Low frequency stimulation of ventral hippocampal commissures reduces seizures in a rat model of chronic temporal lobe epilepsy. *Epilepsia.* (2012) 53:147–56. doi: 10.1111/j.1528-1167.2011.03348.x
20. Elder C, Friedman D, Devinsky O, Doyle W, Dugan P. Responsive neurostimulation targeting the anterior nucleus of the thalamus in 3 patients with treatment-resistant multifocal epilepsy. *Epilepsia Open.* (2019) 4:187–92. doi: 10.1002/epi4.12300
21. Huang L, Luijtelaar G. The effects of acute responsive high frequency stimulation of the subiculum on the intra-hippocampal kainic acid seizure model in rats. *Brain Behav.* (2012) 2:532–40. doi: 10.1002/brb3.70
22. Huang L, van Luijtelaar G. The effects of responsive and scheduled subicular high frequency stimulation in the intra-hippocampal Kainic acid seizure model. *Epilepsy Res.* (2013) 106:326–37. doi: 10.1016/j.eplepsyres.2013.06.010
23. Stefan H, Lopes da Silva HF. Epileptic neuronal networks: methods of identification and clinical relevance. *Front Neurol.* (2013) 4:8. doi: 10.3389/fneur.2013.00008
24. Pittau F, Megevand P, Sheybani L, Abela E, Grouiller F, Spinelli L, et al. Mapping epileptic activity: sources or networks for the clinicians?. *Front Neurol.* (2014) 5:218. doi: 10.3389/fneur.2014.00218
25. Tung JK, Shiu FH, Ding K, Gross RE. Chemically activated luminopsins allow optogenetic inhibition of distributed nodes in an epileptic network for non-invasive and multi-site suppression of seizure activity. *Neurobiol Dis.* (2018) 109:1–10. doi: 10.1016/j.nbd.2017.09.007
26. Cadotte AJ, DeMarse TB, Mareci TH, Parekh MB, Talathi SS, Hwang DU, et al. Granger causality relationships between local field potentials in an animal model of temporal lobe epilepsy. *J Neurosci Methods.* (2010) 189:121–9. doi: 10.1016/j.jneumeth.2010.03.007
27. Seth A K, Barrett A B, Barnett L. Granger causality analysis in neuroscience and neuroimaging. *J Neurosci.* (2015) 35:3293–97. doi: 10.1523/JNEUROSCI.4399-14.2015
28. Park EH, Madsen JR. Granger causality analysis of interictal ieeg predicts seizure focus and ultimate resection. *Neurosurgery.* (2018) 82:99–109. doi: 10.1093/neuros/nyx195
29. Epstein CM, Adhikari BM, Gross R, Willie J, Dhamala M. Application of high-frequency granger causality to analysis of epileptic seizures and surgical decision making. *Epilepsia.* (2014) 55:2038–47. doi: 10.1111/epi.12831
30. Pesaran B, Vinck M, Einevoll GT, Sirota A, Fries P, Siegel M, et al. Investigating large-scale brain dynamics using field potential recordings: analysis and interpretation. *Nat Neurosci.* (2018) 21:903–19. doi: 10.1038/s41593-018-0171-8
31. Zhang F, Zheng Y, Yu C, Wu HC, Zhu J, Xu K. Combined multi-frequency responsive stimulation for effective seizure suppression in temporal lobe epilepsy model. In: *2019 IEEE Biomedical Circuits and Systems Conference (BioCAS).* Nara (2019). p. 1–4. doi: 10.1109/BIOCAS.2019.8919041
32. Zheng Y, Gao H, Zhang J, Wang Y, Zhang S, Xu K, et al. Multi-site closed-loop stimulation strategy for seizure control with a generalized neurostimulator. In: *Neural Engineering (NER), 2017 8th International IEEE/EMBS Conference on IEEE.* Shanghai (2017). doi: 10.1109/NER.2017.8008340
33. Xu K, Zheng Y, Zhang F, Jiang Z, Qi Y, Chen H, et al. An energy efficient adaboost cascade method for long-term seizure detection in portable neurostimulators. *IEEE Trans Neural Syst Rehabil Eng.* (2019) 27:2274–83. doi: 10.1109/TNSRE.2019.2947426
34. Zheng Y, Jiang Z, Ping A, Zhang F, Zhu J, Wang Y, et al. Acute seizure control efficacy of multi-site closed-loop stimulation in a temporal lobe seizure model. *IEEE Trans Neural Syst Rehabil Eng.* (2019) 27:419–28. doi: 10.1109/TNSRE.2019.2894746
35. Otsu N. A threshold selection method from gray-level histograms. *IEEE Trans Syst Man Cybern.* (1979) 1:62–6. doi: 10.1109/TSMC.1979.4310076
36. Sobayo T, Mogul DJ. Should stimulation parameters be individualized to stop seizures: evidence in support of this approach. *Epilepsia.* (2016) 57:131–40. doi: 10.1111/epi.13259

37. Granger CW. Investigating causal relations by econometric models and cross-spectral methods. *Econometrica.* (1969) 37:424–38. doi: 10.2307/1912791
38. Barnett L, Seth AK. The Mvgc multivariate granger causality toolbox: a new approach to granger-causal inference. *J Neurosci Methods.* (2014) 223:50–68. doi: 10.1016/j.jneumeth.2013.10.018
39. Seth AK. A Matlab toolbox for granger causal connectivity analysis. *J Neurosci Methods.* (2010) 186:262–73. doi: 10.1016/j.jneumeth.2009.11.020
40. Upadhya D, Hattiangady B, Castro OW, Shuai B, Kodali M, Attaluri S, et al. Human induced pluripotent stem cell-derived mge cell grafting after status epilepticus attenuates chronic epilepsy and comorbidities via synaptic integration. *Proc Natl Acad Sci USA.* (2019) 116:287–96. doi: 10.1073/pnas.1814185115
41. Zaveri HP, Williams WJ, Sackellares JC. Energy based detection of seizures. *Annu Int Conf IEEE Eng Med Biol.* (1993) 39:363–64.
42. Sobayo T, Fine AS, Gunnar E, Kazlauskas C, Nicholls D, Mogul DJ. Synchrony dynamics across brain structures in limbic epilepsy vary between initiation and termination phases of seizures. *IEEE Trans Biomed Eng.* (2013) 60:821–9. doi: 10.1109/TBME.2012.2189113
43. Gummadavelli A, Zaveri HP, Spencer DD, Gerrard JL. Expanding brain-computer interfaces for controlling epilepsy networks: novel thalamic responsive neurostimulation in refractory epilepsy. *Front Neurosci.* (2018) 12:474. doi: 10.3389/fnins.2018.00474
44. Coben R, Mohammad-Rezazadeh I. Neural connectivity in epilepsy as measured by granger causality. *Front Hum Neurosci.* (2015) 9:194. doi: 10.3389/fnhum.2015.00194
45. Wang Y, Trevelyan AJ, Valentin A, Alarcon G, Taylor PN, Kaiser M. Mechanisms underlying different onset patterns of focal seizures. *PLoS Comput Biol.* (2017) 13:e1005475. doi: 10.1371/journal.pcbi.1005475
46. Bertram EH. Neuronal Circuits in epilepsy: do they matter?. *Exp Neurol.* (2013) 244:67–74. doi: 10.1016/j.expneurol.2012.01.028
47. Li MCH, Cook MJ. Deep brain stimulation for drug-resistant epilepsy. *Epilepsia.* (2018) 59:273–90. doi: 10.1111/epi.13964
48. Desai SA, Rolston JD, McCracken CE, Potter SM, Gross RE. Asynchronous distributed multielectrode microstimulation reduces seizures in the dorsal tetanus toxin model of temporal lobe epilepsy. *Brain Stimul.* (2016) 9:86–100. doi: 10.1016/j.brs.2015.08.008
49. Sun HL, Zhang SH, Zhong K, Xu ZH, Zhu W, Fang Q, et al. Mode-dependent effect of low-frequency stimulation targeting the hippocampal Ca3 subfield on amygdala-kindled seizures in rats. *Epilepsy Res.* (2010) 90:83–90. doi: 10.1016/j.eplepsyres.2010.03.011
50. Wyckhuys T, Raedt R, Vonck K, Wadman W, Boon P. Comparison of hippocampal deep brain stimulation with high (130hz) and low frequency (5hz) on afterdischarges in kindled rats. *Epilepsy Res.* (2010) 88:239–46. doi: 10.1016/j.eplepsyres.2009.11.014
51. Zhong K, Wu DC, Jin MM, Xu ZH, Wang Y, Hou WW, et al. Wide therapeutic time-window of low-frequency stimulation at the subiculum for temporal lobe epilepsy treatment in rats. *Neurobiol Dis.* (2012) 48:20–6. doi: 10.1016/j.nbd.2012.05.011
52. Curia G, Longo D, Biagini G, Jones RS, Avoli M. The pilocarpine model of temporal lobe epilepsy. *J Neurosci Methods.* (2008) 172:143–57. doi: 10.1016/j.jneumeth.2008.04.019
53. Upadhya D, Kodali M, Gitai D, Castro OW, Zanirati G, Upadhya R, et al. A model of chronic temporal lobe epilepsy presenting constantly rhythmic and robust spontaneous seizures, co-morbidities and hippocampal neuropathology. *Aging Dis.* (2019) 10:915–36. doi: 10.14336/AD.2019.0720

9

Refining Planning for Stereoelectroencephalography: A Prospective Validation of Spatial Priors for Computer-Assisted Planning with Application of Dynamic Learning

Vejay N. Vakharia[1,2,3*], *Rachel E. Sparks*[4], *Alejandro Granados*[4], *Anna Miserocchi*[1,2,3], *Andrew W. McEvoy*[1,2,3], *Sebastien Ourselin*[4] *and John S. Duncan*[1,2,3]

[1] Department of Clinical and Experimental Epilepsy, University College London, London, United Kingdom, [2] National Hospital for Neurology and Neurosurgery, London, United Kingdom, [3] Chalfont Centre for Epilepsy, London, United Kingdom, [4] School of Biomedical Engineering and Imaging Sciences, King's College London, London, United Kingdom

***Correspondence:**
Vejay N. Vakharia
v.vakharia@ucl.ac.uk

Objective: Stereoelectroencephalography (SEEG) is a procedure in which many electrodes are stereotactically implanted within different regions of the brain to estimate the epileptogenic zone in patients with drug-refractory focal epilepsy. Computer-assisted planning (CAP) improves risk scores, gray matter sampling, orthogonal drilling angles to the skull and intracerebral length in a fraction of the time required for manual planning. Due to differences in planning practices, such algorithms may not be generalizable between institutions. We provide a prospective validation of clinically feasible trajectories using "spatial priors" derived from previous implantations and implement a machine learning classifier to adapt to evolving planning practices.

Methods: Thirty-two patients underwent consecutive SEEG implantations utilizing computer-assisted planning over 2 years. Implanted electrodes from the first 12 patients (108 electrodes) were used as a training set from which entry and target point spatial priors were generated. CAP was then prospectively performed using the spatial priors in a further test set of 20 patients (210 electrodes). A K-nearest neighbor (K-NN) machine learning classifier was implemented as an adaptive learning method to modify the spatial priors dynamically.

Results: All of the 318 prospective computer-assisted planned electrodes were implanted without complication. Spatial priors developed from the training set generated clinically feasible trajectories in 79% of the test set. The remaining 21% required entry or target points outside of the spatial priors. The K-NN classifier was able to dynamically model real-time changes in the spatial priors in order to adapt to the evolving planning requirements.

Conclusions: We provide spatial priors for common SEEG trajectories that prospectively integrate clinically feasible trajectory planning practices from previous

SEEG implantations. This allows institutional SEEG experience to be incorporated and used to guide future implantations. The deployment of a K-NN classifier may improve the generalisability of the algorithm by dynamically modifying the spatial priors in real-time as further implantations are performed.

Keywords: stereoelectroencephalography, EpiNav, computer-assisted planning, machine learning, spatial priors, epilepsy surgery

INTRODUCTION

Stereotactic neurosurgery requires precise pre-operative trajectory planning and accurate implementation to ensure safety and efficacy. Stereoelectroencephalography (SEEG) is a diagnostic procedure in which multiple electrodes, typically 10–16, are implanted within the brain in patients with drug-refractory focal epilepsy to approximate the epileptogenic zone so that subsequent resective or ablative interventions can render the patient seizure-free. The most significant risk of this procedure is intracerebral hemorrhage, which results in significant morbidity in 2–3% of cases (1). Various surgical techniques are employed for insertion of SEEG electrodes including frame-based, frameless and robotic methods with mean target point accuracies of 2–3 mm (2, 3). To maximize safety, surgeons plan SEEG trajectories to maximize distance from vasculature. Other important considerations include accurate targeting of the regions of interest (ROIs), avoidance of critical structures, maximizing gray-matter sampling, orthogonal drilling angles to the skull, avoidance of other electrodes, optimal spatial sampling of the putative epileptogenic zone and minimizing intracerebral trajectory length. Various computer-assisted planning (CAP) algorithms have been employed to optimize these factors. EpiNav™ is one such stereotactic planning platform that has been applied to SEEG (4–6), laser interstitial thermal therapy (7, 8) and tumor biopsy (9). Previous studies have shown external blinded feasibility ratings of CAP generated trajectories were not significantly different from expert manually planned trajectories, yet due to the wide variation in individual surgeon's planning preferences, these were 62 and 69%, respectively (5). Another potential reason for this is the reliance on whole-brain parcellations to constrain the entry and target points, which in many cases are large structures that require multiple electrodes to pass through them. Furthermore, the algorithms are static without the ability to adapt or learn from previous trajectory planning experience.

Here we present the most extensive series to date of patients that have undergone prospective SEEG planning with CAP. We provide spatial priors to augment CAP by learning from the first 12 patients as a "training set" and subsequently applying this to the prospective planning of a further 20 patients as a "test set." To aid in the generalisability of the algorithm, we additionally utilize K-nearest neighbor (K-NN) clustering as an active learning algorithm to dynamically modify the priors based on individual surgeon's planning preferences.

Abbreviations: CAP, Computer-assisted planning; K-NN, K-nearest neighbor; PET, Positron emission tomography; ROI, Regions of interest; SEEG, Stereoelectroencephalography; SPECT, Single-photon emission computer tomography; WCSS, Within-cluster sum of squares.

METHODS

Patient Inclusion

A total of 32 patients (17 male) with drug-resistant focal epilepsy, in whom SEEG was performed as part of their routine care at The National Hospital for Neurology and Neurosurgery, London, U.K., were included in this prospective validation study. Patients underwent SEEG implantation between February 2017 and March 2019.

All patients underwent a standardized multi-disciplinary assessment consisting of specialist input from neurologists, neurosurgeons, neurophysiologists, neuropsychologists, and psychiatrists. SEEG trajectory target selection was based on an estimation of the seizure onset zone derived from a review of all pre-surgical investigations, including the clinical history and semiology, scalp EEG/video telemetry, neuropsychological and neuropsychiatric evaluations, structural, and functional MRI, PET, and SPECT imaging. Entry regions were also specified for SEEG trajectories where the lateral neocortex was also of electrophysiological interest.

Ethical Approval

Ethical approval for this study was provided by the National Research Ethics Service Committee London, approval reference: 12/LO/0377. Written consent was obtained from all patients before inclusion in the study.

TABLE 1 | Computer-assisted planning parameters.

Parameter	Value
Intracerebral length (mm)	<90
Drilling angle to the skull (deg)	<30 to orthogonal
Gray matter sampling ratio	Maximize
Minimum distance from vasculature (mm)	>3
Risk score	<1
Avoidance of critical structures	Superficial sulcal model
	Vascular model
	Basal ganglia/brainstem
	Frontal and occipital horns of the lateral ventricles.
Distance between electrodes (mm)	>10

EpiNav™

Pre-operative SEEG planning was performed within the EpiNav™ platform (Center for Medical Imaging Computing, University College London/King's College London) which has been described previously (4). In brief, a single gadolinium-enhanced T1 acquisition is used as a reference image to which all other imaging modalities are registered. A whole-brain parcellation was generated, using Geodesic Information Flow version 3.0 (GIF) (10), from which models of the cortex, gray matter and sulci are extracted in an automated fashion. Vascular segmentations were performed following application of a Sato filter to the pre-operative digital subtraction angiography and manual thresholding (11). Digital subtraction angiography was performed 1–2 weeks before SEEG implantation under local anesthesia in the biplanar angiography suite. Depending on the spatial distribution of the SEEG implantation and the patient's individual anatomy, injections of the ipsilateral internal carotid artery and a vertebral artery were performed. The EpiNav™ algorithm generates SEEG trajectories based on optimization of user-defined parameters, which include intracerebral length, drilling angle to the skull, gray matter sampling ratio, minimum distance from vasculature, risk score, and avoidance of critical structures (12). For an in-depth discussion on planning parameter selection see (13). The user-defined parameters applied during this study are shown in **Table 1**.

The risk score is a mathematical representation of the size of the avascular corridor through which the planned trajectory passes in order to reach the target. It is calculated by fitting 128 nodes along the planned trajectory and measuring the distance between the trajectory and vasculature at each node (4, 14). A cumulative score is then provided scaled by the minimum distance defined by the user. In this study, a 3 mm minimum distance from vasculature was applied, resulting in trajectories that pass within 3 mm of a vessel returning a risk score >1. The 3 mm safety margin is a user-defined setting within the software that can be altered based on the planning preferences of the neurosurgeon. Based on our previous implantation accuracies (15) and the recommendations of Cardinale et al. (16), we calculate the minimum permissible distance from vasculature using the following equation:

$$Safety\ Margin\ \ (mm) = Electrode\ radius\ \ (mm) + \frac{\Sigma \left\| i - \hat{i} \right\|}{n} + 3\sigma$$

where, $\frac{\Sigma\left\|i-\hat{i}\right\|}{n}$ represents the mean implantation error and σ the standard deviation of the implantation error.

The user inputs the implantation strategy by typing or selecting the anatomical ROIs. The entry and target regions are based on the segmentation provided by the GIF parcellation. For pragmatic purposes, we define the entry region as the most superficial anatomical structure through which the trajectory enters the brain and the target region as the deepest point of the trajectory. The vector between the entry and target point defines the trajectory vector. We stress that during SEEG procedures all gray matter contact points along the trajectory are considered target structures and hence we extend implantations to deep structures so that as much information as possible can be gained from each implanted electrode. Constraining the automated planning algorithm to the target region alone allows the global minima to be identified for that target region whereas the additional constraint of the entry region returns the local minima. An example of a typical strategy and plan generated from the GIF parcellation is shown in **Figure 1**. The automated planning algorithm first removes trajectories that do not adhere to the length and angle constraints. Next, trajectories that do not pass through the entry region, if specified, or conflict with critical structures are also removed. The remaining trajectories are then optimized for gray matter sampling and returned to the user in a risk-stratified manner, i.e., lowest risk first. For a more detailed description of the computer-assisted planning algorithm please see (4, 6).

After CAP, the user reviews each trajectory to ensure clinical feasibility and safety. The potential trajectories generated for a specific target (or entry-target pair) can be iterated through using

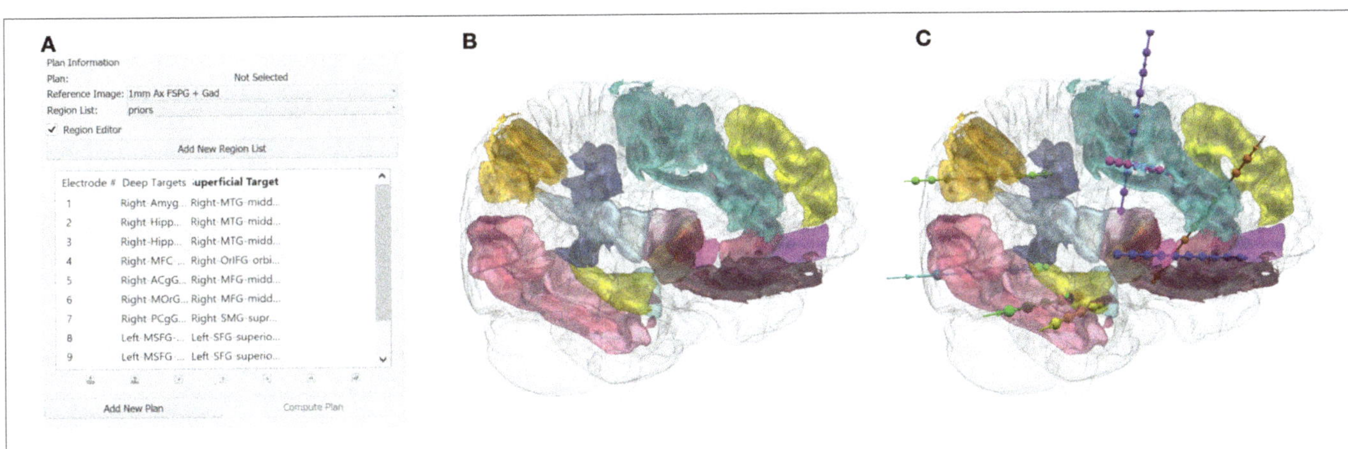

FIGURE 1 | (A) A illustrative example of an anatomy-driven multiple trajectory planning strategy (3), with the target and entry points for the trajectory specified by the user. **(B)** The 3D segmentation of the whole brain structures outlined in the strategy and **(C)** the corresponding CAP trajectories optimizing for the user-defined parameters.

the “Next Entry” or “Next Target” functions. Manual changes to the entry and target points can also be performed by the user if no suitable CAP generated trajectory is found.

Cluster Generation

Following prospective SEEG planning and surgical implantation in the first 12 cases (108 electrodes), each patient’s reference image was normalized to the MNI-152 (ICBM 2009a Non-linear Asymmetric) group template (17). The parameters for transformation were then applied to the electrode trajectories and coordinate points for the entry and target points were extracted. Right and left side trajectories were combined through flipping. Entry point coordinates were taken at the intersection of the planned trajectory and the cortical surface. The cluster centroids for trajectories were calculated from the coordinates in cases in which the ROI was targeted five or more times to form the training set. Trajectories targeting patient-specific abnormalities, such as lesions or PET/SPECT abnormalities were excluded as these were not generalizable. A total of 13 entry and 14 target ROIs were included. Within-cluster sum of squares (WCSS) was calculated to quantify the extent of variance. Based on the normalized trajectories, spatial priors were then generated to constrain the entry and target points.

Prospective Validation

Prospective planning was performed in a further 20 patients (210 electrodes) with spatial priors derived from the training set. The predictive utility of the spatial priors was determined by the proportion of trajectories that passed through both the entry and target priors. In addition, the Euclidean distances between the cluster centroids from the prospective trajectories (test set) and those derived from the first 12 cases (training set) were calculated.

Adaptive Learning

We also implemented a system whereby spatial priors could adapt to evolving SEEG planning practices. The added flexibility would allow the priors to adapt and potentially incorporate new entry or target points outside of the original priors. This would permit external institutions to use the above spatial priors as a starting point and, with subsequent SEEG implantations, enable it to adapt to the individual surgeon’s or institutional preferences. This was accomplished through the implementation of a K-Nearest Neighbor (K-NN) classifier to the prospective validation dataset. The K-NN was deployed using Euclidean distance from 5 uniformly weighted neighbors to determine the classifier assignments.

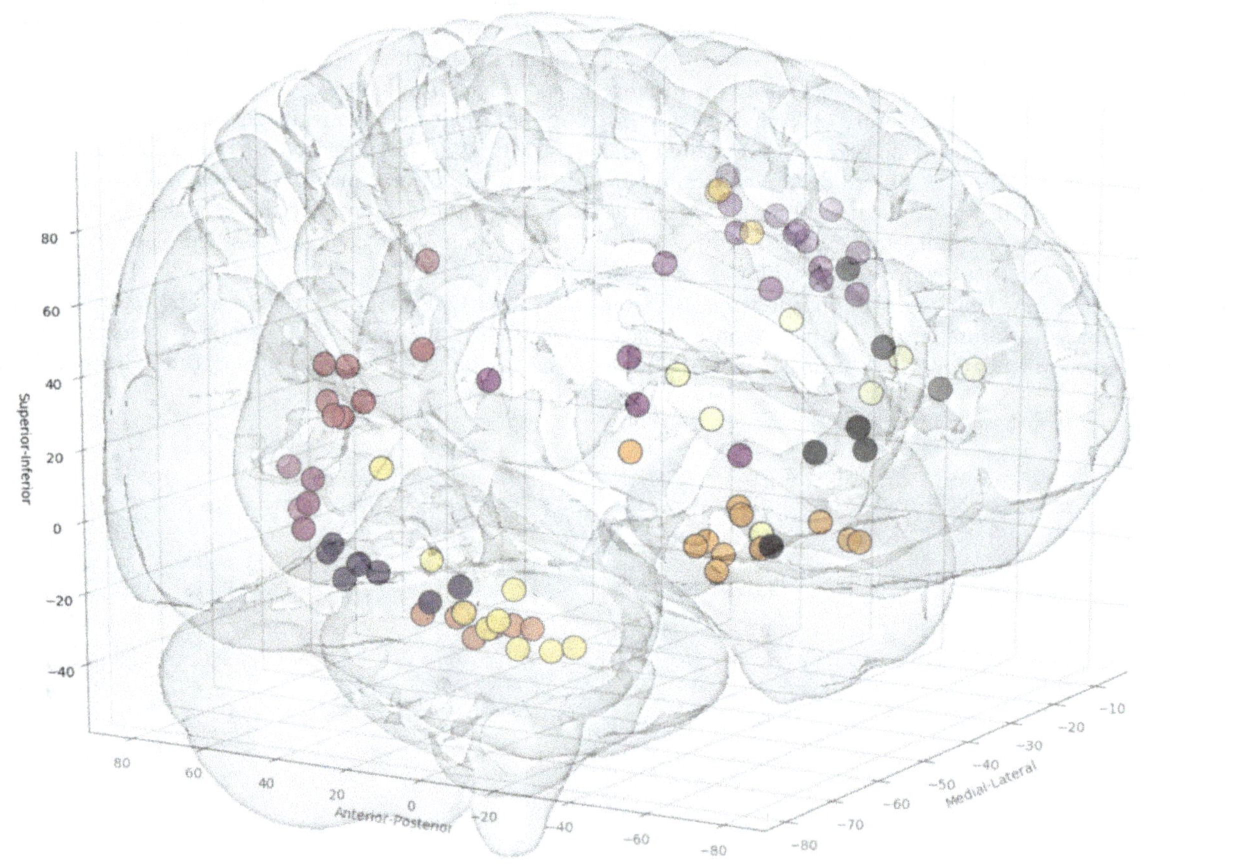

FIGURE 2 | Coordinates of the entry points, shown from a right anterolateral projection for electrode trajectories within the training set (n = 12 patients). **Table 2** outlines the ROIs included for the entry and target points. Greater transparency represents trajectory points closer to the midline.

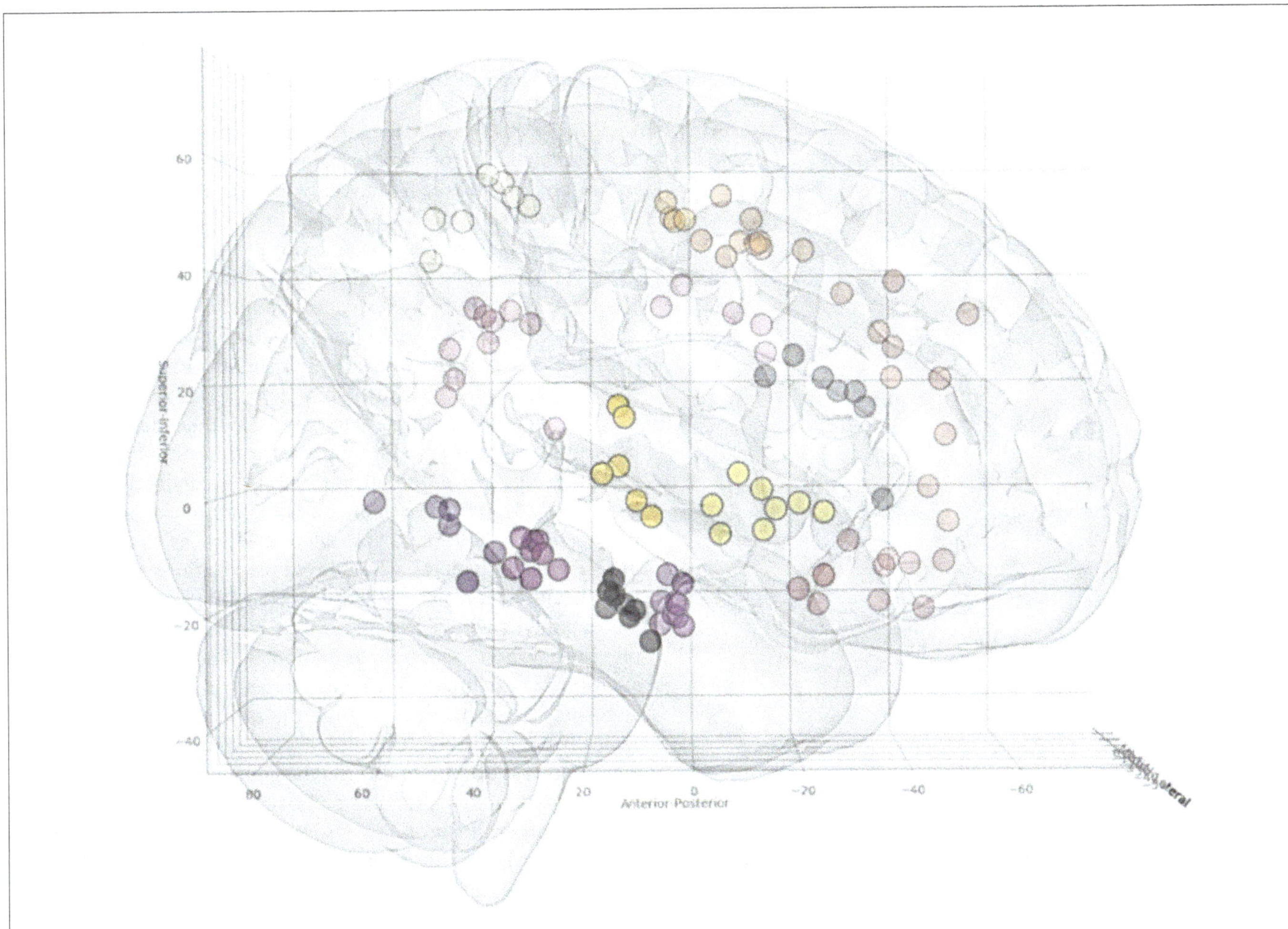

FIGURE 3 | Coordinates of the target points, shown from a right lateral projection, for electrode trajectories within the training set (n = 12 patients). **Table 2** outlines the ROIs included for the entry and target points. Greater transparency represents trajectory points closer to the midline.

Computational analysis was performed with custom scripts utilizing functions from the following python libraries: Pandas, Numpy and SciKit learn. The Matplotlib library was used for data visualization.

RESULTS

Priors Validation

In total, 13 entry and 14 target point clusters were included in the training set derived from the first 12 patients (**Figure 2**). An entry prior for the posterior insula was not generated due to the wide dispersion of selected entry points beyond that of a single GIF parcellation ROI, indicating a lack of consistency during planning. An overview of color coded priors derived from the entry and target regions of the training set are shown in **Figure 3**.

A further 20 patients were then prospectively planned and implanted using the spatial priors derived from the previously implanted trajectories within the training set. Of the prospectively planned trajectories, 79% (129/163) were able to be planned and implanted using the spatial priors to restrict the entry and target regions (see **Table 2** and **Figure 4**). The remaining 21% (34/163) of prospectively implanted trajectories required entry or target points outside of these priors (see **Figure 5**). All prospectively planned and implanted trajectories sampled the intended ROIs and there were no postoperative complications or hemorrhages. Coordinates for the entry and target point cluster centroids from the training set and Euclidean distance to the cluster centroid from the prospective group are shown in **Supplementary Table 1**. On average, the training and test cluster centroids for the majority of entry and target points were 10 mm apart, with the most notable exception being mesial prefrontal cortex electrodes. This most likely reflects the variability of cerebral vasculature between patients and the large anatomical area for electrophysiological sampling.

Adaptive Learning

Given that 21% of the prospectively planned trajectories were outside of the spatial priors, a K-NN machine learning classifier was applied to dynamically refine the boundaries of the entry and target priors based on the data in the training set. Subsequent implantations from the test set were then added to the training set data in 5-folds (random selection of 42 new trajectories with each fold). The K-NN classifier was iteratively re-applied

TABLE 2 | Results of implanted computer-assisted planning electrode in relation to the priors.

	No. trajectories	Through prior	Outside prior
Orbitofrontal	15	13 (87%)	2 (13%)
Amygdala	17	16 (94%)	1 (6%)
Anterior hippocampus	11	8 (73%)	3 (27%)
Posterior hippocampus	13	10 (77%)	3 (23%)
Temporo-occipital junction	6	6 (100%)	0 (0%)
Anterior cingulum	10	10 (100%)	0 (0%)
Middle cingulum	13	7 (54%)	6 (46%)
Posterior cingulum	15	12 (80%)	3(20%)
Mesial pre-frontal cortex	9	8 (89%)	1 (11%)
Anterior SSMA	12	11 (92%)	1 (8%)
Posterior SSMA	8	4 (50%)	4 (50%)
Precuneus	7	4 (57%)	3 (43%)
Anterior insula	17	10 (59%)	7 (41%)
Posterior insula	10	10 (100%)	0 (0%)
Total	163	129 (79%)	34 (21%)

and the dynamic changes in the target priors are shown in **Supplementary Figure 1**.

DISCUSSION

We have previously shown that CAP using the EpiNav^{TM} platform can optimize trajectory planning parameters and return feasible plans in < one-third of the time required for manual planning (6). Computer-assisted planning, however, requires familiarity with the software and algorithms as well as multimodal image processing. In the present study, we undertake a prospective validation of spatial priors to further refine CAP for SEEG electrode trajectories by removing the reliance on ROIs derived from whole-brain parcellations. Based on a training set of 12 patients (108 electrodes) in which the EpiNav^{TM} platform was used for CAP utilizing the GIF parcellation, we generated entry and target spatial priors for common ROIs that were targeted five or more times. Five was chosen as an arbitrary threshold to allow accurate morphological delineation and cluster centroid calculation for the prior. The spatial priors were then prospectively used to restrict the entry and target points instead of the GIF parcellation for CAP in a further 20 patients (210 electrodes). The incorporation of spatial priors allowed feasible trajectories to be returned for 79% of the electrodes. Each of these was subsequently implanted into patients without complication. For the remaining 21%, the implemented entry or target points were outside of the spatial priors. A machine learning classifier was implemented to dynamically modify the priors to account for this. We provide the spatial priors in MNI template space for use by other institutions during CAP or manual planning and as a potential starting point for standardization of SEEG trajectories.

This is the first prospective study describing the utility of spatial priors to refine computer-assisted SEEG trajectory planning. Two main methods for SEEG CAP have been implemented in the literature. The first is where the user defines a target point and the algorithm returns a trajectory with the lowest risk score (18). This has the benefit of ensuring that the precise ROI within the anatomical structure is targeted, but this limits the algorithm to return the local, but not global, minimum risk score. It may also lead to a failure of the CAP algorithm to return a feasible trajectory, especially if the chosen target point is adjacent to a critical structure and therefore contravenes a "hard constraint" within the planning algorithm. Due to this, some groups suggest "roughly" selecting the entry and target point (19–21). The algorithm then returns trajectories within a 1 cm radius allowing for slightly more variation in the entry and target points. This method still requires manual user interaction for rough placement. Another method that has been implemented is to allow the algorithm to define the entry and target points automatically within predefined anatomical structures (4). This is reliant on the anatomical segmentation provided by whole-brain parcellations such as Freesurfer (22) or GIF (10). In general, whole-brain parcellations are developed from healthy controls and the accuracy of the segmentation may fail in patients with gross anatomical abnormalities or following previous surgery. Another limitation is that in some cases the anatomically defined entry and target regions may be very large such as electrodes targeting the anterior cingulum, which typically enter through the middle frontal gyrus. The computer planning algorithm then returns the global minimum risk score, but this may not be practical or feasible. Algorithms have been able to counter this problem to some extent through maximizing spatial distribution but only when multiple electrodes pass through a single ROI (4). One example of this can be seen with temporal implantations. In such a scenario sampling the temporal pole, amygdala, anterior hippocampus, posterior hippocampus and temporo-occipital junction may be required. Unless the clinical scenario dictates otherwise, it is likely that that entry points for all of these electrode trajectories will pass through the middle temporal gyrus. It is beneficial, therefore for the lateral neocortical sampling to be spatially distributed along the anteroposterior axis to prevent electrode conflicts and also aid in the delineation of the lateral neocortical resection margins. More advanced systems also enable the user to iterate through the proposed trajectories in a risk-stratified manner until a feasible trajectory with the lowest risk score is identified (5). Spatial priors can overcome this limitation as the entry and target points are confined to previously implemented trajectories. This removes the reliance on whole-brain parcellations for the entry and target point constraints and ensures reliable spatial sampling. Another benefit is that the risk-stratified trajectories returned to the user are more likely to be clinically acceptable and reduces the need to iterate through the options. In generating these priors, we purposefully excluded trajectories that targeted unique patient-specific abnormalities, such as focal cortical dysplasia, as these would not be generalizable when considering trajectory planning in other patients. In such cases, computer-assisted planning can still be utilized using the segmentation of the lesion as the target and allow the algorithm to choose the most appropriate entry point (12).

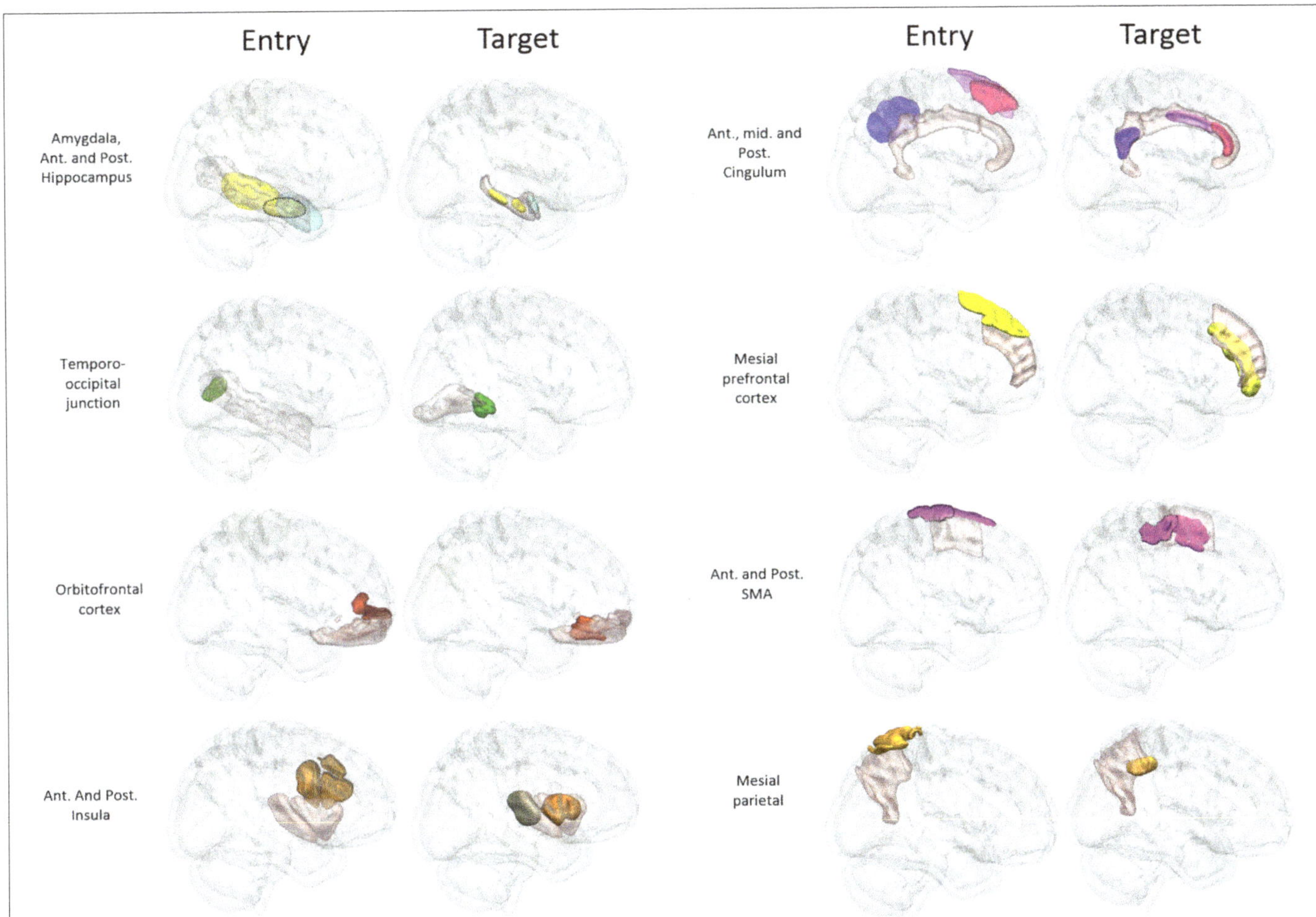

FIGURE 4 | Panel of 3D images shown from right lateral projection with color-coded entry (columns 1 and 3) and target (columns 2 and 4) priors within GIF defined anatomical regions (pink). Color scheme: Amygdala: Cyan, Hippocampus: Yellow, Temporo-occipital junction: Green, Orbitofrontal cortex: Red, Anterior Insula: Brown, Posterior Insula: Gray, Anterior Cingulum: Dark pink, Middle Cingulum: Purple, Posterior Cingulum: Blue, Mesial prefrontal cortex: Yellow, Supplementary sensory-motor area: Magenta, Precuneus: Orange.

As a further analysis, we implemented a K-NN classifier as part of an adaptive learning algorithm. Here the K-NN classifier was used to generate the boundaries that define the priors for the entry and target points of the electrodes in the training set. Electrode entry and target points were then iteratively added in five equal folds, each with randomly selected trajectories. The K-NN classifier then adjusted the priors based on the additional feasible electrode information. The unique benefit of this adaptive technique is the ability to dynamically adapt to changing planning preferences and learn evolving individual surgical preferences. In this implementation, the weighting was uniformly distributed, in that the entry and target points contributed to the classifier equally. Where surgeons prefer entry or target regions within a specific location, weightings could also be applied to favor the distribution. Machine learning has previously been applied retrospectively to SEEG trajectory analysis to identify stereotyped implantation schema (23). In this work, the authors reviewed previous manually planned trajectories from their institution and used a K-NN clustering algorithm to identify that their implantation practices would be distilled down to 8 unique strategies. This work adds further utility as a potential recommendation system i.e., where the algorithm can identify predefined electrode trajectories and suggests where further electrodes are needed. The authors then show that the manually implanted trajectories can be further optimized by applying their computer-assisted planning pipeline once the surgeon has roughly placed an entry and target point within a 1 cm vicinity. It is unclear if these stereotype implantations are generalizable to other institutions that have varying practices. The automated trajectories in their study have also not been prospectively implanted in patients and hence there is no clinical validation of the true safety of the automated trajectories. The work presented in this manuscript, however, is distinct for the following reasons. Firstly, we make no suggestions regarding which targets are included in the implantation strategy as this is defined following the multidisciplinary review of the presurgical evaluation. Instead, we focus on improving the reliability, efficiency and adaptability of precise electrode planning. Secondly, all of

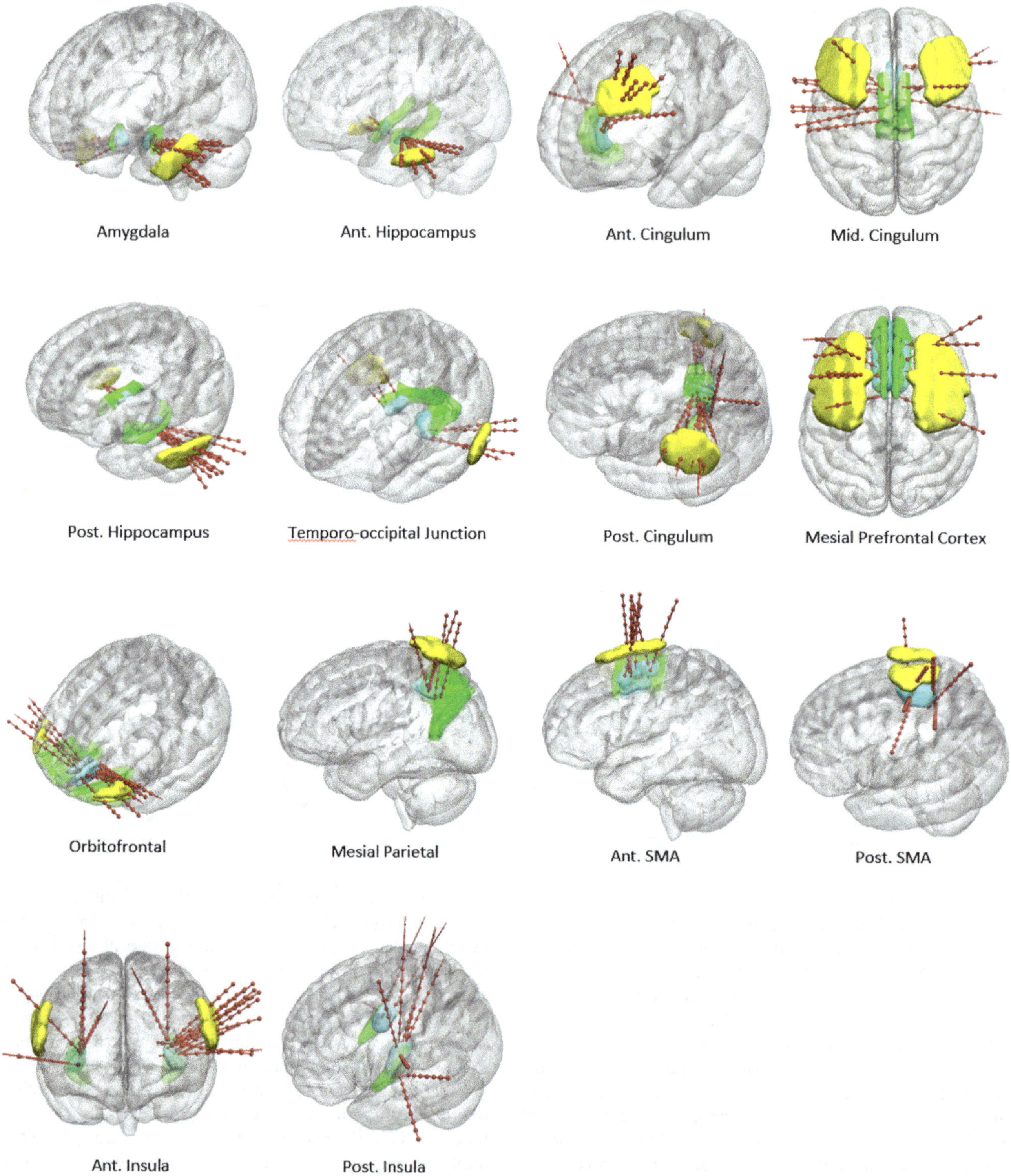

FIGURE 5 | Panel of 3D cortical images shown from various projections with implanted electrode trajectories from the test set (red) passing through the entry priors (yellow) and the target priors (blue) derived from the training set. GIF defined anatomical structures are shown in green.

the automated trajectories were prospectively implanted in our series without complication. Thirdly, the spatial priors generated from the training set leverages our institutional experience and the active learning approach mimics the real-world use of the platform if an external center were to add their implantation trajectories. Additionally, the spatial priors no longer require an anatomical segmentation atlas once generated.

There are limitations to this study. The entry and target priors are derived from a single-center incorporating planning practices from two surgeons. To mitigate this, a K-NN adaptive learning technique was implemented to dynamically modify the priors based on varying surgeon and institutional practices. We also found a considerable variation in the entry points relating to the posterior insula trajectories preventing the generation of an entry prior that was more constrained than the GIF parcellation. The principal reason for this was the between-patient variability in oblique vs. orthogonal (transsylvian) trajectories as a result of vascular constraints. In this study, a K-NN classifier was chosen over other potential learning algorithms as it allows for 3-dimensional clustering in a discriminative non-parametric fashion. Further work should also focus on evaluating other machine learning classifiers. Finally, the spatial prior and prospectively implanted trajectories are based on the pre-operative acquisition of a DSA to guide SEEG trajectory planning, as this is the standard of care at the study institution. The priors are equally applicable, however, to centers that do not use DSA for planning as CAP can be performed with any vascular imaging modality, but conflicts with non-segmented vasculature may be more frequent depending on the minimum clinically significant vessel size considered (24).

CONCLUSION

Spatial priors are a valuable contribution to CAP, allowing future implantations to be guided by previous planning experience. Through the prospective application of spatial priors, we show that feasible trajectories can be planned and implanted in test cases enabling CAP to be performed without the reliance on whole-brain parcellations. In addition, experience from SEEG trajectory planning can be continually refined and used to update the spatial priors dynamically, through the implementation of a K-NN classifier. This opens the possibility of the algorithm adapting to evolving practices as well as dynamically learning individual surgeon's planning preferences from subsequent implantations. Future work will focus on validating this novel preliminary approach through external, multi-center SEEG implantation data.

AUTHOR CONTRIBUTIONS

VV was involved with the conception, design, data acquisition, and analysis as well as manuscript production. All authors critically reviewed the final manuscript prior to submission, contributed to the article, and approved the submitted version. JD was involved with the study design and provided study oversight. SO was involved with computer programing aspects of the EpiNav platform and provided study oversight. AWM was involved with data acquisition. AM was involved with data acquisition. AG was involved with the data acquisition and computer programing aspects of the EpiNav platform. RS was involved with the data acquisition and computer programing aspects of the EpiNav platform.

ACKNOWLEDGMENTS

We acknowledge funding from: NIHR UCLH/UCL Biomedical Research Center, senior investigator schemes and Wellcome Trust (WT106882)/Wellcome/EPSRC (203145Z/16/Z).

SUPPLEMENTARY MATERIAL

Supplementary Figure 1 | MNI coordinate system: K-NN classifier used to define spatial prior boundaries for target points based on the training set and subsequent addition of 5-folds of data from the test set. Dynamic refinement of the spatial priors can be seen with addition of subsequent target point information.

Supplementary Table 1 | Coordinates of training and test set electrode cluster centroids in MNI space.

REFERENCES

1. Mullin JP, Shriver M, Alomar S, Najm I, Bulacio J, Chauvel P, Gonzalez-Martinez J. Is SEEG safe? A systematic review and meta-analysis of stereo-electroencephalography-related complications. *Epilepsia.* (2016) 57:386–401. doi: 10.1111/epi.13298
2. Vakharia VN, Sparks R, O'Keeffe AG, Rodionov R, Miserocchi A, McEvoy A, et al. Accuracy of intracranial electrode placement for stereoencephalography: a systematic review and meta-analysis. *Epilepsia.* (2017) 58:921–32. doi: 10.1111/epi.13713
3. Bourdillon P, Châtillon CE, Moles A, Rheims S, Catenoix H, Montavont A, et al. Effective accuracy of stereoelectroencephalography: robotic 3D versus talairach orthogonal approaches. *J Neurosurg.* (2019) 131:1938–46. doi: 10.3171/2018.7.JNS181164
4. Sparks R, Vakharia V, Rodionov R, Vos SBSB, Diehl B, Wehner T, et al. Anatomy-driven multiple trajectory planning (ADMTP) of intracranial electrodes for epilepsy surgery. *Int J Comput Assist Radiol Surg.* (2017) 12:1245–55. doi: 10.1007/s11548-017-1628-z
5. Vakharia VN, Sparks R, Rodionov R, Vos SB, Dorfer C, Miller J, et al. Computer-assisted planning for the insertion of stereoelectroencephalography electrodes for the investigation of drug-resistant focal epilepsy: an external validation study. *J Neurosurg.* (2018) 130:1–10. doi: 10.3171/2017.10.JNS171826
6. Vakharia VN, Sparks R, Miserocchi A, Vos SB, O'Keeffe A, Rodionov R, et al. Computer-assisted planning for stereoelectroencephalography (SEEG). *Neurotherapeutics.* (2019) 16:1183–97. doi: 10.1007/s13311-019-00774-9
7. Vakharia VN, Sparks R, Li K, O'Keeffe AG, Miserocchi A, McEvoy AW, et al. Automated trajectory planning for laser interstitial thermal therapy in mesial temporal lobe epilepsy. *Epilepsia.* (2018) 59:814–24. doi: 10.1111/epi.14034
8. Li K, Vakharia VN, Sparks R, França LGS, Granados A, McEvoy AW, et al. Optimizing trajectories for cranial laser interstitial thermal therapy using computer-assisted planning: a machine learning approach. *Neurotherapeutics.* (2019) 16:182–91. doi: 10.1007/s13311-018-00693-1
9. Marcus HJ, Vakharia VN, Sparks R, Rodionov R, Kitchen N, McEvoy AW, et al. Computer-assisted versus manual planning for stereotactic brain biopsy: a retrospective comparative pilot study. *Oper Neurosurg (Hagerstown).* (2020) 18:417–22. doi: 10.1093/ons/opz177
10. Cardoso MJ, Modat M, Wolz R, Melbourne A, Cash D, Rueckert D, et al. Geodesic information flows: spatially-variant graphs and their application to segmentation and fusion. *IEEE Trans Med Imaging.* (2015) 34:1976–88. doi: 10.1109/TMI.2015.2418298
11. Zuluaga MA, Rodionov R, Nowell M, Achhala S, Zombori G, Mendelson AF, et al. Stability, structure and scale: improvements in multi-modal vessel extraction for SEEG trajectory planning. *Int J Comput Assist Radiol Surg.* (2015) 10:1227–37. doi: 10.1007/s11548-015-1174-5
12. Nowell M, Sparks R, Zombori G, Miserocchi A, Rodionov R, Diehl B, et al. Comparison of computer-assisted planning and manual planning for

depth electrode implantations in epilepsy. *J Neurosurg.* (2016) 124:1820–8. doi: 10.3171/2015.6.JNS15487
13. Vakharia VN, Duncan JS. Automation advances in stereoelectroencephalography planning. *Neurosurg Clin N Am.* (2020) 31:407–19. doi: 10.1016/j.nec.2020.03.005
14. Sparks R, Zombori G, Rodionov R, Nowell M, Vos SB, Zuluaga MA, et al. Automated multiple trajectory planning algorithm for the placement of stereo-electroencephalography (SEEG) electrodes in epilepsy treatment. *Int J Comput Assist Radiol Surg.* (2017) 12:123–36. doi: 10.1007/s11548-016-1452-x
15. Rodionov R, O'Keeffe A, Nowell M, Rizzi M, Vakharia VN, Wykes V, et al. Increasing the accuracy of 3D EEG implantations. *J Neurosurg.* (2019) 1:1–8. doi: 10.3171/2019.2.JNS183313
16. Cardinale F, Cossu M, Castana L, Casaceli G, Schiariti MP, Miserocchi A, et al. Stereoelectroencephalography: surgical methodology, safety, and stereotactic application accuracy in 500 procedures. *Neurosurgery.* (2013) 72:353–66. doi: 10.1227/NEU.0b013e31827d1161
17. Fonov V, Evans AC, Botteron K, Almli CR, Mckinstry RC, Collins DL. NeuroImage unbiased average age-appropriate atlases for pediatric studies. *Neuroimage.* (2011) 54:313–27. doi: 10.1016/j.neuroimage.2010.07.033
18. Zombori G, Rodionov R, Nowell M, Zuluaga MA, Clarkson MJ, Micallef C, et al. A computer assisted planning system for the placement of sEEG electrodes in the treatment of epilepsy. *Inf Process Comput Interv.* (2011) 8498:118–27. doi: 10.1007/978-3-319-07521-1_13
19. De Momi E, Caborni C, Cardinale F, Castana L, Casaceli G, Cossu M, et al. Automatic trajectory planner for stereoelectroencephalography procedures: a retrospective study. *IEEE Trans Biomed Eng.* (2013) 60:986–93. doi: 10.1109/TBME.2012.2231681
20. De Momi E, Caborni C, Cardinale F, Casaceli G, Castana L, Cossu M, et al. Multi-trajectories automatic planner for StereoElectroEncephaloGraphy (SEEG). *Int J Comput Assist Radiol Surg.* (2014) 9:1087–97. doi: 10.1007/s11548-014-1004-1
21. Scorza D, De Momi E, Plaino L, Amoroso G, Arnulfo G, Narizzano M, et al. Retrospective evaluation and SEEG trajectory analysis for interactive multi-trajectory planner assistant. *Int J Comput Assist Radiol Surg.* (2017) 12:1727–38. doi: 10.1007/s11548-017-1641-2
22. Dale AM, Fischl B, Sereno MI. Cortical surface-based analysis. I. Segmentation and surface reconstruction. *Neuroimage.* (1999) 9:179–94. doi: 10.1006/nimg.1998.0395
23. Scorza D, Amoroso G, Cortes C, Artetxe A, Bertelsen A, Rizzi M, et al. Experience-based SEEG planning: from retrospective data to automated electrode trajectories suggestions. *Healthc Technol Lett.* (2018) 5:167–71. doi: 10.1049/htl.2018.5075
24. Vakharia VN, Sparks R, Vos SB, McEvoy AW, Miserocchi A, Ourselin S, et al. The effect of vascular segmentation methods on stereotactic trajectory planning for drug-resistant focal epilepsy: a retrospective cohort study. *World Neurosurg X.* (2019) 4:100057. doi: 10.1016/j.wnsx.2019.100057

10

Current Conceptual Understanding of the Epileptogenic Network from Stereoelectroencephalography-Based Connectivity Inferences

Kanupriya Gupta[1,2], *Pulkit Grover*[3,4] *and Taylor J. Abel*[1,2,3,5*]

[1] University of Pittsburgh School of Medicine, Pittsburgh, PA, United States, [2] Department of Neurological Surgery, University of Pittsburgh, Pittsburgh, PA, United States, [3] Center for the Neural Basis of Cognition, Carnegie Mellon University/University of Pittsburgh, Pittsburgh, PA, United States, [4] Department of Electrical and Computer Engineering, Carnegie Mellon University, Pittsburgh, PA, United States, [5] Department of Bioengineering, University of Pittsburgh, Pittsburgh, PA, United States

***Correspondence:**
Taylor J. Abel
abeltj@upmc.edu

Localization of the epileptogenic zone (EZ) is crucial in the surgical treatment of focal epilepsy. Recently, EEG studies have revealed that the EZ exhibits abnormal connectivity, which has led investigators to now consider connectivity as a biomarker to localize the EZ. Further, abnormal connectivity of the EZ may provide an explanation for the impact of focal epilepsy on more widespread brain networks involved in typical cognition and development. Stereo-electroencephalography (sEEG) is a well-established method for localizing the EZ that has recently been applied to examine altered brain connectivity in epilepsy. In this manuscript, we review recent computational methods for identifying the EZ using sEEG connectivity. Findings from previous sEEG studies indicate that during interictal periods, the EZ is prone to seizure generation but concurrently receives inward connectivity preventing seizures. At seizure onset, this control is lost, allowing seizure activity to spread from the EZ. Regulatory areas within the EZ may be important for subsequently ending the seizure. After the seizure, the EZ appears to regain its influence on the network, which may be how it is able to regenerate epileptiform activity. However, more research is needed on the dynamic connectivity of the EZ in order to build a biomarker for EZ localization. Such a biomarker would allow for patients undergoing sEEG to have electrode implantation, localization of the EZ, and resection in a fraction of the time currently needed, preventing patients from having to endure long hospital stays and induced seizures.

Keywords: focal epilepsy, SEEG, connectivity, epileptogenic, Granger causality, EZ, biomarker

INTRODUCTION

Focal epilepsy is the most common type of epilepsy (1). Although seizure onset is confined to a focus comprising one or a few areas, several lines of evidence now demonstrate that focal epilepsy is a network disorder with widespread influence rather than a disorder of an isolated area (2, 3). The epileptogenic zone (EZ), often defined theoretically as that part of the cortex which when removed results in seizure freedom, must be localized in order to successfully treat patients with drug-resistant focal epilepsy (4). However, such a definition of the EZ cannot be measured, as it is impossible to know whether a smaller area could have been resected that would have also provided seizure freedom for a patient. Here, we operationalize the EZ as the area of seizure onset and primary seizure organization (5). Neuroimaging modalities such as fMRI and EEG have allowed us to examine how the EZ exhibits abnormal connectivity. By using network models to understand focal epilepsy, we can find new ways to define and identify the EZ. In this manuscript, we describe emerging connectivity methods for identifying the EZ measured by sEEG (**Table 1**) and conceptual advances of the EZ using these methods.

Resting-state EEG connectivity studies have also generated new knowledge about the outward connectivity of the EZ. Whereas, the bilateral posterior cingulate cortex (PCC) has been shown to have the highest outward connectivity in controls during resting state, the ipsilateral hippocampus had the highest outward connectivity in patients with temporal lobe epilepsy (TLE) using electrical source imaging from high-density EEG (19). This finding indicates that the hippocampus (the EZ) seems to be the predominant source of influence outflow in TLE even in the absence of seizures, and it may be disrupting other functional networks, such as those controlled by the PCC. In the immediate period leading up to an interictal discharge, patients with right and left TLE show rapidly increasing outward connectivity from the ipsilateral mesial temporal pole, suggesting that epileptogenic areas recruit other brain regions to generate and spread epileptogenic activity (20).

Localization of the EZ is crucial for patients with drug-resistant focal epilepsy who are candidates for surgery. Stereoelectroencephalography (sEEG), a minimally invasive technique used to record electrical activity directly from the brain, is used frequently in patients with drug-resistant epilepsy in which the EZ cannot be localized using non-invasive modalities. Since sEEG exhibits the fine temporal resolution of intracerebral recordings, it provides an unparalleled opportunity to explore the interictal and ictal network properties of the EZ and may provide opportunities to exploit the network properties of the EZ for localization purposes. Furthermore, if successful algorithms were found using only a short period of interictal data, recording time could be reduced from days to only hours at most, and we would not have to trigger seizures in patients. These improvements would be invaluable for patients with epilepsy, especially children who might not tolerate multiple days in the epilepsy monitoring unit.

sEEG CONNECTIVITY STUDIES

While several studies have examined interictal connectivity using resting-state fMRI (rs-fMRI) and scalp EEG, relatively fewer studies have examined interictal connectivity using sEEG. sEEG offers exquisite spatial and temporal resolution compared to rs-fMRI and scalp EEG, making it well-suited to examine the fine time course of epileptic cortical activity. Unlike scalp EEG, sEEG can measure activity directly from both cortical and subcortical areas and is only limited by the placement of electrodes, which is usually only in areas suspected to be involved in seizure onset or propagation. Whereas, fMRI is reliant on the hemodynamic response, which is a delayed measure associated with brain activation, sEEG provides a real-time measure of electrical brain activity. Compared to subdural grids, another type of invasive monitoring technique which can only be placed on the surface of the cortex, sEEG electrodes can be placed into deep structures of the brain. Although sEEG is more invasive than fMRI and scalp EEG, it does not require a craniotomy like subdural grids and has a good safety profile with a lower rate of postoperative complications and infections compared to grids (21–25). Given that no other technique has the combined high spatiotemporal resolution and safety associated with sEEG, it is an ideal tool for studying epileptogenic networks. Building on a strong premise of previous work, we present connectivity findings from several sEEG papers and provide a framework for a model of ictogenesis that could be used to identify a biomarker for the EZ (26, 27).

FUNCTIONAL CONNECTIVITY METHODS AND FINDINGS

Coherence-Related Undirected Methods

Several methods have been used to analyze the functional connectivity between epileptogenic and non-epileptogenic areas (**Table 1**) during resting-state, pre-ictal, and ictal periods. A recent sEEG study of focal epilepsy measured the Pearson correlation coefficient during resting state and calculated node strength, which measures the average connection between a contact to all other contacts, for each contact (28). The distinguishability between node strength in resected vs. not resected contacts (D_{RS}) was calculated for each patient. Only after correcting for spatial proximity between contacts did the D_{RS} values between seizure-free and not-seizure-free patient groups become significantly different. Patients with seizure-free outcomes had less distinguishability than patients who were not seizure-free, suggesting that resected nodes were more similar to unresected nodes and less epileptogenic in seizure-free patients. This finding also suggests that network properties during resting-state can help differentiate patients who will have better outcomes postoperatively.

In another study, alpha, theta, and delta imaginary coherence within a region and between regions was significantly higher in epileptogenic regions compared to non-epileptogenic regions, with the alpha-frequency band showing the biggest differences (29). Furthermore, several graph theory measures, including nodal betweenness centrality, edge betweenness centrality, and clustering coefficient were significantly higher in epileptogenic regions. The increased edge and nodal betweenness centrality of the EZ indicates that the epileptogenic zone is an important hub for network connectivity. The increased clustering coefficient reflects that the EZ and the nodes that it is connected to occur in a cluster, or segregated group, that are all functionally connected to each other. When all of these network measures were combined into a logistic regression model, the model was able

TABLE 1 | sEEG functional connectivity methods and their advantages and limitations.

Type	Description	Advantages	Limitations
UNDIRECTED, COHERENCE-BASED CONNECTIVITY METHODS			
Pearson correlation coefficient	A measure of the linear relationship between time series.	• Simple to implement	• No directionality (cross-correlation, which measures correlation at different time lags, can measure directionality) • Assumes a linear relationship between time series
Phase locking value	A measure which quantifies the phase synchrony between two different signals in a certain frequency band (6), or the cross-frequency coupling in one time series (7–10).	• Can distinguish between the roles of phase and amplitude in a signal	• No directionality
Imaginary coherence	A measure of functional connectivity that includes first calculating spectral coherence, which measures the explained variance in a sEEG signal by another signal within a specific frequency band (11). Only the imaginary component is used for analysis, which discards coherence that occurs at zero phase lag.	• Avoids false connectivity detection due to volume conduction/field spread	• No directionality [a different measure, Phase Slope Index, can measure directionality (12)]
Type	**Description**	**Advantages**	**Limitations**
DIRECTED CONNECTIVITY METHODS			
Partial directed coherence	A measure of directional connectivity that is based off of the concept of Granger causality. A multivariate autoregressive model is transformed into the frequency domain to perform this analysis (13).	• Each electrode contact's PDC value to another contact is normalized by the sum of the outflow from the contact, which highlights contacts that receive a high degree of inflow.	• Assumes linearity and stationarity of sEEG data • Unclear how Granger causality reflects actual causality
Directed transfer function	A measure of directional connectivity that is based off of Granger causality. A multivariate autoregressive model is transformed into the frequency domain to perform this analysis (14).	• Each value of DTF from electrode contact $x \rightarrow y$ is normalized by the sum of the inflow to y, which highlights contacts that send out a high degree of outflow.	• Assumes linearity and stationarity of sEEG data • Unclear how Granger causality reflects actual causality
Non-linear correlation coefficient (h^2)	A measure of the dependence between time series that takes into account both linear and non-linear relationships.	• Can measure both the strength and direction of connections, since h^2 is asymmetric (h^2_{XY} is not equal to h^2_{YX}) and can be calculated at different time lags (15) • Does not assume a linear relationship between signals	• Heavy computation can be needed (16) • Previously documented small impact of interictal spikes on analysis (17)
Phase transfer entropy	A model-free measure of directed connectivity using phase information (18).	• Can measure directionality • Does not assume a linear relationships between signals • Resistant to spurious connectivity detections due to noise	• A relatively newer measure

to classify epileptogenic regions with an AUC of 0.78. This study suggests that epileptogenic cortex is strongly connected to areas likely involved in primary seizure organization and propagation. Understanding these features of epileptogenic cortex may be exploited to provide a clinically relevant biomarker of the EZ.

Phase-amplitude coupling occurs (PAC) is a connectivity measure based on how the phase of a low-frequency rhythm couples with the amplitude of another high-frequency rhythm. One study used PAC to characterize areas belonging to the ictal core vs. the surrounding penumbra (7). The ictal core was defined as the region of neurons showing hypersynchronous firing in multielectrode array recordings during seizures, whereas the penumbra was defined as a group of areas that show less prominent, unorganized firing. PAC between a low-frequency ictal rhythm and high-gamma frequency amplitude in subdural electrodes was shown to correspond with multiunit firing bursts measured by nearby microelectrode arrays in the ictal core after the onset of seizure activity. However, subdural electrode contacts with low-frequency activity that was not phase-locked to high-gamma amplitude coincided with nearby microelectrode arrays that did not display synchronized firing bursts, suggesting that these contacts are part of the penumbra in which there is a lack of early seizure propagation. The lack of high-frequency oscillations in the penumbra has been thought to be a result of a feedforward inhibitory mechanism, resulting in the penumbra displaying high-amplitude, low-frequency EEG signals without true increases in synchronized neuronal firing (30). Therefore, phase-amplitude coupling between high-frequency oscillations and low-frequency ictal activity appears to be a biomarker for the epileptogenic zone, which can be targeted for resection while sparing the ictal penumbra. Another study used Phase Locking Value (PLV) to identify the seizure onset zone using ictal data in 10 patients with focal epilepsy (8). In seizure-free patients, resected electrodes displayed greater PLV right before seizure onset, and higher PLV peak and power just after seizure onset. This finding further suggests that PAC between low and high-frequency rhythms could be a reflection of the mechanism leading to seizure generation and propagation. Several measures calculated from the PLV were combined into a logistic regression model to classify electrode contacts as belonging to either the seizure onset zone (SOZ) or non-SOZ. Ninety-six percent of the electrodes classified as belonging to the SOZ were within the resection area in seizure-free patients. In patients that were not seizure-free, the more electrodes that were labeled by the algorithm as in the SOZ that were not resected, the worse the patient's seizure outcome.

Directional Connectivity Methods

Granger causality is a concept that has been used to develop several connectivity measures and is a favorable connectivity analysis method given that it can provide directional inferences of influence. In a study using generalized Partial Directed Coherence (PDC), a Granger causality-based method, on resting-state sEEG data, the region of the highest inflow colocalized with the EZ in nine patients with temporal lobe epilepsy (31). In-degree, a graph theory measure of the number of inward connections to a node, was similarly found to be effective at localizing the EZ in another study when applied to PDC analyses from pre-ictal sEEG data (5 s before seizure onset), as epileptogenic regions had the highest in-degree (32). Together, these studies indicate that there is possibly a control mechanism preventing seizures during seizure-free periods and that during a seizure such influence may be lost. Another study using non-linear regression, an alternative to Granger causality-based methods for studying directed network connectivity, found that in pre-ictal sEEG data (8 s before seizure onset), the total number of connections was found to be better at localizing the epileptogenic zone than the number of inward or outward connections, suggesting that the pre-ictal period could be a transition point between the inward influence received during resting-state and the outward connectivity demonstrated during seizure onset (33). However, it is also possible that inward connectivity toward the EZ drives the EZ to send outward ictogenic connectivity. Epileptogenic structures in patients with mesial TLE also show increased synchronization in the pre-ictal period, which may be a seizure generation mechanism (34).

Contrary to the inward influence received during interictal and pre-ictal periods, the EZ shows a switch in connectivity patterns during seizure onset. At the start of a seizure, the EZ can be identified as the region containing the contact with the highest out-degree (35) or the most causal outflow (36). Using Directed Transfer Function (DTF) connectivity, nodes with high betweenness centrality, a graph theory marker for hubs in a network, during seizures have also been shown to coincide with the seizure onset zone (37). This finding was modulated by frequency, as overlap with the SOZ was greater for nodes with large betweenness centrality values in higher frequency gamma and beta networks compared to theta and alpha networks. The high betweenness centrality of nodes thought to be involved in seizure activity was shown to decrease during a seizure and reach a minimum 1 min after a seizure, perhaps because Granger causal influence is spreading more distally from the EZ as the seizure progresses and cortical activity is synchronizing. However, after a seizure, the betweenness centrality rose to pre-ictal levels in just 5 min after a seizure, emphasizing the need to understand the dynamics of EZ connectivity.

In patients who were seizure-free postsurgery, the SOZ colocalized more with nodes with high betweenness centrality in the gamma band during seizures compared to those of patients who still had seizures after surgery (37). This finding suggests that regions involved in generating epileptogenic activity display high gamma band connectivity in ictal periods, which is supported by phase-amplitude coupling studies mentioned earlier and studies showing that fast gamma band activity and suppression of lower frequency activity during seizure onset can localize the EZ (38, 39). However, the relative contribution of connectivity in higher frequencies during ictal periods, with that in alpha band during resting-state, to the epileptogenicity of the EZ remains to be investigated. Furthermore, patients who did not have seizure freedom after surgery have been shown to have a greater percentage of nodes with high betweenness centrality preoperatively, highlighting that as more regions in the brain are highly connected, and likely to spread epileptogenicity, the less likely the patient will be seizure-free (40). However, if the resected area has nodes with high betweenness centrality during the middle to after the end of the seizure, the patient is less likely to be seizure-free. Hence, within or near the EZ, there may be nodes that should be spared from resection, as they are likely involved in suppressing seizures. Another sEEG study using phase transfer entropy found that the ratio of out/in connections increased from the interictal to ictal state but declined drastically from the late-ictal to post-ictal state, suggesting a need to study the possible role of inward connectivity in seizure control (41).

In a sEEG study using non-linear regression, brain regions were classified as belonging to the EZ, propagation zone (PZ), or non-involved zone (NIZ) using ictal data (42). Then, resting-state connectivity was measured between zones and within a zone itself. This analysis revealed that resting-state connectivity was greater within the EZ compared to the NIZ, and greater within the PZ vs. the NIZ, illustrating that the more epileptogenic the area, the more that area is connected within itself, which could be a mechanism for seizure generation. Furthermore, the connectivity between EZ-PZ was higher than the connectivity between EZ-NIZ, and the connectivity within the EZ was significantly higher than connectivity between the EZ-NIZ but not higher than connectivity between the EZ-PZ. Therefore, the EZ seems to be highly connected to itself and the PZ, but not the NIZ. Whereas, high internal connectivity in the EZ could allow for generation of epileptogenic activity, enhanced EZ-PZ connectivity could allow for quick propagation of epileptogenic

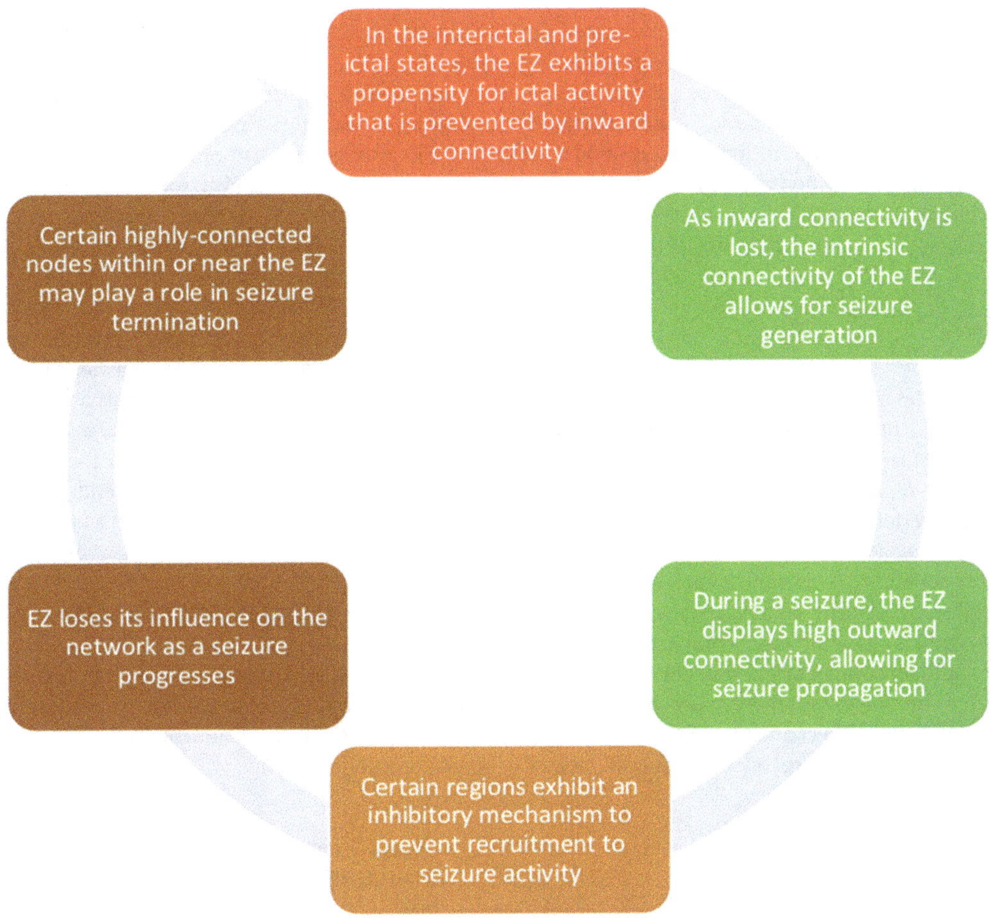

FIGURE 1 | Connectivity of the epileptogenic zone changes between interictal, pre-ictal, and ictal time periods. During interictal periods, the EZ displays both high outward connectivity, which is likely related to the EZ's seizure-generating activity, and inward connectivity, which is possibly preventing a seizure from starting. During seizure onset, we propose that such inward control is lost and that the internal connectivity of the EZ allows for seizure generation. Epileptogenic influence spreads from the EZ via its high connectivity to propagation zones. However, the EZ becomes less influential in the network over time, and regions in or near the EZ may be involved in seizure cessation.

activity during a seizure. The EZ was also shown to be the source of outward connectivity toward the PZ and NIZ. Although this seems contradictory to an earlier finding that inflow was able to localize the EZ during resting state, it is possible that the EZ could be receiving inward connectivity while also producing outward connectivity toward propagation zones.

Cortico-Cortico-Evoked Potentials

Another method that uses directional connectivity to localize the EZ is based on cortico-cortico-evoked potentials (CCEPS). In patients with cortical electrodes, stimulation is applied at one electrode and the resulting evoked potential is measured at other electrode sites. One study illustrated that the amplitude of local CCEPs after stimulation in the SOZ is greater than the amplitude of local CCEPs after stimulation in a region near the SOZ that is not active at seizure onset, suggesting that the epileptogenic cortex is more responsive to excitation due to increased connectivity compared to non-epileptogenic areas (43). A recent study of patients with drug-resistant epilepsy used CCEPs to study directional connectivity between different areas of the brain (44). A large amplitude response evoked from stimulation was taken as a marker for the presence of a directed connection from the stimulation site to the recording site. After constructing connectivity matrices, the authors used graph theory measures to compare the connectivity of the EZ vs. non-EZ. When stimulation was applied to a contact located in the EZ, other electrode contacts in the EZ had a large amplitude evoked potential, reiterating that areas within the EZ are highly connected. Furthermore, the EZ was shown to have higher degree centrality, illustrating that it is highly connected to other nodes in the network (45). Another CCEP paper on patients with focal epilepsy found that contacts in the SOZ had increased out-degree, indicating a higher number of outward connections, as well as increased structural and functional connectivity toward areas of seizure propagation (46).

FUTURE DIRECTIONS

There are several promising topics for future investigation. sEEG studies showing the dynamic nature of directional connectivity of the EZ between interictal, pre-ictal, and ictal time periods are needed to demonstrate how the EZ may be prevented from producing seizures during interictal periods and subsequently becomes uncontrollable just before seizure onset. The dynamic connectivity of the EZ could be used to build an individualized model of epileptogenicity for each patient that identifies the number and location of epileptogenic foci, as well as the optimal area of resection that spares regions that may be involved in seizure control.

DISCUSSION

Findings from sEEG studies have allowed us to better understand how focal epilepsy has widespread effects on brain network connectivity. Taken together, sEEG connectivity findings have shed light on a model of ictogenesis (**Figure 1**): (1) during interictal and pre-ictal periods, the EZ, which may be sending outward connectivity to generate a seizure, is also controlled by inflow from other regions; (2) during seizure onset, the EZ is no longer controlled by inward connectivity and generates epileptiform activity via its high intrinsic connectivity; (3) the EZ sends epileptic influence to propagation zones; (4) areas that are not invaded by seizure activity may be protected by a feedforward inhibition mechanism; (5) as a seizure progresses, the EZ loses its influence on the network, which then builds up again post-ictally; and (6) seizure termination may be partly a result of internal regulation within or near the EZ.

Barriers to implementation of automated resting-state sEEG analysis in the clinic include several parameters that still need to be explored fully and optimized, such as the effect of type of focal epilepsy on suitability for connectivity-based analyses and the amount of resting-state data that would need to be analyzed to localize the EZ confidently. However, the sEEG studies discussed in this paper showing connectivity-based differences between the EZ and non-EZ have been performed on patients with different types of focal epilepsy, and even a few minutes of data has been shown to be sufficient for these analyses. These results show the promise of implementing sEEG-based localization methods of the EZ into clinical practice. Hence, it is exciting that soon we could have automated, intraoperative localization and removal of the EZ that prevents patients from enduring long hospital stays and multiple seizures and gives them a better chance at long-term seizure freedom.

AUTHOR CONTRIBUTIONS

KG wrote the initial and revised drafts of the manuscript. PG and TA are equally responsible for reading and editing of the manuscript. All authors contributed to the article and approved the submitted version.

REFERENCES

1. Beghi E. The epidemiology of epilepsy. *Neuroepidemiology.* (2020) 54:185–91. doi: 10.1159/000503831
2. van Diessen E, Diederen SJ, Braun KP, Jansen FE, Stam CJ. Functional and structural brain networks in epilepsy: what have we learned? *Epilepsia.* (2013) 54:1855–65. doi: 10.1111/epi.12350
3. Spencer DD, Gerrard JL, Zaveri HP. The roles of surgery and technology in understanding focal epilepsy and its comorbidities. *Lancet Neurol.* (2018) 17:373–82. doi: 10.1016/S1474-4422(18)30031-0
4. Luders HO, Najm I, Nair D, Widdess-Walsh P, Bingman W. The epileptogenic zone: general principles. *Epileptic Disord.* (2006) 8(Suppl.2):S1–9
5. Kahane P, Landre E, Minotti L, Francione S, Ryvlin P. The bancaud and talairach view on the epileptogenic zone: a working hypothesis. *Epileptic Disord.* (2006) 8(Suppl.2):S16–26.
6. Lachaux JP, Rodriguez E, Martinerie J, Varela FJ. Measuring phase synchrony in brain signals. *Hum Brain Mapp.* (1999) 8:194–208. doi: 10.1002/(SICI)1097-0193.1999.8:4<194::AID-HBM4>3.0.CO;2-C
7. Weiss SA, Banks GP, McKhann GM, Jr., Goodman RR, Emerson RG, et al. Ictal high frequency oscillations distinguish two types of seizure territories in humans. *Brain.* (2013) 136:3796–808. doi: 10.1093/brain/awt276
8. Elahian B, Yeasin M, Mudigoudar B, Wheless JW, Babajani-Feremi A. Identifying seizure onset zone from electrocorticographic recordings: a machine learning approach based on phase locking value. *Seizure.* (2017) 51:35–42. doi: 10.1016/j.seizure.2017.07.010
9. Mormann F, Fell J, Axmacher N, Weber B, Lehnertz K, Elger CE, et al. Phase/amplitude reset and theta-gamma interaction in the human medial temporal lobe during a continuous word recognition memory task. *Hippocampus.* (2005) 15:890–900. doi: 10.1002/hipo.20117
10. Penny WD, Duzel E, Miller KJ, Ojemann JG. Testing for nested oscillation. *J Neurosci Methods.* (2008) 174:50–61. doi: 10.1016/j.jneumeth.2008.06.035
11. Bastos AM, Schoffelen JM. A tutorial review of functional connectivity analysis methods and their interpretational pitfalls. *Front Syst Neurosci.* (2015) 9:175. doi: 10.3389/fnsys.2015.00175
12. Nolte G, Ziehe A, Nikulin VV, Schlogl A, Kramer N, Brismar T, et al. Robustly estimating the flow direction of information in complex physical systems. *Phys Rev Lett.* (2008) 100:234101. doi: 10.1103/PhysRevLett.100.234101
13. Baccala LA, Sameshima K. Partial directed coherence: a new concept in neural structure determination. *Biol Cybern.* (2001) 84:463–74. doi: 10.1007/PL00007990
14. Kaminski MJ, Blinowska KJ. A new method of the description of the information flow in the brain structures. *Biol Cybern.* (1991) 65:203–10. doi: 10.1007/BF00198091
15. Lopes da Silva F, Pijn JP, Boeijinga P. Interdependence of EEG signals: linear vs. nonlinear associations and the significance of time delays and phase shifts. *Brain Topogr.* (1989) 2:9–18. doi: 10.1007/BF01128839
16. Wang HE, Benar CG, Quilichini PP, Friston KJ, Jirsa VK, Bernard C. A systematic framework for functional connectivity measures. *Front Neurosci.* (2014) 8:405. doi: 10.3389/fnins.2014.00405
17. Bettus G, Wendling F, Guye M, Valton L, Regis J, Chauvel P, et al. Enhanced EEG functional connectivity in mesial temporal lobe epilepsy. *Epilepsy Res.* (2008) 81:58–68. doi: 10.1016/j.eplepsyres.2008.04.020
18. Lobier M, Siebenhuhner F, Palva S, Palva JM. Phase transfer entropy: a novel phase-based measure for directed connectivity in networks coupled by oscillatory interactions. *Neuroimage.* (2014) 85:853–72. doi: 10.1016/j.neuroimage.2013.08.056
19. Coito A, Genetti M, Pittau F, Iannotti GR, Thomschewski A, Holler Y, et al. Altered directed functional connectivity in temporal lobe epilepsy in the absence of interictal spikes: a high density EEG study. *Epilepsia.* (2016) 57:402–11. doi: 10.1111/epi.13308
20. Coito A, Plomp G, Genetti M, Abela E, Wiest R, Seeck M, et al. Dynamic directed interictal connectivity in left and right temporal lobe epilepsy. *Epilepsia.* (2015) 56:207–17. doi: 10.1111/epi.12904
21. Mullin JP, Shriver M, Alomar S, Najm I, Bulacio J, Chauvel P, et al. Is SEEG safe? A systematic review and meta-analysis of stereo-electroencephalography-related complications. *Epilepsia.* (2016) 57:386–401. doi: 10.1111/epi.13298
22. Remick M, Ibrahim GM, Mansouri A, Abel TJ. Patient phenotypes and clinical outcomes in invasive monitoring for epilepsy: an individual patient data meta-analysis. *Epilepsy Behav.* (2020) 102:106652. doi: 10.1016/j.yebeh.2019.106652
23. Yan H, Katz JS, Anderson M, Mansouri A, Remick M, Ibrahim GM,

et al. Method of invasive monitoring in epilepsy surgery and seizure freedom and morbidity: a systematic review. *Epilepsia.* (2019) 60:1960–72. doi: 10.1111/epi.16315

24. Katz JS, Abel TJ. Stereoelectroencephalography versus subdural electrodes for localization of the epileptogenic zone: what is the evidence? *Neurotherapeutics.* (2019) 16:59–66. doi: 10.1007/s13311-018-00703-2
25. Abel TJ, Varela Osorio R, Amorim-Leite R, Mathieu F, Kahane P, Minotti L, et al. Frameless robot-assisted stereoelectroencephalography in children: technical aspects and comparison with Talairach frame technique. *J Neurosurg Pediatr.* (2018) 22:37–46. doi: 10.3171/2018.1.PEDS17435
26. Panzica F, Varotto G, Rotondi F, Spreafico R, Franceschetti S. Identification of the epileptogenic zone from stereo-eeg signals: a connectivity-graph theory approach. *Front Neurol.* (2013) 4:175. doi: 10.3389/fneur.2013.00175
27. Bartolomei F, Lagarde S, Wendling F, McGonigal A, Jirsa V, Guye M, et al. Defining epileptogenic networks: contribution of SEEG and signal analysis. *Epilepsia.* (2017) 58:1131–47. doi: 10.1111/epi.13791
28. Wang Y, Sinha N, Schroeder GM, Ramaraju S, McEvoy AW, Miserocchi A, et al. Interictal intracranial electroencephalography for predicting surgical success: the importance of space and time. *Epilepsia.* (2020) 61:1417–26. doi: 10.1111/epi.16580
29. Goodale SE, Gonzalez HFJ, Johnson GW, Gupta K, Rodriguez WJ, Shults R, et al. Resting-State SEEG may help localize epileptogenic brain regions. *Neurosurgery.* (2020) 86:792–801. doi: 10.1093/neuros/nyz351
30. Schevon CA, Weiss SA, McKhann G Jr, Goodman RR, Yuste R, Emerson RG, et al. Evidence of an inhibitory restraint of seizure activity in humans. *Nat Commun.* (2012) 3:1060. doi: 10.1038/ncomms2056
31. Vlachos I, Krishnan B, Treiman DM, Tsakalis K, Kugiumtzis D, Iasemidis LD. The concept of effective inflow: application to interictal localization of the epileptogenic focus from iEEG. *IEEE Trans Biomed Eng.* (2017) 64:2241–52. doi: 10.1109/TBME.2016.2633200
32. Li YH, Ye XL, Liu QQ, Mao JW, Liang PJ, Xu JW, et al. Localization of epileptogenic zone based on graph analysis of stereo-EEG. *Epilepsy Res.* (2016) 128:149–57. doi: 10.1016/j.eplepsyres.2016.10.021
33. Courtens S, Colombet B, Trebuchon A, Brovelli A, Bartolomei F, Benar CG. Graph measures of node strength for characterizing preictal synchrony in partial epilepsy. *Brain Connect.* (2016) 6:530–9. doi: 10.1089/brain.2015.0397
34. Bartolomei F, Wendling F, Regis J, Gavaret M, Guye M, Chauvel P. Pre-ictal synchronicity in limbic networks of mesial temporal lobe epilepsy. *Epilepsy Res.* (2004) 61:89–104. doi: 10.1016/j.eplepsyres.2004.06.006
35. van Mierlo P, Carrette E, Hallez H, Raedt R, Meurs A, Vandenberghe S, et al. Ictal-onset localization through connectivity analysis of intracranial EEG signals in patients with refractory epilepsy. *Epilepsia.* (2013) 54:1409–18. doi: 10.1111/epi.12206
36. Wilke C, van Drongelen W, Kohrman M, He B. Neocortical seizure foci localization by means of a directed transfer function method. *Epilepsia.* (2010) 51:564–72. doi: 10.1111/j.1528-1167.2009.02329.x
37. Wilke C, Worrell G, He B. Graph analysis of epileptogenic networks in human partial epilepsy. *Epilepsia.* (2011) 52:84–93. doi: 10.1111/j.1528-1167.2010.02785.x
38. Bartolomei F, Chauvel P, Wendling F. Epileptogenicity of brain structures in human temporal lobe epilepsy: a quantified study from intracerebral EEG. *Brain.* (2008) 131:1818–30. doi: 10.1093/brain/awn111
39. Grinenko O, Li J, Mosher JC, Wang IZ, Bulacio JC, Gonzalez-Martinez J, et al. A fingerprint of the epileptogenic zone in human epilepsies. *Brain.* (2018) 141:117–31. doi: 10.1093/brain/awx306
40. Grobelny BT, London D, Hill TC, North E, Dugan P, Doyle WK. Betweenness centrality of intracranial electroencephalography networks and surgical epilepsy outcome. *Clin Neurophysiol.* (2018) 129:1804–12. doi: 10.1016/j.clinph.2018.02.135
41. Wang MY, Wang J, Zhou J, Guan YG, Zhai F, Liu CQ, et al. Identification of the epileptogenic zone of temporal lobe epilepsy from stereo-electroencephalography signals: a phase transfer entropy and graph theory approach. *Neuroimage Clin.* (2017) 16:184–95. doi: 10.1016/j.nicl.2017.07.022
42. Lagarde S, Roehri N, Lambert I, Trebuchon A, McGonigal A, Carron R, et al. Interictal stereotactic-EEG functional connectivity in refractory focal epilepsies. *Brain.* (2018) 141:2966–80. doi: 10.1093/brain/awy214
43. Iwasaki M, Enatsu R, Matsumoto R, Novak E, Thankappen B, Piao Z, et al. Accentuated cortico-cortical evoked potentials in neocortical epilepsy in areas of ictal onset. *Epileptic Disord.* (2010) 12:292–302. doi: 10.1684/epd.2010.0334
44. Zhao C, Liang Y, Li C, Gao R, Wei J, Zuo R, et al. localization of epileptogenic zone based on cortico-cortical evoked potential (CCEP): a feature extraction and graph theory approach. *Front Neuroinformatics.* (2019) 13:31. doi: 10.3389/fninf.2019.00031
45. Liu J, Li M, Pan Y, Lan W, Zheng R, Wu F-X, et al. Complex brain network analysis and its applications to brain disorders: a survey. *Complexity.* (2017) 2017:8362741. doi: 10.1155/2017/8362741
46. Parker CS, Clayden JD, Cardoso MJ, Rodionov R, Duncan JS, Scott C, et al. Structural and effective connectivity in focal epilepsy. *Neuroimage Clin.* (2018) 17:943–52. doi: 10.1016/j.nicl.2017.12.020

11

Transfer Function Models for the Localization of Seizure Onset Zone from Cortico-Cortical Evoked Potentials

Golnoosh Kamali[1]*, Rachel June Smith*[2]*, Mark Hays*[3]*, Christopher Coogan*[4]*, Nathan E. Crone*[4]*, Joon Y. Kang*[5*†] *and Sridevi V. Sarma*[1,2*†]

[1] Neuromedical Control Systems Laboratory, Department of Electrical and Computer Engineering, Institute of Computational Medicine, Johns Hopkins University, Baltimore, MD, United States, [2] Neuromedical Control Systems Laboratory, Department of Biomedical Engineering, Institute of Computational Medicine, Johns Hopkins University, Baltimore, MD, United States, [3] Cognitive Research, Online Neuroengineering and Electrophysiology Laboratory, Department of Biomedical Engineering, Johns Hopkins University, Baltimore, MD, United States, [4] Cognitive Research, Online Neuroengineering and Electrophysiology Laboratory, Department of Neurology-Epilepsy, Johns Hopkins School of Medicine, Baltimore, MD, United States, [5] Department of Neurology-Epilepsy, Johns Hopkins School of Medicine, Baltimore, MD, United States

***Correspondence:**
Sridevi V. Sarma
ssarma2@jhmi.edu
Joon Y. Kang
jkang50@jhmi.edu

Surgical resection of the seizure onset zone (SOZ) could potentially lead to seizure-freedom in medically refractory epilepsy patients. However, localizing the SOZ can be a time consuming and tedious process involving visual inspection of intracranial electroencephalographic (iEEG) recordings captured during passive patient monitoring. Cortical stimulation is currently performed on patients undergoing invasive EEG monitoring for the main purpose of mapping functional brain networks such as language and motor networks. We hypothesized that evoked responses from single pulse electrical stimulation (SPES) can also be used to localize the SOZ as they may express the natural frequencies and connectivity of the iEEG network. To test our hypothesis, we constructed patient specific transfer function models from the evoked responses recorded from 22 epilepsy patients that underwent SPES evaluation and iEEG monitoring. We then computed the frequency and connectivity dependent "peak gain" of the system as measured by the $\mathcal{H}_\infty$ norm from systems theory. We found that in cases for which clinicians had high confidence in localizing the SOZ, the highest peak gain transfer functions with the smallest "floor gain" (gain at which the dipped $\mathcal{H}_\infty$ 3dB below DC gain) corresponded to when the clinically annotated SOZ and early spread regions were stimulated. In more complex cases, there was a large spread of the peak-to-floor (PF) ratios when the clinically annotated SOZ was stimulated. Interestingly for patients who had successful surgeries, our ratio of gains, agreed with clinical localization, no matter the complexity of the case. For patients with failed surgeries, the PF ratio did not match clinical annotations. Our findings suggest that transfer function gains and their corresponding frequency responses computed from SPES evoked responses may improve SOZ localization and thus surgical outcomes.

Keywords: epilepsy, CCEPs, stimulation, SPES, seizure

INTRODUCTION

Epilepsy is a widespread neurological disease that affects nearly 1% of the world's population (1). First-line treatment for epilepsy is anti-epileptic medication, however up to 30% of patients do not respond to the drugs and thus are considered to have medically refractory epilepsy (MRE) (2, 3). However, for MRE patients with well-defined seizure onset zones (SOZ) and early spread regions, seizure freedom may be possible with surgical resection, disconnection of, or electrical stimulation of the SOZ. Localization of the SOZ often requires invasive monitoring with intracranial (iEEG) recordings, but even with such techniques surgical success rates remain highly variable ranging 30–70% (4, 5).

Current SOZ localization methods rely on clinicians inspecting abnormalities on individual channels from iEEG recordings, despite the fact that the epileptic brain is a complex network wherein individual channels interact dynamically (6); therefore, novel tools that investigate epilepsy with a network model may serve as a superior framework for identifying the SOZ. A clinical tool developed to analyze brain networks *in vivo* is single-pulse electrical stimulation (SPES), which elicits an evoked response potential (ERP) in regions that are connected to the stimulation site, known as cortico-cortical evoked potentials (CCEPs) (7, 8).

SPES evokes CCEPs (9, 10) to define effective, or directed, connections to map the human brain (10). The mechanisms of CCEPs induced by SPES are still not fully certain (10), but it is hypothesized that the earliest sensory response is a depolarization in the middle laminae (N1 response), followed by complex patterns of excitatory and inhibitory post-synaptic potentials to form the N2 response (11). The technique was first used to map inter-areal connectivity of the language (9) and motor cortices (12), but has been extended to evaluate functional connections of the frontal-temporal lobe (13), the parietal-frontal lobe (14), the limbic network (15), the insula (16, 17), and deeper brain structures (18, 19). In the last decade SPES has been gaining traction as a tool to probe functional and pathological connectivity in epilepsy and to localize the epileptic networks (20).

SPES has been used as an investigational tool in epilepsy by probing seizure networks as well as investigating cortical excitability (20). A decreased threshold of excitability, as measured by the presence or strength of CCEPs in the stimulating or surrounding regions, possibly indicates seizure-prone tissue (20). This increased excitability is hypothesized to be evident when features of CCEPs differ when stimulated or recorded in the SOZ regions as compared to in healthy tissue. For example, the amplitude of the CCEP response was found to be higher in the SOZ regions when compared to outside regions (21–23) as well as in early ictal propagation sites (24, 25). A second marker of epileptogenicity induced by CCEPs are "delayed responses," neuronal activities that resemble spikes or slow waves that occur 100 ms to 1 s after the stimulation onset that are more likely to be present in SOZ regions (26–28). Additionally, it was shown that removal of areas that consistently exhibited these delayed responses resulted in good outcomes (29–31). High frequency activity during the CCEP (32, 33) or suppression of high-frequency activity after stimulation (34) have been investigated for their SOZ localizing power. Specifically high frequency oscillations were found to colocalize with CCEP responses (35–37), in one study as much as 40% of the time (38). Lastly, graph theoretical properties of the networks generated from CCEP response amplitudes revealed that networks are more bi-directionally connected in the SOZ than in non-SOZ regions (39–41).

Current computational approaches to analyzing seizure networks from CCEPs either compute iEEG features on individual channels, such as the N1 peak amplitudes and signal latencies (21, 25, 36, 42, 43), or they compute static pairwise correlations, organize these correlations into adjacency matrices, and derive graph-theoretic measures (44, 45). These approaches are limited in their ability to capture the underlying network dynamics of the disease. Computing iEEG features such as N1 peak amplitudes forgoes the network aspect of epilepsy by inspecting individual channels instead of its connections to others. While graph theoretic approaches can compute summary statistics of interest such as nodal centralities and network hubs, such measures are not based on well-formulated hypotheses of the role of the SOZ in the iEEG network, and worse many different networks (adjacency matrices) can have identical summary statistics. The interpretations of such measures are thus ambiguous. In contrast, dynamical network models can reveal the natural frequencies of the epileptic network, its connectivity properties, and the underlying dynamics of seizure generation.

We hypothesized that the SOZ is distinguishable from other brain regions in that it generates the "largest" network response to the "smallest" pulse input or "kick." To test this hypothesis, we investigated a property of transfer functions that reflected the epileptogenic nature of the EEG network. Specifically, we calculated the system gain defined by the $\mathcal{H}_\infty$ norm of a transfer function, a notion that describes the amplification and spread of the CCEPs in the network, and the corresponding input "size" required to achieve the system gain. Our approach consisted of building patient specific transfer function models for every stimulation pair. System gains were then computed by calculating the $\mathcal{H}_\infty$ norm of the single input-multi output (SIMO) model, the "peak," for each stimulation pair. For each system model, the 2-norm or "energy" of the associated frequency response a the roll-off, defined to be 3dB below DC gain, was also computed and denoted as the "floor" gain. Finally, we calculated the peak-to-floor (PF) gain ratio. We then defined a confidence statistic that was computed for each patient to assess the level of agreement between the PF ratio, the stimulated SOZ contacts, and surgical outcome. We found that the PF ratio correlates well with clinically annotated SOZ and early spread regions for more straightforward clinical cases and with greater accuracy than current visual assessment approaches. This computational tool may aid clinicians in the identification of the epileptogenic network and thereby improve surgical outcomes.

MATERIALS AND METHODS

Patients

We used a retrospective dataset of 22 MRE patients who underwent iEEG monitoring and SPES for localization of seizures

TABLE 1 | Summary of patient clinical data.

Patient	Gender	Age	Seizure type	MRI	SOZ	Surgery	Pathology	CC	ES	# of SOZ contacts	Total # of stimulated contacts
1	M	25	FocalA, FocalA to BilateralTC	Non-lesional	Left frontal, involving the premotor and motor cortex	Resection	Non-specific, inflammatory changes	High	3	3	7
2	F	43	Focal_IA	Non-lesional	Left posterior basal temporal-occipital region	Resection	Normal	High	3	3	8
3	F	35	Focal-IAsensory Focal_IA	Cystic multilobulated cortically based mass in left temporal lobe	Left temporal	Resection	DNET vs. oliogodendroglioma	High	2	1	5
4	F	18	FocalA to BilateralTC	Subtle thickening in the right middle frontal gyrus	Right frontal	Resection	Cortical dysplasia	Low	1	3	11
5	M	32	Focal-Asensory Focal-Amotor Focal_IA	Gliososis in the posterior superior left parietal lobe	Left superior parietal lobule	Resection	Cortical dysplasia	High	4	8	25
6	M	38	Focal_IA with occasional TC	Mild asymmetric thickening in the dorsal left para-hippocampal gyrus	Left mesial and para-hippocampal gyrus	MRgLiTT	N/A	Low	1	4	5
7	F	32	Focal_IA	Left frontal encephalomalacia	Left posterior cingulate	MRgLiTT	N/A	High	4	3	26
8	F	27	Focal_IA	Bilateral occipital lissencephaly	Bilateral mesial temporal structures	RNS	N/A	High	3	8	13
9	F	24	Focal_IA	Left temporal encephalomalacia	Left temporal lobe	Resection	Non-specific, inflammatory changes	Low	1	2	9
10	F	27	Focal_IA to BilateralTC	Left periventricular hetertopia and left frontal encephalamalacia	Left inferior frontal region	Resection	Non-specific, inflammatory changes	High	1	4	19
11	F	51	Focal_IA BilateralTC	Right MTS	Right mesial temporal structures	MRgLiTT	N/A	Low	N/A	2	6
12	M	48	Focal_IA	Periventricular bilateral nodular heterotopa and diffuse cortical dysgensis	Left mesial temporal structures	MRgLiTT	N/A	High	2	2	17
13	F	23	Focal_IA	Left temporal encephalomalacia	Left temporal lobe, mesial and neocortical	RNS	N/A	Low	3	5	18
14A	F	23	Focal_IA	Non-lesional	Right posterior temporal region	Awaiting surgery	N/A	High	N/A	3	25
14B	F	23	Focal_IA	Non-lesional	Right posterior temporal region	Awaiting surgery	N/A	High	N/A	3	10
15	M	32	Focal_IA with and without BilateralTC	Non-lesional	Right temporal lobe (neocortex)	Awaiting surgery	N/A	High	N/A	1	9
16	M	32	Focal_IA	Right parietal encephalomalacia	Right temporal and parietal region	Awaiting surgery	N/A	High	N/A	5	14

(Continued)

TABLE 1 | Continued

Patient	Gender	Age	Seizure type	MRI	SOZ	Surgery	Pathology	CC	ES	# of SOZ contacts	Total # of stimulated contacts
17	M	19	Focal_IA with occasional TC	Non-lesional	Left mesial temporal structures	Awaiting surgery	N/A	Low	N/A	4	17
18	F	35	Focal_IA	Right MTS	Bilateral mesial temporal structures	MRgLiTT	N/A	Low	1	4	19
19	M	58	Focal_IA	Non-lesional	Left mesial temporal structures	Awaiting surgery	N/A	High	N/A	2	17
20	M	41	Focal_IA	Enlargement of the left amygdala	Left temporal neocortex	Awaiting surgery	N/A	High	N/A	5	18
21	F	32	Focal_A Focal_IA	Left occipital periventricular nodules	Left occipital and right posterior temporal region	Awaiting surgery: Possible RNS	N/A	High	N/A	2	15
22	F	53	Focal_IA with secondary generalization	Non-lesional	Left temporal lobe (temporal pole and mesial temporal structures	Awaiting surgery	N/A	Low	N/A	7	25

FocalA, Focal Awareness Seizure; Focal_IA, Focal Impaired Awareness Seizures; TC, Tonic Clonic Seizures; MRgLiTT, MRI guided laser interstitial thermal therapy; RNS, Responsive Neurostimulator.

at the Johns Hopkins Hospital (JHH) Epilepsy Monitoring Unit (EMU) with patient's consent as part of the Studies of Patients with Implanted Intracranial Electrodes (IRB 00044461). At least two board-certified epileptologists reviewed the iEEG during the patient's seizures and identified electrodes involved in regions of seizure onset (SOZ), early spread (EP), and irritative (IZ). Seizure onset was defined as the first consistent presence of rhythmic spikes, rhythmic sharp waves, regular or low amplitude activity in the beta range, or recruiting gamma activity that was either prior or coinciding with the clinical manifestation of the seizure. The early spread regions were defined as those areas to which the seizure activity spread before secondary generalization occurred, and irritative zones were marked where there were epileptic spikes only (46).

Patients were classified as having successful surgical outcomes if they experienced seizure freedom one-year after surgery (Engel class I) or nearly seizure freedom (Engel class II) and failed outcomes if they experienced seizure recurrence (Engel classes III-IV) (47) (**Table 1**). However, in instances where a responsive neurostimulation device (RNS) was used rather than resection or ablation, Engel class III was a surgical success. Thirteen of the 22 patients underwent surgical intervention and were evaluated for surgical outcome. Due to the lack of outcome data in the remaining 9 patients, we categorized all patients by a custom "clinical complexity (CC)" score (**Figure 1**) (42, 43). Patients with lesional or focal epilepsy in the temporal lobe were classified as CCLow and those patients with non-lesional or multifocal epilepsy outside of the temporal or that were non-localizable were classified as CCHigh (**Figure 1**). These categories were developed in light of previous outcome studies that showed that patients with visible lesions on MRI (lesional) have higher surgical success rates (~70%), while non-lesional, extratemporal, and multifocal epilepsies have much lower success rates (48–50) (**Figure 1**).

Single-Pulse Electrical Stimulation

SPES was conducted in a bipolar fashion of adjacent electrode pairs clinically annotated in the SOZ and early spread regions as well some outside of the SOZ using a Blackrock acquisition system at a sampling rate of 1 or 2 kHz (51). A monophasic, alternating polarity, 0.3 ms width square wave pulse at a fixed frequency of 0.5 Hz was delivered to all the electrode pairs an average of 50 times. Current intensity was titrated until manifestations of local/distant evoked response potentials (ERPs), discharges/seizures, or a maximum intensity of 12 mA was reached. A 5 mA stimulus intensity was most often used. Responses were recorded from all channels during the 50 trials. The data was digitized and stored in an IRB-approved database compliant with the Health Insurance Portability and Accountability Act regulations. Data was then preprocessed as .dat files for analysis in MATLAB (52). The research protocol was approved by the Institutional Review Board and informed consent was obtained from all participants.

iEEG Preprocessing

The average evoked response was computed for every contact in 2 s epochs. We included 500 ms of data before stimulus onset and 1,500 ms post stimulus onset. We calculated the distribution of

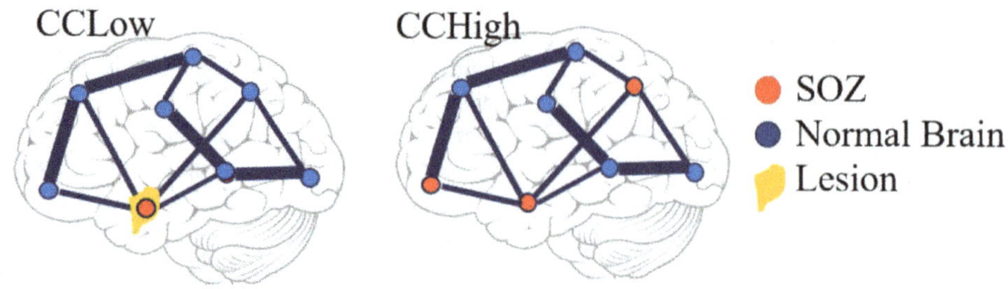

FIGURE 1 | Pictorial representation of clinical complexity. CCLow was defined as cases that were lesional, only one seizure focus, or solely confined to the temporal lobe. CCHigh was defined as cases of multi-focal epilepsy, a seizure focus outside the temporal lobe, and/or no lesions on imaging.

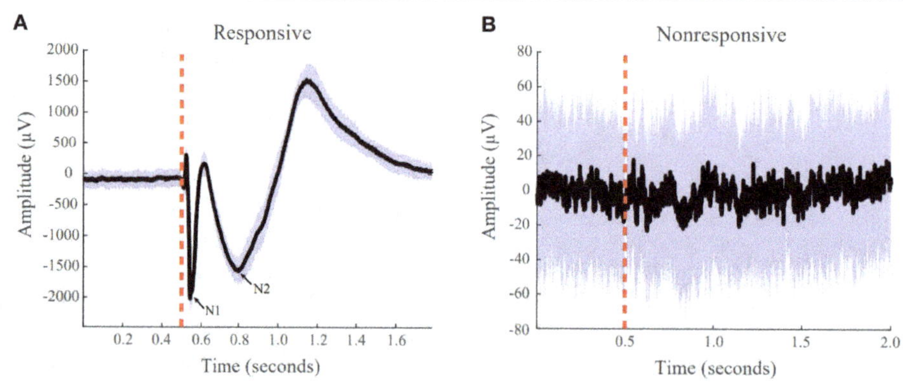

FIGURE 2 | Examples of responsive and non-responsive waveforms from patient iEEG data. **(A)** Responsive CCEPs were defined as an absolute value of the post-stimulus amplitude >100 uV from the baseline. The N1 and N2 peak are labeled. **(B)** Non-responsive CCEP that does not meet the 100 uV post-stimulus amplitude threshold. The black line indicates the average evoked response, the purple boundaries denote one standard deviation, and the red vertical dotted line indicates the stimulation onset.

the 50 time series responses for each 2 s window and marked channels as artifactual if the median standard deviation of the sample distributions was >1,000. These artifactual channels were then removed from the dataset. Next, artifacts due to electrical stimulation were removed by replacing the data 2 ms before and 8 ms after stimulus onset with a linearly spaced vector between those voltage values. We classified channels as responsive and non-responsive if the absolute value of the maximum post-stimulus amplitude was $>100\mu V$ from the baseline (**Figure 2**). Non-responsive channels were removed from the dataset before model construction.

Transfer Function Model Construction

SIMO transfer functions were constructed for each subject and each stimulating electrode pair to estimate the behavior of the CCEPs. To construct our transfer function models, we first built stable, discrete, linear time invariant (LTI) state space models of the following form for each stimulating contact pair:

$$\boldsymbol{x}(t+1) = \boldsymbol{A}\boldsymbol{x}(t) + \boldsymbol{B}u(t) \tag{1}$$

where $\boldsymbol{x}(t) \in \mathbb{R}^{N\times 1}$ is the state vector, $\boldsymbol{A} \in \mathbb{R}^{N\times N}$ is the state transition matrix, $u(t) \in \mathbb{R}$ is the input stimulation pulse, and $\boldsymbol{B} \in \mathbb{R}^{N\times 1}$ is the input matrix, with N representing the total number of contacts for each dataset. $\boldsymbol{A}$ and $\boldsymbol{B}$ were calculated via least-squares estimation as described in (53), and the state vector was comprised of the responsive iEEG signals (**Figure 3**). The models were stimulated with input signal $(t) = 0$ or 1, where the first non-zero element corresponded to the iEEG stimulation onset, with a pulse duration of 2 ms, and t is the index for each millisecond. The pair of stimulation electrodes were not included in the models as state variables and were instead characterized as providing the exogenous input $u\,(t)$. Next, to improve our model fits, we established a scaling factor, α, based on the range of data $\mathbf{x}(t)$ in relation to the range of the model reconstruction $\hat{\mathbf{x}}(t)$ for every contact, k:

$$\alpha_k = \frac{\max x_k\,(t) - \min x_k(t)}{\max \hat{x_k}\,(t) - \min \hat{x_k}\,(t)} \tag{2}$$

We then scaled our $\boldsymbol{A}$ and $\boldsymbol{B}$ by this factor, giving us the following:

$$\overline{\boldsymbol{x}}(t+1) = \overline{\boldsymbol{A}}x(t) + \overline{\boldsymbol{B}}u(t) \tag{3}$$

where $\overline{\boldsymbol{A}} = \alpha\boldsymbol{A}$ and $\overline{\boldsymbol{B}} = \alpha\boldsymbol{B}$.

Once the state space models were created, we calculated the SIMO transfer function model from $u(t)$ to $\boldsymbol{x}(t)$ via the formula

$$\boldsymbol{H}\,(z) = \left(zI - \overline{\boldsymbol{A}}\right)^{-1}\overline{\boldsymbol{B}} \tag{4}$$

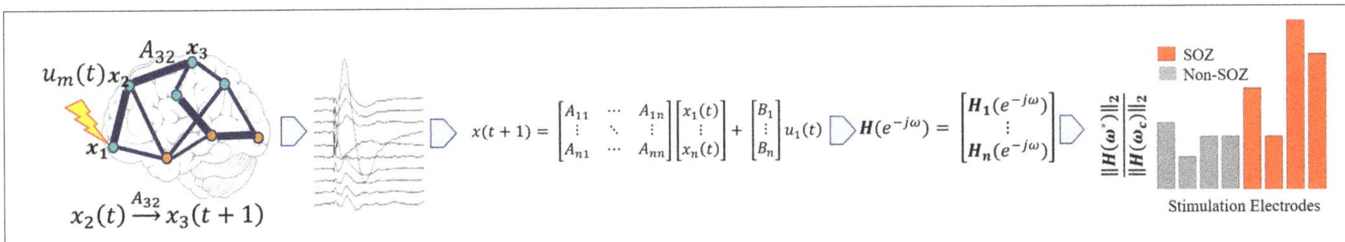

FIGURE 3 | Pipeline to obtain system gain $\boldsymbol{H}_\infty$- to- input norm ratio from individual patients' SPES iEEG data. Starting from top left, a brain region is stimulated. Then a stereotyped response is extracted for each electrode, from which the average evoked CCEP is calculated. The CCEPs are used to construct a state-space model. From the state space model, a SIMO transfer function vector is constructed via $\boldsymbol{H}(z) = \boldsymbol{C}(zI - \boldsymbol{A})^{-1}\boldsymbol{B}$. Then the maximum system gain is calculated for every stimulation pair through $\|\boldsymbol{H}(\omega)\|_\infty = sup\ \omega\epsilon R\sigma_{\max}(\boldsymbol{H}(e - i\omega))$ and the 2-norm of the associated frequency response at the cutoff frequency, is computed resulting in the PF ratio. The expectation is that the true SOZ contacts will have the largest PF ratios.

which is derived by taking the z-transform of (1). These transfer function models represent the input-output behavior of CCEPs under SPES. The SIMO transfer function models characterize how each iEEG node (channel) *dynamically* influences the rest of the network and how the network responds to an exogenous stimulus, like SPES.

Investigating Model Properties

After constructing the SIMO transfer function models for each stimulating pair for each subject, we investigated whether properties of these transfer functions correlated to clinically annotated SOZ regions. Specifically, we investigated the peak system gain and the magnitude of the frequency response at the roll-off frequency defined to be the frequency at which the magnitude dipped 3dB below the DC gain (gain at 0 frequency) for each model. The *system gain* of a transfer function, a metric that quantifies how much ERPs can be amplified and spread in the iEEG network, may reveal epileptogenic zone (EZ) regions. The larger the gain, the more influence the node has on spreading activity throughout the network. We also hypothesized that the peak of the frequency response should be followed by a steep roll-off since seizures happen infrequently, which is likely a consequence of resonance in the iEEG network. Consistent with the theory of "fragility" in epileptic brain networks (54), we further hypothesized that the SOZ should produce the largest network responses with the smallest input size.

We therefore proposed a metric which can capture the large system responses and its fast magnitude drop-off through a ratio of peak-to-floor gains, the PF ratio. Epileptogenic regions when stimulated should result in a high PF ratio. To compute the PF ratio for a given stimulation pair, we calculated the system gain of all the SIMO transfer function as quantified by the $\mathcal{H}_\infty$ norm. The $\mathcal{H}_\infty$ norm of each stimulation electrode pair j was calculated, as follows:

$$\left\|\boldsymbol{H}_j\right\|_\infty = sup\ \omega\epsilon R\sigma_{\max}(\boldsymbol{H}_j(e - i\omega)) = sup\ \omega\epsilon R\left\|\boldsymbol{H}_j(e - i\omega)\right\|_2 \quad (5)$$

where $\sup_{\omega\in\mathbb{R}}$ denotes the supremum or least upper bound over all real frequencies ω and σ_{max} denotes the maximum singular value of the vector $\boldsymbol{H}_j$. The third equality is due to the fact $\boldsymbol{H}_j(e - i\omega)$ that is a column vector.

For each system gain there is a frequency ω^* at which this maximum gain was achieved, $\left\|\boldsymbol{H}_j(\omega^*)\right\|_\infty$. To quantify the "quick" magnitude drop, we calculated the cut-off frequency at which this occurred, ωc. The cutoff frequency in electrical engineering is the boundary where th energy flowing through a system begins to reduce (55). From here, we then calculated the 2-norm of the frequency response evaluated at this cut-off frequency ωc, $\left\|\boldsymbol{H}_j(\omega c)\right\|_2$, and finally the PF ratio as follows:

$$PF_j = \frac{\left\|\boldsymbol{H}_j(\omega*)\right\|_2}{\left\|\boldsymbol{H}_j(\omega c)\right\|_2} \quad (6)$$

where j represents each stimulation electrode pair ω^* is the peak frequency at which the maximum system gain was attained, and ωc is the cut-off frequency at which the magnitude response begins to drop (**Figure 4**).

Correlating PF Ratios to Epileptogenic Regions

Once the PF ratio was computed for each stimulating pair for each subject, we measured the agreement between our PF ratios and the clinical annotations through a confidence statistic (CS). We defined the CS to be the ratio of the mean of the PF ratios of stimulation pairs in the clinically annotated SOZ and early spread (EP) to the mean of the PF ratios of all other stimulation pairs:

$$CS = \frac{\frac{1}{m}\sum_{SOZ\&EP} PF_j}{\frac{1}{n-m}\sum_{Other} PF_j} \quad (7)$$

where m is the number of stimulation pairs in the SOZ and EP regions, n is the total number of stimulation pairs, and *other* is all the stimulation pairs not in the SOZ or EP. We expected the highest GN ratios to closely match the clinical annotated SOZ in patients with a lower clinical complexity score (CCLow). That is we expected higher confidence statistics in patients with lower clinical complexity. On the other hand, patients with a higher clinical complexity score (CCHigh) may show more disagreement between the model results and the clinical notations, resulting in lower and more variable confidence statistics.

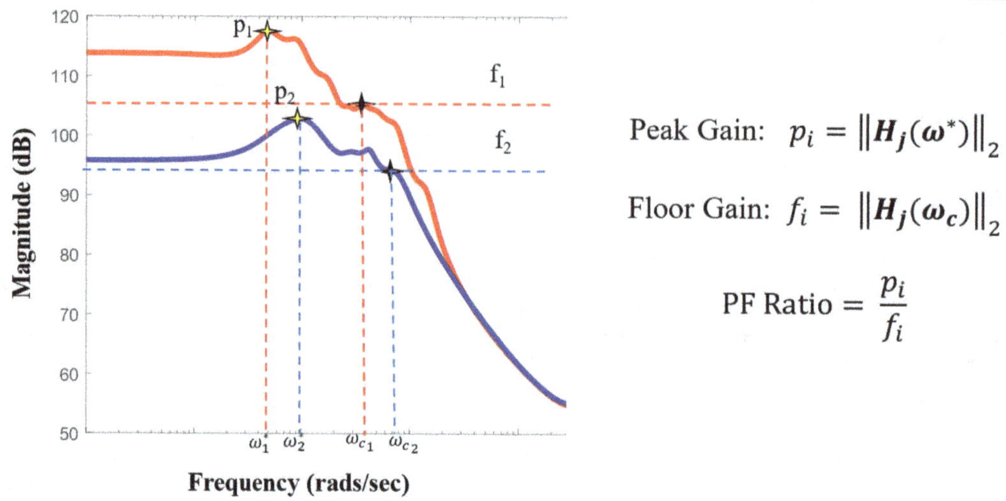

FIGURE 4 | Pictorial representation of the PF ratio and its calculation. Representative bode plot of two transfer function models, where red denotes a clinically annotated SOZ dataset and blue denotes a dataset stimulated that is not part of the epileptogenic region, with their labeled peak and cutoff frequencies, ω^* and ωC, respectively. The cutoff frequency is defined as the frequency for which the magnitude is 3dB less than the gain at frequency 0, $\omega = 0$ (DC gain).

Correlating CCEPs Amplitude to Epileptogenic Regions

In the current SPES literature, there are numerous methods for CCEP analysis. The most common practice is visual inspection of the peak response amplitude, more precisely, the N1 response. The N1 responses are early sharp negative responses occurring anywhere from 10 to 30 ms post stimulation and are believed to reflect the direct structural connections (**Figure 2**) (11). For our study, to be able to compare the N1 response with our PF ratio, we calculated the N1 peak for all evoked potentials. This was done after the preprocessing of our data in which we looked at a window 10 ms before and 30 ms after the onset of stimulation. Within that time frame, the maximum absolute peak amplitude was calculated, which we called the N1 peak for all output contacts. We then calculated our confidence statistic using the N1 peak as well.

RESULTS

Transfer Function Models Reconstruct CCEPs

We first assessed whether the SIMO transfer function models were able to accurately reconstruct CCEPs by calculating the percentage of data points that lied within the 95% confidence interval of the mean from the 50 stimulation trials. This resulted in an average concordance of 92.96% indicating that our models were able to accurately reconstruct the mean waveforms of our data, capturing the input-output behavior of CCEPs under SPES (**Figure 5**).

Higher PF Ratios in the Seizure Onset Zone for Low Clinical Complexity Cases

In cases of low clinical complexity, our expectation was that our models would agree with the clinical annotations, and in cases of high clinical complexity there would be high variability of agreement between our model statistics and clinical annotations. We further hypothesized that successful surgical outcomes will show high agreement regardless of clinical complexity.

Patient 13 is an example of a low clinical complexity case (CCLow) and Patient 14 is an example of a high clinical complexity case (CCHigh) (**Figure 6**). These two cases show alignment with our hypothesis in the low clinical complexity cases, our PF ratios are the highest in the areas of the clinical annotated SOZ as well as early spread regions resulting in a higher confidence statistic, while in the higher complexity case, the highest PF ratios are not in areas deemed to be part of the epileptogenic network.

In Patient 13, the largest PF ratios were associated with stimulation pairs that were in the SOZ (**Figure 6A**). Further, most other contact pairs in the EP (orange) also yielded high PF ratios, while the two electrodes pairs believed to not be part of the epileptic network (gray) had the smallest PF ratios. The high degree of agreement between our model gains and the clinical annotations resulted in a CS of 1.034.

In Patient 14, the largest PF ratios were in areas outside of the clinical annotations (**Figure 6B**), where the average PF ratio of 27.550 for the SOZ and EP electrodes and an average GN ratio of 80.2357 in all other electrode pairs.

Faster Magnitude Roll-Offs in Successful Patient Outcomes

In successful surgical outcomes, where clinicians were able to accurately localize the SOZ, we anticipated frequency response plots similar to the ones in **Figure 4**, where the SOZ stimulated dataset would have a high peak gain and a roll-off in magnitude compared to the non-SOZ stimulated datasets. The mean frequency response plot of the SOZ and EP stimulated datasets of Patient 18, a surgical success, had a high peak gain and a big

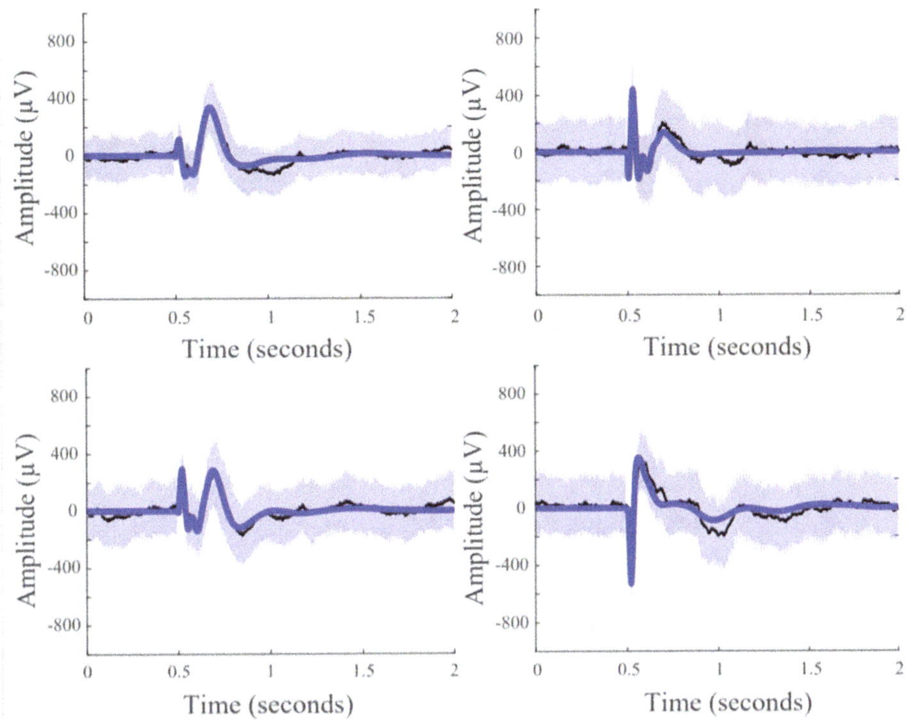

FIGURE 5 | Model fits of four representative responsive channels from patient data showing SIMO transfer function models capture CCEP responses in recording electrodes. Black lines are the average the evoked responses, blue lines are the model reconstruction, and the purple boundaries denotes one standard deviation.

roll-off compared to the non-EZ stimulated datasets (**Figure 7A**). In the failed surgical outcome case of Patient 2 (**Figure 7B**), the SOZ stimulated datasets not only had a very small peak gain, but a rather slow roll-off as well. However, the non-SOZ stimulated datasets had overall the highest peak gains and incredibly fast roll-offs, suggesting that these datasets may be part of the epileptogenic region.

Correlating Surgical Outcomes to PF Ratios

We have summarized our findings for all 22 patients with three different scatter plots (**Figure 8**). The first plot displays the confidence statistic for all patients classified in terms of their clinical complexity, confidence statistic, and surgical outcome if available (**Figure 8A**). The second plot displays the confidence statistic for only those patients with surgical outcome classified in terms of their confidence statistic and either surgical failure or success (**Figure 8B**). Finally, the last scatter plot again displays the confidence statistic for patients with surgical outcome but has now separated outcomes in terms of the Engel Score (**Figure 8C**). The dotted line indicates the degree of agreement boundary, where CS values above the line indicate patients whose highest PF ratios agreed most with the clinically annotated SOZ and EP regions, and thereby implying a greater chance of surgical success, while those CS values below the line indicate patients whose highest PF ratios varied most with clinical annotations, and potentially imply a greater chance of surgical failure.

We tested whether the transfer function models were able to not only localize the SOZ, but also anticipate the surgical outcome for seizure freedom. Overall, in the MRE patients who underwent resective surgery and had a successful outcome (ES I and ES II), indicating the clinicians were able to successfully localize the SOZ, our models had the highest PF ratios in the clinically annotated SOZ and therefore a high confidence statistic (CS $\geq$ 1), irrespective of the clinical complexity (**Figure 8C**). In the surgical resection cases that resulted in poor seizure outcomes (ES III and ES IV), suggesting the clinicians were unable to precisely and accurately localize the SOZ, our models exhibited low PF ratios in the clinically annotated SOZ and larger PF ratio values in areas that were not part of the clinically annotated SOZ (CS $<$ 1) (**Figure 8C**). Thus, we conjecture that in patients that have undergone surgical resection/ablation, a high concordance between our models and clinical annotations would suggest seizure freedom, while large variations between our models and annotations would suggest a poor surgical outcome.

PF Ratios vs. N1 Peaks

To determine the efficacy of our system metric over the current CCEP analysis through visual inspection of the N1 amplitude, we analyzed the correlation between PF ratio and peak amplitude as well as the confidence statistic for N1. The confidence statistic for N1 demonstrated slightly poorer performance in the classification of surgical outcomes than the PF ratio (**Figure 8B**). In the CCLow cases, one of the datasets (Patient 4) which has a successful surgical outcome has a CS $<$ 1, while in the CCHigh

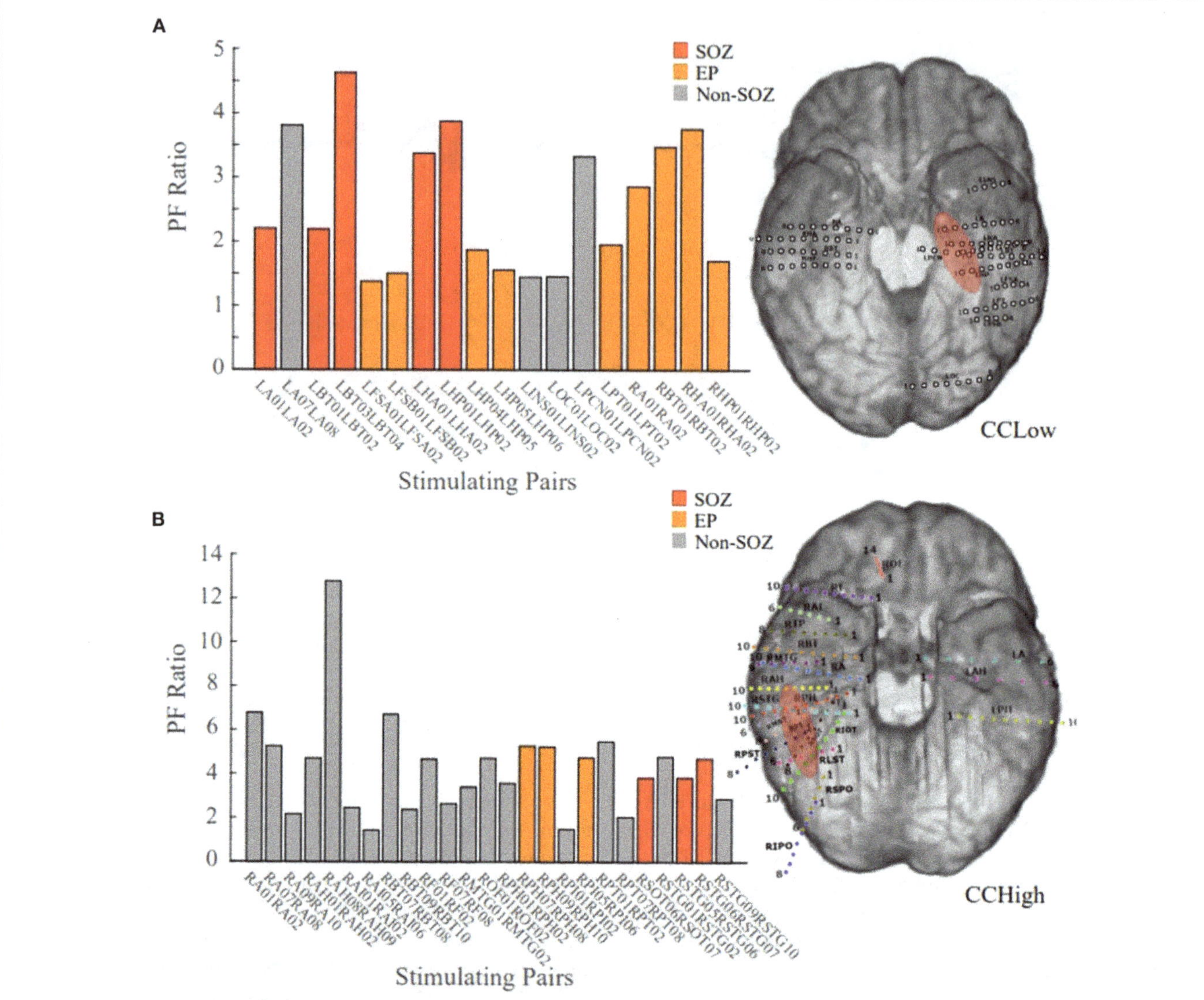

FIGURE 6 | Bar plot of the PF ratios, where red indicates electrode pairs in the clinically annotated seizure onset zone (SOZ), orange indicates early spread (EP), and gray represents all others. To the right of the bar graphs are the electrode implantation maps for each patient with the clinical annotated SOZ denoted in red. **(A)** PF ratios of representative "model success" Patient 13 dataset; high PF ratio values closely correspond with SOZ and EP regions. **(B)** PF ratios of representative "model disagreement" Patient 14A dataset; SOZ and EP PF ratios are indistinguishable from non-epileptogenic regions.

case Patient 2, which had an unsuccessful surgical result, has a CS > 1 (**Figure 8B**). Additionally, the Pearson correlation between PF ratios and N1 peak amplitude for all datasets averaged 0.1515 ± 0.1676, indicating little correspondence between the metrics (**Supplementary Figure 1**).

DISCUSSION

Patient specific dynamical network models were built from SPES data and analyzed for a population of medically refractory epilepsy patients that were admitted to the Johns Hopkins Hospital. These patients were admitted for the localization of their seizure network for the possibility of seizure freedom via surgical resection. As epileptic seizures are believed to result from a pathologically connected brain network with epileptic foci (56), we conjectured that the analysis of intracranial EEG data in response to stimulation in the context of dynamic networks would provide an advantage to current localization techniques that are based on passive iEEG. SPES provides an opportunity to actively perturb the brain, and then capture and analyze the rich dynamics of the iEEG network to localize the SOZ.

Dynamical Network Models for the Localization of the SOZ

Work done by A. Li et al. (54) showed that an epileptic brain can be modeled as a network that is on the verge of instability,

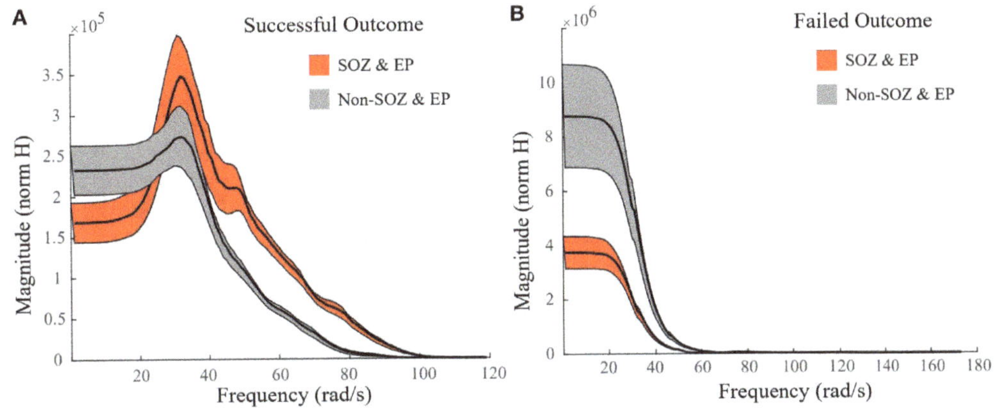

FIGURE 7 | Representative frequency response plots of a successful and failed surgical outcome where red denotes SOZ and EP stimulated datasets, grey denotes non-SOZ and EP stimulated datasets, black is the mean frequency response, and the shaded regions denote ±2 standard error. **(A)** Frequency response plot of the SOZ & EP stimulated datasets vs the non-SOZ & EP stimulated datasets for successful surgical outcome Patient 18. The SOZ & EP stimulated datasets show a larger peak gain and a bigger roll off than the non-SOZ & EP counterparts. **(B)** Frequency response plot of the SOZ & EP stimulated datasets vs the non-SOZ & EP stimulated datasets for failed surgical outcome Patient 2.

where a small perturbation can result in the manifestation of a seizure. There are nodes within this network that are potentially more "fragile" than others, corresponding to the brain regions associated with the onset of the seizure. The fragility of these network nodes makes them susceptible to small perturbations, evoking a significant response or disturbance in the network, possibly initiating a seizure. We hypothesized that these "fragile" nodes should produce large responses, responses larger than the other nodes within the network. It is also known that seizure spread is specified by impaired excitation and inhibition balance, suggesting that large responses may be a potential biomarker of this imbalance (57–59).

We used transfer function models to analyze the responses of the network to SPES. One performance metric of these models that can quantify and characterize this notion is the peak gain of the system and the cutoff frequency at which the magnitude drops by half. This can be calculated through a ratio of the $\mathcal{H}_\infty$ norm and the 2-norm of the associated frequency response evaluated at the cutoff frequency. Our conjecture was that those electrode pairs with the highest PF ratio of peak gain to cutoff gain to input norm would correspond to the electrode pairs in the clinically annotated SOZ, particularly for patients with low clinical complexity and successful surgical outcomes.

PF Ratios Correlate to Clinical Annotations

We hypothesized that the areas involved in the epileptogenic region, such as SOZ and EP, when stimulated, would produce the largest system gains and the biggest response drop-offs as compared to areas not involved in the epileptogenic network. We further conjectured that for those patients whose epilepsy was due to a lesion, had a focal onset, or originated solely in the temporal region (CCLow), the clinicians would be able to identify the SOZ accurately and completely. This would suggest that, in our models, those electrode pairs in the clinically annotated SOZ and EP, should have large gain values *and* small floor gain values, when compared to other electrode pairs. Therefore, we expected to see a higher degree of agreement between our PF ratios and the clinical annotations, resulting in a confidence statistic ≥ 1. However, for those patients whose epilepsy was non-lesional, multifocal, and extratemporal, (CCHigh), we speculated that the clinicians had a more difficult time precisely locating the SOZ and early spread regions. Thus, we expected in these cases for our PF ratios to have more variations and potential disagreements with the clinical annotations (more variable CS), possibly highlighting areas that may have been overlooked or that could not be captured with the current localization methods. Our models may also be able to predict which patients will have surgical success and which will fail, depending on the level of disagreement between the model and the clinical annotations. A larger discordance would indicate a more complex case and the increased likelihood of a failed outcome.

We explored the relationship between the ratio of the system gains and the input norms of our transfer function models to regions of epileptogenic interest. Overall, we found that the patient cases classified of lower clinical complexity tended to have the highest PF ratio in the electrodes clinically marked as SOZ. If not in the SOZ, often electrode pairs with higher PF ratios belonged to locations that were of interest, such as the EP. For example, Patient 13 had been classified as CCLow because the patient presented with a focal encephalomalacia of the inferior temporal lobe. This lesion, in conjunction with the patient's seizure semiology and iEEG recordings made the localization of the SOZ and early spread regions more straightforward for the clinicians.

On the other hand, as the clinical complexity increased, the discrepancies between the model PF ratios and the clinically annotated SOZs also increased. In Patient 14, the electrode pairs in the clinically annotated SOZ and EP, yielded some of the smallest PF ratio values (**Figure 6B**). However, this patient has been admitted to the JHH EMU on two separate occasions for

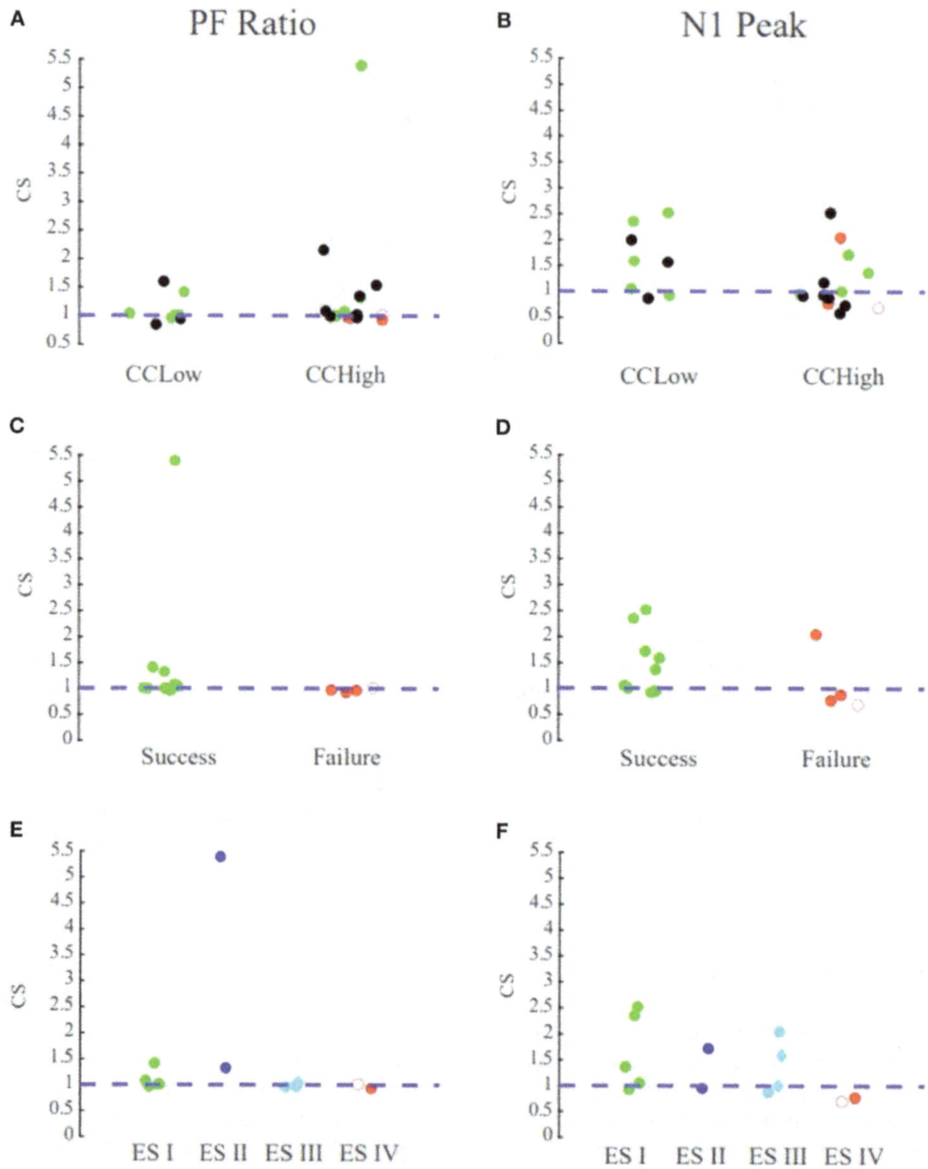

FIGURE 8 | PF ratio confidence statistic reflects surgical outcome. Green circles denote those patients with successful surgical outcomes, red denotes those with failed surgical outcomes, and black denotes datasets that currently have no surgical outcome. The blue dotted line denotes the boundary for the degree of agreement between clinical annotations and the performance metrics. Diamond shape indicates RNS patients and open circle indicates outlier Patient 5. Top row contains the confidence statistic plots for all datasets. Middle row are the confidence statistic plots for surgical patients categorized by surgical success and failures. Bottom row has the confidence statistic plots for surgical patients categorized by Engel Score. **(A)** The confidence statistic plot for the PF ratio for all datasets. CCLow patients often have CS > 1, and surgical success nearly always have CS values >1. **(B)** The confidence statistic plot for N1 peak for all datasets. Less distinction is provided between groups according to the N1 amplitude as compared to system gain. **(C,D)** Confidence statistic plots for surgical patients categorized by surgical success/failure for **(C)** PF ratio **(D)** and N1 peak. **(E,F)** Confidence statistic plot for surgical patients categorized by Engel score for **(E)** PF ratio and **(F)** N1 peak.

localization of seizure onset. During both stays, the clinicians were unable to localize the SOZ, requiring a third visit with the implantation of a grid. The inability to localize this patient's seizures implies that though there is disagreement between the clinical annotations and the PF ratios, our model may be identifying regions of interest that the clinicians were unable to identify through individual iEEG channel inspection.

Large Magnitude Drop Offs Correlate to Epileptogenic Regions

Studying the mean frequency responses of our systems, we explored properties that may indicate the epileptogenic zone. We observed that the frequency responses of the SOZ stimulated datasets in successful surgical outcomes, had not only some of the largest system gains, but also some of the quickest and biggest

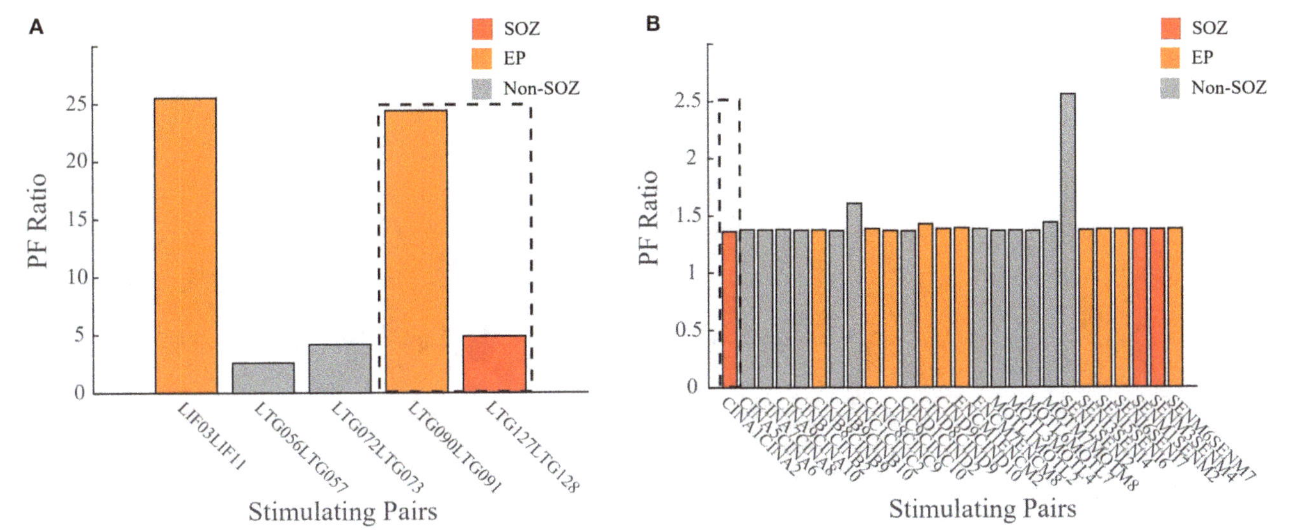

FIGURE 9 | Bar plot of the PF ratio transfer functions for two patient datasets with surgical outcome data. Dashed lines indicate the areas of resection. **(A)** CCLow Patient 3 who now is seizure free (ESII), **(B)** CCHigh Patient 7 who still has seizures (ES IV). Red indicates electrode pairs in the clinically annotated seizure onset zone (SOZ), orange is early spread (EP), and gray are all others. In surgical success, the resected regions closely matched the clinically annotated SOZ regions with high PF ratio values.

magnitude drops, especially when compared to their non-SOZ counterparts (**Figure 7A**). This difference became even more striking when comparing the mean SOZ stimulated datasets vs the mean non-SOZ stimulated datasets for a failed surgical outcome case. In this instance, the clinically annotated SOZ stimulated datasets had some of the smallest peak gains and some of the slower, smaller magnitude drop offs, while the non-SOZ stimulated datasets had very high peak gains and steep drop offs (**Figure 7B**). This may suggest a resonance-like property of cortical networks that can generate seizures if triggered by a periodic stimulation at a particular frequency. This is certainly the case for photosensitive epilepsy (60), where flashing stimuli (in time or space) at a particular frequency may cause a seizure. Our findings suggest that resonance may be more prevalent in all types of epilepsy.

PF Ratios Reflect Surgical Outcomes

A true test for SOZ localization algorithms is in their ability to predict surgical outcomes. We defined a successful surgical outcome to be those patients with an Engel score or I and II, or if a responsive neurostimulation (RNS) device was implanted, an Engel score of III was considered a success. A failed surgical outcome was defined as those patients who had surgical resection or ablation and received an Engel score of III or IV. Patient 3 was categorized as CCLow and now has seizure freedom (ES II) (**Figure 9A**). The clinicians identified electrode pairs LIF03/11, LTG09/91 and LTG127128 as those they believed to be the in the EP (orange) and SOZ (red), respectively. Our model revealed that LTG90/91 and LIF03/11 had the highest PF ratios out of all electrode pairs. The resected areas included the SOZ contact LTG127/128 and EP contact LTG90/91, which had one of the highest PF ratios. Which had the two highest PF ratios. Given the surgical outcome of ES II, this demonstrates the agreement between our model and clinical annotations in patient cases of low clinical complexity and the correlation to successful surgical outcomes.

In unsuccessful surgical outcomes (ES III and ES IV), we hypothesized the highest PF ratios would be in regions not labeled as the SOZ. Patient 7 was a difficult case (CCHigh) who, despite a laser ablation at contact CINA1-2, had no improvement in their seizure frequency (ES IV) (**Figure 9B**). The low PF ratio in CINA1-2 indicates that our algorithm identified this region of the brain as non-epileptogenic. Moreover, our algorithm identified SENI1-2 as a region that may possibly show epileptogenicity due to the high PF ratio values in that region.

There were instances where our model agreed with the clinical annotations resulting in a high confidence statistic, however, the surgical outcome did not result in seizure freedom. Outlier Patient 5 is a patient whose clinically annotated SOZ and EP contacts resulted in high PF ratios which would normally suggest a success (**Figure 10**). The regions that were resected were those in the SOZ pairs LPPS1/2 and LSPS1/2, which resulted in an unsuccessful surgical outcome (ES IV). However, despite the poor surgical results, the confidence statistic for this patient (Patient 5) was high (CS = 1.0263). Due to part of the SOZ (electrode pair LFP63/64) being located in a language area of the cortex, it was not surgically removed to prevent a functional deficit. The next highest PF ratios not resected were in the EP pairs LFPG33/34 and LFPG35/36, which were also located in the eloquent cortex (motor), making the tissue not viable for resection. Failing to remove the entire SOZ likely caused the failed outcome. This is just one of several examples demonstrating the complexity of diagnosing and treating these

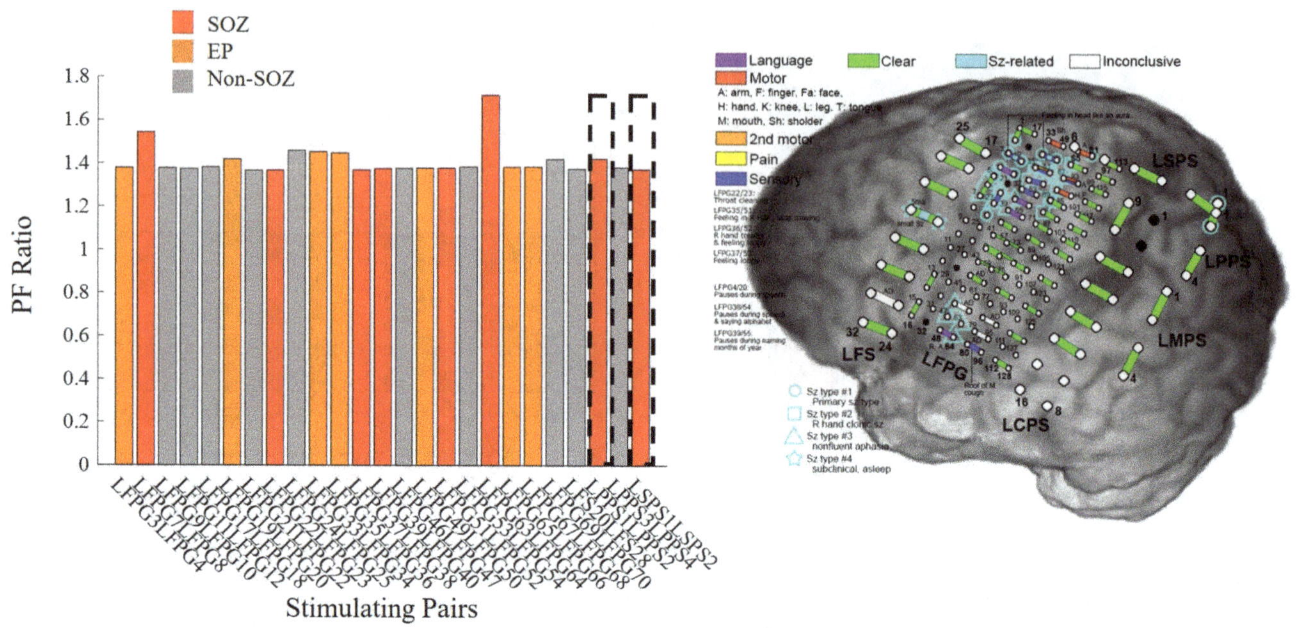

FIGURE 10 | Bar plot of PF ratios for Patient 5 with a high confidence statistic value according to the model, but an unsuccessful surgical outcome. The dotted boxes represent the regions that were resected. Red indicates electrode pairs in the clinically annotated seizure onset zone (SOZ), orange is early spread (EP), and gray are all others. Regions with high PF ratios were not resected because they were in eloquent cortex, possibly explaining the seizure persistence.

patients and more importantly the difficulty of evaluating computational algorithms.

Study Limitations

The major limitation of this study is the low number of study subjects, particularly those with surgical outcomes. Extending this study to more patients with varying pathologies and epilepsy etiologies, particularly those with surgical outcomes, would increase the power of this study. The inclusion of more surgical outcome data would help to prove the efficacy of the PF ratio and its advantages over the N1 peak. There are also other properties of the transfer function models that need to be explored, such as the phase delay, and pole-zero locations. Potentially, analysis and inclusion of these additional metrics may help more accurately and fully characterize the epileptic network and show the advantage of using the PF ratio for localization of the SOZ, particularly in cases of high clinical complexity.

AUTHOR CONTRIBUTIONS

GK, RS, SS, NC, and JK designed the study. NC, JK, MH, and CC conducted the experiments and collected the data. GK and RS implemented the algorithms, preprocessed the data, performed the data analysis, and wrote the manuscript. SS and JK provided the research ideas and revised the manuscript. All authors revised and approved the final version of the manuscript.

ACKNOWLEDGMENTS

The authors would like to thank the members of the Neuromedical Control Systems Lab (NCSL) and the Crone Lab for their helpful discussions regarding this work.

REFERENCES

1. Singh A, Trevick S. The epidemiology of global epilepsy. *Neurol Clin.* (2016) 34:837–47. doi: 10.1016/j.ncl.2016.06.015
2. Berg AT, Kelly MM. Defining intractability: comparisons among published definitions. *Epilepsia.* (2006) 47:431–6. doi: 10.1111/j.1528-1167.2006.00440.x
3. Kwan P, Brodie MJ. Definition of refractory epilepsy: defining the indefinable? *Lancet Neurol.* (2010) 9:27–9. doi: 10.1016/S1474-4422(09)70304-7
4. Bulacio JC, Jehi L, Wong C, Gonzalez-Martinez J, Kotagal P, Nair D, et al. Longterm seizure outcome after resective surgery in patients evaluated with intracranial electrodes. *Epilepsia.* (2012) 53:1722–30. doi: 10.1111/j.1528-1167.2012.03633.x
5. Gonzalez-Martinez JA, Srikijvilaikul T, Nair D, Bingaman WE. Long-term seizure outcome in reoperation after failure of epilepsy surgery. *Neurosurgery.* (2007) 60:873–80. doi: 10.1227/01.NEU.0000255438.13871.FA
6. Holmes MD, Tucker DM. Identifying the epileptic network. *Front Neurol.* (2013) 4:84. doi: 10.3389/fneur.2013.00084
7. Wilson CL, Isokawa M, Babb TL, Crandall PH. Functional connections in the human temporal lobe. *Exp Brain Res.* (1990) 82:279–92. doi: 10.1007/BF00231248
8. Wilson CL, Isokawa M, Babb TL, Crandall PH, Levesque MF, Engel J Jr. Functional connections in the human temporal lobe. II. Evidence for a loss of functional linkage between contralateral limbic structures. *Exp Brain Res.* (1991) 85:174–87. doi: 10.1007/BF00229999
9. Matsumoto R, Nair DR, LaPresto E, Najm I, Bingaman W, Shibasaki H, et al. Functional connectivity in the human language system: a cortico-cortical evoked potential study. *Brain.* (2004) 127:2316–30. doi: 10.1093/brain/awh246
10. Keller CJ, Honey CJ, Entz L, Bickel S, Groppe DM, Toth E, et al. Corticocortical evoked potentials reveal projectors and integrators in human brain networks. *J Neurosci.* (2014) 34:9152–63. doi: 10.1523/JNEUROSCI.4289-13.2014

11. Keller CJ, Honey CJ, Mégevand P, Entz L, Ulbert I, Mehta AD. Mapping human brain networks withcortico-ortical evoked potentials. *Philos Trans Royal Soc B.* (2014) 369:20130528. doi: 10.1098/rstb.2013.0528
12. Matsumoto R, Nair DR, LaPresto E, Bingaman W, Shibasaki H, Lüders HO. Functional connectivity in human cortical motor system: a cortico-cortical evoked potential study. *Brain.* (2007) 130:181–97. doi: 10.1093/brain/awl257
13. Lacruz ME, García Seoane JJ, Valentin A, Selway R, Alarcón G. Frontal and temporal functional connections of the living human brain. *Eur J Neurosci.* (2007) 26:1357–70. doi: 10.1111/j.1460-9568.2007.05730.x
14. Matsumoto R, Nair DR, Ikeda A, Fumuro T, Lapresto E, Mikuni N, et al. Parieto-frontal network in humans studied by cortico-cortical evoked potential. *Human Brain Mapping.* (2012) 33:2856–72. doi: 10.1002/hbm.21407
15. Enatsu R, Gonzalez-Martinez J, Bulacio J, Kubota Y, Mosher J, Burgess RC, et al. Connections of the limbic network: a corticocortical evoked potentials study. *Cortex.* (2015) 62:20–33. doi: 10.1016/j.cortex.2014.06.018
16. Almashaikhi T, Rheims S, Jung J, Ostrowsky-Coste K, Montavont A, De Bellescize J, et al. Functional connectivity of insular efferences. *Human Brain Mapping.* (2014) 35:5279–94. doi: 10.1002/hbm.22549
17. Dionisio S, Mayoglou L, Cho SM, Prime D, Flanigan PM, Lega B, et al. Connectivity of the human insula: a cortico-cortical evoked potential (CCEP) study. *Cortex.* (2019) 120:419–42. doi: 10.1016/j.cortex.2019.05.019
18. Kubota Y, Enatsu R, Gonzalez-Martinez J, Bulacio J, Mosher J, Burgess RC, et al. *In vivo* human hippocampal cingulate connectivity: a corticocortical evoked potentials (CCEPs) study. *Clin Neurophysiol.* (2013) 124:1547–56. doi: 10.1016/j.clinph.2013.01.024
19. Mégevand P, Groppe DM, Bickel S, Mercier MR, Goldfinger MS, Keller CJ, et al. The hippocampus and amygdala are integrators of neocortical influence: a corticocortical evoked potential study. *Brain Connectivity.* (2017) 7:648–60. doi: 10.1089/brain.2017.0527
20. Matsumoto R, Kunieda T, Nair D. Single pulse electrical stimulation to probe functional and pathological connectivity in epilepsy. *Seizure.* (2017) 44:27–36. doi: 10.1016/j.seizure.2016.11.003
21. Iwasaki M, Enatsu R, Matsumoto R, Novak E, Thankappen B, Piao Z, et al. Accentuated cortico-cortical evoked potentials in neocortical epilepsy in areas of ictal onset. *Epileptic Disord.* (2010) 12:292–302. doi: 10.1684/epd.2010.0334
22. Zhang N, Zhang B, Rajah GB, Geng X, Singh R, Yang Y, et al. The effectiveness of cortico-cortical evoked potential in detecting seizure onset zones. *Neurol Res.* (2018) 40:480–90. doi: 10.1080/01616412.2018.1454092
23. Enatsu R, Piao Z, O'Connor T, Horning K, Mosher J, Burgess R, et al. Cortical excitability varies upon ictal onset patterns in neocortical epilepsy: a cortico-cortical evoked potential study. *Clin Neurophysiol.* (2012) 123:252–60. doi: 10.1016/j.clinph.2011.06.030
24. Lega B, Dionisio S, Flanigan P, Bingaman W, Najm I, Nair D, et al. Cortico-cortical evoked potentials for sites of early versus late seizure spread in stereoelectroencephalography. *Epilepsy Res.* (2015) 115:17–29. doi: 10.1016/j.eplepsyres.2015.04.009
25. Enatsu R, Jin K, Elwan S, Kubota Y, Piao Z, O'Connor T, et al. Correlations between ictal propagation and response to electrical cortical stimulation: a cortico-cortical evoked potential study. *Epilepsy Res.* (2012) 101:76–87. doi: 10.1016/j.eplepsyres.2012.03.004
26. Kokkinos V, Alarcón G, Selway RP, Valentín A. Role of single pulse electrical stimulation (SPES) to guide electrode implantation under general anaesthesia in presurgical assessment of epilepsy. *Seizure.* (2013) 22:198–204. doi: 10.1016/j.seizure.2012.12.012
27. Nayak D, Valentín A, Selway RP, Alarcón G. Can single pulse electrical stimulation provoke responses similar to spontaneous interictal epileptiform discharges? *Clin Neurophysiol.* (2014) 125:1306–11. doi: 10.1016/j.clinph.2013.11.019
28. Valentin A, Anderson M, Alarcón G, García-Seoane JJ, Selway R, Binnie CD, et al. Responses to single pulse electrical stimulation identify epileptogenesis in the human brain *in vivo. Brain.* (2002) 125:1709–18. doi: 10.1093/brain/awf187
29. Flanagan D, Valentín A, García Seoane JJ, Alarcón G, Boyd SG. Single-pulse electrical stimulation helps to identify epileptogenic cortex in children. *Epilepsia.* (2009) 50:1793–803. doi: 10.1111/j.1528-1167.2009.02056.x
30. Valentín A, Alarcón G, García-Seoane JJ, Lacruz ME, Nayak SD, Honavar M, et al. Single-pulse electrical stimulation identifies epileptogenic frontal cortex in the human brain. *Neurology.* (2005) 65:426–35. doi: 10.1212/01.wnl.0000171340.73078.c1
31. Valentín A, Alarcón G, Honavar M, García Seoane JJ, Selway RP, Polkey CE, et al. Single pulse electrical stimulation for identification of structural abnormalities and prediction of seizure outcome after epilepsy surgery: a prospective study. *Lancet Neurol.* (2005) 4:718–26. doi: 10.1016/S1474-4422(05)70200-3
32. Kobayashi K, Matsumoto R, Matsuhashi M, Usami K, Shimotake A, Kunieda T, et al. High frequency activity overriding cortico-cortical evoked potentials reflects altered excitability in the human epileptic focus. *Clin Neurophysiol.* (2017) 128:1673–81. doi: 10.1016/j.clinph.2017.06.249
33. Mouthaan BE, Van't Klooster MA, Keizer D, Hebbink GJ, Leijten FSS, Ferrier CH, et al. Single Pulse Electrical Stimulation to identify epileptogenic cortex: clinical information obtained from early evoked responses. *Clin Neurophysiol.* (2016) 127:1088–98. doi: 10.1016/j.clinph.2015.07.031
34. Davis TS, Rolston JD, Bollo RJ, House PA. Delayed high-frequency suppression after automated single-pulse electrical stimulation identifies the seizure onset zone in patients with refractory epilepsy. *Clin Neurophysiol.* (2018) 129:2466–74. doi: 10.1016/j.clinph.2018.06.021
35. Jacobs J, Zijlmans M, Zelmann R, Olivier A, Hall J, Gotman J, et al. Value of electrical stimulation and high frequency oscillations (80-500 Hz) in identifying epileptogenic areas during intracranial EEG recordings. *Epilepsia.* (2010) 51:573–82. doi: 10.1111/j.1528-1167.2009.02389.x
36. Van'T Klooster MA, Zijlmans M, Leijten FSS, Ferrier CH, Van Putten MJAM, Huiskamp GJM. Time-frequency analysis of single pulse electrical stimulation to assist delineation of epileptogenic cortex. *Brain.* (2011) 134:2855–66. doi: 10.1093/brain/awr211
37. Van 't Klooster MA, van Klink NEC, van Blooijs D, Ferrier CH, Braun KPJ, Leijten FSS, et al. Evoked versus spontaneous high frequency oscillations in the chronic electrocorticogram in focal epilepsy. *Clin Neurophysiol.* (2017) 128:858–66. doi: 10.1016/j.clinph.2017.01.017
38. Donos C, Mîndruţă I, Malîia MD, Raşină A, Ciurea J, Barborica A. Co-occurrence of high-frequency oscillations and delayed responses evoked by intracranial electrical stimulation in stereo-EEG studies. *Clin Neurophysiol.* (2017) 128:1043–52. doi: 10.1016/j.clinph.2016.11.028
39. Boido D, Kapetis D, Gnatkovsky V, Pastori C, Galbardi B, Sartori I, et al. Stimulus-evoked potentials contribute to map the epileptogenic zone during stereo-EEG presurgical monitoring. *Human Brain Mapping.* (2014) 35:4267–81. doi: 10.1002/hbm.22516
40. Zhao C, Liang Y, Li C, Gao R, Wei J, Zuo R, et al. Localization of epileptogenic zone based on cortico-cortical evoked potential (CCEP): a feature extraction and graph theory approach. *Front Neuroinform.* (2019) 13:1–9. doi: 10.3389/fninf.2019.00031
41. Van Blooijs D, Leijten FSS, van Rijen PC, Meijer HGE, Huiskamp GJM. Evoked directional network characteristics of epileptogenic tissue derived from single pulse electrical stimulation. *Human Brain Mapping.* (2018) 39:4611–22. doi: 10.1002/hbm.24309
42. Bulacio JC, Chauvel P, McGonigal A. Stereoelectroencephalography: interpretation. *J Clin Neurophysiol.* (2016) 33:503–10. doi: 10.1097/WNP.0000000000000305
43. Sheikh S, Thompson N, Bingaman W, Gonzalez Martinez J, Najm I, Jehi L. Redefining success in epilepsy surgery: the importance of relative seizure reduction in patient reported quality of life. *Epilepsia.* (2019) 60:2078–85. doi: 10.1111/epi.16327
44. Farahani FV, Karwowski W, Lighthall NR. Application of graph theory for identifying connectivity patterns in human brain networks: a systematic review. *Front Neurosci.* (2019) 13:585. doi: 10.3389/fnins.2019.00585
45. Bernhardt C, Bonilha L, Gross DW. Network analysis for a network disorder: the emerging role of graph theory in the study of epilepsy. *Epilepsy Behav.* (2015) 50:162–70. doi: 10.1016/j.yebeh.2015.06.005
46. Gotz-Trabert K, Hauck C, Wagner K, Fauser S, Schulze- Bonhage A. Spread of ictal activity in focal epilepsy. *Epilepsia.* (2008) 49:1594–601. doi: 10.1111/j.1528-1167.2008.01627.x
47. Engel J. *Surgical Treatment of the Epilepsies.* Lippincott Williams and Wilkins. (1993).

48. Vakharia VN, Duncan JS, Witt JA, Elger CE, Staba R, Engel J. Getting the best outcomes from epilepsy surgery. *Ann Neurol.* (2018) 83:676–90. doi: 10.1002/ana.25205
49. Chen H, Agostini M, Ding K, Gupta P, Madden C, Mickey B, et al. Predictors of seizure recurrence and longitudinal outcome after epilepsy surgery. *Neurology.* (2013) 80:4. doi: 10.1155/2016/7982494
50. Ryvlin P, Cross JH, Rheims S. Epilepsy surgery in children and adults. *Lancet Neurol.* (2014) 13:1114–26. doi: 10.1016/S1474-4422(14)70156-5
51. Blackrock Microsystems LLC. Salt Lake City, UT.
52. MATLAB. *9.7.0.1296695 (R2019b) Update 4, [computer program].* Natick, MA: The Mathworks, Inc. (2019).
53. Proctor JL, Brunton SL, Kutz JN. Dynamic mode decomposition with control. *SIAM J Appl Dyn Syst.* (2016) 15:142–61. doi: 10.1137/15M1013857
54. Li A, Inati S, Zaghlou K, Sarma S. Fragility in epileptic networks: the epileptogenic zone. In: *2017 American Control Conference.* Seattle, WA (2017). p. 2817–22. doi: 10.23919/ACC.2017.7963378
55. Oppenheim AV, Willsky AS, Nawab SH. *Signals and Systems.* Upper Saddle River, NJ: Prentice Hall. (1997).
56. Khambhati AN, Davis KA, Oommen BS, Chen SH, Lucas TH, Litt B, et al. Dynamic network drivers of seizure generation, propagation and termination in human neocortical epilepsy. *PLoS Comput Biol.* (2015) 11:1–19. doi: 10.1371/journal.pcbi.1004608
57. Blume WT. Clinical intracranial overview of seizure syn- chrony and spread. *Can J Neurol Sci.* (2009) 36:55–7.
58. Chagnac-Amitai Y, Connors BW. Horizontal spread of synchronized activity in neocortex and its control by GABA- mediated inhibition. *J Neurophysiol.* (1989) 61:747–58. doi: 10.1152/jn.1989.61.4.747
59. Connors BW, Pinto DJ, Telfeian AE. Local pathways of seizure propagation in neocortex. *Int Rev Neurobiol.* (2001) 45:527–46. doi: 10.1016/S0074-7742(01)45027-6
60. Martins da Silva A, Leal B. Photosensitivity and epilepsy: Current concepts and perspectives-A narrative review. *Seizure.* (2017) 50:209218. doi: 10.1016/j.seizure.2017.04.001

12

Classification of Stereo-EEG Contacts in White Matter vs. Gray Matter Using Recorded Activity

Patrick Greene[1*], *Adam Li*[1], *Jorge González-Martínez*[2] *and Sridevi V. Sarma*[1]

[1] *Neuromedical Control Systems Lab, Institute for Computational Medicine, Biomedical Engineering, Johns Hopkins University, Baltimore, MD, United States,* [2] *Neurosurgery, Cleveland Clinic, Cleveland, OH, United States*

***Correspondence:**
Patrick Greene
pagreene@jhu.edu

For epileptic patients requiring resective surgery, a modality called stereo-electroencephalography (SEEG) may be used to monitor the patient's brain signals to help identify epileptogenic regions that generate and propagate seizures. SEEG involves the insertion of multiple depth electrodes into the patient's brain, each with 10 or more recording contacts along its length. However, a significant fraction ($\approx$ 30% or more) of the contacts typically reside in white matter or other areas of the brain which can not be epileptogenic themselves. Thus, an important step in the analysis of SEEG recordings is distinguishing between electrode contacts which reside in gray matter vs. those that do not. MRI images overlaid with CT scans are currently used for this task, but they take significant amounts of time to manually annotate, and even then it may be difficult to determine the status of some contacts. In this paper we present a fast, automated method for classifying contacts in gray vs. white matter based only on the recorded signal and relative contact depth. We observe that bipolar referenced contacts in white matter have less power in all frequencies below 150 Hz than contacts in gray matter, which we use in a Bayesian classifier to attain an average area under the receiver operating characteristic curve of 0.85 $\pm$ 0.079 (SD) across 29 patients. Because our method gives a probability for each contact rather than a hard labeling, and uses a feature of the recorded signal that has direct clinical relevance, it can be useful to supplement decision-making on difficult to classify contacts or as a rapid, first-pass filter when choosing subsets of contacts from which to save recordings.

Keywords: stereo-electroencephalography, SEEG, white matter, classification, power spectrum, bipolar reference

1. INTRODUCTION

Over 15 million epilepsy patients worldwide and 1 million in the US suffer from drug-resistant epilepsy (1–4). Approximately 50% of such patients have focal drug-resistant epilepsy, where a specific region or set of regions in the brain is the source of the abnormal electrical activity resulting in seizures. This region, termed the epileptogenic zone (EZ), is the area of cortex that is necessary and sufficient for initiating seizures and whose removal or disconnection is necessary for complete abolition of seizures (5–8). When successful, surgical resection treatments stop seizures or allow them to be controlled with medications. Outcomes depend critically on the clinician's ability to accurately identify the EZ.

In cases where standard methods such as EEG are inconclusive in determining the EZ, a more invasive modality called stereo-electroencephalography (SEEG) may be used. With SEEG, multiple depth electrodes are inserted into a patient's brain, each with 10 or more contacts along its length. This allows relatively high resolution mapping of the electrical activity in both shallow and deep structures of the brain. One drawback however is that a significant fraction of the contacts will reside in white matter or other areas of the brain which can not be epileptogenic themselves (although they can contribute to propagation of seizures). Thus, accurate localization of the EZ begins with determining which electrode contacts provide useful information about brain activity. Generally these are contacts which reside in gray matter or close to it. Especially in cases where patients have a large number of electrodes implanted, it is highly convenient for the SEEG reader to have such contacts readily identified. If a contact in gray matter is ignored because it is incorrectly believed to be in white matter, a part of the EZ may be missed. On the other hand, if a contact in white matter is assumed to be in gray matter, it may confound localization. Further, in studies that use network-based analysis to assist in identification of the epileptogenic zone, it is important to have a complete labeling of all contacts with information about which are likely to be in gray vs. white matter (9–12).

Another aspect of presurgical planning is functional mapping of the patient's brain to determine the borders of highly important areas such as those used for speech or movement which should be avoided as much as possible during surgery. Functional mapping involves sub-threshold stimulation of both white matter and gray matter regions of the patient's brain and observing the electrical and behavioral response. Stimulation parameters in white matter must be tuned differently than those for gray matter, and the results of the stimulation are interpreted differently as well. An incorrect label of a contact as being white matter will result in the wrong stimulation settings and potentially errors in functional mapping.

Many epilepsy treatment centers, including those not invested in research and data analysis such as the aforementioned network analysis methods, have resource and time constraints in both the presurgical planning and functional mapping stages which do not allow gray/white matter labeling of all recording contacts. Instead, labels are identified for only a fraction of contacts around the likely EZ or perhaps even for no contacts at all. The latter approach, while taking little time, relies heavily on physician experience and is potentially prone to errors in localization. For those contacts which are labeled however, whether this is a full or partial labeling, the standard approach uses co-registration of MRIs with CT scans, which are overlaid onto brain atlases to anatomically identify regions including white matter (13). Contacts are then classified based on majority-voting or distance measures using white matter voxel masks derived from segmentations of the T1 MRI (e.g., FreeSurfer) (14, 15). However, MRI-based methods, including those that combine other modalities like diffusion tensor imaging, take significant amounts of time to analyze and annotate, hence the tendency toward partial labeling in many centers, and accuracy depends highly on the quality of images (13, 16, 17). While software exists to assist with and automate parts of the segmentation and gray/white matter classification process, to our knowledge all such software is based on MRI and CT images (15). A method which requires minimal time and uses non-imaging data would give clinicians an additional source of information that may be helpful, especially at centers where labeling is currently not done at all or in cases of contacts whose position is uncertain.

In this paper we present a fast, automated Bayesian method for estimating the probability that an electrode contact is in white matter based only on the spectral content of the recorded signal and the relative contact depth. We tested our method using SEEG recordings from 29 drug resistant epilepsy patients who underwent invasive monitoring for treatment purposes. We found that our classifier achieved an average area under the receiver operating characteristic curve of 0.845 ± 0.079 (SD) across patients. Our method is accurate enough that it can be used to supplement MRI-based approaches to further improve accuracy and reduce the time needed to find an informative subset of recording contacts. In particular, for treatment centers where electrode contact labeling is not done due to time or resource limitations, or is done for only a small subset of contacts, our method can be thought of as identifying contacts which have strong, lower correlation signals relative to their neighbors—typically gray matter contacts—without requiring any additional work or scans on the part of the clinician and very little additional time. As one step within a larger automation pipeline for aiding identification of the EZ, we believe that such a method may prove useful in increasing speed and localization accuracy regardless of whether the center uses a full, partial, or no labeling.

2. MATERIALS AND METHODS

2.1. Data Collection

EEG data from 29 epilepsy patients who underwent intracranial EEG monitoring, which included depth electrodes with stereotactic EEG (SEEG) were selected from the Cleveland Clinic. Patients exhibiting the following criteria were excluded: patients with no seizures recorded, pregnant patients, patients less than 5 years of age, and patients with an EEG sampling rate less than 1000 Hz. For each patient, we aggregated interictal data where the patient was not seizing. **Figure 1** shows an example SEEG implantation with common reference voltage data from white and gray matter contacts.

Data were recorded using a Nihon Kohden (Tokyo, Japan) acquisition system with a typical sampling rate of 1,000–2,000 Hz. Signals were referenced to a separate, common electrode placed subcutaneously on the scalp. The clinicians then clipped snapshots of SEEG data and passed it through a secure transfer for analysis in the form of the European Data Format (EDF) (18). We discarded electrodes from further analysis if they were deemed excessively noisy by clinicians, or were not relevant (for example: reference, or EKG, or not attached to the brain). We stored data in the BIDS-iEEG format and performed processing using Python 3.6, MNE-Python, and MNE-BIDS, as well as MATLAB (19–23). Figures were generated using MATLAB and Matplotlib (24). An implementation of our classifier is available at https://github.com/Patrick-Greene/WM-classifier.

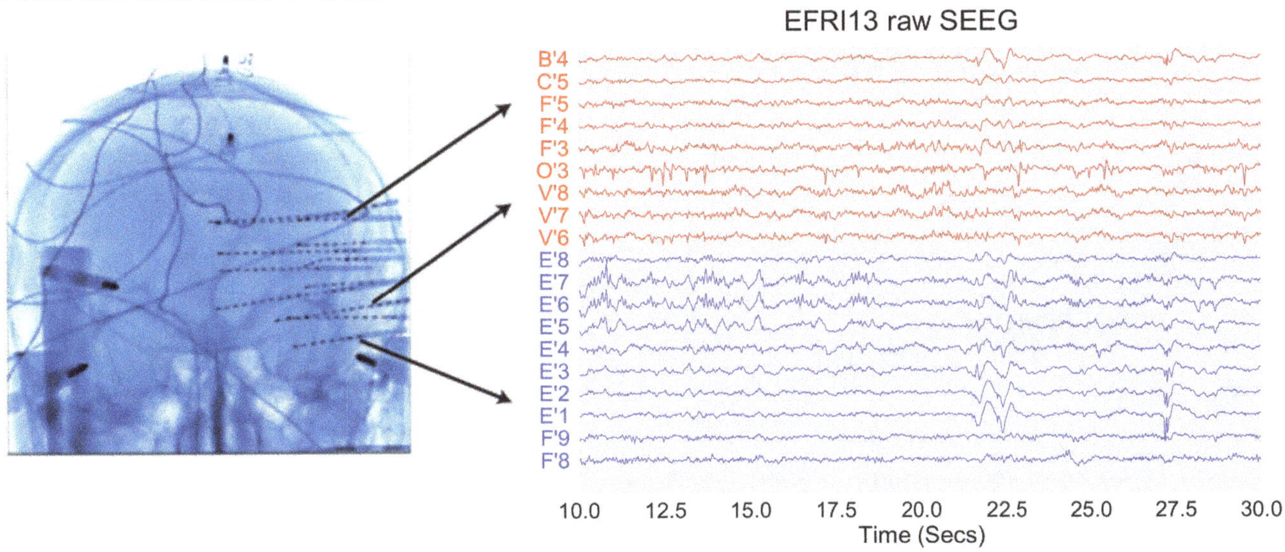

FIGURE 1 | Example of SEEG electrode placement and raw voltage data for sample subject EFRI13 over a 20 s snapshot. Blue traces denote gray matter and red traces denote white matter. Each trace has a scale of 400 uV and has a monopolar reference.

Decisions regarding the need for invasive monitoring and the placement of electrode arrays were made independently of this work and part of routine clinical care. All data were acquired with approval of the local Institutional Review Board (IRB) at each clinical institution. The acquisition of data for research purposes was completed with no impact on the clinical objectives of the patient stay. Digitized data were stored in an IRB-approved database compliant with Health Insurance Portability and Accountability Act (HIPAA) regulations.

2.2. Feature Extraction

For each electrode contact, the raw, common reference SEEG data were bipolar referenced by subtracting off the signal from the adjacent contact closer to the tip of the shank (i.e., the next deeper or more mesial electrode). The contact at the end of the shank had the previous contact subtracted. White matter contacts were those identified by the treating physician as being in white matter using the standard MRI and CT coregistration procedure described previously. Ambiguous electrodes were labeled according to which class the clinician felt was most correct (i.e., if an electrode appeared to be more in gray matter than white matter, it would be labeled as gray matter), and this was the "ground truth" used in our training set and for computing test set error rates. For the purposes of this study, we simplified the analysis by removing all contacts which were not in either white or gray matter, for example contacts in ventricles or outside the cortical surface, during preprocessing.

We chose two features for each electrode contact which preliminary exploration and conversations with clinicians identified as potentially useful in classification. Feature one was the average vertical shift in the contact's power spectrum (in log scale) relative to the average power spectrum over all contacts within that patient. This was computed as the average difference across all frequencies from 1 to 150 Hz between each contact's power spectral density and the average power spectral density. This feature takes into account the fact that white matter contacts tend to have both smaller and more correlated signals because they are further from the neural source of the signal, the gray matter. **Figure 2** shows examples of the average power spectrum for white and gray matter contacts under both common and bipolar referencing schemes. The lower overall power in white matter contacts can clearly be seen, particularly in the bipolar referenced data. We subtract off the average power spectral density across contacts within each patient in order to account for across-patient differences in mean power.

Between 1 and 150 Hz the difference between the gray and white matter power spectra in log scale can be closely approximated by a simple downward shift, allowing us to reduce the relevant information in the spectrum to a single dimension—the size of the shift relative to the average spectrum. For significantly higher frequencies (250+ Hz), both spectra have almost equally low power and thus do not contribute much to classification while also violating the simple shift described above, requiring a higher dimensional feature space. For smaller frequency ranges, the estimate of the shift amount is slightly less accurate because it is averaged over fewer frequencies. We thus use roughly the largest frequency range in which the simple shift approximation still holds. The exact cutoff at 150 Hz is not important though; one can vary the upper frequency limit by 50 Hz in either direction with minimal change in accuracy. The power spectral density was estimated using Welch's method in 10 equally spaced 10 s windows, then averaged across the windows. The spectrum in a 4 Hz band around 60 and 120 Hz was omitted due to line noise. The use of multiple windows helped to average out temporary changes in the spectrum due to movement or other artifacts. The number and length of windows was

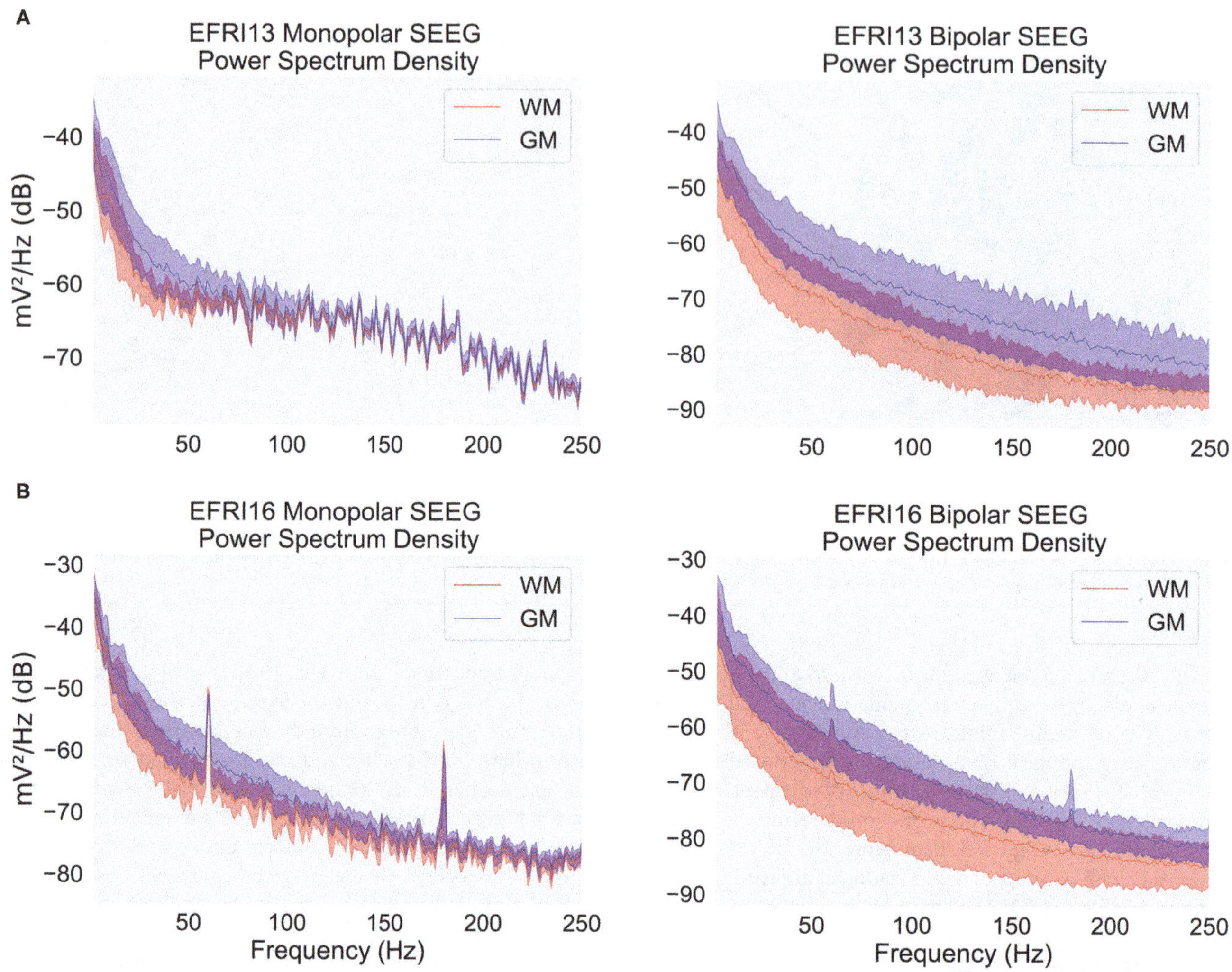

FIGURE 2 | Power spectral density (PSD) plots for two example patients over a snapshot of 10 s with monopolar and bipolar referencing. EFRI13 **(A)**, and EFRI16 **(B)** are shown with PSD segregated based on contacts in white matter (red traces) or gray matter (blue traces). Shaded regions denote one standard deviation. Spikes at multiples of 60 Hz are due to line frequency noise.

chosen to balance running time and accuracy of the estimated spectrum. Longer or more windows did not significantly change the estimated feature values.

The second feature for each contact was the contact's distance from the most peripheral electrode shank, where the distance between contacts was normalized to 1. We will refer to this as the contact depth or distance along the shank. The most peripheral contact was defined as the first contact that was not outside the brain. For example, if the first 3 contacts on a shank were outside the brain, contact 4 would have a depth value of 0, contact 5 would have a value of 1, and so forth. The normalization was simply for convenience because all our patients had the same distance between contacts; if applying the method on a heterogeneous set of electrodes, one would use the actual distance along the shank instead. This feature takes into account the spatial distribution of white matter along the electrode.

2.3. Bayesian Classification

Our overall goals is, for each contact on an electrode in the test set, to classify it as either being in white or gray matter. We approach this classification problem from a Bayesian perspective, which allows us to give class probabilities for each contact that explicitly take into account its feature values, the overall structure of the brain, and uncertainty in our parameter estimates.

With the features described above, we use a kernel density estimator to estimate the continuous feature distributions for both white and gray matter on the training data D. The value of the density at any point is given by a distance-weighted average of feature values at nearby training points, where the weighting function is a gaussian K_{α} centered at the evaluation point and parameterized by the vector of kernel widths $\boldsymbol{\alpha}_{wm} = (\alpha_{wm,1}, \alpha_{wm,2})$ or $\boldsymbol{\alpha}_{gm} = (\alpha_{gm,1}, \alpha_{gm,2})$ for the white and gray matter distributions, respectively. For a new contact in the test set, we use these distributions to evaluate the probability of

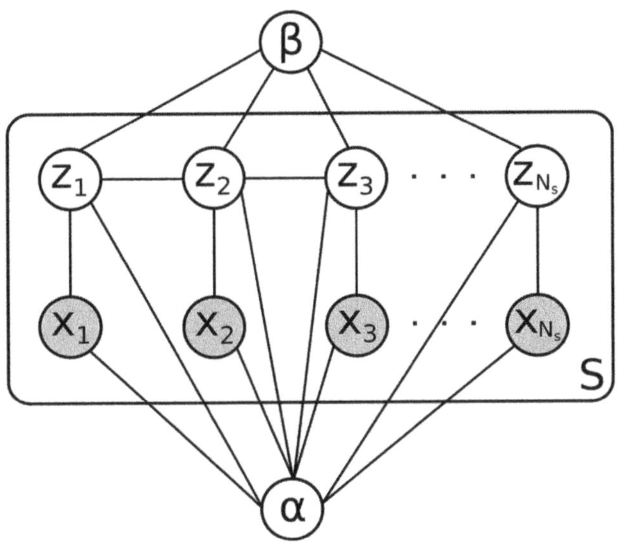

FIGURE 3 | Graphical model for a patient in the test set. There are S electrode shanks to be classified, each with N_s electrode contacts. The contact label is given by z_i, and the observed features are given by x_i. α and β are parameters whose distribution is estimated using the training set D, which is not shown here.

observing the contact's feature values, given that it is either in white matter or gray matter (the *likelihood* of the contact's data). This likelihood is calculated for each contact on an electrode shank and, under the assumption that each contact's data is independent conditioned on the class assignment (gray or white matter), the likelihood of the electrode shank as a whole is computed by multiplying together the individual contact probabilities. This independence assumption, along with several others used in the derivation of our classifier, is shown graphically in **Figure 3**.

We now wish to take into account the large-scale distribution of white and gray matter in the brain. Given the physical structure of the brain, we would find it unlikely for an electrode to have contacts that alternate between white matter and gray matter in rapid succession. More typical would be to have several gray matter contacts in a row, followed by several white matter contacts in a row, perhaps followed by another chunk of gray matter contacts. This tendency for neighboring contacts to have the same classification is captured by our *prior* distribution on labelings, which consists of an exponentially increasing function of a sum of pairwise products between neighboring contact classes. Since the classes are denoted -1 for gray matter and 1 for white matter, neighboring contacts that have the same class assignment increase the prior probability, while contacts that have different assignments decrease the probability, resulting in a tendency toward fewer gray/white matter transitions on each electrode. This prior is a one-dimensional version of an Ising-type prior used for example in image de-noising, where neighboring pixels in an image are assumed more likely to have the same color (25). The degree to which gray/white matter transitions are penalized is determined by a parameter β. For a fixed choice of parameters $\boldsymbol{\alpha}$ and β, the product of this prior distribution with the likelihood gives, after normalization, the *posterior* probability of a particular labeling of all the contacts on an electrode shank.

We now turn to the problem of determining our unknown parameters. We allow the user to explicitly choose the kernel width $\boldsymbol{\alpha}_2 = (\alpha_{wm,2}, \alpha_{gm,2})$ in the second feature dimension corresponding to the contact depth. This is because the appropriate kernel width depends on the physical distance between contacts relative to the size of white matter or gray matter structures in the brain. Larger kernel widths mean that the spatial distribution of white or gray matter varies slowly from contact to contact, while smaller widths allow for more rapid variation. For example, if it is known that contacts are spaced several cm apart, the spatial distribution of white or gray matter varies relatively rapidly with respect to this distance, and hence a smaller kernel width would be called for. In our patients, the contacts are 5 mm apart, so we expect the spatial distribution of white or gray matter to be fairly similar between neighboring contacts. We thus use a larger kernel width equal to the spacing between contacts.

Our data set contains only regularly-spaced electrodes, however, electrodes with irregular spacing can also be accommodated by our method. Rather than using normalized units for the contact positions along the shank (feature two), one would use the actual positions in mm. The estimated white and gray matter densities would automatically scale. The limits of the integral used to compute the likelihood (see **Supplementary Equation 5**) should be modified accordingly, going from halfway between the previous and next contact positions. The $\boldsymbol{\alpha}_2$ kernel width can be chosen according to the smallest set of spacings on the electrode. Cross validation on the training set could also be used to choose $\boldsymbol{\alpha}_2$ if a more hands-off approach is desired.

Similarly to the classification problem itself, for the remaining parameters $\boldsymbol{\alpha}_1$ and β we estimate their posterior distribution in a Bayesian way by calculating the likelihood of the data given the parameters and multiplying it by a prior distribution. In this case we use a diffuse exponential distribution because we do not have any prior knowledge about parameter values.

Finally, we integrate the posterior probability distribution for each electrode shank's labeling with respect to the posterior distribution of the parameters to form the *posterior predictive* distribution. This takes into account uncertainty in our parameter estimates by forming a weighted average of the class probabilities for various possible parameter values, with weights determined by how probable the parameter values are given the training data. In practice, we estimate this integral by using a truncated gaussian approximation to the posterior parameter distribution (truncated because the parameters must be positive), and average the posterior class probability with respect to samples drawn from this distribution. In the results shown, we average across 100 samples. To compute the probability that any individual contact is in white matter, we sum the posterior predictive over all possible labelings of the other contacts. A detailed mathematical exposition of our method can be found in the **Supplementary Material**.

2.4. Training and Testing

We primarily used leave-one-out cross validation to train and test our method, although we also report results for four-fold cross validation. For a given test patient, the remaining 28 patients were used as training data to estimate the feature distributions for both the white and gray matter classes. We measure overall accuracy by calculating a receiver operating characteristic (ROC) curve and measuring the area under the curve (AUC). A point on the ROC curve is found by picking a probability threshold between 0 and 1, then classifying all contacts on all electrode shanks by whether their estimated probability of being in white matter falls above or below the probability threshold. Contacts with estimated probability above the threshold are classified as being in white matter, and those below the threshold are classified as being in gray matter. The resulting true positive rate—the number of correctly identified white matter contacts divided by the total number of true white matter contacts, and the false positive rate—the number of contacts identified as white matter which were actually in gray matter, divided by the total number of true gray matter contacts, is then calculated. Plotting the true positive rate vs. the false positive rate for various values of the threshold probability produces the ROC curve. Higher threshold probabilities result in fewer false positives but also fewer true positives, and vice versa for lower thresholds, so that ROC curves increase from $(0, 0)$ to $(1, 1)$ as the threshold is lowered. The area under an ROC curve is a summary measure of how efficiently the classifier trades off false positives for true positives, with a maximum value of 1.

3. RESULTS

The normalized histograms of the white and gray matter training data are shown together in **Figure 4A**. We then use kernel density estimators as described previously to give smoothed estimates of each of these distributions. Overlaid contour plots of the density estimates are shown in **Figure 4B**. In estimating the posterior parameter distributions, we found the average mean of the α_1 kernel width posterior distributions to be 0.135 for gray matter and 0.156 for white matter (averaged across patients), and the average standard deviations of these posterior distributions to be 0.012 and 0.015, respectively (averaged across patients). The larger kernel width for the white matter distribution is expected given that there are fewer contacts in white matter than gray matter, resulting in fewer data points to estimate the feature distribution. For β, the average mean of its posterior distribution was 7.738 across patients, with an average standard deviation of its distribution of 0.249. The small standard deviations of the posterior distributions relative to their means indicates that the parameters are well-estimated with a 28 patient training set.

Figure 5 shows example outputs for six patients: the two patients with highest overall accuracy, two patients at the median level of accuracy, and the two least accurate patients. For the high accuracy patients, we see that nearly all gray and white matter contacts are correctly identified with high confidence - probability near 1 for true white matter contacts and probability near 0 for true gray matter contacts. For the median accuracy patients we see some mislabelings, particularly near the transitions between white and gray matter. In patient LA24 a section of white matter spanning three contacts is missed completely, and in patient LA08 sections of gray matter on two electrodes are indicated as likely to be in white matter. Labelings are also done with lower confidence, shown by the lighter reds and blues, particularly in LA24, which denote probabilities closer to 0.5. However, the estimated probabilities still do a good job of tracking the white matter distribution overall. In the patient with the second worst AUC, EFRI17, most of the white matter contacts are missed and a spurious white matter region is found on one of the electrodes. Within this spurious region, the U'5, U'4, and U'3 contacts were labeled by clinicians as being in Heschl's gyrus, which is used for acoustic processing and has a high density of white matter tracts through its center (26). To the classifier's credit, most of the missed contacts are indicated with higher white matter probability than surrounding contacts, albeit still below 0.5. In LA01, the patient with the lowest AUC, we see that this poor accuracy is due almost completely to a low true positive rate. There are only five white matter contacts in this patient, and our classifier fails to find any of them. Nearly all the gray matter contacts are correctly identified however. The two worst patients are somewhat outliers in that the third worst patient has an AUC of 0.74, nearly 10 percentage points better. Only 5 patients had an AUC under 0.8, meaning that the median patients with 0.86 AUC are well representative of most patients.

Figure 6 shows the ROC curves for all 29 patients using two different approaches to setting the prior smoothing parameter β. When we integrate over the posterior distribution of β given the training set as described in the section 2, we obtain the set of ROC curves in **Figure 6A**. The mean AUC in this case was 0.845 ± 0.079 (SD). If instead we choose a particular value of β for each patient by explicitly maximizing the AUC over the training set, we obtain the set of curves in **Figure 6B**. Although choosing the AUC-maximizing β predictably results in a slightly higher average AUC (0.859 ± 0.097), the difference is quite small and choosing β in this way is much slower, as it requires running the classifier on the entire training set for multiple values of β. The AUC-maximizing β is approximately 3 on average, while the mean of the posterior distribution of β in our usual approach is 7.7 on average as stated above. While this higher value reduces overall AUC slightly, it also decreases the variance across patients. This can most clearly be seen in the least accurate patient LA01, where the mislabeled white matter contacts are less confidently mislabeled.

The dotted line in **Figure 6** with slope 1 represents the average performance for a random classifier that, given a threshold $\tau \in [0, 1]$, labels a contact as white matter with probability τ. For reference, the deterministic classifier that guesses gray matter for all contacts is the same as the random classifier with a threshold of 0, and would be at the point $(0, 0)$ on the graph. This demonstrates why we use ROC curves rather than a simple percentage correct out of the total number of contacts. We might think that if only about 30% of contacts are in white matter, a "dumb" classifier that labels everything as gray matter should have 70% accuracy. In fact it does, but yet it fails as a useful classifier because it has no ability to detect true positives, and its position at $(0, 0)$ on the ROC graph reflects this.

In four-fold cross validation, the training sets are reduced by 25% compared to leave-one-out, resulting in a slightly decreased

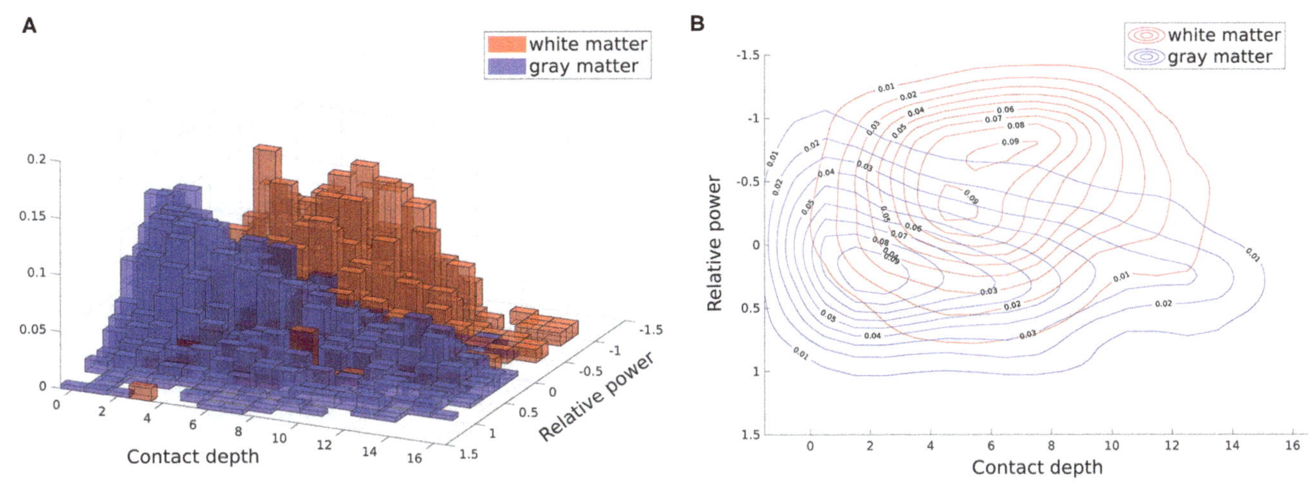

FIGURE 4 | Two dimensional white and gray matter distributions of features: power spectrum difference from average (relative power) and contact depth. These distributions (specifically the training subsets of them) form our white and gray matter likelihoods. All contacts from all patients are shown here, with the feature distribution of white matter contacts shown in red and the distribution for gray matter contacts shown in blue. **(A)** Histogram. **(B)** Overlaid contour plots of estimated kernel densities.

average AUC of 0.790 ± 0.115 (SD) when integrating over the posterior distribution of β. The low dimensionality of our method and integration over parameters helps to minimize the drop in performance, although we can see that having more training data is generally beneficial.

Given the fact that the electrical signals produced by gray matter regions propagate some distance into neighboring white matter rather than stopping abruptly at the boundary, we would expect white matter contacts to have signals that are more similar to gray matter the closer they are to the boundary. Our classifier should therefore be less confident (i.e., assign probabilities closer to 0.5) for contacts near a gray/white matter boundary, and more confident for contacts that are deeper in white matter. A similar argument applies to gray matter contacts, as those close to a white matter region receive less signal from the white matter direction, and thus should have lower signal power overall. One place where we know gray/white matter boundaries occur is where there are transitions in the electrode labeling from gray to white or vice versa. **Figure 7** shows how our classifier's output probabilities change as a function of distance from these transition points. As expected, contacts near the transition between a gray matter and white matter region tend to be more uncertain, as shown by the median value closer to 0.5, and less accurately assigned, as shown by the larger spread in probabilities, while contacts deeper within white or gray matter are more confidently and accurately assigned.

4. DISCUSSION

4.1. Feature Selection

In preliminary testing, we investigated several potential features, including the difference in white and gray matter power spectra in the common (also called monopolar) reference signal. The common reference signal is taken relative to one common reference used by all contacts (not to be confused with common average referencing). It is often used by clinicians in conjunction with the bipolar reference signal when examining epilepsy patients and thus seems like an obvious feature candidate. While we found that white and gray matter had somewhat different power spectral densities in the common reference signal, this difference was often much less pronounced than in the bipolar signal and varied more depending on the frequency. This can be seen in **Figure 2**. We believe this is because the bipolar reference signal takes advantage of the fact that signals in white matter are both smaller and more correlated due to their increased distance from neural sources.

Specifically, if we view the signal on each contact as a combination of a shared source detected across neighboring contacts with some amplitude decay from one contact to the next and an independent local source detected on only the nearest contact, then contacts in white matter will tend to be farther from both their shared and local sources (since the sources must be located in gray matter). If the signal from these sources decays inversely with distance, then the local contributions in white matter contacts will tend to be smaller, and the shared portion of the signal will be closer in magnitude across neighboring electrodes because the rate of decay in signal strength is slower further from the source. Subtracting the signals on neighboring electrodes therefore tends to reduce the signal strength on white matter contacts relatively more than on gray matter contacts, resulting in a larger contrast between the two. We refer the reader to the **Supplementary Material** for a more in-depth exposition of this argument. Although we expect this to be the typical situation, there can be scenarios where the bipolar signal on white matter contacts remains large due to the geometry of the sources. For example, two contacts within a narrow channel of white matter

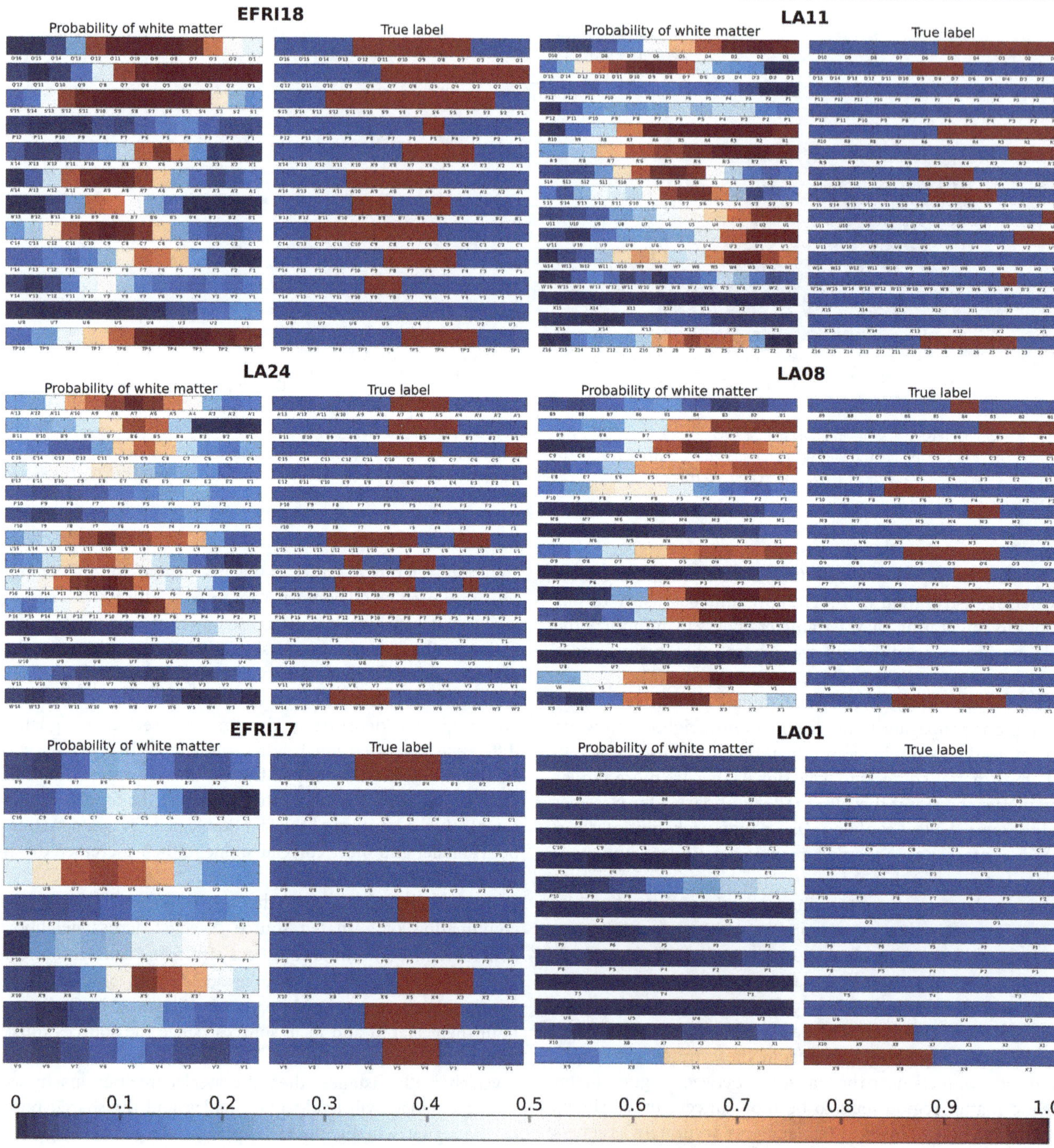

FIGURE 5 | Examples of estimated white matter probabilities for several patients. For each patient, the left column is the probabilities estimated by our classifier, while the right column is the reference labeling done by clinicians using MRI+CT. Each row represents one electrode shank, with individual contacts labeled below. In the reference labeling, red indicates that the contact was labeled as white matter, blue indicates gray matter. In the estimated probabilities, red indicates higher probability of a contact being in white matter according to our classifier. First row: Two of the best patients (EFRI18, LA11), each with > 0.9 AUC. Second row: Two median patients (LA24, LA08), each with 0.86 AUC. Third row: The two worst patients (EFRI17, LA01), representing 0.65 and 0.62 AUC, respectively.

may have sizable local contributions from separate patches of adjacent gray matter, resulting in a bipolar signal that remains relatively large.

In practice we found that out of 29 patients analyzed, 19 had better AUC when using bipolar referencing, while the remaining 10 patients had better AUC under common referencing. For

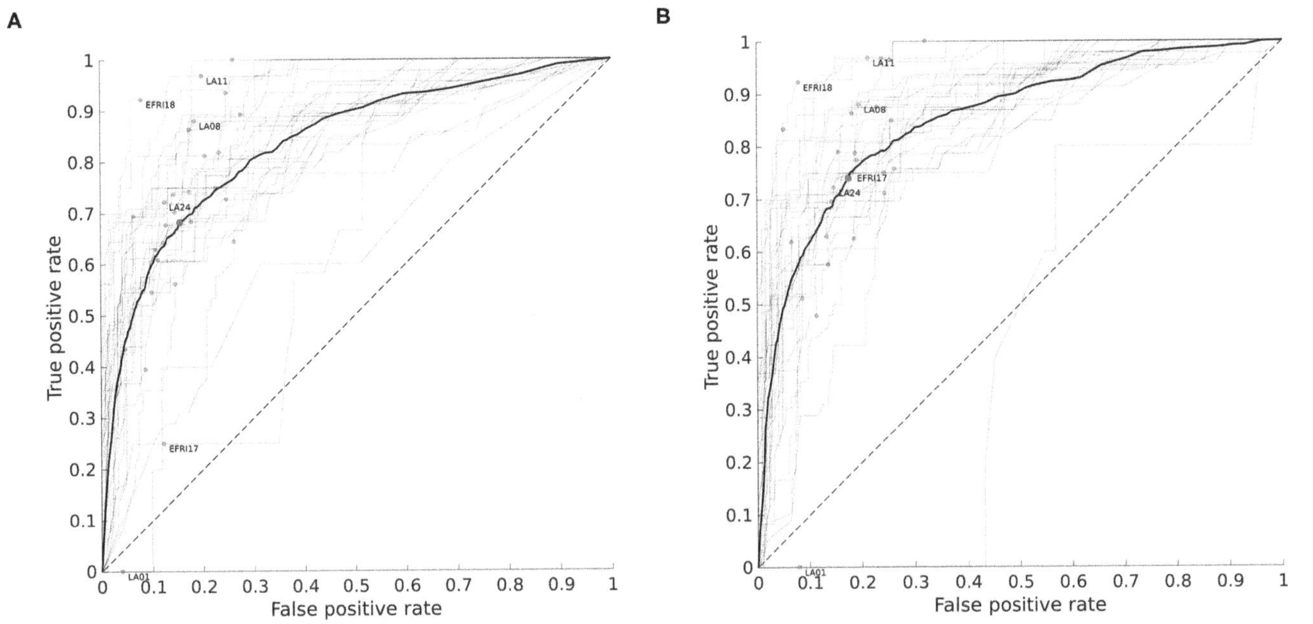

FIGURE 6 | Receiver operating characteristic (ROC) curves for all patients. For a given threshold value p_{thresh}, a contact is classified as white matter if the probability computed by the classifier is above that threshold. Each curve shows how the fraction of false positives (gray matter contacts incorrectly classified as white matter) and true positives (white matter contacts correctly identified) varies with the threshold level. The red dots indicate the point on the curve obtained when $p_{thresh} = 0.5$. The area under the curve (AUC) is the integral of the ROC curve and measures overall performance. **(A)** ROC curves when prior smoothing parameter β is automatically integrated over with respect to its estimated posterior distribution (see section 2). Mean AUC = 0.845 ± 0.079 (SD). Patients shown in **Figure 5** are labeled. The mean ROC curve is shown in bold. **(B)** ROC curves when β is chosen to maximize AUC over the training set. Mean AUC = 0.859 ± 0.097 (SD).

those patients who did better under common referencing, the difference was often slight. As a result, we did not find an improvement in average AUC when using both common and bipolar referenced features, as opposed to using only bipolar referenced features.

Our second feature, the contact depth, was less important than the first feature, increasing AUC by about 3 percentage points over using the first feature alone. However, it still contributed positively to overall accuracy by encoding the coarse spatial distribution of white and gray matter along an electrode. When an electrode is inserted, it must first pass through the cortex before entering white matter, resulting in the outermost electrodes almost always being in gray matter. The next set of electrodes toward the middle are then more likely to be in white matter, although there can be substantial variation depending on the brain region and angle of insertion due to the anatomy of gyri and sulci. The contacts at the end of an electrode are often used to record from deeper brain areas, and thus are more likely to be in gray matter again. These general tendencies are reflected in the distribution shown in **Figure 4**.

4.2. Uncertainty Quantification

One significant aspect of our classifier is that, rather than giving a single labeling for each electrode, as would be the case in a maximum likelihood classifier or support vector machine, it gives a marginal probability for each contact, and this probability is computed with respect to a flexible and explicit distribution (the kernel density estimate), unlike for example logistic regression where probabilities can be computed but the underlying distribution is implicit and restricted to the exponential family. Furthermore the probabilities take into account uncertainty in the parameter estimates through the posterior predictive calculation, which none of the above methods do and which can be important for small training sets.

For clinical use, we consider giving accurate uncertainty estimates nearly as important as giving the right answer. Any classification method will result in errors, but when the uncertainty in a labeling is given accurately, it allows the clinician to ignore a large fraction of those. Defining the "confidence" that our classifier has in a labeling by $2|p - 0.5|$, where p is the estimated probability of white matter, we find that on mislabelings (defined as $p > 0.5$ for a gray matter contact or $p < 0.5$ for a white matter contact), our classifier had an average confidence level of 54.7, vs. 76.6% for correct labelings. Giving useful probabilities means accurately estimating the underlying data distributions, which becomes increasingly difficult as the number of features increases. This is related to overfitting and can occur even when test set accuracy is very good. Neural networks for example, will typically use hundreds of features and obtain good accuracy, but at the cost of output layer "probabilities" that may not correspond to real error rates or can vary wildly with small perturbations of the input.

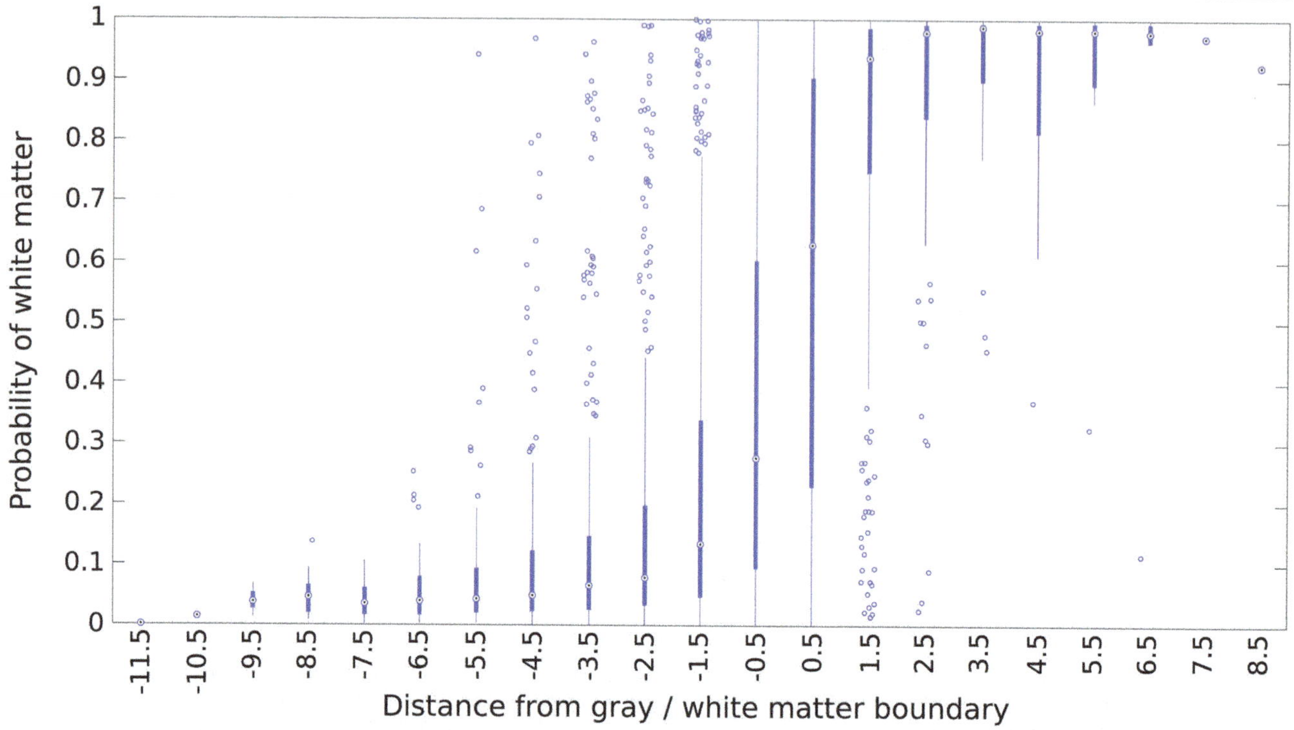

FIGURE 7 | Estimated probability of white matter for electrode contacts as a function of distance from the nearest white matter/gray matter transition. The transition point is defined to be at $x = 0$, and the first contact on the white matter side is at $x = 0.5$, the second contact is at $x = 1.5$, and so forth in unit increments. Positive distances indicate that the contact is deeper into a white matter region, while negative distances indicate the same for gray matter regions. The center circle of each box plot is the median, the thick line indicates the first and third quartiles, and the thin line represents an additional 1.5 times the interquartile range. Points outside this are plotted individually as circles.

4.3. Interpretability

Interpretability of features is another aspect we feel is relevant for clinical usefulness. Because of our decision to use features that are explicitly related to the end goal of selecting a subset of informative channels for seizure localization, our classifier's mistakes tend to be clinically acceptable. A white matter contact that has an above-average signal power has a higher chance of being mislabeled as gray matter, but the fact that it is capturing a strong signal means that clinicians may want to keep this channel anyway as it is likely to be picking up signal from an adjacent gray matter region. It is also possible that there are errors in the clinician-labeled ground truth classifications, and that in some cases it may be the clinician labeling which is wrong rather than our classifier. Several patients had files which indicated uncertainty about some of the labeled white matter contacts, showing that even with MRI and CT, it can be difficult to determine whether some contacts are in white or gray matter, and that a signal-based classifier may be useful as an independent reference.

4.4. Computational Efficiency

Our classifier takes less than 5 min to run per patient, much faster than the typical hand-labeling process using MRI and CT which can take several hours. In theory, the evaluation of the likelihood in the posterior predictive requires a sum over a number of terms that grows quadratically with the size of the number of contacts in the data set, due to the use of a gaussian kernel estimator to evaluate the distribution rather than a parametric model. For large datasets, one can reduce this somewhat by using a kernel with finite support rather than a gaussian. As the number of data points increases, the estimated kernel width will become narrower, reducing the growth in the number of points within the support of the kernel. For very large datasets we recommend simply using a subset as the training data; since our model is low-dimensional, it is not necessary to use vast amounts of data to estimate the feature distributions, and using a random training subset of a few dozen patients will likely yield nearly identical results.

The run time of our classifier can also be adjusted by changing the number of samples drawn from the posterior distribution of the parameters when computing the posterior predictive. With our truncated gaussian approximation, drawing samples is fast but evaluating the posterior probability of a labeling is slow due to having to recalculate the normalizing constant for each sample. In our case, we have sufficient training data that our posterior parameter distributions are tightly peaked, and thus relatively few samples are needed. The required number of samples depends on the desired amount of variance in the posterior predictive estimate. If one has less than 20 or so patients, more extensive sampling will likely be needed, with total computation time increasing linearly with the number of samples.

4.5. Future Work

One limitation of our current approach is the way in which we compute the distribution of our second feature, the location of white or gray matter along the electrode. For simplicity we pool the data from all electrodes, giving us a coarse average distribution which ignores the differences between electrodes inserted in different brain regions or at different angles. An improvement on this would be to estimate separate distributions as functions of the brain region and other implantation variables, which would allow more detailed structure to be captured and improve the usefulness of this feature. Further testing would be needed to explore the trade-off between accuracy and the amount of extra data needed to estimate the distributions.

Additional refinements to our method are possible, for example the sample-based estimation of the posterior predictive could be parallelized to further increase speed. Another avenue for improvement would be the use of common reference data in addition to bipolar reference data. As described above, although the majority of contacts are better distinguished using bipolar data, there are undoubtedly a fraction of contacts which can be more accurately classified using the common reference. Simply adding the common reference power as a third feature does not improve accuracy by a useful amount however. What is needed is an additional feature that determines whether a contact is more likely to benefit from using the bipolar or common reference. The previous discussion (also see **Supplementary Material**) suggests some possibilities which we leave for future work, such as estimating the fraction of common vs. local variance.

AUTHOR CONTRIBUTIONS

PG developed the method with support from SS and implemented it. PG wrote the manuscript with contributions from AL, SS, and JG-M. JG-M provided clinical information and raw patient data. AL organized the data into the BIDS format. All authors contributed to the article and approved the submitted version.

ACKNOWLEDGMENTS

We would like to thank Professor of Neurology Joon Kang at Johns Hopkins for helpful discussion on how white matter signals differ from those in gray matter, as well as professor Pierre Sacré at University of Liège for providing annotated data for the EFRI patients.

REFERENCES

1. Brodie MJ, Shorvon SD, Canger R, Halasz P, Johannessen S, Thompson P, et al. Commission on European affairs: appropriate standards of epilepsy care across Europe. *Epilepsia.* (1997) 38:1245–50.
2. Berg AT, Kelly MM. Defining intractability: comparisons among published definitions. *Epilepsia.* (2006) 47:431–6. doi: 10.1111/j.1528-1167.2006.00440.x
3. Kwan P, Brodie MJ. Early identification of refractory epilepsy. *N Engl J Med.* (2000) 342:314–9. doi: 10.1056/NEJM200002033420503
4. Berg AT. Identification of pharmacoresistant epilepsy. *Neurol Clin.* (2009) 27:1003–13. doi: 10.1016/j.ncl.2009.06.001
5. Lüders HO, Najm I, Nair D, Widdess-Walsh P, Bingman W. The epileptogenic zone: general principles. *Epileptic Disord.* (2006) 8(Suppl. 2):S1–9. Available online at: https://www.jle.com/en/revues/epd/revue.phtm
6. Jehi L. *The Epileptogenic Zone: Concept and Definition.* American Epilepsy Society (2018). Available online at: http://www.ncbi.nlm.nih.gov/pubmed/29844752 http://www.pubmedcentral.nih.gov/articlerender.fcgi?artid=PMC5963498.
7. Penfield W. Epileptogenic lesions. *Acta Neurol Psychiatr Belgica.* (1956) 56:75–88.
8. Penfield W, Jasper H. *Epilepsy and the Functional Anatomy of the Human Brain.* Vol. 155. 1st ed. Boston, MA: Little Brown (1954).
9. Sritharan D, Sarma SV. Fragility in dynamic networks: application to neural networks in the epileptic cortex. *Neural Comput.* (2014) 26:2294–327. doi: 10.1162/NECO_a_00644
10. Li A, Inati S, Zaghloul K, Sarma S. Fragility in epileptic networks : the epileptogenic zone. In: *American Control Conference* (Seattle, WA) (2017). p. 1–8.
11. Li A, Chennuri B, Subramanian S, Yaffe R, Gliske S, Stacey W, et al. Using network analysis to localize the epileptogenic zone from invasive EEG recordings in intractable focal epilepsy. *Netw Neurosci.* (2018) 2:218–40. doi: 10.1162/netn_a_00043
12. Li A, Fitzgerald Z, Hopp J, Johnson E, Crone N, Bulacio J, et al. Virtual cortical stimulation mapping of epilepsy networks to localize the epileptogenic zone. In: *Proceedings of the Annual International Conference of the IEEE Engineering in Medicine and Biology Society.* Institute of Electrical and Electronics Engineers (Berlin:IEEE) (2019). p. 2328–2331.
13. Oostenveld R, Fries P, Maris E, Schoffelen JM. FieldTrip: open source software for advanced analysis of MEG, EEG, and invasive electrophysiological data. *Comput Intell Neurosci.* (2011) 2011:156869. doi: 10.1155/2011/156869
14. Fischl B. FreeSurfer. *Neuroimage.* (2012) 62:774–81. doi: 10.1016/j.neuroimage.2012.01.021
15. Narizzano M, Arnulfo G, Ricci S, Toselli B, Tisdall M, Canessa A, et al. SEEG assistant: a 3DSlicer extension to support epilepsy surgery. *BMC Bioinform.* (2017) 18:124. doi: 10.1186/s12859-017-1545-8
16. Fisher RS. Therapeutic devices for epilepsy. *Ann Neurol.* (2012) 71:157–68. doi: 10.1002/ana.22621
17. Mercier MR, Bickel S, Megevand P, Groppe DM, Schroeder CE, Mehta AD, et al. Evaluation of cortical local field potential diffusion in stereotactic electro-encephalography recordings: a glimpse on white matter signal. *Neuroimage.* (2017) 147:219–32. doi: 10.1016/j.neuroimage.2016.08.037
18. Kemp B, Värri A, Rosa AC, Nielsen KD, Gade J. A simple format for exchange of digitized polygraphic recordings. *Electroencephalogr Clin Neurophysiol.* (1992) 82:391–3.
19. Holdgraf C, Appelhoff S, Bickel S, Bouchard K, D'Ambrosio S, David O, et al. iEEG-BIDS, extending the Brain Imaging Data Structure specification to human intracranial electrophysiology. *Sci Data.* (2019) 6:102. doi: 10.1038/s41597-019-0105-7
20. Gorgolewski KJ, Auer T, Calhoun VD, Craddock RC, Das S, Duff EP, et al. The brain imaging data structure, a format for organizing and describing outputs of neuroimaging experiments. *Sci Data.* (2016) 3:160044. doi: 10.1038/sdata.2016.44
21. Gramfort A, Luessi M, Larson E, Engemann DA, Strohmeier D, Brodbeck C, et al. MEG and EEG data analysis with MNE-Python. *Front Neurosci.* (2013) 7:267. doi: 10.3389/fnins.2013.00267
22. Gramfort A, Luessi M, Larson E, Engemann DA, Strohmeier D, Brodbeck C, et al. MNE software for processing MEG and EEG data. *Neuroimage.* (2014) 86:446–60. doi: 10.1016/j.neuroimage.2013.10.027
23. MATLAB. *(R2019a).* Natick, MA: The MathWorks Inc. (2019).
24. Hunter JD. Matplotlib: a 2D graphics environment. *Comput Sci Eng.* (2007) 9:99–104. doi: 10.1109/MCSE.2007.55
25. Besag J. On the statistical analysis of dirty pictures. *J R Stat Soc Ser B.* (1986) 48:259–79.

13

Indications, Techniques and Outcomes of Robot-Assisted Insular Stereo-Electro-Encephalography

Amaury De Barros [1], Julien Francisco Zaldivar-Jolissaint [2], Dominique Hoffmann [2], Anne-Sophie Job-Chapron [3], Lorella Minotti [3], Philippe Kahane [3], Emmanuel De Schlichting [2] and Stephan Chabardès [2]*

[1] Department of Neurosurgery, Toulouse University Hospital, Toulouse, France, [2] CHU Grenoble Alpes, Clinical University of Neurosurgery, Grenoble, France, [3] CHU Grenoble Alpes, Clinical University of Neurology, Grenoble, France

***Correspondence:**
Amaury De Barros
amaurydebarros@yahoo.fr

Stereo-electro-encephalography (SEEG) is an invasive, surgical, and electrophysiological method for three-dimensional registration and mapping of seizure activity in drug-resistant epilepsy. It allows the accurate analysis of spatio-temporal seizure activity by multiple intraparenchymal depth electrodes. The technique requires rigorous non-invasive pre-SEEG evaluation (clinical, video-EEG, and neuroimaging investigations) in order to plan the insertion of the SEEG electrodes with minimal risk and maximal recording accuracy. The resulting recordings are used to precisely define the surgical limits of resection of the epileptogenic zone in relation to adjacent eloquent structures. Since the initial description of the technique by Talairach and Bancaud in the 1950's, several techniques of electrode insertion have been used with accuracy and relatively few complications. In the last decade, robot-assisted surgery has emerged as a safe, accurate, and time-saving electrode insertion technique due to its unparalleled potential for orthogonal and oblique insertion trajectories, guided by rigorous computer-assisted planning. SEEG exploration of the insular cortex remains difficult due to its anatomical location, hidden by the temporal and frontoparietal opercula. Furthermore, the close vicinity of Sylvian vessels makes surgical electrode insertion challenging. Some epilepsy surgery teams remain cautious about insular exploration due to the potential of neurovascular injury. However, several authors have published encouraging results regarding the technique's accuracy and safety in both children and adults. We will review the indications, techniques, and outcomes of insular SEEG exploration with emphasis on robot-assisted implantation.

Keywords: epilepsy, SEEG (stereoelectroencephalography), stereotaxic, epilepsy surgery planning, robot-assisted surgery (RAS)/computer assisted surgery (CAS)

INTRODUCTION

The insular cortex is anatomically located deep inside the lateral sulcus, enclosed and covered by the frontoparietal and temporal opercula. Its hidden location inspired Gray to name this deep cortical structure the "Island of Reil," in tribute to the seminal description of the insula by Christian Reil (1). The neurofunctional role of the insula remained poorly understood, and its role in brain network organization and connectivity was underestimated until pioneers like Penfield and Faulk in Montreal (2), and Guillaume and Mazars in Paris (3), who both described the involvement of the insula in refractory epilepsy using electrocorticography during anterior temporal lobectomy surgeries. But before the advent of modern presurgical investigations and microsurgical techniques, insular surgery in addition to anterior temporal resection was considered at risk with high morbidity and poor effectiveness to increase epileptic control (4). This explains why the issue of insular investigation and resection entered a silent period of almost four decades, with the exception of very few studies of lesion cases.

A major breakthrough occurred in 2000, when Isnard et al. using stereo-electro-encephalography (SEEG), demonstrated that some failures of temporal lobectomy could be related to seizures originating in the insular cortex (5). Since then, the role of the insula in surgically focal epilepsy has been extensively investigated (6), showing first that insular (or insulo-opercular) cortex epilepsy may mimic temporal, frontal, or parietal epilepsy, and second that the insula can be part of widely extended epileptogenic zones such as in the case of temporal "plus" epilepsies (7). Overall, the complexity of focal epilepsies involving the insula makes the precise determination of the ictal topographical culprit of paramount importance, especially when a surgical treatment is envisioned. In this context, SEEG recordings are especially well-suited to giving access directly to deep brain structures that cannot be recorded using subdural grids or strips. Recent developments in imaging, computer-assisted planning (particularly image fusion algorithms and planning software), and robotic assistance currently allow safer and more accurate electrode insertion for performing electrophysiological recordings. Still, robotics has gained interest in the epilepsy surgery field due to their reliable, reproducible, safe, accurate, and time-saving electrode insertion potential and their versatility for orthogonal and oblique electrode insertions.

We will review here the indications, techniques and outcomes of insular SEEG exploration, emphasizing the current role of computational-image guidance and robot-assistance.

INDICATIONS FOR INSULAR SEEG

As a general rule, SEEG indications in insular epilepsy do not significantly differ from those proposed for other drug-resistant focal epilepsy, the clinical data—corroborated by ictal scalp-EEG and neuroimaging findings—being among the most important features. In the specific context where the insula can be part of the epileptogenic zone, two situations must be distinguished: either (i) the seizures are suspected to originate from the insula before they spread to other cortical areas (including the contralateral insula), therefore mimicking perisylvian, frontal, temporal, and even parietal seizures (8) or (ii) the insula is part of a more diffuse epileptogenic network as in temporo-insular epilepsy, which is the most frequent form of temporal "plus" epilepsies (9). In these scenarios, auras are of paramount importance, such as painful somatosensory sensations (10), olfactory, gustatory, auditory, and vestibular manifestations (11); or breathlessness, laryngeal discomfort, and perioral paresthesiae (12). Other clinical features, such as a reflex component of the seizures (13), or an ictal bradycardia/asystole (14–16) can also suggest an insular involvement. For Nguyen and colleagues (17), the insula should be explored whenever a clinical pattern other than the one expected to emerge from the ictal onset zone comes to the fore, especially in MRI negative cases. The combination of some of the "specific" insular (or insulo-opercular) fingerprints described above, as well as their occurrence with hypermotor behavior (18), somato-motor signs, temporal-like automatism or spasm-like behavior, should lead to consideration of the insula (or insulo-opercular complex) as a possible seizure onset zone.

In addition to these clinical cues, SEEG should include an insular exploration when (i) there exists an insular lesion likely responsible for the seizure, in order to precisely delineate the borders of the resection, to perform a functional mapping (e.g., the dominant hemisphere for language) or to apply radiofrequency thermocoagulation; (ii) there is a cortical anomaly on standard MRI imaging in the close vicinity of the insula (e.g., supra- or infra-sylvian operculum, posterior part of the orbito-frontal cortex); or (iii) there is a suspicion of insular involvement in EEG-HD, MEG, fMRI, or PET studies (19).

Implantation Strategy in Suspected Insular Cases

The complexity of the insular cortex and the many forms of insular lobe seizures make SEEG implantation a challenge whenever insular epilepsy is suspected. The basic principle, however, remains the same as for any SEEG study: the number, targets, and trajectories of insular as well as extra-insular electrodes being personalized according to patients' specific profiles. While most patients have an epileptogenic zone extending beyond the insula, some may have a very focal seizure onset, which first needs a large insulo-opercular coverage. The best approach therefore combines an oblique approach through the frontal or parietal cortices to allow a larger insular sampling, with a lateral orthogonal trajectory through the fronto-parietal and temporal operculum in order to disentangle the insula from operculum involvement in seizure generation (see below). A bilateral insulo-opercular implantation has to be considered whenever the seizure lateralization is unclear. To better evaluate the extent of the future resection and to exclude any extra-insular onset, seizure spread must also be evaluated, which requires an appropriate sampling of the extra-insular regions to which the insula is closely connected. This extra-insular spread, which occurs often, early, and rapidly after the seizure onset, accounts for the majority of the semiological features and can therefore be anticipated from clinical seizure analysis (frontal vs. perisylvian vs. temporal semiology).

Robot-Assisted SEEG

Historical Perspective and Hardware Development

Robot is derived from the root of the Czech word "robota" which means "forced labor." That resumes the human desire to delegate tiring, difficult, and repetitive tasks to technology. In this way, robot-assisted surgery has been developed in almost the entire field of surgery, including neurosurgery (20, 21). With the exponential development of robotics, stereotactic neurosurgeons rapidly recognized their potential for clinical use.

The first robot-aided neurosurgical procedure (a stereotactic biopsy) was carried out in 1985, making use of an industrial robot (PUMA 200) (22). A few years later, Benabid et al. in Grenoble, France, began to develop dedicated neurosurgical robots for general micro-neurosurgical procedures (using a Surgiscope microscope) and stereotactic procedures (Neuromate).

The Neuromate® robot (Renishaw-mayfield; Nyon, Switzerland) was developed and used successfully for brain biopsies, deep-brain stimulation, and SEEG (23, 24) and approved by the Food and Drug Administration for commercialization, leading to its worldwide diffusion and utilization for stereotactic procedures including SEEG. The ROSA® (Medtech SAS, Zimmer Biomet, Montpellier, France) robotic arm was later developed in the 2000's in France, based on an industrial robotic arm. It differed from the Neuromate in its built-in haptic capabilities, allowing the intuitive mobilization of the arm by the surgeon as an extension of herself. It also possesses a user-friendly graphical interface with a touch-screen monitor that can be used intraoperatively. The ROSA® is additionally more mobile (six movement axes as compared to five for the Neuromate).

The last-born commercial robotic arm is the iSYS1® (iSYS Medizintechnik, Kitzbühel, Austria), a novel miniature robotic arm with four axes of freedom that attaches to a classic three-pin headholder such as the Mayfield clamp (25). Neuromate® and ROSA® offer the possibility to perform both frame-based or frameless techniques while the iSYS1® offers a frameless technique only.

Other robotic arms had been developed over the years but were never used for SEEG or broadly commercialized.

Frame-Based Robot-Assisted SEEG Technique

The original Talairach's frame-based technique used an external fixed-grid system coupled with intraoperative teleangiography and ventriculography in order to allow the positioning of orthogonal electrodes in the desired place using two-dimensional imagery (26).

Nowadays, MRI and image fusion with digital subtraction angiography (DSA) have become the gold standard for SEEG pre-operative planning, as they are accurate and reliable.

Using a classical manual Leksell stereotactic frame, several epilepsy centers have described techniques of orthogonal and oblique depth-electrode insertion in the insula with good accuracy and few complications (27–29).

The first automatic robot-assisted techniques followed the same basic principles and used a cranial frame fixed on a robot (24). Robot assistance made oblique trajectories much easier due to robot reliability, versatility (multiple movement axes), and insertion-axis rigidity (30). Several groups have published their experience with frame-based robot-assisted methods (31–34), which have proven to be safe and accurate. Recently, frameless techniques have emerged in order to gain time without compromising accuracy.

Frameless Robot-Assisted SEEG Technique

The development of frameless insertion techniques aimed to simplify the process, with gains in time and procedural simplicity. These methods require a referencing step in order to match the patient's anatomy with the radiological images and pre-surgical planning. Laser-based facial referencing is possible with the ROSA® robot. As with current neuronavigation systems, several facial and skull landmarks are collected by the laser system in order to accurately superimpose the 3-D radiological exams on the patient's real anatomy. It is worth noting that using a CT exam for the laser referencing process appears to be much more accurate than using MRI, thus adding an additional step of CT/MRI image fusion (35). In our center, we use bone fiducial markers and intraoperative CT imaging (O-Arm®, Medtronic, Minneapolis, USA) for the referencing process and fuse the images with our MRI target plan and angiography. Trajectories are planned a week before the surgery on the ROSA® software. The resulting trajectories are executed by the ROSA® robot once the referencing accuracy has been carefully checked with the patient's anatomy (**Figure 1**). This technique was compared to frame-based methods on SEEG in term of complications but not accuracy (36). Our accuracy data published on DBS with sub-millimetric accuracy highlight the precision of this method (37). Dorfer et al. (25) used bone fiducial markers with the iSYS1® robot for SEEG, reporting millimetric accuracy. In Milan, Cardinale et al. (38) used the Neuromate® dedicated fiducial markers (Neurolocate) developed by Renishaw (Mayfield, Nyon, Switzerland) and mounted on the robot arm, rendering the use of bone or skin fiducial markers unnecessary with a gain of time and simplicity. Neuromate® offers another possibility of referencing based on ultrasound registration and is used by other teams (39) (**Figure 2**).

Insular SEEG Electrode Trajectories: Advantages and Limitations

Orthogonal approach (Figure 3)

The first papers describing insular SEEG sampling used an orthogonal trans-opercular approach (5, 40). The entire perysylvian area can be recorded with information from either opercula and insula. However, the orthogonal approach imposes sampling limitations, with few contacts per electrode that are actually in the insular cortex, requiring the multiplication of trajectories with presumed greater vascular risk.

Oblique approach (Figure 3)

Oblique approaches were developed through frontal and parietal entry points, in order to allow more extensive insular sampling while also limiting the vascular risks (30). A larger number of insular contacts are achieved through a less vascular intraparenchymal route. Oblique bone drilling, however, represents a technical challenge because of bone ripping, and the planned trajectories have to be longer. Both of these factors can result in target point inaccuracy. The second main pitfall is the occasional proximity of the entry point to the superior sagittal sinus, leading to possible transection of venous Trolard's lakes, but this problem is encountered in practice only exceptionally.

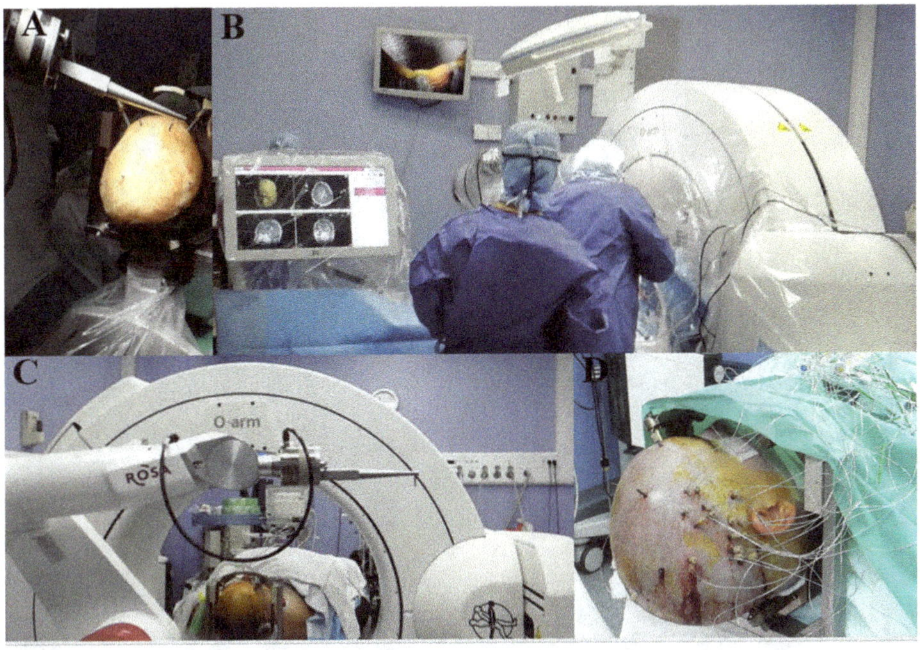

FIGURE 1 | Example of ROSA-robot system in the operating room in Grenoble. **(A)** Five bone fiducials markers anchored in the patient skull in non-coplanar manner. **(B)** ROSA-robot system with sterile touchscreen easy to use interface and intraoperative CT. **(C)** ROSA-robot dedicated bone fiducials markers system for referencing process. **(D)** Immediate postoperative view of a right SEEG.

Posterior parasagittal trans-insular approach

As with the oblique approach, the posterior approach allows insular sampling that is widely distributed, and electrodes can reach the amygdala (28). However, when the implantation scheme is not planned specifically for posterior implantation, the multiplicity of electrodes placed in standard SEEG makes the use of this trajectory challenging as the posterior parieto-occipital entry point can be difficult to access, even with robotic assistance. Furthermore, as with the oblique approach, the length of the trajectory can be a factor for inaccuracy. Finally, the Sylvian cistern can be transected in the posterior part of the peri-insular sulcus.

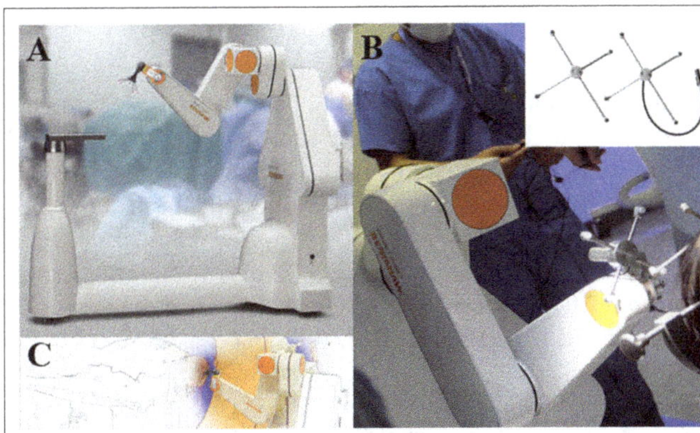

FIGURE 2 | Neuromate-Robot system by Renishaw. **(A,C)** Neurolocate® system used for frameless registration. **(B)** Registration with Ultrasound technology. Images provided by RENISHAW with permission for publication (Renishaw-mayfield; Nyon, Switzerland).

Insular SEEG accuracy

Few studies exist on the accuracy of SEEG electrode implantation relative to planned trajectories, and the specific literature on insular trajectories is even more scarce. **Table 1** summarizes the different studies published and available at the date of this review.

Different methods have been used to calculate trajectory accuracy. Most authors have used the 3D Euclidean distance for assessing electrode divergence from the initial target plan in the three spatial planes at both the entry point and the final target using the formula

$$Ed\ (a,b) = \sqrt{(Xa - Xb)^2 + \left(Ya - Yb\right)^2 + \left(Za - Zb\right)^2}$$

It is noteworthy that the lateral deviation, the radial error in a given plane, gave shorter distances compared to the Euclidean distance as emphasized by Ho et al. (46) with, at the target point, a lateral deviation estimate of 1.75 mm compared to 3.39 mm for the Euclidean distance (without insular electrodes).

Globally, entry-point errors range from 0.5 to 1.5 mm with either frame-based or frameless robot-assisted methods. Laser-based facial referencing with MRI appears to have a larger error margin (35). Entry-point errors seem to be dependent on the temporal pole position during surgery, the thickness of the scalp and the angle of the trajectory relative to the tangential plane of the skull (33). Inaccuracies at the entry point and distance to

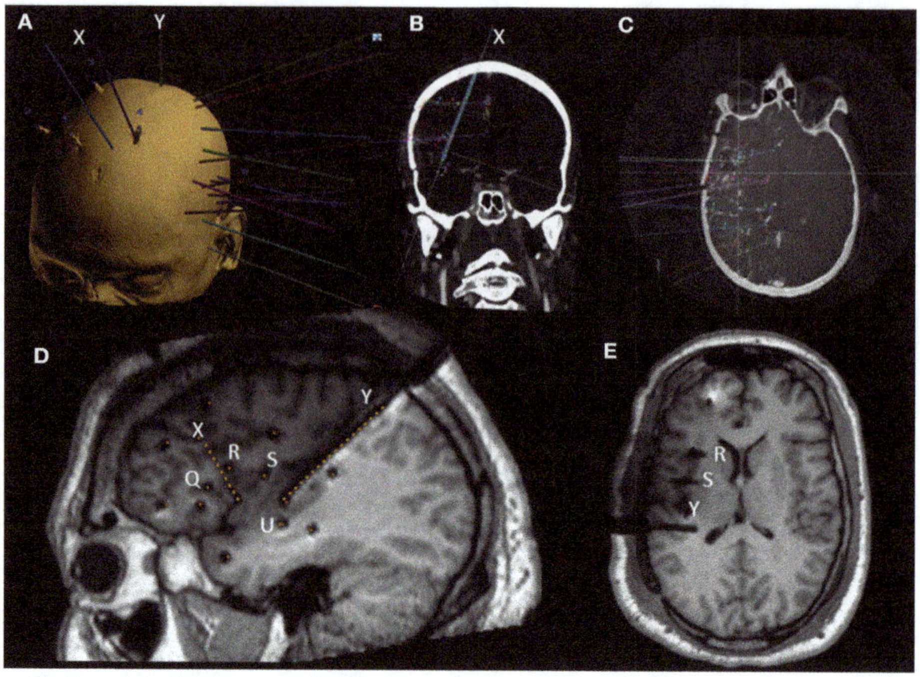

FIGURE 3 | Example of preoperative SEEG planning on ROSA software and postoperative MRI with mixed orthogonal and oblique trajectories. **(A)** 3D view of a left SEEG planning along with bone fiducials markers. **(B)** In plane view along oblique anterior insular (X) trajectory. **(C)** Example of SEEG planning fused with 3D angiography. **(D)** Postoperative sagittal T1 MRI with dark shadows representing electrodes with yellow dots superimposed representing planned trajectories. Note the oblique trajectories (X and Y) and four orthogonal trajectories (Q, R, S, and U). **(E)** Postoperative axial T1 MRI with dark shadows representing electrodes. Note the end location of contacts in the upper insula of orthogonal electrodes (R and S).

the target logically have a negative impact on target accuracy. An angle > 30° between the skull and the trajectory can lead to significant target deviations (45). Globally, target errors are in a range from 1.0 to 3.0 mm with 0.5 to 1.5 mm of difference between oblique and orthogonal trajectories. For comparison, with conventional frame-based SEEG (**Tables 1, 2**), target errors range from 2.0 to 4.0 mm. Neuronavigation systems have smaller accurate results in accordance with Vakharia et al. (51).

SEEG planning, vascular avoidance, and vascular complications

Clinicians fear vascular complications, as hemostatic control is impossible given the percutaneous nature of the technique, and the consequences of intracranial bleeding can be ominous.

During SEEG planning, particular care must be taken to avoid vascular structures. A vessel-free safety radius of 2 mm is often considered around the planned trajectory. Angiography has remained the gold standard vascular examination for trajectory planning. With advances in MRI, CT, and computer-assisted fusion and planning techniques over the past two decades, some groups have drifted toward other means of vascular imaging for preoperative trajectory planning in order to reduce the length of the workflow. Intraoperative vascular imaging possibilities have also emerged, such as injected angio-CT with O-Arm (52). Whether these changes provide substantial advantages remains to be clearly determined.

In **Table 3**, we have summarized the vascular complications, SEEG technique, and type of vascular imagery used for referencing in the currently available literature on insular targeting with robot or non–robot-assisted techniques. Major bleeding complications have been defined as those causing death, needing surgical treatment, or leaving permanent sequelae. In a recent meta-analysis revising all sampling trajectories, hemorrhagic risk was estimated to be around 1.0%. The most frequent type of hemorrhagic complication was intraparenchymal hematoma followed by subdural and epidural hematomas. In comparison, infections, hardware-related complications, and permanent neurologic deficits were, respectively, estimated at 0.8, 0.4, and 0.6% (64).

Interestingly, in the series from Milan (59), no major bleeding events were observed since robotic assistance was adopted, using a frameless technique. In the series from Cleveland (61), it appears that the adoption of robotic assistance has also had a beneficial effect, with a tendency for a lower hemorrhagic risk when comparing the technique to the conventional frame-based method. The Cleveland Group also described a higher hemorrhagic risk when MRI was used for vascular assessment compared to angiography, and they have currently added computed tomographic angiography (CTA) to their planning workflow, resulting in a decrease in hemorrhagic events (34).

In the consideration of vascular imaging for trajectory planning, another question arises. Should we also consider the

TABLE 1 | Relevant literature about insular robot-assisted SEEG accuracy.

Epilepsy center/study	Patients	Method	Frameless referencing process	Number of procedures/number of electrodes/ number of insular electrodes	Error measure	Entry point	Target point
Milan (Italy) Cardinale et al. (33) Cardinale et al. (38)	A and P	Neuromate frameless vs. neuromate frame-based vs. conventional frame-based method	Neurolocate	8/127/NR vs. 81/1,050/NR vs. 37/517/NR	Euclidean distance	All electrodes 0.59 vs. 0.78 vs. 1.43	All electrodes 1.49 vs. 1.77 vs. 2.69
Cleveland (USA) Gonzalez-Martinez et al. (41)	A and P	Rosa Frameless vs. conventional frame-based method	Laser-based facial scanning	101/1,245/NS vs. 103/1,367/NR	Euclidean distance	All electrodes 1.2 vs. 1.1	All electrodes 1.7 vs. NR
Vienna (Austria) Dorfer et al. (25)	A and P	iSys1 frameless	6 bone fiducial markers	16/93/13 5 of the 16/31/NR with K-wire	Lateral deviation	All electrodes 1.3 1.54–1.18 with K-wire[a]	All electrodes 1.5 1.82–1.66 with K-wire[a]
Strasbourg (France) Ollivier et al. (42)	A and P	ROSA frameless	Laser-based facial scanning	66/901/NR	Euclidean distance	All electrodes Orthogonal:1.39 Oblique:1.63	All electrodes Orthogonal:2.61 Oblique:3.29
Roma (Italy) De Benedictis et al. (43)	P	ROSA frameless	Laser-based facial scanning	36/386/NR	Euclidean distance	All electrodes 1.50	All electrodes 1.96
Barcelona (Spain) Candela-Canto et al. (39)	P	Neuromate	Ultrasound co-registration	14/164/NR	Planning software (formula not described)	All electrodes 1.57	All electrodes 1.77
Lyon (France) Bourdillon et al. (32)	A and P	Neuromate Frame-based vs. conventional frame-based method	/	50/565/96 vs. 50/628/NR	Euclidean distance	NR	All electrodes 1.15 vs. 4.00
Great ormond street hospital London (UK) Sharma et al. (44)	P	Neuromate frame-based vs. optical neuro-navigation (ON)	/	20 (14 robot; 6 ON)/218/NS	Euclidean distance	All electrodes Robot: 0.71 ON: 5.5	All electrodes Robot: 1.07 ON: 4.5
London (Canada) Bottan et al. (31)	A	Neuromate frame-based (+ 1 bone fiducial marker)	/	41/98/98	Euclidean distance	**Insular electrodes** Orthogonal: 1.5 Oblique: 1.5 Parasagittal: 1.3	**Insular electrodes** Orthogonal: 1.9 Oblique: 2.4 Parasagittal: 1.5
Frankfurt (Germany) Spyrantis et al. (35)	A	ROSA frame-based vs. ROSA frameless	CT laser-based facial scanning vs. MRI laser-based facial scanning	19/171/15 CT-frame: 4/49/8 CT- laser: 7/60/1 3T MRI-laser: 7/56/6 1.5T MRI-laser: 1/6/0	Euclidean distance	**Insular electrodes:** CT-frame: 0.88 3T MRI-laser: 3.36 **All electrodes:** CT-frame: 0.86 CT-laser: 1.85 3T MRI-laser: 3.02 1.5T MRI-laser: 0.97	**Insular electrodes:** CT-frame: 1.99 3T MRI-laser: 4.07 **All electrodes:** CT-frame: 2.28 CT-laser : 2.41 3T MRI-laser: 3.51 1.5T MRI-laser: 1.71
Munt Sinaï; New York (USA) Iordanou et al. (45)		ROSA frameless	CT laser-based facial scanning or bone fiducials	25/319/NR	Lateral deviation (LD) and depth error (DE)	**All electrodes: Oblique electrodes** LD:1.76 **Orthogonal electrodes** LD:1.32	**All electrodes: Oblique electrodes** LD: 2.05 DE: 2.32 **Orthogonal electrodes:** LD: 1.45 DE: 2.33

A, Adults; EP, Entry point error; NR, Not reported; P, Pediatric; TP, Target point error.

[a] The authors developed a technique for skull drilling based on pre-drill with a K-wire with an improved accuracy.

TABLE 2 | Relevant literature about non robot-assisted SEEG accuracy for insular trajectories.

Epilepsy center/study	Patients	Technique	Number of patient/number of electrodes/number of insular electrodes	Error measure	EP (mm)	TP (mm)
National hospital for neurology and neurosurgery; London (UK) Nowell et al. (47)	A	Frameless neuronavigation	22/187/15	Lateral deviation	NR	**All:** 3.66 **Insula:** 2.83
Rouen (France) Gilard et al. (48)	A and P	Conventional frame-based	10/106/10	Euclidean distance	NR	**All:** 2.06
Amsterdam (The Netherlands) Verburg et al. (49)	A and P	Frameless neuronavigation	7/99/5	Euclidean distance	NR	**All:** 3.5
Maastricht (The Netherlands) van der Loo et al. (50)	A and P	Conventional Frame-based	76/902/NR	Euclidean distance	**All:** 1.54	**All:** 2.93

EP, Entry point error; NR, Not reported; TP, Target point error.

smallest vessels as potential hazards? Are larger vessels more prone to be injured or more resistant to traction?

In studies made on susceptibility weighted imaging (SWI) or digital subtraction angiography (DSA), it appears that trajectories at the vicinity of vessels of a caliber < 1.5 mm in the brain parenchyma (not at the cortical entry) could not be hazardous (65). Other authors suggest that SWI may overestimate the vasculature and thus limit the number of trajectories without influencing the bleeding incidence (66). The topic is still a matter of debate with some authors considering that "the better we can see the enemy, the better we can plan to avoid it" (67).

In the currently available literature, insular trajectories do not seem to be associated with higher hemorrhagic complications, at least for orthogonal trajectories (55). In our experience, neither oblique nor orthogonal trajectories seem to be associated with an overexposure risk of bleeding.

Outcomes after insular SEEG

The main challenge in interpreting insular SEEG tracings consists in differentiating primary insular involvement from early secondary involvement. In the case of temporo-insular epilepsy (temporal plus epilepsy—TPE), non-recognition of primary insular involvement can lead to resective surgery failure (7, 68). On the other hand, resection of the insula, when its involvement is a secondary event, does not improve resective surgery outcomes but exposes the patient to unnecessary surgical risks (53). The utility of SEEG is thus self-evident in these complex situations.

Isnard et al. (12) described insular or operculo-insular epilepsy in 10% of the patients from their cohort. In one patient (2%), the EZ was temporo-insular (TPE). In the vast majority of their series (86% of patients), the insular involvement was secondary to a temporal onset zone. Afif et al. (30) similarly showed 17% of primary insular epileptic involvement and 50% of secondary insular involvement. Alomar et al. (62) found 17% of primary involvement but only 0.37% of secondary involvement. Desai et al. (27) described 10% of primary and 25% of secondary insular involvement. Salado et al. (29) showed 41% of primary and 22% of secondary insular.

Whether these differences emerge from a high variability of epileptic syndromes, a topographical or genetic fingerprint or simply differences in SEEG sampling strategies and techniques remains unclear. This should be resolved as the amount of available data increase.

In the papers previously cited, resective surgery was the most frequently proposed therapeutic option, except when eloquent areas were in the EZ or when bilateral epilepsy was the culprit.

In cases where resective surgery is functionally impossible, vagal nerve stimulation can be proposed. An alternative approach has emerged with focal EZ ablation by thermal therapy. Laser-interstitial thermal therapy (LITT) has indeed been proposed by some authors (62, 69) with encouraging results. However, its availability across the world is still limited due to its cost, its highly complex technical platform, and its expertise requirement. In Europe, radio-frequency thermocoagulation (RF-TC) has been developed to address cases of non-resectable EZs, and sometimes as a primary treatment strategy when an extremely focal EZ is detected on SEEG.

Radio-frequency thermo-coagulation in the insula

Stereotactic lesion formation in epilepsy is not a novel approach, but the use of SEEG electrodes for RF-TC was published by Guénot et al. (70) in Lyon. They used this strategy in the insula in two patients with an 80% decrease in seizure events and no permanent adverse events (one patient suffered from transient oral paresthesia).

In our experience, based on 23 patients, seven RF-TC procedures were performed on the insula. Two patients had beneficial effects from the procedure (71). In the biggest insular RFTC-dedicated series published by Saint Anne's group (Paris), 89% of their 19 patients were good responders with 10 Engels's class I, 4 class II, and 3 class III patients (72). RFTC was performed as a separate procedure after SEEG. Transient postoperative deficits were observed in 42% (eight patients) with

TABLE 3 | Overview of insular SEEG literature regarding vascular imaging reference and vascular complications.

Epilepsy center/ study period	Number of patients	Vascular imaging reference	Method	Insular trajectory	Direct vascular related complication[a]
Grenoble (France)					
Afif et al. (30) *1998–2005*	30	Angiography	Frame-based Robot-assisted	Oblique	One major bleeding after electrode removal not related to insula
Blauwblomme et al. (53) *2001–2010*	17	Angiography	Frame-based Robot-assisted	Orthogonal Oblique	No vascular complications
Gras-Combes et al. (54) *2009–2013*	6	Angiography Angiography	Frame-based Robot-assisted Frameless robot-assisted	Orthogonal Oblique	No vascular complications
Abel et al. (36) *2013–2017*	17	Angiography Angiography	Frameless Robot-assisted vs.	Orthogonal Oblique	4 minor bleedings not related to insula
< 2013	18		Frame-based robot-assisted		2 minor bleeding not related to insula
Lyon (France)					
Isnard et al. (12) *1996–2001*	50	Angiography	Conventional Frame-based	Orthogonal	NR
Bourdillon et al. (55) *1995–2015*	459	Angiography	Conventional Frame-based and Frame-based robot-assisted	Orthogonal	7 major bleedings not related to insula with conventional frame-based method (1 death)
Bourdillon et al. (32) *2012–2015*	100	Angiography with O-arm	Conventional frame-based method and Frame-based robot-assisted	Orthogonal	No vascular complications
Fondation Rotschild, Paris (France)					
Dorfmüller et al. (56) Dylgjeri et al. (57) *2009–2012*	19 10	MRI Gado	Frameless robot-assisted	Orthogonal Oblique	No vascular complications
Pitié-Salpétrière, Paris (France)					
Mathon et al. (58) *1991–2014*	157	MRI Gado (+ TOF Gado)	Conventional Frame-based	NR	2 minor bleedings 3 major bleedings Not related to insula 1 stroke of the insula (temporal electrode insertion)
Montpellier (France)					
Gil Robles et al. (28) *<2009*	9	MRI Gado	Conventional Frame-based	Parasagittal posterior	No vascular complications
Strasbourg (France)					
Ollivier et al. 62 *2010–2016*	66	MRI Gado	Frameless Robot-assisted	Oblique	8 minor bleedings 1 major bleeding (Not specified if insular trajectory involved)
Nancy (France)					
Salado et al. (29) *2008–2016*	99	MRI Gado (double injection)	Conventional frame-based	Orthogonal (97.3%) Oblique (2.7%)	6 minor bleedings 1 major bleeding (Not related to insula)
Rouen (France)					
Gilard et al. (48) *<2016*	10	CTA	Conventional frame-based	NR	No vascular complications
Milan (Italy)					
Cardinale et al. (59) *1996–2018*	713	Angiography (+/- with O-arm)	Conventional frame-based Frame-based robot-assisted Frameless robot-assisted since 2016	NR	5 major bleedings with conventional frame-based method. 0 major bleeding with robot (Not specified if insular trajectory involved)
Roma (Italy)					
De Benedictis et al. (43) *2011–2016*	116	MRI Gado	Frameless robot-assisted	NR	No vascular complications

(Continued)

TABLE 3 | Continued

Epilepsy center/ study period	Number of patients	Vascular imaging reference	Method	Insular trajectory	Direct vascular related complication[a]
Barcelona (Spain)					
Candela-Canto et al. (39) *2016–2018*	14	CTA (bi-phasic injection)	Frameless robot-assisted	NR	1 major bleeding not related to insula
Vienna (Austria)					
Desai et al. (25) *2014–2015*	16	MRI Gado	Frameless robot-assisted	Oblique	No vascular complications
Frankfurt (Germany)					
Spyrantis et al. (35) *2012–2018*	19	MRI Gado	Frameless robot-assisted	NR	No vascular complications
Sofia (Bulgary)					
Minkin et al. (60) *2013-2015*	34	MRI Gado (double injection) and MRA	Conventional Frame-based	Orthogonal (75%) Oblique (25%)	1 minor bleeding
Amsterdam (The Netherlands)					
Verburg et al. (49)	7	MRI Gado	Frameless Neuronavigation	NR	1 major bleeding after electrode removal (Not specified if insular trajectory involved)
Maastricht (The Netherlands)					
van der Loo et al. (50) *2008–2016*	71	MRI Gado	Conventional Frame-based	Orthogonal Oblique	2 major bleedings 4 minor bleedings
Great ormond street hospital, London (UK)					
Sharma et al. (44) *2014–2017*	14 6	CTA	Frame-based robot-assisted Frameless Neuronavigation	NR	No vascular complications
National hospital for neurology and neurosurgery, London (UK)					
Nowell et al. (47) *<2014*	22	CTA and 3D phase contrast MRI	Frameless Neuronavigation	Oblique	1 minor bleeding (Not specified if insular trajectory involved)
London (Canada)					
Bottan et al. (31) *2017-2018*	41	MRI Gado (double injection)	Frame-based robot-assisted	Orthogonal (15.3%) Oblique (82.7%) Parasagittal (2%)	No vascular complications
Cleveland (USA)					
McGovern et al. (61) *2009–2017*	526	Angiography MRI Gado alone or + CTA	Conventional frame-based method and frame-based robot-assisted and frameless robot-assisted since 2013	Orthogonal Oblique	93 minor bleedings[b] 12 major bleedings (9 transient deficit 2 permanent deficits 1 death)
Alomar et al. (62) 2009–2013	135 with insular trajectories	Angiography (27 patients) MRI Gado + CTA (108 patients)	Conventional frame-based method (27) Frameless robot-assisted (108)	Orthogonal (88.5%) Oblique (11.5%)	1 minor bleeding not related to insula
Lebanon (USA)					
Desai et al. (27) *2001–2009*	20	MRI Gado	Conventional frame-based method	Frontal oblique	No vascular complications
Saint Louis (USA)					
Miller et al. (63) *2016*	11	CTA	Frameless robot-assisted	NR	1 minor bleeding
Munt Sinaï; New York (USA)					
Iordanou et al. (45) *<2018*	25	MRI Gado	Frameless robot-assisted	Orthogonal Oblique	No vascular complications reported

CTA, Computed tomographic angiography; Gado, Gadolinium; MRI, Magnetic resonance imaging; NR, Not reported; TOF, Time of flight.
[a]Major bleeding refer to potential fatal or permanent sequelae bleeding or the need for surgical removal.
[b]The authors described all form of bleedings including subarachnoid minimal bleedings always excluded from other reports.

mild hemiparesis, hypoesthesia, dysgeusia, or dysarthria. Only one remained in a permanent mild dysarthria.

Finally, RF-TC can be used alone or in combination with insular or extra-insular corticectomy (29) and can be repeated in case of relapse (73) at the cost of a new lead implantation. Of note, performing RF-TC does not contraindicate subsequent surgery and can even be used as a strong predictive factor of postsurgical outcome (74).

CONCLUSION

The potential of preoperative SEEG exploration for planning effective and safe epilepsy surgeries has been recognized and established over the past decades. The technique has proven to be particularly useful when the insula needs to be explored as symptoms of insular epilepsy are harder to recognize or detect on a standard EEG. With the advances in robotic-assisted surgery, SEEG techniques have been simplified, and their accuracy has increased, thus diminishing the intervention risks and time constraints.

The future of the technique will most probably rely on computer-assisted planning strategies in order to reduce the time needed for trajectory planning and will probably employ artificial intelligence-based software (75). Further developments could come from accuracy registration verification in the operating room, with real-time augmented reality allowing an increase in accuracy (76).

While the dawn of SEEG seems to have passed and the technique has established itself as an essential tool for surgical planning in epilepsy surgery, the future of the technique appears brighter than ever, as robotics and software automatization aid neurosurgeons in this complex task.

AUTHOR CONTRIBUTIONS

AD wrote the manuscript and built the figures. JZ-J revised the manuscript and co-built the figures. DH, A-SJ-C, PK, and LM revised the manuscript. ED co-wrote the manuscript. SC co-wrote the manuscript and provided final manuscript revision. All authors contributed to the article and approved the submitted version.

REFERENCES

1. Fusar-Poli P, Howes O, Borgwardt S. Johann cristian reil on the 200th anniversary of the first description of the insula (1809). *J Neurol Neurosurg Psychiatr.* (2009) 80:1409. doi: 10.1136/jnnp.2009.185884
2. Penfield W, Faulk ME. The insula: further observations on its function. *Brain.* (1955) 78:445–70. doi: 10.1093/brain/78.4.445
3. Guillaume JMM, Mazars G. Techniques de résection de l'insula dans les épilepsies insulaires. *Revue Neurol.* (1949) 461–501.
4. Silfvenius H, Gloor P, Rasmussen T. Evaluation of insular ablation in surgical treatment of temporal lobe epilepsy. *Epilepsia.* (1964) 5:307–20. doi: 10.1111/j.1528-1157.1964.tb03338.x
5. Isnard J, Guénot M, Ostrowsky K, Sindou M, Mauguière F. The role of the insular cortex in temporal lobe epilepsy. *Ann Neurol.* (2000) 48:614–23. doi: 10.1002/1531-8249(200010)48:4<614::AID-ANA8>3.0.CO;2-S
6. Jobst BC, Gonzalez-Martinez J, Isnard J, Kahane P, Lacuey N, Lahtoo SD, et al. The insula and its epilepsies. *Epilepsy Curr.* (2019) 19:11–21. doi: 10.1177/1535759718822847
7. Kahane P, Barba C, Rheims S, Job-Chapron AS, Minotti L, Ryvlin P. The concept of temporal 'plus' epilepsy. *Revue Neurol.* (2015) 171:267–72. doi: 10.1016/j.neurol.2015.01.562
8. Isnard J, Hagiwara K, Montavont A, Catenoix H, Mazzola L, Ostrowsky-Coste K, et al. Semiology of insular lobe seizures. *Revue Neurol.* (2019) 175:144–9. doi: 10.1016/j.neurol.2018.12.002
9. Barba C, Minotti L, Job A-S, Kahane P. The insula in temporal plus epilepsy. *J Clin Neurophysiol.* (2017) 34:324–7. doi: 10.1097/WNP.0000000000000389
10. Montavont A, Mauguiere F, Mazzola L, Garcia-Larrea L, Catenoix H, Ryvlin P, et al. On the origin of painful somatosensory seizures. *Neurology.* (2015) 84:594–601. doi: 10.1212/WNL.0000000000001235
11. Barba C, Barbati G, Minotti L, Hoffmann D, Kahane P. Ictal clinical and scalp-EEG findings differentiating temporal lobe epilepsies from temporal "plus" epilepsies. *Brain.* (2007) 130:1957–67. doi: 10.1093/brain/awm108
12. Isnard J, Guenot M, Sindou M, Mauguiere F. Clinical manifestations of insular lobe seizures: a stereo-electroencephalographic study. *Epilepsia.* (2004) 45:1079–90. doi: 10.1111/j.0013-9580.2004.68903.x
13. Xiao H, Tran TPY, Pétrin M, Boucher O, Mohamed I, Bouthillier A, et al. Reflex operculoinsular seizures. *Epileptic Disord.* (2016) 18:19–25. doi: 10.1684/epd.2016.0801
14. Catenoix H, Mauguière F, Guénot M, Isnard J, Ryvlin P. Recording the insula during ictal asystole. *Int J Cardiol.* (2013) 169:e28–30. doi: 10.1016/j.ijcard.2013.08.100
15. Seeck M, Zaim S, Chaves-Vischer V, Blanke O, Maeder-Ingvar M, Weissert M, et al. Ictal bradycardia in a young child with focal cortical dysplasia in the right insular cortex. *Eur J Paediatr Neurol.* (2003) 7:177–81. doi: 10.1016/S1090-3798(03)00051-5
16. Tayah T, Savard M, Desbiens R, Nguyen DK. Ictal bradycardia and asystole in an adult with a focal left insular lesion. *Clin Neurol Neurosurg.* (2013) 115:1885–7. doi: 10.1016/j.clineuro.2013.04.011
17. Nguyen DK, Nguyen DB, Malak R, Leroux J-M, Carmant L, Saint-Hilaire J-M, et al. Revisiting the role of the insula in refractory partial epilepsy. *Epilepsia.* (2009) 50:510–20. doi: 10.1111/j.1528-1167.2008.01758.x
18. Ryvlin P, Minotti L, Demarquay G, Hirsch E, Arzimanoglou A, Hoffman D, et al. Nocturnal hypermotor seizures, suggesting frontal lobe epilepsy, can originate in the insula. *Epilepsia.* (2006) 47:755–65. doi: 10.1111/j.1528-1167.2006.00510.x
19. Minotti L, Montavont A, Scholly J, Tyvaert L, Taussig D. Indications and limits of stereoelectroencephalography (SEEG). *Neurophysiol Clin.* (2018) 48:15–24. doi: 10.1016/j.neucli.2017.11.006
20. Leal Ghezzi T, Campos Corleta O. 30 years of robotic surgery. *World J Surg.* (2016) 40:2550–7. doi: 10.1007/s00268-016-3543-9
21. Nathoo N, Çavuşoglu MC, Vogelbaum MA, Barnett GH. In Touch with robotics: neurosurgery for the future. *Neurosurgery.* (2005) 56:421–33. doi: 10.1227/01.NEU.0000153929.68024.CF
22. Kwoh YS, Hou J, Jonckheere EA, Hayati S. A robot with improved absolute positioning accuracy for CT guided stereotactic brain surgery. *IEEE Trans Biomed Eng.* (1988) 35:153–60. doi: 10.1109/10.1354
23. Benabid AL, Cinquin P, Lavalle S, Le Bas JF, Demongeot J, de Rougemont J. Computer-driven robot for stereotactic surgery connected to CT scan and magnetic resonance imaging. Technological design and preliminary results. *Appl Neurophysiol.* (1987) 50:153–4. doi: 10.1159/000100701
24. Benabid AL, Hoffmann D, Ashraf A, Koudsie A, Esteve F, Le Bas JF. Robotics in neurosurgery: current status and future prospects. *Chirurgie.* (1998) 123:25-31. doi: 10.1016/s0001-4001(98)80035-4
25. Dorfer C, Minchev G, Czech T, Stefanits H, Feucht M, Pataraia E, et al. A novel miniature robotic device for frameless implantation of depth electrodes in refractory epilepsy. *J Neurosurg.* (2016) 126:1622-8. doi: 10.3171/2016.5.JNS16388

26. Talairach J, Bancaud J. Stereotaxic approach to epilepsy. In: Karger AG, editor. *Progress in Neurological Surgery*. Basel (1973). p. 297–354. doi: 10.1159/000394343
27. Desai A, Jobst BC, Thadani VM, Bujarski KA, Gilbert K, Darcey TM, et al. Stereotactic depth electrode investigation of the insula in the evaluation of medically intractable epilepsy. *J Neurosurg.* (2011) 114:1176–86. doi: 10.3171/2010.9.JNS091803
28. Gil Robles S, Gelisse P, El Fertit H, Tancu C, Duffau H, Crespel A, et al. Parasagittal transinsular electrodes for stereo-EEG in temporal and insular lobe epilepsies. *Stereo Funct Neurosurg.* (2009) 87:368–78. doi: 10.1159/000249818
29. Salado AL, Koessler L, De Mijolla G, Schmitt E, Vignal J-P, Civit T, et al. sEEG is a safe procedure for a comprehensive anatomic exploration of the insula: a retrospective study of 108 procedures representing 254 transopercular insular electrodes. *Oper Neurosurg.* (2018) 14:1–8. doi: 10.1093/ons/opx106
30. Afif A, Chabardes S, Minotti L, Kahane P, Hoffmann D. Safety and usefulness of insular depth electrodes implanted via an oblique approach in patients with epilepsy. *Oper Neurosurg.* (2008) 62:471–80. doi: 10.1227/01.neu.0000326037.62337.80
31. Bottan JS, Rubino PA, Lau JC, MacDougall KW, Parrent AG, Burneo JG, et al. Robot-assisted insular depth electrode implantation through oblique trajectories: 3-dimensional anatomical nuances, technique, accuracy, and safety. *Oper Neurosurg.* (2019) 18:278–83. doi: 10.1093/ons/opz154
32. Bourdillon P, Châtillon C-E, Moles A, Rheims S, Catenoix H, Montavont A, et al. Effective accuracy of stereoelectroencephalography: robotic 3D versus Talairach orthogonal approaches. *J Neurosurg.* (2018) 131:1938–46. doi: 10.3171/2018.7.JNS181164
33. Cardinale F, Cossu M, Castana L, Casaceli G, Schiariti MP, Miserocchi A, et al. Stereoelectroencephalography: surgical methodology, safety, and stereotactic application accuracy in 500 procedures. *Neurosurgery.* (2013) 72:353–66. doi: 10.1227/NEU.0b013e31827d1161
34. McGovern RA, Butler RS, Bena J, Gonzalez-Martinez J. Incorporating new technology into a surgical technique: the learning curve of a single surgeon's stereo-electroencephalography experience. *Neurosurgery.* (2020) 86:E281-9. doi: 10.1093/neuros/nyz498
35. Spyrantis A, Cattani A, Woebbecke T, Konczalla J, Strzelczyk A, Rosenow F, et al. Electrode placement accuracy in robot-assisted epilepsy surgery: A comparison of different referencing techniques including frame-based CT versus facial laser scan based on CT or MRI. *Epilepsy Beha.* (2019) 91:38–47. doi: 10.1016/j.yebeh.2018.11.002
36. Abel TJ, Varela Osorio R, Amorim-Leite R, Mathieu F, Kahane P, Minotti L, et al. Frameless robot-assisted stereoelectroencephalography in children: technical aspects and comparison with Talairach frame technique. *J Neurosurg Pediatr.* (2018) 22:37-46. doi: 10.3171/2018.1.PEDS17435
37. Liu L, Mariani SG, De Schlichting E, Grand S, Lefranc M, Seigneuret E, et al. Frameless ROSA® robot-assisted lead implantation for deep brain stimulation: technique and accuracy. *Oper Neurosurg.* (2019) 19:57–64. doi: 10.1093/ons/opz320
38. Cardinale F, Rizzi M, d'Orio P, Casaceli G, Arnulfo G, Narizzano M, et al. A new tool for touch-free patient registration for robot-assisted intracranial surgery: application accuracy from a phantom study and a retrospective surgical series. *Neurosurg Focus.* (2017) 42:E8. doi: 10.3171/2017.2.FOCUS16539
39. Candela-Cantó S, Aparicio J, López JM, Baños-Carrasco P, Ramírez-Camacho A, Climent A, et al. Frameless robot-assisted stereoelectroencephalography for refractory epilepsy in pediatric patients: accuracy, usefulness, and technical issues. *Acta Neurochirurgi.* (2018) 160:2489-500. doi: 10.1007/s00701-018-3720-8
40. Frot M, Mauguière F. Timing and spatial distribution of somatosensory responses recorded in the upper bank of the sylvian fissure (SII Area) in humans. *Cereb Cortex.* (1999) 9:854–63. doi: 10.1093/cercor/9.8.854
41. González-Martínez J, Bulacio J, Thompson S, Gale J, Smithason S, Najm I, et al. Technique, results, and complications related to robot-assisted stereoelectroencephalography. *Neurosurgery.* (2016) 78:169-80. doi: 10.1227/NEU.0000000000001034
42. Ollivier I, Behr C, Cebula H, Timofeev A, Benmekhbi M, Valenti MP, et al. Efficacy and safety in frameless robot-assisted stereo-electroencephalography (SEEG) for drug-resistant epilepsy. *Neurochirurgie.* (2017) 63:286-90. doi: 10.1016/j.neuchi.2017.03.002
43. De Benedictis A, Trezza A, Carai A, Genovese E, Procaccini E, Messina R, et al. Robot-assisted procedures in pediatric neurosurgery. *Neurosurg Focus.* (2017) 42:E7. doi: 10.3171/2017.2.FOCUS16579
44. Sharma JD, Seunarine KK, Tahir MZ, Tisdall MM. Accuracy of robot-assisted versus optical frameless navigated stereoelectroencephalography electrode placement in children. *J Neurosurg Pediatr.* (2019) 23:297–302. doi: 10.3171/2018.10.PEDS18227
45. Iordanou JC, Camara D, Ghatan S, Panov F. Approach angle affects accuracy in robotic stereoelectroencephalography lead placement. *World Neurosurg.* (2019) 128:e322-8. doi: 10.1016/j.wneu.2019.04.143
46. Ho AL, Muftuoglu Y, Pendharkar AV, Sussman ES, Porter BE, Halpern CH, et al. Robot-guided pediatric stereoelectroencephalography: single-institution experience. *J Neurosurg Pediatr.* (2018) 22:489–96. doi: 10.3171/2018.5.PEDS17718
47. Nowell M, Rodionov R, Diehl B, Wehner T, Zombori G, Kinghorn J, et al. A novel method for implementation of frameless StereoEEG in epilepsy surgery. *Oper Neurosurg.* (2014) 10:525–34. doi: 10.1227/NEU.0000000000000544
48. Gilard V, Proust F, Gerardin E, Lebas A, Chastan N, Fréger P, et al. Usefulness of multidetector-row computerized tomographic angiography for the surgical planning in stereoelectroencephalography. *Diagnost Interven Imag.* (2016) 97:333-7. doi: 10.1016/j.diii.2015.10.001
49. Verburg N, Baayen JC, Idema S, Klitsie MAJ, Claus S, de Jonge CS, et al. *In vivo* accuracy of a frameless stereotactic drilling technique for diagnostic biopsies and stereoelectroencephalography depth electrodes. *World Neurosurg.* (2016) 87:392-8. doi: 10.1016/j.wneu.2015.11.041
50. van der Loo LE, Schijns OEMG, Hoogland G, Colon AJ, Wagner GL, Dings JTA, et al. Methodology, outcome, safety and *in vivo* accuracy in traditional frame-based stereoelectroencephalography. *Acta Neurochir.* (2017) 159:1733–46. doi: 10.1007/s00701-017-3242-9
51. Vakharia VN, Sparks R, O'Keeffe AG, Rodionov R, Miserocchi A, McEvoy A, et al. Accuracy of intracranial electrode placement for stereoencephalography: A systematic review and meta-analysis. *Epilepsia.* (2017) 58:921–32. doi: 10.1111/epi.13713
52. Cardinale F, Pero G, Quilici L, Piano M, Colombo P, Moscato A, et al. Cerebral angiography for multimodal surgical planning in epilepsy surgery: description of a new three-dimensional technique and literature review. *World Neurosurg.* (2015) 84:358–67. doi: 10.1016/j.wneu.2015.03.028
53. Blauwblomme T, David O, Minotti L, Job A-S, Chassagnon S, Hoffman D, et al. Prognostic value of insular lobe involvement in temporal lobe epilepsy: a stereoelectroencephalographic study. *Epilepsia.* (2013) 54:1658–67. doi: 10.1111/epi.12260
54. Gras-Combe G, Minotti L, Hoffmann D, Krainik A., Kahane P, Chabardes S. Surgery for nontumoral insular epilepsy explored by stereoelectroencephalography. *Neurosurgery.* (2016) 79:578-88. doi: 10.1227/NEU.0000000000001257
55. Bourdillon P, Ryvlin P, Isnard J, Montavont A, Catenoix H, Mauguière F, et al. Stereotactic electroencephalography is a safe procedure, including for insular implantations. *World Neurosurg.* (2017) 99:353-61. doi: 10.1016/j.wneu.2016.12.025
56. Dorfmüller G, Ferrand-Sorbets S, Fohlen M, Bulteau C, Archambaud F, Delalande O, et al. Outcome of surgery in children with focal cortical dysplasia younger than 5 years explored by stereo-electroencephalography. *Child Nervous Syst.* (2014) 30:1875-83. doi: 10.1007/s00381-014-2464-x
57. Dylgjeri S, Taussig D, Chipaux M, Lebas A, Fohlen M, Bulteau C, et al. Insular and insulo-opercular epilepsy in childhood: an SEEG study. *Seizure.* (2014) 23:300-8. doi: 10.1016/j.seizure.2014.01.008
58. Mathon B, Clemenceau S, Hasboun D, Habert M-O, Belaid H, Nguyen-Michel V-H, et al. Safety profile of intracranial electrode implantation for video-EEG recordings in drug-resistant focal epilepsy. *J Neurol.* (2015) 262:2699-712. doi: 10.1007/s00415-015-7901-6
59. Cardinale F, Rizzi M, Vignati E, Cossu M, Castana L, d'Orio P, et al. Stereoelectroencephalography: retrospective analysis of 742 procedures in a single centre. *Brain.* (2019) 142:2688-704. doi: 10.1093/brain/awz196
60. Minkin K, Gabrovski K, Penkov M, Todorov Y, Tanova R, Milenova Y, et al. Stereoelectroencephalography using magnetic resonance angiography

for avascular trajectory planning: technical report. *Neurosurgery.* (2017) 81:688–95. doi: 10.1093/neuros/nyx166

61. McGovern RA, Ruggieri P, Bulacio J, Najm I, Bingaman WE, Gonzalez-Martinez JA. Risk analysis of hemorrhage in stereo-electroencephalography procedures. *Epilepsia.* (2019) 60:571-80. doi: 10.1111/epi.14668
62. Alomar S, Mullin JP, Smithason S, Gonzalez-Martinez J. Indications, technique, and safety profile of insular stereoelectroencephalography electrode implantation in medically intractable epilepsy. *J Neurosurg.* (2018) 128:1147-57. doi: 10.3171/2017.1.JNS161070
63. Miller BA, Salehi A, Limbrick DD, Smyth MD. Applications of a robotic stereotactic arm for pediatric epilepsy and neurooncology surgery. *J Neurosurg Pediatr.* (2017) 20:364–70. doi: 10.3171/2017.5.PEDS1782
64. Mullin JP, Shriver M, Alomar S, Najm I, Bulacio J, Chauvel P, et al. Is SEEG safe? A systematic review and meta-analysis of stereo-electroencephalography-related complications. *Epilepsia.* (2016) 57:386–401. doi: 10.1111/epi.13298
65. Li K, Vakharia VN, Sparks R, Rodionov R, Vos SB, McEvoy AW, et al. Stereoelectroencephalography electrode placement: detection of blood vessel conflicts. *Epilepsia.* (2019) 60:1942-8. doi: 10.1111/epi.16294
66. Barros G, Lang MJ, Mouchtouris N, Sharan AD, Wu C. Impact of trajectory planning with susceptibility-weighted imaging for intracranial electrode implantation. *Opera Neurosurg.* (2018) 15:60-5. doi: 10.1093/ons/opx215
67. Feng AY, Ho AL, Kim LH, Sussman ES, Pendharkar AV, Iv M, et al. Utilization of novel high-resolution, MRI-based vascular imaging modality for preoperative stereoelectroencephalography planning in children: a technical note. *Stereot Funct Neurosurg.* (2020) 98:1-7. doi: 10.1159/0005 03693
68. Barba C, Rheims S, Minotti L, Guénot M, Hoffmann D, Chabardès S, et al. Temporal plus epilepsy is a major determinant of temporal lobe surgery failures. *Brain.* (2016) 139:444–51. doi: 10.1093/brain/awv372
69. Hale AT, Sen S, Haider AS, Perkins FF, Clarke DF, Lee MR, et al. Open resection versus laser interstitial thermal therapy for the treatment of pediatric insular epilepsy. *Neurosurgery.* (2019) 85:E730-6. doi: 10.1093/neuros/nyz094
70. Guénot M, Isnard J, Ryvlin P, Fischer C, Mauguière F, Sindou M. SEEG-guided RF thermocoagulation of epileptic foci: feasibility, safety, and preliminary results. *Epilepsia.* (2004) 45:1368-74. doi: 10.1111/j.0013-9580.2004.17704.x
71. Dimova P, de Palma L, Job-Chapron A-S, Minotti L, Hoffmann D, Kahane P. Radiofrequency thermocoagulation of the seizure-onset zone during stereoelectroencephalography. *Epilepsia.* (2017) 3:381-92. doi: 10.1111/epi.13663
72. Mullatti N, Landre E, Mellerio C, Oliveira AJ, Laurent A, Turak B, et al. Stereotactic thermocoagulation for insular epilepsy: lessons from successes and failures. *Epilepsia.* (2019) 60:1565–79. doi: 10.1111/epi.16092
73. Isnard J, Taussig D, Bartolomei F, Bourdillon P, Catenoix H, Chassoux F, et al. French guidelines on stereoelectroencephalography (SEEG). *Neurophysiol Clin.* (2018) 48:5–13. doi: 10.1016/j.neucli.2017.11.005
74. Bourdillon P, Isnard J, Catenoix H, Montavont A, Rheims S, Ryvlin P, et al. Stereo electroencephalography–guided radiofrequency thermocoagulation (SEEG-guided RF-TC) in drug-resistant focal epilepsy: results from a 10-year experience. *Epilepsia.* (2017) 58:85–93. doi: 10.1111/epi.13616
75. Vakharia VN, Sparks R, Miserocchi A, Vos SB, O'Keeffe A, Rodionov R, et al. Computer-assisted planning for stereoelectroencephalography (SEEG). *Neurotherapeutics.* (2019) 16:1183–97. doi: 10.1007/s13311-019-00774-9
76. Zeng B, Meng F, Ding H, Wang G. A surgical robot with augmented reality visualization for stereoelectroencephalography electrode implantation. *Int J Comp Assist Radiol Surg.* (2017) 12:1355-68. doi: 10.1007/s11548-017-1634-1

14

Analysis of Interictal Epileptiform Discharges in Mesial Temporal Lobe Epilepsy Using Quantitative EEG and Neuroimaging

Elaine Keiko Fujisao, Karen Fernanda Alves, Thais O. P. Rezende and Luiz Eduardo Betting*

Departamento de Neurologia, Psiquiatria e Psicologia, Faculdade de Medicina de Botucatu, UNESP - Universidade Estadual Paulista, Botucatu, Brazil

***Correspondence:**
Elaine Keiko Fujisao
elaine.keiko@gmail.com

Objective: Investigate areas of correlation between gray matter volumes by MRI and interictal EEG source maps in subtypes of mesial temporal lobe epilepsy (MTLE).

Method: 71 patients and 36 controls underwent 3T MRI and and routine EEG was performed. Voxel-based morphometry (VBM) was used for gray matter analysis and analysis of interictal discharge sources for quantitative EEG. Voxel-wise correlation analysis was conducted between the gray matter and EEG source maps in MTLE subtypes.

Results: The claustrum was the main structure involved in the individual source analysis. Twelve patients had bilateral HA, VBM showed bilateral hippocampal. Twenty-one patients had right HA, VBM showed right hippocampal and thalamic atrophy and negatively correlated involving the right inferior frontal gyrus and insula. Twenty-two patients had left HA, VBM showed left hippocampal atrophy and negatively correlated involving the left temporal lobe and insula. Sixteen patients had MTLE without HA, VBM showed middle cingulate gyrus atrophy and were negatively correlated involving extra-temporal regions, the main one located in postcentral gyrus.

Conclusions: Negative correlations between gray matter volumes and EEG source imaging. Neuroanatomical generators of interictal discharges are heterogeneous and vary according to MTLE subtype.

Significance: These findings suggest different pathophysiological mechanisms among patients with different subtypes of MTLE.

Keywords: mesial temporal lobe epilepsy, magnetic ressonance imaging, eletroencepalogram, hippocampal atrophy, quantitative EEG, quantitative MR analysis

INTRODUCTION

Interictal spikes in the EEG of patients with mesial temporal lobe epilepsy (MTLE) critically contribute to the diagnosis and lateralization of the epileptogenic zone (1, 2). Seizures can originate from one or more anatomical structures of the temporal lobe and spread inward (temporal) or outward (extratemporal) through connected neural networks (3).

Anatomical generators of epileptiform discharges in MTLE have not yet been accurately identified. The maximal negativity of epileptiform activity is in middle and posterior temporal electrodes suggesting a possible onset in the temporal neocortex (4). Intracranial recordings and magnetoencephalograpy (MEG) also support a temporal origin and indicate that conventional noninvasive EEG and MEG cannot identify true mesial temporal spikes (5).

Using quantitative EEG one investigation demonstrated that 62% of MTLE patients had dipole source localization in the epileptogenic temporal lobe (6). Two main types of dipole orientation were described, one with vertical orientation corresponding to inferior or basal temporal spikes and the second with horizontal orientation corresponding to lateral temporal spikes. The second showed widespread cortical thinning when compared to the fisrt one: in the left hemisphere involving cingulate, supramarginal, occipitotemporal an parahippocampal gyri, precuneus and parietal lobule; in the right hemisphere, frontomedial, central and basal gyri and precuneus was envolved. These findings suggest that a large cortical network in this group is affected and showed that the distribution of interictal spikes was associated with widespread cortical thinning beyond the mesiotemporal region (7, 8).

MTLE pathophysiology is not limited to the amygdalo-hippocampal system. Quantitative MRI revealed an extensive network of abnormal neural structure in these patients (9). In-depth investigation showed that in unilateral MTLE the ipsilateral hippocampus is markedly abnormal, and extrahippocampal cortical regions (including the precentral and paracentral gyri) show decreased thickness (10).

The relationship between structural and neurophysiological observations is not completely understood. The objective of the present study was to investigate correlations between gray matter volumes and interictal EEG source maps in subtypes of MTLE. It was hypothesized that this correlation may be present and would change according to subtypes of MTLE. This observation could help to map the epileptogenic circuitry involved in the pathophysiology of MTLE and improve understanding of the mechanisms of interictal epileptiform discharges observed in these patients.

METHODS

Subjects

Seventy-one patients with MTLE (51 women, mean age 46.2 ± 12.6 years) and 36 control subjects (18 women, mean age 32 ± 7 years) with no history of epilepsy or neurological diseases were investigated. Patients were selected at the Outpatient Epilepsy Clinic of the Hospital das Clínicas of Botucatu Medical School. The diagnosis of MTLE was assigned according to clinical and

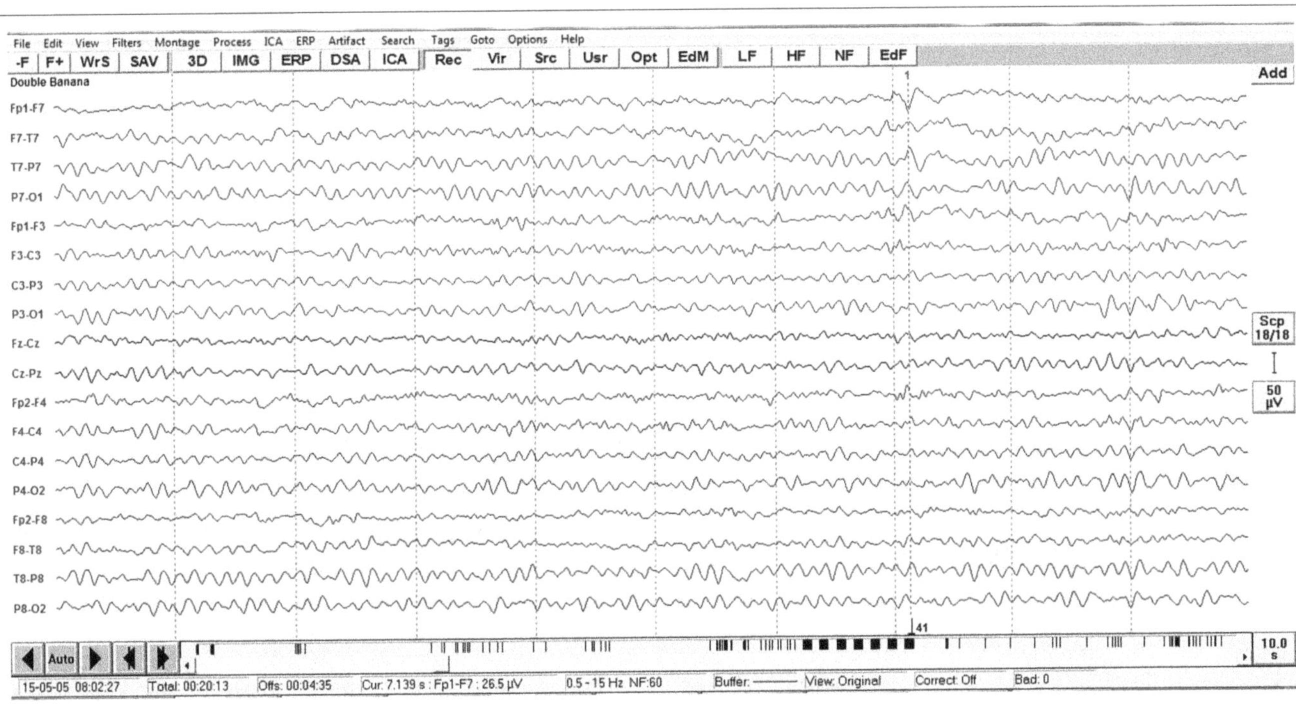

FIGURE 1 | Example of EEG imported to the software BESA with the left temporal epileptiform activity with phase reversal with equipotentiality F7 -T1. For each individual, all epileptiform discharges were manually selected.

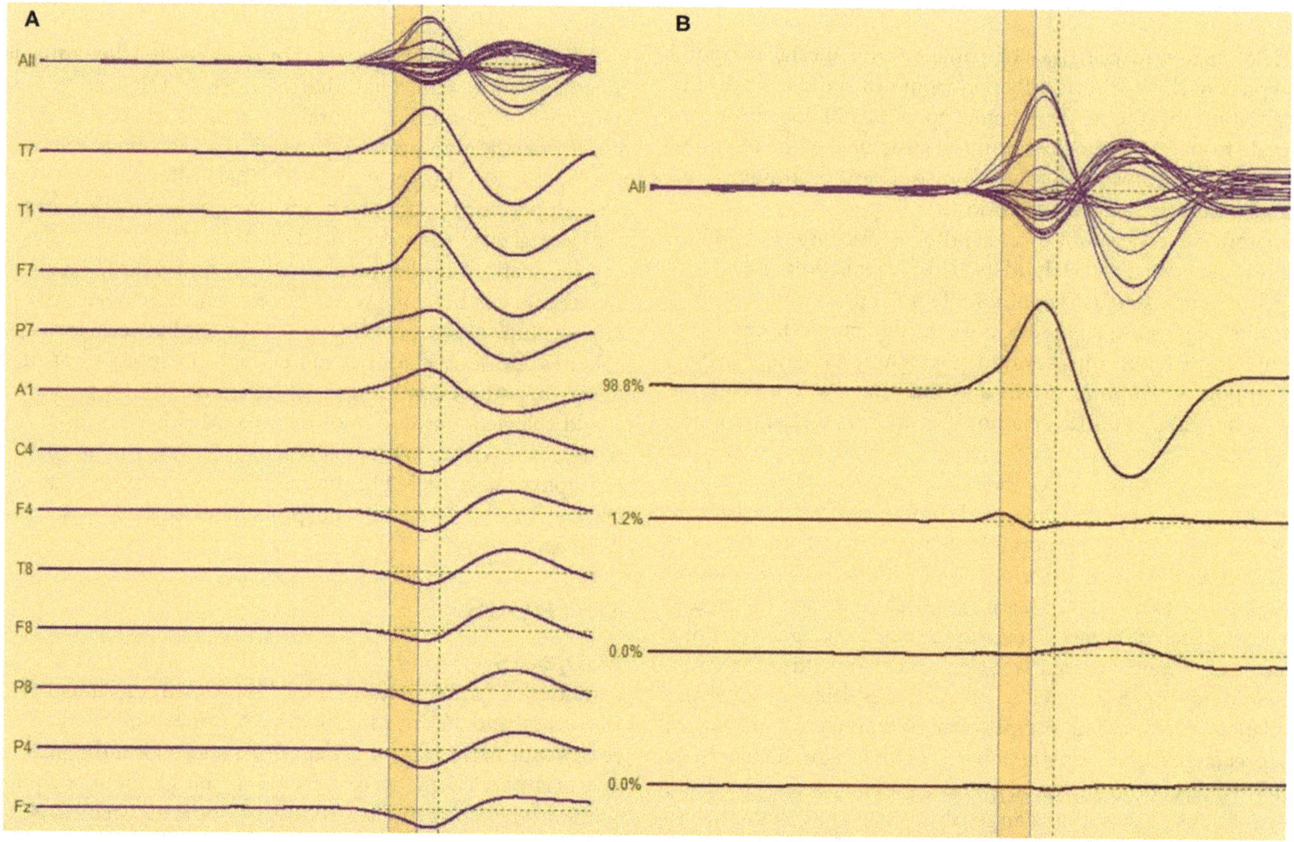

FIGURE 2 | (A,B) Analysis of interictal discharge for each individual all epileptiform discharges were averaged. A 10 ms segment in the ascending portion of the averaged epileptiform activity was then selected.

electroencephalographic criteria (1). All patients had at least one typical EEG with temporal epileptiform discharges. Patients with extra-temporal pathology, double pathology or non-epileptic seizures were excluded. Controls were randomly recruited from the local community. All participants signed an informed consent form approved by the local Ethics Committee.

Electroencephalography Acquisition

Patients were submitted to EEG with a 32-channel Nihon-Kohden (Tokyo, Japan) system. EEG acquisition used the international 10-20 electrode placement system and 1,000 Hz sample rate, with additional Silverman T1 and T2 electrodes. In all 23 electrodes impedance was kept below 10 kΩ and duration of EEG was approximately 20 min including photostimulation and hyperventilation.

Analysis of Interictal Discharges

Analysis of interictal discharge sources was performed using BESA Research 6.0 software (BESA GmbH, Gräfelfing, Germany). EEG was imported to the software and for each individual all epileptiform discharges were manually selected and averaged (**Figure 1**). A 10 ms segment in the ascending portion of the averaged epileptiform activity was then selected, guided by principal component analysis, and was maintained with an average of 97.7% for left discharges and 97.3% for right discharges, which means that the analysis represents the majority of the spikes in both sides (**Figure 2**). For patients with more than one EEG or bilateral discharges the exams were individually analyzed and the discharges were grouped by side and also separately analyzed. Classical LORETA Analysis Recursively Applied (CLARA) algorithm included in the BESA package was used to generate epileptiform discharges source maps using a realistic approximation model for adult patients. Peak locations of the discharges maps were extracted according to Tailarach coordinates (11). Source images were exported as three-dimensional high resolution files (1 mm) in ANALYZE format (**Figure 3**). These images were used to calculate mean and overlap images for the MTLE subgroups (12).

Magnetic Resonance Imaging Acquisition

All subjects underwent MRI. Images were acquired using a 3T scanner (Siemens, Verio, Erlangen, Germany) with a 12-channel head coil. The acquisition protocol included magnetization-prepared rapid gradient-echo (MPRAGE) with 0.5 × 0.5 mm voxels, acquired with 1 mm thickness in the sagittal plane; excitation angle 9°; TR (repeat time) 2,300 ms; TE (excitation time) 2.47 ms; TI (inversion time) 1,100 ms; matrix 256 × 256 and field of view (FOV) 256 mm; Axial FLAIR (Fluid

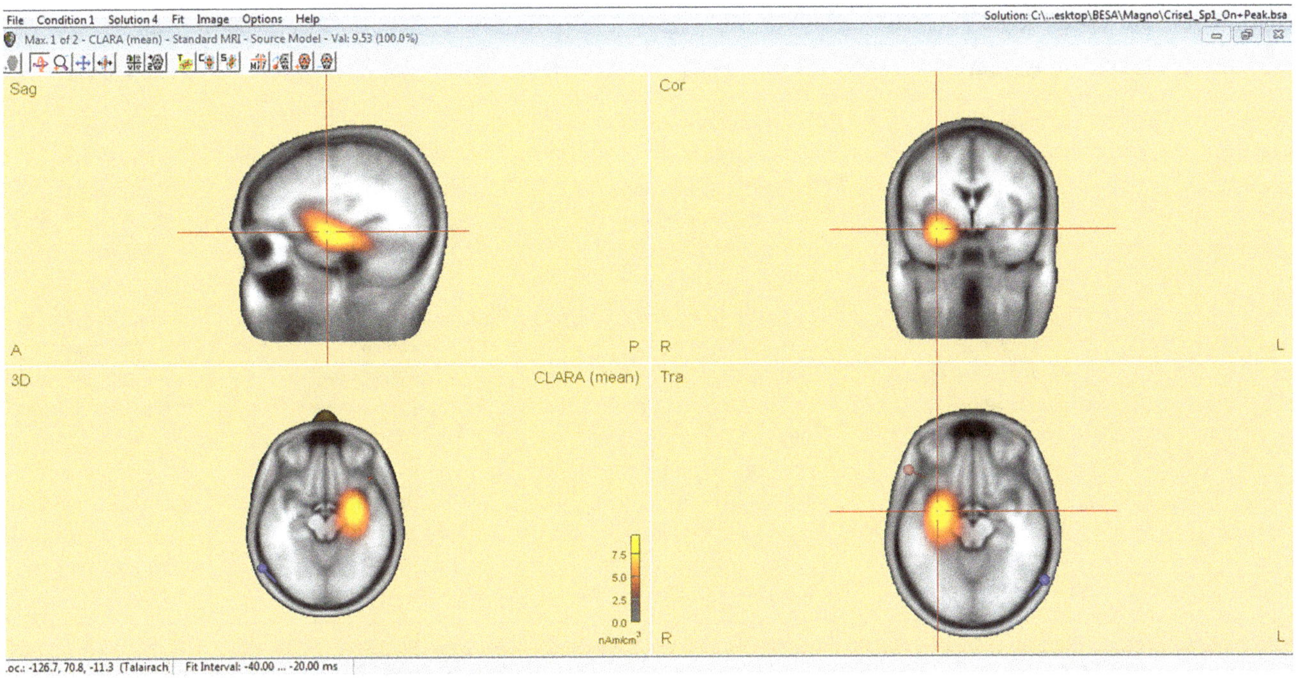

FIGURE 3 | Classical LORETA analysis recursively applied (CLARA) algorithm included in the BESA package used to generate epileptiform discharges source maps from a realistic approximation model for adult patients, according to Tailarach coordinates extracted as three- dimensional high-resolution files (1 mm) in ANALYZE format.

Attenuated Inversion Recovery) 4.0 mm thick; excitation angle 150°; TR 9,000 ms; TE 80 ms; TI 2,500 ms; 208 × 256 matrix and FOV 220 mm; Coronal T2 perpendicular to the long axis of the hippocampus with 2.2 mm of thickness; excitation angle 120°; TR 4,000 ms; TE 135 ms; matrix 230 × 256 and FOV 180 mm; coronal T1 STIR (Short TI Inversion Recovery) perpendicular to the long axis of the hippocampus with 2.2 mm thickness; excitation angle 150°; TR 2,100 ms; TE 9.5 ms; TI 499 ms; matrix 230 × 256 and FOV 180 mm; coronal T2 STIR perpendicular to the long axis of the hippocampus with 2.2 mm of thickness; excitation angle 150°; TR 4,300 ms; TE 74 ms; matrix 128 × 128 and FOV 180 mm. Quantitative structural analysis was performed using the T1 volumetric sequence. Qualitative assessment of hippocampus and evaluation of other cerebral lesions was performed with the remainder sequences.

MRI Quantitative Analysis

Automatic volumetry was conducted using standard routines within FreeSurfer software (version 6.0, https://surfer.nmr.mgh.harvard.edu/) (13, 14). This program automatically normalizes intensity, corrects for movement artifacts, removes extra-cerebral tissues, registers the images into Talairach space, and segments subcortical structures including hippocampus (15). For each subject, hippocampal volume was normalized to total intracranial volume (16). Across groups, hippocampal volumes were normalized to those of controls (yielding a z score). Asymmetry index was calculated as 2 × (right hippocampal volume – left hippocampal volume) / (right hippocampal volume + left hippocampal volume). HA was defined as when the standardized volumes were at least 2 standard deviations (SDs) less than the mean, or when the asymmetry index was at least 2 SDs from the mean in either direction.

Based on the volumetry findings, patients were divided into four groups: bilateral HA (BHA), right HA (RHA), left HA (LHA) and without HA (normal). Voxel-based morphometry (VBM) was performed using the SPM12 program (http://www.fil.ion.ucl.ac.uk) running on MATLAB® R2012b platform. This program performs a unified segmentation (17). Initially the gray matter of all subjects was automatically segmented. Then, using the Diffeomorphic Anatomical Registration Through Exponentiated Lie Algebra (DARTEL) algorithm, a template was created based on all individuals included in the study. This template was registered into standard ICBM-152 (International Consortium for Brain Mapping) space. The final step was to register the segmented images with the template. Structural images were also modulated with the objective of preserving gray matter and minimizing distortions due to normalization. A Gaussian filter (8 mm Full Width at Half Maximum) was applied to all segmented images and EEG maps in order to reduce variation and normally distribute the intensity of the voxels.

Correlation and Statistical Analysis

Voxel wise comparisons were made by full factorial design, looking for areas of increased or decreased gray matter. The four

TABLE 1 | Clinical, electroencephalographic, and neuroimaging features of the four groups of patients with mesial temporal lobe epilepsy (bilateral, right and left hippocampal atrophy, and without hippocampal atrophy).

	Bilateral	Right	Left	Normal
n (%)	12 (16.9%)	21 (29.6%)	22 (30.9%)	16 (22.6%)
Refractory (%)	11 (91.7%)	20 (95.2%)	21 (95.4%)	11 (68.75%)
First seizure	10.3 ± 9.6 (1–24)	12.0 ± 10.2 (1–39)	19.2 ± 16.5 (1–55)	31.4 ± 16.5 (10–75)
Duration	31.0 ± 13.8 (10–55)	34.1 ± 15.8 (10–60)	32.6 ± 16.7 (4–55)	17.3 ± 15.5 (1–48)
Frequency	4.25 ± 5.8 (0–20)	10.9 ± 20.2 (0–90)	7.7 ± 10.0 (0–36)	3.1 ± 5.6 (0–20)
AEDs	1.9 ± 0.5 (1–3)	2.1 ± 0.6 (1–3)	2.4 ± 1 (1–5)	1.2 ± 0.4 (1–2)
Age	41.2 ± 14.6 (18–61)	45.0 ± 12.0 (20–60)	46.3 ± 10.9 (30–61)	51.2 ± 13.3 (31–80)
Gender	8 women	15 women	15 women	12 women
Vol RH	2522 ± 421 (1949–3504)	2603 ± 379 (1888–3526)	3510 ± 338 (3000–4260)	3508 ± 522 (2671–4245)
z RH	−4.2 ± 1.4 (−6.9 to−2.2)	−3.8 ± 1.6 (−6.9–0.7)	1.3 ± 2.3 (−1.4–7.1)	0.8 ± 1.8 (−1.5–4.3)
Vol LH	2248.3 ± 555.7 (1828 – 3674)	3506.3 ± 181.7 (3108 – 3868)	2584.6 ± 346.2 (1961 – 3409)	3408.5 ± 467.0 (2767 – 4039)
z LH	−5.6 ± 1.9 (−8.0 to −2.0)	1.0 ± 1.4 (−1.5–4.1)	−3.5 ± 1.9 (−7.3 to −0.5)	0.7 ± 1.9 (−1.6–4.1)
z AIS	3.1 ± 3.9 (−2.0–10.3)	−9.5 ± 4.04 (−19.5 to −2.1)	8.4 ± 3.7 (1.9–15.5)	0.2 ± 0.9 (−1.6–1.6)
EEG/patient	1 ± 0 (1–1)	1.2 ± 0.4 (1–2)	1.4 ± 0.7 (1–4)	1.2 ± 0.5 (1–3)
Discharges	11.3 ± 13.4 (1–37)	36.7 ± 55.8 (5–234)	4.2 ± 3 (2–7)	12.3 ± 19 (1–55)
Right Left	37.7 ± 54.7 (2–155)	6.6 ± 18.4 (2–70)	44.9 ± 80.6 (1–359)	7.4 ± 4.8 (1–16)

n, number of subjects in group; Refractory (%): patients remaining with at least one monthly seizure despite appropriate use of antiepileptic medications; First seizure, age of first seizure in years; Duration, time of epilepsy since the first recurrent seizure; Frequency, estimated number of monthly seizure; AEDs, number of antiepileptic medications currently in use by the patients; Age, in years; Vol RH, right (non-normalized) hippocampal volume in cubic millimeters; z RH - z, right hippocampus score; Vol LH, left hippocampal volume (non-normalized) in cubic millimeters; z RH – z, left hippocampus score; z AIS, z - asymmetry index score; EEG/patient, number of EEGs analyzed per patient; Discharges, number of epileptiform discharges analyzed by patients. Data demonstrated in the mean ± standard deviation (minimum value - maximum value).

patient groups were compared to controls. A p value < 0.05, corrected for multiple comparisons (Bonferroni correction), was the threshold for statistical significance. Age, sex, and total intracranial volume were introduced as covariates.

For the four groups, voxel by voxel correlation analysis was also performed between the interictal discharge source maps and gray matter volume maps using SPM5 and BPM program (18). Regions of interest analysis were also performed for VBM and for correlation analysis, using the same parameters. Three analyzes were performed, the first global analysis, the second involving the temporal lobes and the third including only the hippocampi. The regions were selected according to the AAL (Automatic Anatomic Labeling) atlas (19–21).

RESULTS

Clinical Features

Of the 71 MTLE patients studied, average age of seizure onset was 18.4 ± 15.7 years and frequency of seizures was 7.1 ± 13 seizures per month. Twelve patients had bilateral HA (8 females, 41.1 ± 14.6 years) with standardized mean volumes of −5.6 ± 1.9 SDs and −4.2 ± 1.4 for the left and right hippocampus, respectively. Twenty-one patients had right HA (15 women, mean age 45 ± 12 years) with mean hippocampal volumes of 1.0 ± 1.4 SDs (left) and −3.8 ± 1.6 (right). Twenty-two patients had left HA (15 women, mean age 46.3 ± 10.9 years), mean normalized volumes were −3.5 ± 1.9 SDs for the left and 1.3 ± 2.3 for the right hippocampus. Sixteen patients had normal MRI without HA (12 females, 51.2 ± 13.3 years), and standardized mean hippocampal volumes of 0.7 ± 1.9 SDs and 0.8 ± 1.8 for the left and right hippocampus, respectively. Additional characteristics can be found in **Table 1** and **Appendix**.

Electroencephalographic Features

Eighty-six EEGs were investigated. Eleven patients had two records, one patient had three records, and one patient four records (mean of 1.2 ± 0.5 records per patient). Thirty patients had right discharges only, 33 had left discharges only, and 8 had bilateral discharges. In total, 2,366 epileptiform discharges were observed, 1,367 left (33 ± 62 discharges per patient, range 1–359) and 959 right (25 ± 44 discharges per patient, range 1–234).

In BHA group, 264 discharges on left (37.7 ± 54.7 discharges, range 2–155) and 79 discharges on right (11.3 ± 13.4 discharges, range 1–37) were analyzed. In RHA group, 139 discharges on left (6.6 ± 18.4 discharges, range 2–70) and 771 discharges on right were analyzed (36.7 ± 55.8 discharges, range 5–234). In LHA group, 897 discharges were analyzed on left (44.9 ± 80.6 discharges, 1–359) and 21 on right (4.2 ± 3 discharges, 2–7). In normal group, 67 discharges on left (7.4 ± 4.8 discharges, 1–16) and 88 discharges on right (12.3 ± 19 discharges, 1–55) were analyzed.

Source analysis of the discharges showed 95 foci distributed over 16 areas. The main areas were claustrum (22%), inferior frontal region (16%), insula (12%) and superior temporal gyrus (12%). For BHA patients, the three main locations were claustrum (23%), inferior frontal gyrus (23%), and lentiform nucleus (15%). For RHA patients the three main locations were claustrum (20%), insula (20%), and inferior frontal gyrus (16%).

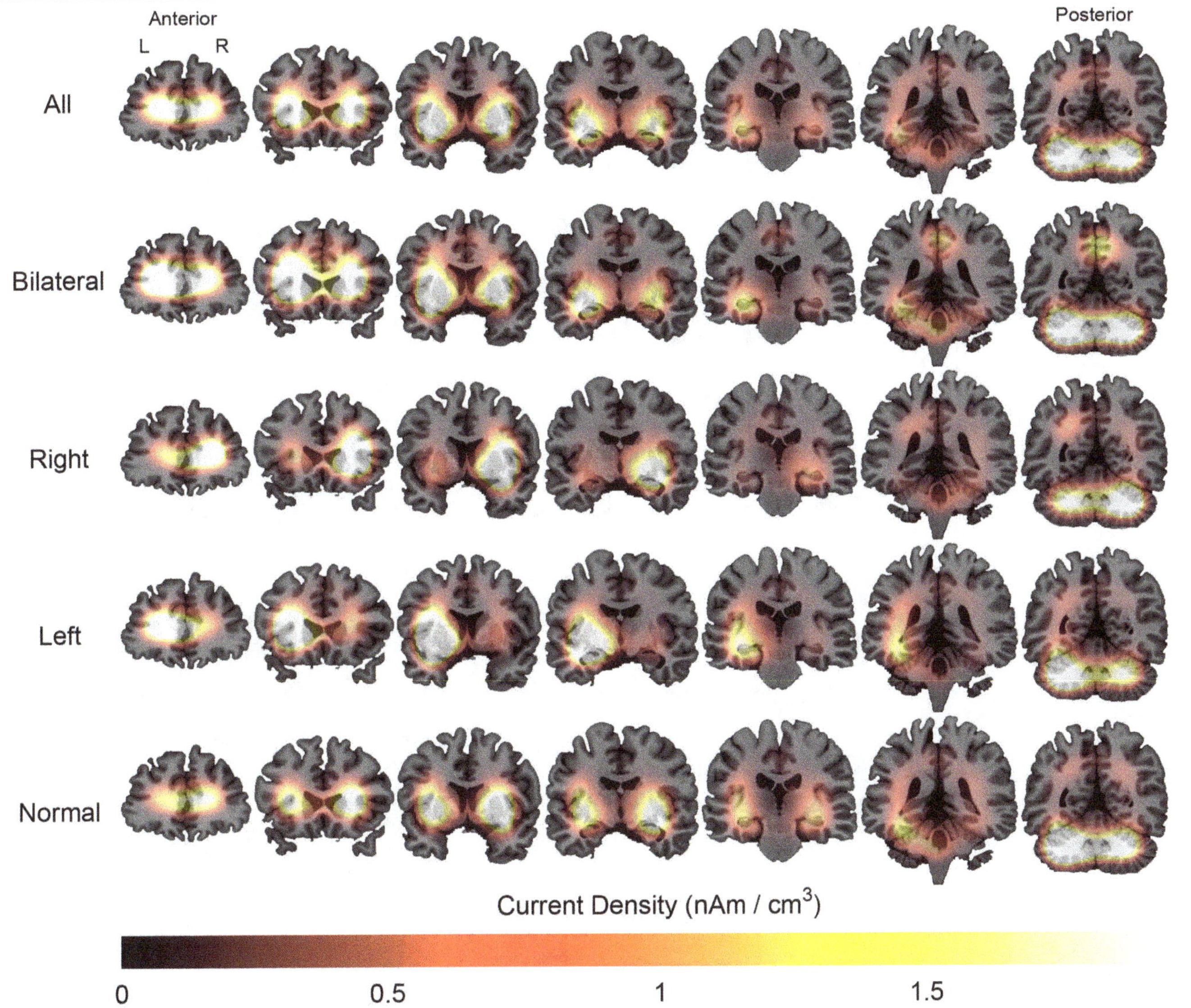

FIGURE 4 | Average maps of the localization of interictal epileptiform discharges of patients with mesial temporal lobe epilepsy. The figure is color-coded according to the current density and overlaid on an MRI model (coronal section). The orientation is in neurological convention (right on right). The slices on left are anteriorly located than those to right.

For LHA patients the three main locations were claustrum (19%), superior temporal gyrus (19%), and inferior frontal gyrus (15%). For the normal group, the three main locations were claustrum (33%), lentiform nucleus (22%), and parahipocampal gyrus, lentiform gyrus, and precentral gyrus (11% each). Maps of discharges can be observed in **Figure 4** (average) and **Figure 5** (overlap of all patients).

Table 1 summarizes the clinical and electroencephalographic features, **Table 2** shows the source location for all patients and **Supplementary Tables** shows the source location for the subgroups.

Voxel-Based Morphometry Analysis

The BHA group, as compared to controls, showed atrophy in seven main regions (totaling 166,853 mm^3), the most significant region being right hippocampus. For the RHA group, only one cluster was significantly atrophied (hippocampus; 6,819 mm^3). Two clusters of atrophy were observed in the LHA group, the most significant being left hippocampus (total 5,863 mm^3). In the normal group, six clusters were atrophied, the main one located in middle cingulate gyrus (totaling 6,5076 mm^3). All clusters are listed in **Table 3**.

No areas of increased gray matter volumes were observed.

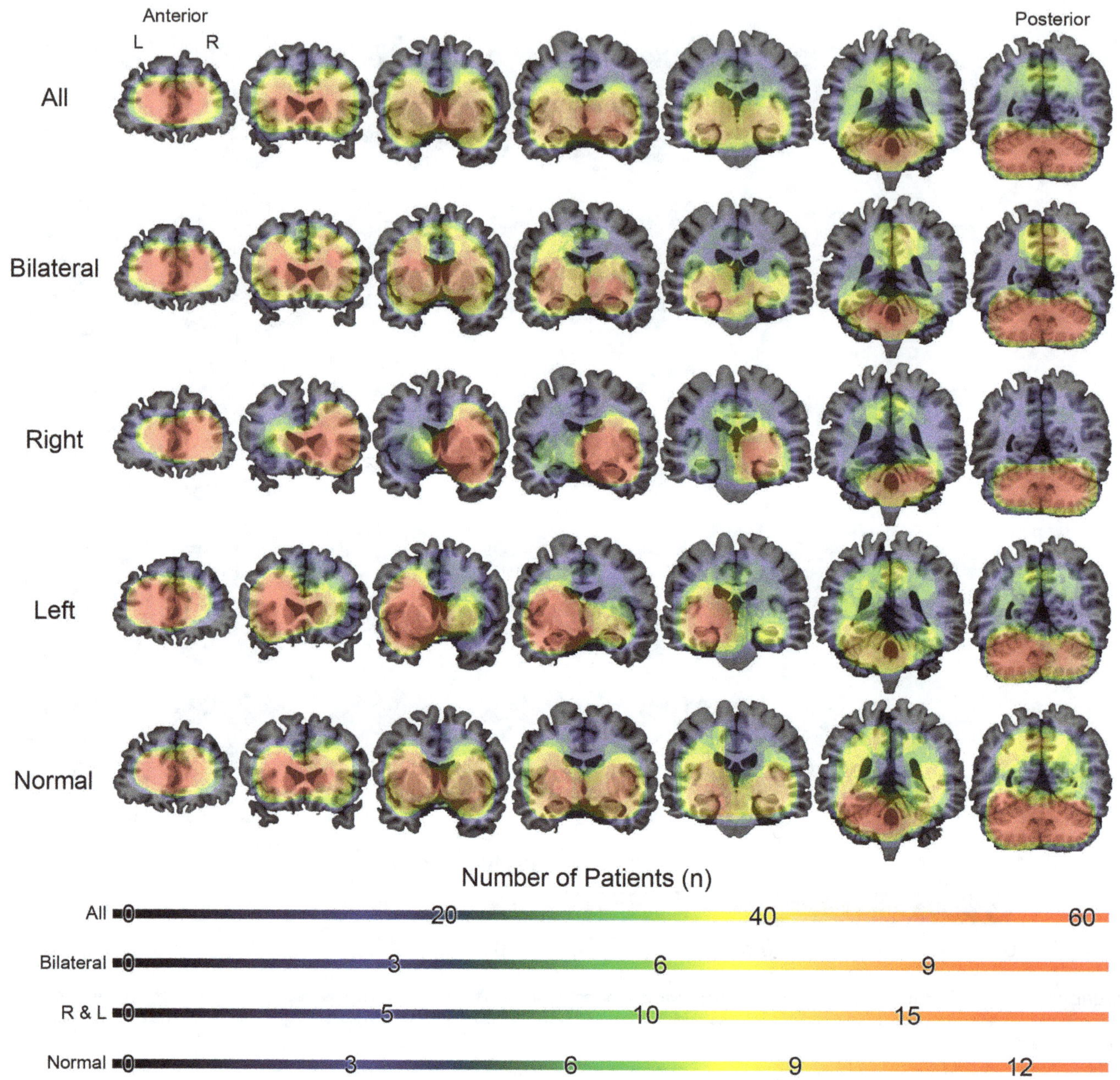

FIGURE 5 | Overlap maps of the localization of interictal epileptiform discharges of patients with mesial temporal lobe epilepsy. The figure is color-coded according to the number of individuals and overlaid on a magnetic resonance model (coronal section). The figure is in the neurological orientation (right on right). The slices on left are anteriorly located than those to right.

Correlation Analysis

Correlations were drawn between source maps of interictal epileptiform discharges and gray matter maps. For the BHA group, a strong negative correlation was observed in right insula ($r = -0.87$, $p < 0.0001$). In RHA group, the right inferior frontal gyrus was significant ($r = 0.70$, $p = 0.020$). In the LHA group, left hippocampus was negatively correlated ($r = -0.56$, $p = 0.001$). For the normal group two clusters of correlated regions were observed, the main one located in postcentral gyrus ($r = -0.86$, $p < 0.0001$). No areas of positive correlations were observed. Detailed results of these analyses can be seen in **Table 3** and **Figure 6**.

DISCUSSION

Using quantitative EEG source imaging the present study demonstrated that at an individual level, interictal epileptiform discharges involved the claustrum of patients with MTLE. This behavior occurred in all subgroups (BHA, RHA, LHA, and normal). Voxel wise structural analysis revealed a different pattern of gray matter atrophy for each subgroup. Correlation analysis between gray matter and interictal spike source imaging revealed that there was not a perfect overlap between major structural abnormalities and source distribution.

The claustrum is a thin, irregular neural structure located on the inner surface of the insula with connections to nearly all cortical regions, and its function is thought to include synchronization of disparate perceptual, cognitive, and motor modalities (22). Bilateral abnormalities in the claustrum were associated with refractory status epilepticus, focal motor seizures, and myoclonic seizures (23). Physiological properties of the claustrum may help to explain the propagation and synchronization of abnormal epileptic activity from various cortical regions, since claustro-cortical fibers connect the claustrum with several cortical areas including the prefrontal cortex, pre- and postcentral gyri, and orbitofrontal and medial temporal cortices (24).

The claustrum is composed of GABA-ergic interneurons, damage to which could promote a state of hypersynchronization in connections with distant cortical regions. The frontal piriform cortex was found in the evaluation of IED in patients with focal epilepsy in one study. Because of their location close to the claustrum, they may be responsible for the origin and spread of epileptiform activity (25).

Several theories have been proposed to explain the impairment of consciousness that occurs during focal seizures: reduction of cerebral blood flow to areas responsible for consciousness in response to hyperflow in temporal regions; bilateral activation of hippocampus after unilateral seizure and, more recently, a loss of activity of the default mode network with bilateral deactivation of posterior cingulate (26). The involvement of insular cortex and claustrum could be related to impairment of consciousness and the frequent involvement of orofacial musculature in focal seizures (23).

Other regions identified as sources for interictal epileptiform discharges were inferior frontal region, insula, and superior temporal gyrus. Interictal spikes may be related to cognitive decline, as observed in experimental models (27). A more widespread distribution of epileptogenic discharges as observed in some patients may influence cognition via frontal and temporal lobes and limbic system that are especially involved in cognition.

One investigation of 22 patients with HA and 12 patients without HA used equivalent dipole source localization to analyze interictal epileptiform discharges obtained during pre-surgical video-EEG monitoring. This investigation showed no differences between patients with or without HA suggesting the same etiology for these discharges (6). Using similar source analysis methodology to that used here, a study with 15 patients applied the low-resolution electromagnetic tomography (LORETA) algorithm and observed that this technique can aid in detection of discharge propagation (28).

TABLE 2 | Results of the source localization using the CLARA algorithm for all patients with mesial temporal lobe epilepsy.

Anatomy	Right	Left	Total
Claustrum	11	10	21
Inferior frontal	8	7	15
Insula	6	6	12
Superior temporal	5	7	12
Parahhipocampal	5	3	8
Lentiform	5	2	7
Cingulate	2	3	5
Culmen	1	2	3
Caudate	0	3	3
Middle frontal	1	1	2
Precentral	0	2	2
Middle temporal	0	1	1
Inferior temporal	0	1	1
Sub-lobar	0	1	1
Thalamus	1	0	1
White matter	1	0	1

Therefore, precise determination of the epileptogenic zone is vital for surgical planning, and the possibility of noninvasive tests being used in the preoperative routine may benefit these patients. Coito et al. (29) evaluated IED routine EEG with electrical source analysis in 34 patients (20 temporal lobe epilepsy and 14 extra temporal epilepsy) before and after surgery. The efficiency were concordant with the presumed epileptic zone in 76% of the patients, showing the importance of these findings.

Regarding the morphometric evaluation, patients with BHA presented diffuse atrophy with a centrifugal pattern compared to the other groups. In the groups with unilateral HA, the evaluation by VBM demonstrated ipsilateral atrophy, as expected. When comparisons were made, we observed that the group with right HA exhibits changes related to the right lower frontal gyrus, lower right temporal and left hippocampus in the three analyzes, respectively. Such changes could be related to anterior, mesial and contralateral spread of epileptiform discharges in the group with HA on the right. On the other hand, in the group with left HA the correlation changes were restricted to the mesial structures on the left, in the three analyzes: left parahipocampal gyrus, left upper temporal gyrus and left hippocampus. Thus, the more limited pattern of correlation on the left indicates a higher current density with a greater degree of atrophy in these structures. Thus, a different neuroanatomical involvement was discovered in patients with left or right epileptiform discharges.

Moreover, for groups with lateralized HA, VBM revealed that patients with LHA had more anterior hippocampal involvement and patients with RHA had a more posterior involvement. A previous investigation described similar findings (30). Abnormalities outside the mesial temporal lobe were also observed. Patients in LHA group presented a slightly

TABLE 3 | Results of voxel-based morphometry (VBM) and correlation analysis between gray matter volumes and interictal discharges source maps (EEG) for patients with mesial temporal lobe epilepsy (bilateral, right and left hippocampal atrophy, and without hippocampal atrophy) with normal controls.

Group	Method	p (FWE)/r	Size (mm)	T or Z	Coordinates	Anatomy
Bilateral	VBM	0	67,203	8.57	30 −16 −18	Hippocampus
	VBM	0	7,298	5.31	52 −25 8	Superior temporal
	VBM	0	6,9073	5.22	7 −12 42	Middle cingulate
	VBM	0.015	3,518	4.86	34 −78 39	Middle occipital
	VBM	0.011	3,783	4.57	36 46 31	Middle frontal
	VBM	0.041	2,675	4.42	25 48 −13	Anterior orbital
	VBM	0.000	13,303	4.34	−23 −70 −24	Cerebellum
	EEG	0.000/−0.87	4,932	3.49	29 1 8	Putamen/insula
Right	VBM	0.001	6,819	5.37	26 −32 −2	Hippocampus
	EEG	0.020/−0.70	1,038	3.46	32 33 8	Inferior frontal/insula
Left	VBM	0.035	2,810	4.95	−29 −15 −20	Hippocampus
	VBM	0.026	3,053	4.31	−17 14 −3	Putamen
	EEG	0.001/−0.56	1,717	2.64	−28 −5 −19	Hippocampus/insula
Normal	VBM	0	7,302	5.46	−2 −24 31	Middle cingulate
	VBM	0	10,153	5.36	44 −21 10	Superior temporal
	VBM	0	32,290	5.29	−23 12 −12	Anterior insula
	VBM	0.022	3,208	4.68	−9 −94 19	Occipital pole
	VBM	0	8,153	4.63	−4 −10 16	Thalamus
	VBM	0.009	3,970	4.34	−34 8 −36	Temporal pole
	EEG	0.000/−0.86	4,335	3.98	53 −21 56	Pre/postcentral
	EEG	0.000/−0.78	5,335	3.31	18 61 6	Superior and medial frontal

more diffuse pattern involving bilateral basal ganglia and thalamus. The literature related to MTLE laterality and atrophy is controversial. One investigation found more structural abnormalities in patients with right MTLE, especially in ipsilateral insula and contralateral thalamus (31). Another study observed a higher degree of cerebral atrophy, longer duration of disease, and worse control of seizures in patients with left HA (32).

Patients without HA showed widespread area of atrophy involving the amygdala, cingulate, temporal, and frontal cortex. This observation is in line with other studies suggesting that MRI-negative temporal lobe epilepsy is a different condition involving separate networks (33).

Negative correlations were observed between gray matter volumes and source maps; i.e., increased current densities were associated with reduced gray matter. For unilateral MTLE, differential network involvement was found in patients with left (hippocampal region and insula) or right (inferior frontal gyrus) HA. Once again these findings align with connectivity studies to point to distinct patterns for right or left HA (34). These results show how a focal pathology can influence diffuse neural networks differently depending on the affected hemisphere. Patients with bilateral HA had areas of correlation localized to the basal ganglia, insula, and mesial frontal regions. Finally, patients without any hippocampal atrophy had an extensive area of extra-temporal correlations. This suggests that the irritative zone does not always contain the epileptogenic zone. It also indicates that neuroanatomical generators and pathways of interictal discharges are heterogeneous and vary according to MTLE subtype.

Scalp EEG has a very precise temporal resolution, but limited spatial resolution for source analysis. The number of electrodes in this study was modest; currently, there are EEG studies with a greater number of electrodes and channels, and thus greater accuracy of source detection (35). However, the methodology used here is very similar to that of daily clinical practice and should be relatively easy to implement in clinical settings in the future.

Associated anatomopathological studies may help to confirm diagnosis and elucidate the relationship between HA and epileptogenic networks in MTLE (36). Future investigations using dense array EEG, with a higher number of subjects and prospectively evaluating these patients after surgical procedure should be performed in order to confirm these findings.

CONCLUSIONS

At the individual level, interictal epileptiform discharges localized mainly to the claustrum of patients with MTLE. Quantitative analysis of MRI showed a heterogeneous and distinct pattern for MTLE subtypes. Finally, correlation analysis between quantitative EEG and structural MRI failed to demonstrate overlap with the epileptogenic zone but illustrated different networks involved in each MTLE subgroup. The

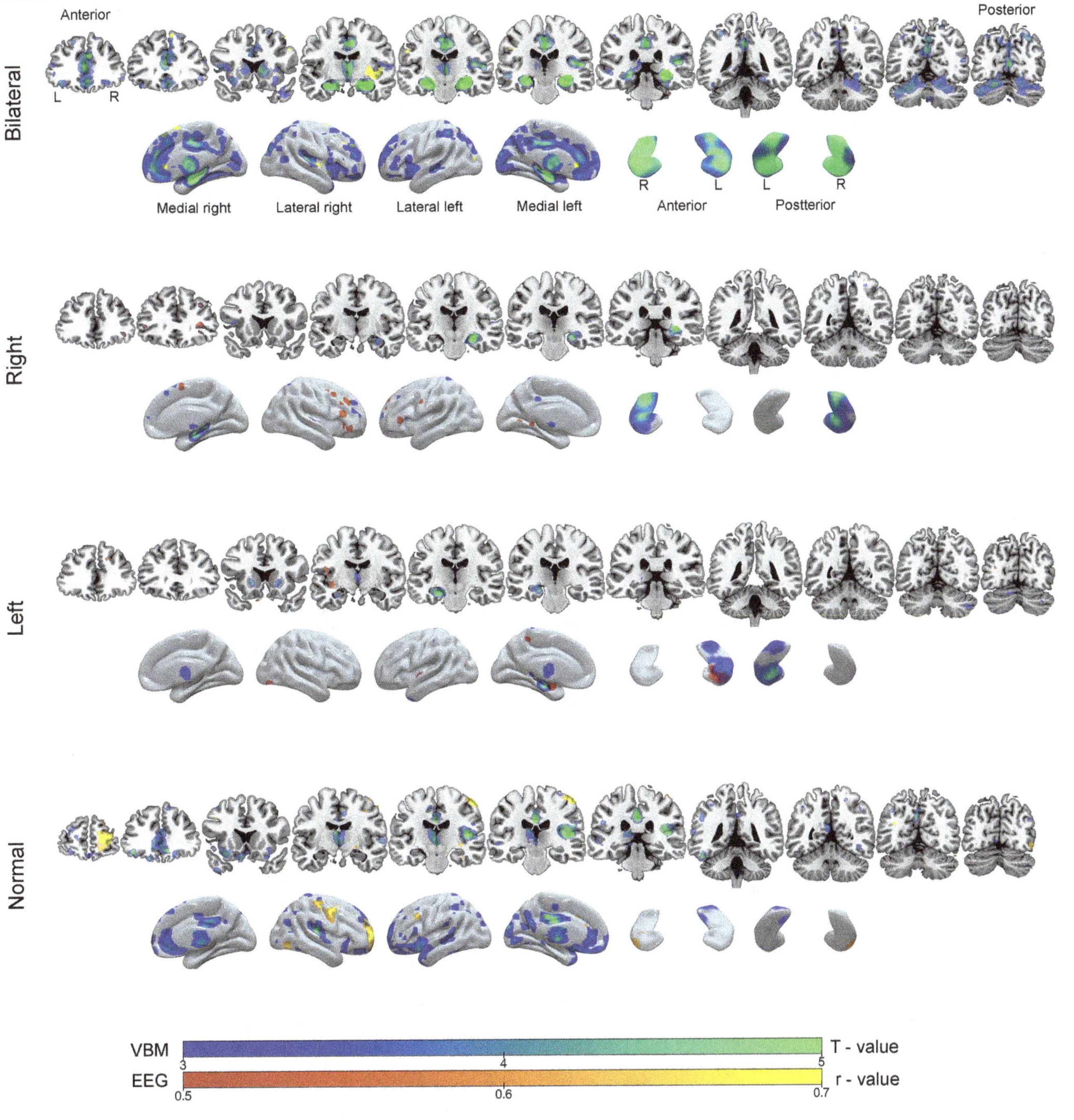

FIGURE 6 | Results of the voxel-based morphometry (VBM, blue-green color scale) and correlation analysis between EEG source images and gray matter maps (red-yellow color scale) according to groups of mesial temporal lobe epilepsy. The results are overlaid on coronal MRI model slices in neurological orientation (right to right) and in three-dimensional models of the brain and hippocampus. The color scale in the figure indicates the results of statistical analysis for VBM (T - value) and correction analysis between EEG and gray matter (r - value, negative correlations).

observations of the present investigation suggest different pathophysiological mechanisms for interictal epileptiform discharges even among patients with unilateral HA. These findings may contribute to a better understanding of the MTLE pathophysiology, the extent of abnormalities and, in the future, to a more individualized approach for surgical therapy.

AUTHOR CONTRIBUTIONS

EF took the lead in writing the manuscript. All authors provided critical feedback and helped shape the research, analysis and manuscript. EF and LB designed the model and the computational framework and analyzed the data.

REFERENCES

1. Scheffer IE, Berkovic S, Capovilla G, Connolly MB, French J, Guilhoto L, et al. ILAE classification of the epilepsies: position paper of the ILAE Commission for Classification and Terminology. *Epilepsia.* (2017) 58:512–21. doi: 10.1111/epi.13709
2. Alvim MKM, Morita ME, Yasuda CL, Damasceno BP, Lopes TM, Coan AC, et al. Is inpatient ictal video-electroencephalographic monitoring mandatory in mesial temporal lobe epilepsy with unilateral hippocampal sclerosis? A prospective study. *Epilepsia.* (2018) 59:410–9. doi: 10.1111/epi.13977
3. Kahane P, Bartolomei F. Temporal lobe epilepsy and hippocampal sclerosis: lessons from depth EEG recordings. *Epilepsia.* (2010) 51:59–62. doi: 10.1111/j.1528-1167.2009.02448.x
4. Sadler M, Desbiens R. Scalp EEG in temporal lobe epilepsy surgery. *Can J Neurol Sci.* (2000) 27 (Suppl. 1):S22–8. doi: 10.1017/S0317167100000603
5. Wennberg R, Valiante T, Cheyne D. EEG and MEG in mesial temporal lobe epilepsy: where do the spikes really come from? *Clin Neurophysiol.* (2011) 122:1295–313. doi: 10.1016/j.clinph.2010.11.019
6. Oliva M, Meckes-Ferber S, Roten A, Desmond P, Hicks RJ, O'Brien TJ, et al. EEG dipole source localization of interictal spikes in non-lesional TLE with and without hippocampal sclerosis. *Epilepsy Res.* (2010) 92:183–90. doi: 10.1016/j.eplepsyres.2010.09.006
7. Engel J, Pedley TA. *Epilepsy: A Comprehensive Textbook.* 2nd ed. Philadelphia: Wolters Kluwer/Lippincott Williams & Wilkins (2008).
8. Reinsberger C, Tanaka N, Cole AJ, Lee JW, Dworetzky BA, Bromfield EB, et al. Current dipole orientation and distribution of epileptiform activity correlates with cortical thinning in left mesiotemporal epilepsy. *Neuroimage.* (2010) 52:1238–42. doi: 10.1016/j.neuroimage.2010.04.264
9. Yasuda CL, Betting LE, Cendes F. Voxel-based morphometry and epilepsy. *Expert Rev Neurother.* (2010) 10:975–84. doi: 10.1586/ern.10.63
10. Whelan CD, Altmann A, Botia JA, Jahanshad N, Hibar DP, Absil J, et al. Structural brain abnormalities in the common epilepsies assessed in a worldwide ENIGMA study. *Brain.* (2018) 141:391–408. doi: 10.1093/brain/awx341
11. Talairach J, Tournoux P. Co-Planar Stereotaxic Atlas of the Human Brain: 3-Dimensional Proportional System: An Approach to Cerebral Imaging. Vol. viii, Stuttgart; New York, NY: Thieme Medical Publishers (1988). p. 122.
12. Rorden C, Brett M. Stereotaxic display of brain lesions. *Behav Neurol.* (2000) 12:191–200. doi: 10.1155/2000/421719
13. Dale AM, Fischl B, Sereno MI. Cortical surface-based analysis. I Segmentation and surface reconstruction. *Neuroimage.* (1999) 9:179–94. doi: 10.1006/nimg.1998.0395
14. Fischl B, Sereno MI, Dale AM. Cortical surface-based analysis. II: Inflation, flattening, and a surface-based coordinate system. *Neuroimage.* (1999) 9:195–207. doi: 10.1006/nimg.1998.0396
15. Fischl B, van der Kouwe A, Destrieux C, Halgren E, Ségonne F, Salat DH, et al. Automatically parcellating the human cerebral cortex. *Cereb Cortex.* (2004) 14:11–22. doi: 10.1093/cercor/bhg087
16. Jack CR Jr, Twomey CK, Zinsmeister AR, Sharbrough FW, Petersen RC, Cascino GD. Anterior temporal lobes and hippocampal formations: normative volumetric measurements from MR images in young adults. *Radiology.* (1989) 172:549–54. doi: 10.1148/radiology.172.2.2748838
17. Ashburner J, Friston KJ. Unified segmentation. *Neuroimage.* (2005) 26:839–51. doi: 10.1016/j.neuroimage.2005.02.018
18. Casanova R, Srikanth R, Baer A, Laurienti PJ, Burdette JH, Hayasaka S, et al. Biological parametric mapping: a statistical toolbox for multimodality brain image analysis. *Neuroimage.* (2007) 34:137–43. doi: 10.1016/j.neuroimage.2006.09.011
19. Maldjian JA, Laurienti PJ, Burdette JB, Kraft RA. An automated method for neuroanatomic and cytoarchitectonic atlas-based interrogation of fMRI data sets. *NeuroImage.* (2003) 19:1233–9. doi: 10.1016/S1053-8119(03)00169-1
20. Maldjian JA, Laurienti PJ, Burdette JH. Precentral gyrus discrepancy in electronic versions of the talairach atlas. *Neuroimage.* (2004) 21:450–5. doi: 10.1016/j.neuroimage.2003.09.032
21. Tzourio-Mazoyer N, Landeau B, Papathanassiou D, Crivello F, Etard O, Delcroix N, et al. Automated anatomical labeling of activations in SPM using a macroscopic anatomical parcellation of the MNI MRI single-subject brain. *Neuroimage.* (2002) 15:273–89. doi: 10.1006/nimg.2001.0978
22. Crick FC, Koch C. What is the function of the claustrum? *Philos Trans R Soc Lond B Biol Sci.* (2005) 360:1271–9. doi: 10.1098/rstb.2005.1661
23. Meletti S, Giovannini G, d'Orsi G, Toran L, Monti G, Guha R, et al. New-onset refractory status epilepticus with claustrum damage: definition of the clinical and neuroimaging features. *Front Neurol.* (2017) 8:111. doi: 10.3389/fneur.2017.00111
24. Milardi D, Bramanti P, Milazzo C, Finocchio G, Arrigo A, Santoro G, et al. Cortical and subcortical connections of the human claustrum revealed *in vivo* by constrained spherical deconvolution tractography. *Cereb Cortex.* (2015) 25:406–14. doi: 10.1093/cercor/bht231
25. Laufs H, Richardson MP, Salek-Haddadi A, Vollmar C, Duncan JS, Gale K, et al. Converging PET and fMRI evidence for a common area involved in human focal epilepsies. *Neurology.* (2011) 77:904–10. doi: 10.1212/WNL.0b013e31822c90f2
26. Danielson NB, Guo JN, Blumenfeld H. The default mode network and altered consciousness in epilepsy. *Behav Neurol.* (2011) 24:55–65. doi: 10.1155/2011/912720
27. Kleen JK, Scott RC, Holmes GL, Lenck-Santini PP. Hippocampal interictal spikes disrupt cognition in rats. *Ann Neurol.* (2010) 67:250–7. doi: 10.1002/ana.21896
28. Zumsteg D, Friedman A, Wieser HG, Wennberg RA. Propagation of interictal discharges in temporal lobe epilepsy: correlation of spatiotemporal mapping with intracranial foramen ovale electrode recordings. *Clin Neurophysiol.* (2006) 117:2615–26. doi: 10.1016/j.clinph.2006.07.319
29. Coito A, Biethahn S, Tepperberg J, Carboni M, Roelcke U, Seeck M, et al. Interictal epileptogenic zone localization in patients with focal epilepsy using electric source imaging and directed functional connectivity from low-density EEG. *Epilepsia Open.* (2019) 4:281–92. doi: 10.1002/epi4.12318
30. Keller SS, Mackay CE, Barrick TR, Wieshmann UC, Howars MA, Roberts N. Voxel-based morphometric comparison of hippocampal and extrahippocampal abnormalities in patients with left and right hippocampal atrophy. *Neuroimage.* (2002) 16:23–31. doi: 10.1006/nimg.2001.1072
31. Pail M, Brazdil M, Marecek R, Mikl M. An optimized voxel-based morphometric study of gray matter changes in patients with left-sided and right-sided mesial temporal lobe epilepsy and hippocampal sclerosis (MTLE/HS). *Epilepsia.* (2010) 51:511–8. doi: 10.1111/j.1528-1167.2009.02324.x
32. Coan AC, Appenzeller S, Bonilha L, Li LM, Cendes F. Seizure frequency and lateralization affect progression of atrophy in temporal lobe epilepsy. *Neurology.* (2009) 73:834–42. doi: 10.1212/WNL.0b013e3181b783dd
33. Vaughan DN, Rayner G, Tailby C, Jackson GD. MRI-negative temporal lobe epilepsy: a network disorder of neocortical connectivity. *Neurology.* (2016) 87:1934–42. doi: 10.1212/WNL.0000000000003289
34. Besson P, Dinkelacker V, Valabregue R, Thivard L, Leclerc X, Baulac M, et al. Structural connectivity differences in left and right temporal lobe epilepsy. *Neuroimage.* (2014) 100:135–44. doi: 10.1016/j.neuroimage.2014.04.071
35. Lantz G, Grave de Peralta R, Spinelli L, Seeck M, Michel CM. Epileptic source localization with high density EEG: how many electrodes are needed? *Clin Neurophysiol.* (2003) 114:63–9. doi: 10.1016/S1388-2457(02)00337-1
36. Breedlove J, Nesland T, Vandergrift WA 3rd, Betting LE, Bonilha L. Probabilistic ictal EEG sources and temporal lobe epilepsy surgical outcome. *Acta Neurol Scand.* (2014) 130:103–10. doi: 10.1111/ane.12253

15

Contributions of Robotics to the Safety and Efficacy of Invasive Monitoring with Stereoelectroencephalography

Amir H. Faraji[1,2], *Madison Remick*[2] *and Taylor J. Abel*[2,3*]

[1] *Department of Neurological Surgery, Houston Methodist Hospital, Houston, TX, United States,* [2] *Department of Neurological Surgery, University of Pittsburgh, Pittsburgh, PA, United States,* [3] *Department of Bioengineering, University of Pittsburgh, Pittsburgh, PA, United States*

Correspondence:
Taylor J. Abel
abeltj@upmc.edu

The purpose of this review is to provide a discussion of the history and utility of robotics in invasive monitoring for epilepsy surgery using stereoelectroencephalography (sEEG). The authors conducted a literature review of available sources to describe how the advent of surgical robotics has improved the efficacy and ease of performing sEEG surgery. The sEEG method integrates anatomic, electrographic, and clinical information to test hypotheses regarding the localization of the epileptogenic zone (EZ) and has been used in Europe since the 1950s. One of the primary benefits of robot-assisted sEEG implantation techniques is the ability to seamlessly transition between both orthogonal and oblique trajectory types using a single technique. Based on available information, it is our view that, when applied appropriately, robotic sEEG can have a low rate of complications and many advantages over both non-robotic sEEG implantation and traditional craniotomy-based invasive monitoring methods.

Keywords: robotics, stereoelectroencephalography, frameless technique, epilepsy surgery, neurosurgery

INTRODUCTION

The utilization of surgical robots has improved the precision and accuracy of a given procedure. Robots have predetermined, reproducible, and exact paths that limit error, excursions, and the potential for injury to nearby structures if utilized properly (1). Neurosurgeons recognized the utility of robotic assistance more than 30 years ago with the Minerva CT-guided biopsy (University of Lausanne) and PUMA (Advance Research and Robotics) systems, introduced in 1985 (2–4). These systems demonstrated high rates of malfunction and safety concerns related to a lack of operational safeguards and clinical experience. Additional operative robotic systems were subsequently introduced, including the NeuroMate (Integrated Surgical Systems) in 1987, an MRI-compatible system in 1995, and the Cyberknife system (Accuray Incorporated) in 1998 (5–7). The utilization of surgical robotics has improved the utility and performance of several neurosurgical procedures (3, 5, 8–16).

More recently, operative robotic systems for neurosurgical procedures have been increasingly adopted in the United States following the demonstration of their utility in Europe (17–22). Benabid et al. initially described a computer-driven technique for stereotaxy connected to CT and MR imaging in 1987 (5). Moreover, the neurosurgical center in Grenoble, France has utilized a stereotactic robot since 1989 and a microscope robot since 1995 for various surgical procedures

(23). Their team further expanded the indications for robotic-assisted stereotaxy to include deep brain stimulation (DBS), stereoelectroencephalography (sEEG), and tumor biopsies or resections (17, 24). Finally, the ROSA-Brain system (Medtech, Zimmer Biomet) was released in 2007 and gained FDA approval in 2012 for cranial surgery (12, 25–27). The ROSA system is used typically for sEEG implantation; however, it is increasingly being applied to deep brain stimulation as well. While the ROSA system is widely utilized, there are now several other cranial robotic systems also in use for cranial surgery, including the Neuromate (Renishaw) and Renaissance (Mazor) systems (6, 16, 28–33). It is also noteworthy that much of the robust data on complications and surgical outcomes following robotic-assisted sEEG are performed using the ROSA system, which is again reflective of its widespread use specifically at large-volume epilepsy centers. Furthermore, non-robotic systems such as the FHC microtargeting epilepsy platform, may also play a role in some centers with limited patient volume or where robotic purchases may not be permissible (34, 35). These systems are less bulky and require less initial economic investment, but do not allow for a stereotactic plan which can be simultaneously modified during surgical placement. This review will describe how the advent of surgical robotics has improved the efficacy and ease of performing sEEG surgery. A timeline of important events in the history of robotics in sEEG surgery can be found in **Figure 1**.

ROBOTIC VERSATILITY FOR BOTH OBLIQUE AND ORTHOGONAL SEEG TRAJECTORIES

The epileptogenic zone (EZ) is commonly defined as the region of brain tissue that results in seizure freedom when removed. However, it is further described as the area of cortex which is indispensable for the generation of clinical seizures, taking into account both the anatomical location of the origin of the seizures as well as the associated regions of discharge which give rise to their accompanying clinical symptoms (36, 37). Therefore, it is essential to fully delineate the EZ prior to effective epilepsy surgery (37–39). Epileptologists attempt to identify the EZ via non-invasive methods, such as video electroencephalography (EEG) and advanced imaging studies such as magnetic resonance imaging (MRI) (40). In many instances, however, invasive monitoring is required to adequately understand and characterize the EZ (41, 42). Stereoelectroencephalography (sEEG) is a method of planning and implanting percutaneous intracerebral electrodes based upon a customized patient-specific anatamo-electro-clinical hypothesis (43). In other words, the sEEG method integrates anatomic, electrographic, and clinical information to test hypotheses regarding the localization of the EZ and has been used in Europe since the 1950s (44).

Orthogonal placement of sEEG electrodes is heavily influenced by the Talairach method (45). First described by neurosurgeons Talairach and Szikla in 1967, this method creates a standardized grid for neurosurgical procedures, whereby distances to lesions were proportional to the overall brain size (46). In 1988, a second edition of the Talairach Atlas was coauthored by Tournoux and was based upon a postmortem dissection of a human brain (47). The Talairach coordinate system is defined by making two anchors—the anterior commissure (AC) and posterior commissure (PC)—lie on a straight horizonal line in the midsagittal plane. Originally, this method used pneumoencephalograms to identify these two anatomical anchor points. Bancaud, a neurologist, collaborated with Talairach to develop a collaborative approach to sEEG implantation. Therefore, sEEG allowed not only the recording of deep brain structures but also the possibility of a three-dimensional analysis of seizure spread and distribution as well as its correlation to a patient's clinical characteristics. Orthogonal sEEG implantations are standardized to enable electrographic information to be obtained from both the cortical surface and deep targets.

One of the great advantages of robot-assisted implantation techniques is the ability to seamlessly transition between both orthogonal and oblique trajectory types using a single technique. Previously, neurosurgeons would use a Talairach frame, which provided the capability of rapid implantation of orthogonal sEEG electrodes, but was unable to place oblique electrodes (48). When the Talairach frame was used, a Leksell frame could then be used secondarily if an oblique trajectory was necessary. A recent study by Bourdillon et al., which compared the traditional orthogonal Talairach approach to a frame-based robotic technique, concluded that while both procedures are safe and sufficient, the effective accuracy (96.5 vs. 13.7%; 95% CI, −0.863 to −0.781; $p < 0.001$; $t = -39.92$) and absolute accuracy (1.15 vs. 4.00 mm; 95% CI, 2.597–3.183; $p < 0.001$; $t = 19.73$) was significantly higher in cases utilizing the robotic technique (49). These findings highlight the added value of robotics in the precision and accuracy of implantation. In contrast, the Leksell frame can be used to place both oblique and orthogonal trajectories but is limited by a need to manually configure each trajectory intraoperatively and also the Leksell frame "no-fly zone," which sometimes necessitates replanning of trajectories intraoperatively based on Leksell frame placement (50). Robotic devices circumvent these limitations and enable a platform through which sEEG trajectories can be planned entirely before entering the operating room.

While the discussion of oblique vs. orthogonal implantation trajectories is subjective and heavily dependent on individual surgeon training and experience, it is our view that orthogonal or quasi-orthogonal implantation trajectories (in relation to the midline sagittal plane as defined by the AC–PC) are preferred for most sEEG targets. We would like to emphasize that surgical robotics allow for the safe and accurate implantation of sEEG electrodes in any direction; however, oblique trajectories play a crucial role for some targets (see below). There are three primary conceptual justifications, in our view, for favoring orthogonal implantations for the majority of sEEG trajectories:

1) Coverage volume reasons: Numerous functional networks are distributed and organized along an orthogonal orientation vs. the mid-sagittal plane. For example, the orientation of the cortical and subcortical perisylvian areas are principally

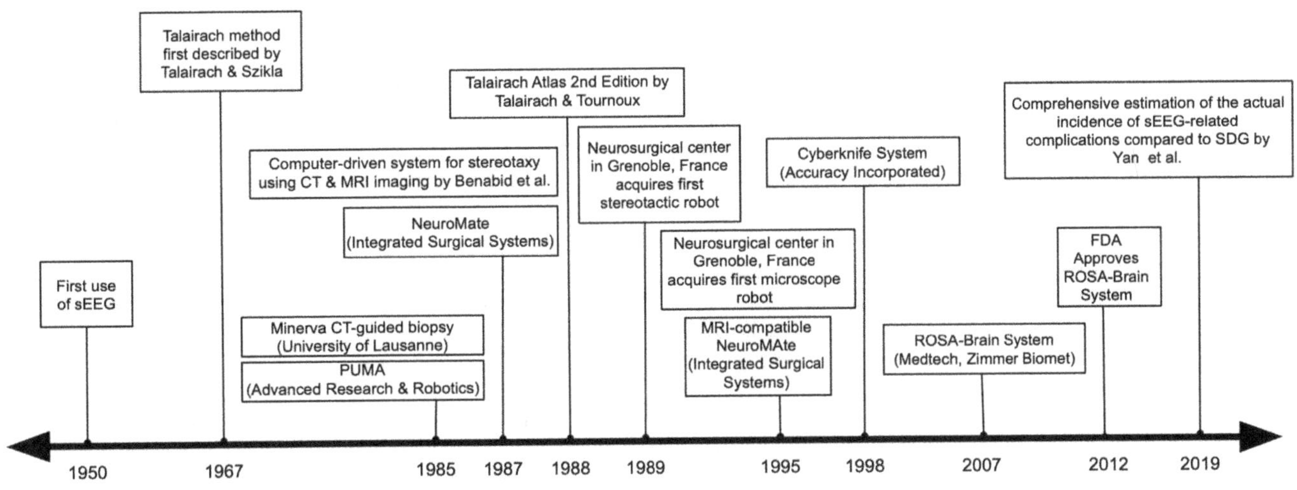

FIGURE 1 | A timeline of important events in the history of robotics in sEEG surgery.

distributed along a rostral–caudal orientation. Therefore, systematic orthogonal electrode implantation facilitates an understanding of the target structure(s) and also its interaction with surrounding brain pathways. While there are many networks in the brain that are not organized orthogonally, many relevant to the mesial temporal lobe, for example, can be investigated in an orthogonal approach to record activity of the amygdala or hippocampus, while more superficial trajectories can record from the temporal neocortex. In relation to SEEG electrode implantation, the Talairach method also aims to successively place anteroposterior and dorsoventral depth electrodes, thus obtaining broad electrophysiological coverage that reconstitutes the three-dimensional brain volume. In addition, this technique remains uniquely suited for the rational investigation of longitudinal and transversal cortical connections. If oblique trajectories are applied as the primary manner of exploration, this three-dimensional understanding may be overlooked or underrepresented.

2) Surgical reasons: The three-dimensional anatomical definition of the EZ is conceptualized in orthogonal planes (axial, coronal, and sagittal) during surgical resections (51). Thus, neurosurgeons typically appreciate neuroanatomy in orthogonal orientations that are constructed within the surgeon's mind, as these orthogonal planes and their anatomic relationships are constant and predictable and routinely parallel with imaging studies. Upon introduction of an oblique plane, this necessary predictability is lost, and the anatomical relationships between structures is increasingly obscured (52). With the advent of surgical robotics, oblique trajectories have become increasingly prevalent. This ultimately results in significantly increased complexity in interpreting SEEG recordings. Finally, a comprehensive neuroimaging pipeline allows for the direct visualization of sEEG anatomical targets and electrodes. The quality of imaging studies and the overlay between a fiducial-based scan and the planning scan allows the stereotactic robot arm to maximize precision via an accurate registration, safely place sEEG electrodes, and provide for meaningful interpretation of clinical information. As the technology evolves, image registration may eventually become an automated process; however, it will still rely on selection of fiducials until real-time imaging feedback can be incorporated into the surgical workflow.
3) Technical reasons: Orthogonal implantations may be safer and more precise when compared to oblique trajectories (53). Oblique trajectories in relation to the skull may generate lead deflections, which may factor into placement inaccuracies (such as epidural electrodes, for example) or predispose a patient to complications, such as intracranial hemorrhage. In addition, long oblique trajectories (e.g., the medial–lateral insular trajectory) may have decreased accuracy due to long span. Orthogonal implantations are shorter and moreover less prone to deflections.

Oblique implantations are conducted in specific situations, where the targeted cortical areas are truly and more efficiently explored via such trajectories, as described:

1) Ventromedial prefrontal cortex (vmPFC): Significant portions of vmPFC, which includes the gyrus rectus and the orbital gyri, can be difficult to investigate via standard orthogonal sEEG trajectories. The bony structure of the orbital cavity necessitates oblique trajectories. As mentioned, attempts at low orthogonal approaches to the gyrus rectus may also lead to a subdural deflection of the sEEG electrode. The preferred implantation method for this region is obtained via oblique orientation electrodes with an entry point located in the frontal areas (at the hair line) in converging orientation and targeting the most posterior and medial aspect of the vmPFC in the gyrus rectus.
2) Dorsal frontal and parietal areas: The dorsal frontal areas are also challenging to investigate via orthogonal SEEG

trajectories. The skull is curved in this topography, thus making orthogonal implantations imprecise and perhaps less safe (53). Oblique implantations are more suitable when placed along the coronal plane while preserving orthogonality in the sagittal plane. The dorsal parietal areas are equally as difficult for orthogonal electrode implantation for similar reasons. In these situations, oblique SEEG trajectories that are nearly perpendicular to the skull are preferred to avoid deflection.

3) Skull defects preventing orthogonal trajectories: Skull defects, such as from prior surgical intervention, may prevent typical lead placement if the bony defect is in the orthogonal projection of the intended target. In this scenario, oblique implantations are preferred and perhaps the only alternative. This may further apply to trajectories where bone may be too thin to accommodate an anchor post, or in the presence of air cells, bony emissary vessels, etc. However, there are unique situations in which oblique trajectories are warranted. For example, in some cases of temporal corticectomy, an oblique trajectory may be required to reach mesial structures.
4) Insula: The insular cortex can be explored with either orthogonal or oblique SEEG trajectories (54, 55). However, a medial to lateral oblique trajectory maximizes gray matter coverage of the insular gyri. Trajectories originating from the frontal bone can target the anterior short gyri and conversing a parietal bone entry site can be used to approach the posterior long insular gyri. A combination of both trajectories is commonly used, depending on the pre-implantation hypothesis. These oblique trajectories maximize insular coverage by providing several contacts within the insula, whereas orthogonal approaches provide only one or two insular electrodes per trajectory (56). The disadvantage of oblique approaches is the lack of opercular coverage. With an orthogonal approach, a single SEEG electrode may explore the insula with its distal contacts and also explore the adjacent opercular cortex with its most superficial contacts. Since the insulo-opercular regions are often involved together in the EZ, the simultaneous evaluation of both cortical areas has distinct advantages in understanding the organization of the EZ and provides a functional assessment of the opercular areas, which may ultimately require resection to gain surgical access to the insular cortex. However, this subtle disadvantage of oblique investigations can be overcome with the addition of orthogonally placed electrodes in the opercular areas in addition to oblique insular electrodes, albeit this approach requires added electrodes.

COMPLICATIONS AND PATTERNS OF USE IN SEEG IMPLANTATION: CONTRIBUTIONS OF ROBOTICS

While different invasive monitoring techniques offer distinct philosophical approaches, as well as unique advantages and disadvantages, sEEG stands apart as a less invasive approach (57). Furthermore, sEEG provides an exclusive opportunity to sample and record from deep cortical structures with unparalleled accuracy to provide surgeons and clinicians with high-powered, three-dimensional mappings of epileptic networks that are used to meticulously guide resection (58). As the use of sEEG for invasive monitoring becomes increasingly popular, both within the United States and across the globe, its relative safety and efficacy has been well-documented and its rate of complications are reported to be the lowest amongst all methods of invasive monitoring in both adult and pediatric patient populations (59–64). Though sEEG has been in use in France since the 1950s, the advent of robotics and recent neuroimaging techniques have led to its proliferation and acceptance throughout North America (65).

The largest sEEG series ever reported, by Cardinale et al., described the 20-year single-institution experience of seizure freedom rates, outcome predictors, and complication rates from 742 sEEG procedures in 713 patients conducted between May 1996 and July 2018 (66). Seizure freedom outcomes were compared to 1,128 patients who underwent surgical intervention after non-invasive evaluation. Furthermore, 185 of the sEEG cases (25.9%) were pediatric patients with the average total cohort age of 26.2 ± 11.8 years. The institutional surgical workflow consisted of the traditional Talairach approach until 2009, after which time the center adopted an image-guided workflow utilizing 3D imaging and robotic assistance (3DIRA). Among sEEG patients, resective surgery was indicated in 79.9% of the total cohort, with 59.4% of patients ultimately achieving seizure freedom at 2 years. With regards to medical and procedural complications, these were present in 13 (1.8%) procedures of which 4 (0.5%) were classified as major events (i.e., one death, two permanent contralateral hemiplegic conditions, and one unilateral leg compartment syndrome with permanent deficit). Although statistically insignificant, it is noteworthy that the overall complication rate was lower following implementation of the 3DIRA workflow (0.9 vs. 2.4%; $p = 0.16$), and no major procedure-related complications were reported out of 5,181 3DIRA-implanted electrodes. These findings substantially support the efficacy and safety of sEEG in both adult and pediatric patients. Furthermore, the decreased rate of complications following implementation of a 3DIRA workflow emphasizes the value and utility of new robotic technologies in neurosurgery.

In 2016, Mullin et al. published a meta-analysis of observational data describing the rates of sEEG complications in 2,624 patients aged between 1 and 69 years (average age, 24 years) from 30 previously published studies (62). Additionally, the review included 124 pediatric patients (4.7%) from four previously published studies examining the efficacy and safety of sEEG in children (67–70). The pooled prevalence rate of 1.3% (95% CI 0.9–1.7%) for all complications demonstrates a remarkably low complication rate in sEEG surgery. While the most common risk is hemorrhagic complications (pooled prevalence 1.0%, 95% CI 0.6–1.4%), the hemorrhage rate was significantly lower when compared to a meta-analysis of patients monitored with subdural grid electrodes (SDG; pooled prevalence 4.0%, 95% CI 3.2–4.8%) (61). Furthermore, a lower overall rate of infection in sEEG monitored patients (pooled prevalence 0.8%, 95% CI 0.3–1.2%) was demonstrated when compared to the reported infection rate (pooled prevalence 2.3%, 95% CI 1.5–3.1%) in the previously mentioned meta-analysis. The overall pooled prevalence of either transient or permanent neurological deficits was 0.6% (95% CI, 0.2–1.0%); however, it was noted that the causes of permanent neurological deficit were not always attributable to sEEG. Of the 2,624 patients in the pooled meta-analysis, there were five reported mortalities: two from intracerebral hemorrhage (ICH), two from preimplantation ventriculography (which is no longer performed routinely at most centers), and one from severe cerebral edema from a likely underlying metabolic derangement. The meta-analysis also noted a total of 11 hardware complications, including one patient who required an additional craniotomy for removal of a retained electrode.

When comparing the complication rates of the two most common methods of invasive monitoring, sEEG and SDG, the relative safety and efficacy of sEEG becomes increasingly clear. A systematic review published by Yan et al. in 2019 examined rates of epilepsy surgery-associated morbidity and subsequent seizure freedom in patients with drug-resistant epilepsy (DRE) monitored with either sEEG or SDG (59). The review included 48 observational studies that captured 1,973 sEEG patients and 2,036 SDE patients, of which 29 examined both adult and pediatric patients and 8 were pediatric-only studies. While none of the included studies performed direct head-to-head comparisons between the two monitoring techniques, sEEG was associated with 4.8% morbidity compared to a rate of 15.5% with SDG (WMD, −10.6%; 95% CI, −11.6–19.6%; $p =$ 0.001). Reported complications included hemorrhage, infection, cerebrospinal fluid (CSF) leak, lead fracture, transient and permanent neurological deficits, and medical complications. Rates of subdural and epidural hematoma (0.7% sEEG; 3.4% SDG; WMD, −2.6%; 95% CI, −2.8 to −2.4%; $p = 0.01$), cerebrospinal fluid leak (0% sEEG; 0.6% SDG; WMD, −1.0%; 95% CI, −1.1 to −0.9%; $p = 0.01$), lead fracture (0.4% sEEG; 1.0% SDG; WMD, −0.5%; 95% CI, −0.7 to −0.2%; $p = 0.01$), transient neurological deficit (1.9% sEEG; 5.7% SDG; WMD, −1.4%; 95% CI, −1.7 to −1.1%; $p = 0.01$), and medical complications (0.7% sEEG; 2.6% SDG; WMD, −1.4%; 95% CI, −1.7 to −1.2%; $p =$ 0.01) were significantly lower among sEEG patients compared to SDG. The rate of infection was also significantly lower among sEEG patients (0.9% sEEG; 1.6% SDG; WMD, −1.6%; 95% CI, −1.7 to −1.5%; $p = 0.01$). Although sEEG can be technically difficult in very young children (i.e., before the age of 2 years), it provides a means of extended recording time coupled with a lower risk of infection compared to SDG (71). While intraparenchymal hemorrhage was significantly more common in sEEG (2.3% sEEG; 1.4% SDG; WMD, 1.5%; 95% CI, 1.4 to −1.7%; $p = 0.01$), the results suggest an overall lower complication profile compared to SDG. The pooled prevalence of mortality was 0.2% among sEEG patients and 0.4% among SDG (WMD, −10.6%; 95% CI, −11.6 to −9.6%; $p = 0.01$) with all mortalities attributed to the method of invasive monitoring itself.

Additional benefits of sEEG with regards to low complication rates can be seen at the individual patient level. A recently published individual patient data (IPD) meta-analysis by Remick et al. was the first to simultaneously examine individual patient phenotypes and their outcomes following invasive monitoring with either sEEG or SDG (63). The review analyzed 595 patients from 33 studies, of which 15 examined both adult and pediatric patients and nine included pediatric patients only. Morbidities such as infection, hemorrhage, and transient and permanent neurological deficits were used as dependent variables in a regression analysis aimed at identifying their associations with patient phenotypes. The results indicate that clinical profiles of patients undergoing sEEG significantly differ from their SDG counterparts. For example, sEEG was a dominant contributor to patient phenotypes associated with low morbidity, while patient phenotypes involving multiple subpial transections, anterior temporal lobectomy, amygdalectomy, and hippocampectomy disproportionately contributed to greater morbidity and were strongly colinear with SDG. As a result, complication rates may be associated with the unique epileptic etiologies that invasive monitoring is used to explore. The authors conclude that while sEEG is associated with a lower rate of resection (82.0%; 95% CI, 78.8–84.2%) compared with SDG (92.7%; 95% CI, 91.1–94.4%; $p = 0.0002$), the clinical phenotypes of sEEG patients were also associated with lower rates of complication, suggesting that the nature of the invasive monitoring technique itself may contribute to patient morbidities. As a minimally invasive approach, sEEG may provide patients with a lower risk approach to successful localization of the EZ.

Finally, there may be spatial and temporal trends in sEEG utilization that contribute to complications in its use. For example, sEEG electrodes were first used to study epilepsy in France during the 1950s; however, the technique did not emerge in practice in the United States until the mid-1970s, where it has been slow to gain popularity (72). While sEEG usage has exponentially increased in recent decades, it is still considered a relatively novel technique when compared to traditional North American methods such as SDG (64). As a result, differences in both institution- and surgeon-level education, training, and experience may contribute to observed rates of complications and decrease over time as sEEG becomes a more widely utilized approach. Furthermore, while modern robotic placement is gaining traction as a valuable enhancement to the precision and accuracy of traditional stereotaxy, many centers continue to utilize manual frame-based and frameless techniques for electrode insertion.

While many of the studies discussed in this review are reflective of adult data, a great number included children in their analyses. This is not surprising as pediatric cases represent a large proportion of sEEG implantations, especially at high volume epilepsy centers. However, the safety profile of robotic sEEG usage in children is comparable to adults in pediatric-only studies (48, 70, 71, 73–76). Furthermore, some studies have examined differences in the utility of frameless robotic technique as opposed to the traditional Talairach frame approach, suggesting that pediatric patients specifically benefit from the swift precision and accuracy that is gained through the use of surgical robots in sEEG surgery. A recent observational study described the technical aspects of and comparison between frameless robot-assisted vs. Talairach frame-based sEEG in 17 children with DRE at an institution with over 30 years of sEEG experience (48). The authors report that, while there were no significant differences in complication rates regardless of a robotic approach, the frameless robot-assisted technique was more efficient, as it required less operating room time and time under anesthesia.

CONCLUSION

The contributions of robotics to the safety and efficacy of invasive monitoring in epilepsy surgery have grown substantially in recent decades. Although sEEG has been in use in France since the 1950s, the advent of robotics and recent neuroimaging techniques have led to its proliferation and acceptance throughout North America. The traditional Talairach frame approach provided the capability of rapid implantation of orthogonal sEEG electrodes; however, it falls short of allowing placement of oblique electrodes. One of the great advantages of robot-assisted implantation techniques is the ability to seamlessly transition between both orthogonal and oblique trajectory types using a single technique. Furthermore, while there are a variety of factors that contribute to both the rates and types of complications observed in sEEG patients, sEEG surgery demonstrates an inherently low complication profile, especially when compared to traditionally held methods of invasive monitoring, such as SDG.

AUTHOR CONTRIBUTIONS

AF, MR, and TA equally contributed to the literature review, drafting, and final version of the manuscript in its entirety. All authors read and approved the final manuscript.

ACKNOWLEDGMENTS

This is a short text to acknowledge the contributions of specific colleagues, institutions, or agencies that aided the efforts of the authors.

REFERENCES

1. Davies B. A review of robotics in surgery. *Proc Inst Mech Eng H.* (2000) 214:129–40. doi: 10.1243/0954411001535309
2. Drake JM, Joy M, Goldenberg A, Kreindler D. Computer- and robot-assisted resection of thalamic astrocytomas in children. *Neurosurgery.* (1991) 29:27–33. doi: 10.1109/ICAR.1991.240561
3. Kwoh YS, Hou J, Jonckheere EA, Hayati S. A robot with improved absolute positioning accuracy for CT guided stereotactic brain surgery. *IEEE Trans Biomed Eng.* (1988) 35:153–60. doi: 10.1109/10.1354
4. Glauser D, Fankhauser H, Epitaux M, Hefti J-L, Jaccottet A. Neurosurgical robot minerva: first results and current developments. *J Image Guid Surg.* (1995) 1:266–72. doi: 10.1002/(sici)1522-712x(1995)1:5<266::aid-igs2>3.0.co;2-8
5. Benabid AL, Cinquin P, Lavalle S, Le Bas JF, Demongeot J, de Rougemon J. Computer-driven robot for stereotactic surgery connected to ct scan and magnetic resonance imaging: technological design andpreliminary results. *Stereotact Funct Neurosurg.* (1987) 50:153–4. doi: 10.1159/000100701
6. Masamune K, Kobayashi E, Masutani Y, Suzuki M, Dohi T, Iseki H, et al. Development of an MRI-compatible needle insertion manipulator for stereotactic neurosurgery. *Comput Aided Surg.* (1995) 1:242–8. doi: 10.3109/10929089509106330
7. Adler JR, Murphy MJ, Chang SD, Hancock SL. Image-guided robotic radiosurgery. *Neurosurgery.* (1999) 44:1299–307. doi: 10.1227/00006123-199906000-00079
8. McBeth PB, Louw DF, Rizun PR, Sutherland GR. Robotics in neurosurgery. *Am J Surg.* (2004) 188:68S–75S. doi: 10.1016/j.amjsurg.2004.08.004
9. Cardinale F. Stereoelectroencephalography: application accuracy, efficacy, and safety. *World Neurosurg.* (2016) 94:570–1. doi: 10.1016/j.wneu.2016.07.070
10. Cardinale F. Letter to the editor: stereoelectroencephalography for insular-opercular/perisylvian epilepsy. *J Neurosurg Pediatr.* (2017) 19:271–2. doi: 10.3171/2016.8.PEDS16450
11. Cardinale F, Casaceli G, Raneri F, Miller J, Lo Russo G. Implantation of stereoelectroencephalography electrodes: a systematic review. *J Clin Neurophysiol.* (2016) 33:490–502. doi: 10.1097/WNP.0000000000000249
12. González-Martínez J, Bulacio J, Thompson S, Gale J, Smithason S, Najm I, et al. Technique, results, and complications related to robot-assisted stereoelectroencephalography. *Neurosurgery.* (2016) 78:169–79. doi: 10.1227/NEU.0000000000001034
13. Calisto A, Dorfmüller G, Fohlen M, Bulteau C, Conti A, Delalande O. Endoscopic disconnection of hypothalamic hamartomas: safety and feasibility of robot-assisted, thulium laser-based procedures. *J Neurosurg Pediatr.* (2014) 14:563–72. doi: 10.3171/2014.8.PEDS13586
14. Gonzalez-Martinez J, Vadera S, Mullin J, Enatsu R, Alexopoulos AV, Patwardhan R, et al. Robot-assisted stereotactic laser ablation in medically intractable epilepsy: operative technique. *Neurosurgery.* (2014) 10:167–73. doi: 10.1227/NEU.0000000000000286
15. Procaccini E, Dorfmüller G, Fohlen M, Bulteau C, Delalande O. Surgical management of hypothalamic hamartomas with epilepsy: the stereoendoscopic approach. *Neurosurgery.* (2006) 59:ONS336–46. doi: 10.1227/01.NEU.0000233900.06146.72
16. Varma TRK, Eldridge P. Use of the neuroMate stereotactic robot in a frameless mode for functional neurosurgery. *Int J Med Robot Comput Assist Surg.* (2006) 2:107–13. doi: 10.1002/rcs.88
17. Lefranc M, Le Gars D. Robotic implantation of deep brain stimulation leads, assisted by intra-operative, flat-panel CT. *Acta Neurochir.* (2012) 154:2069–74. doi: 10.1007/s00701-012-1445-7
18. Neudorfer C, Hunsche S, Hellmich M, El Majdoub F, Maarouf M. Comparative study of robot-assisted versus conventional frame-based deep brain stimulation stereotactic neurosurgery. *Stereotact Funct Neurosurg.* (2018) 96:327–34. doi: 10.1159/000494736
19. Eljamel MS. Robotic neurological surgery applications: accuracy and consistency or pure fantasy? *Stereotact Funct Neurosurg.* (2009) 87:88–93. doi: 10.1159/000202974
20. Eljamel MS. Validation of the pathFinder^{TM} neurosurgical robot using a phantom. *Int J Med Robot Comput Assist Surg.* (2007) 3:372–7. doi: 10.1002/rcs.153
21. Lefranc M, Capel C, Pruvot AS, Fichten A, Desenclos C, Toussaint P, et al. The impact of the reference imaging modality, registration method and intraoperative flat-panel computed tomography on the accuracy of the ROSA® stereotactic robot. *Stereotact Funct Neurosurg.* (2014) 92:242–50. doi: 10.1159/000362936
22. Candela S, Vanegas MI, Darling A, Ortigoza-Escobar JD, Alamar M, Muchart J, et al. Frameless robot-assisted pallidal deep brain stimulation surgery in pediatric patients with movement disorders: precision and short-term clinical results. *J Neurosurg Pediatr.* (2018) 22:416–25. doi: 10.3171/2018.5.PEDS1814
23. Benabid AL, Hoffmann D, Ashraf A, Koudsie A, Esteve F, Le-Bas JF. The robotization of neurosurgery: state of the art and future outlook. *Bull Acad Natl Med.* (1997) 181:1625–36.
24. Lefranc M, Zouitina Y, Tir M, Merle P, Ouendo M, Constans JM, et al. Asleep robot-assisted surgery for the implantation of subthalamic electrodes provides the same clinical improvement and therapeutic window as awake surgery. *World Neurosurg.* (2017) 106:602–8. doi: 10.1016/j.wneu.2017.07.047

25. Gonzalez-Martinez J, Bulacio J, Alexopoulos A, Jehi L, Bingaman W, Najm I. Stereoelectroencephalography in the "difficult to localize" refractory focal epilepsy: early experience from a North American epilepsy center. *Epilepsia.* (2013) 54:323–30. doi: 10.1111/j.1528-1167.2012.03672.x
26. Vadera S, Chan A, Lo T, Gill A, Morenkova A, Phielipp NM, et al. Frameless stereotactic robot-assisted subthalamic nucleus deep brain stimulation: case report. *World Neurosurg.* (2017) 97:762.e11–4. doi: 10.1016/j.wneu.2015.11.009
27. Faraji AH, Kokkinos VK, Sweat JC, Crammond DJ, Richardson RM. Robotic-assisted stereotaxy for deep brain stimulation lead implantation in awake patients. *Oper Neurosurg.* (2020) 19:444–52. doi: 10.1093/ons/opaa029
28. Li G, Su H, Cole GA, Shang W, Harrington K, Camilo A, et al. Robotic system for MRI-guided stereotactic neurosurgery. *IEEE Trans Biomed Eng.* (2015) 62:1077–88. doi: 10.1109/TBME.2014.2367233
29. Lang M, Greer A, Sutherland G. Intra-operative robotics: neuroArm. *Acta Neurochir Suppl.* (2011) 109:231–236. doi: 10.1007/978-3-211-99651-5_36
30. Ho M, McMillan AB, Simard JM, Gullapalli R, Desai JP. Toward a meso-scale SMA-actuated MRI-compatible neurosurgical robot. *IEEE Trans Robot.* (2012) 28:213–22. doi: 10.1109/TRO.2011.2165371
31. Comber DB, Barth EJ, Webster RJ. Design and control of an magnetic resonance compatible precision pneumatic active cannula robot. *J Med Device.* (2014) 8:011003. doi: 10.1115/1.4024832
32. Yang B, Tan UX, McMillan AB, Gullapalli R, Desai JP. Design and control of a 1-DOF MRI-compatible pneumatically actuated robot with long transmission lines. *IEEE ASME Trans Mechatronics.* (2011) 16:1040–8. doi: 10.1109/TMECH.2010.2071393
33. Iordanou JC, Camara D, Ghatan S, Panov F. Approach angle affects accuracy in robotic stereoelectroencephalography lead placement. *World Neurosurg.* (2019) 128:e322–8. doi: 10.1016/j.wneu.2019.04.143
34. Yu H, Pistol C, Franklin R, Barborica A. Clinical accuracy of customized stereotactic fixtures for stereoelectroencephalography. *World Neurosurg.* (2018) 109:82–8. doi: 10.1016/j.wneu.2017.09.089
35. D'Agostino E, Kanter J, Song Y, Aronson JP. Stereoencephalography electrode placement accuracy and utility using a frameless insertion platform without a rigid cannula. *Oper Neurosurg.* (2020) 18:409–16. doi: 10.1093/ons/opz200
36. Rosenow F, Luders H. Presurgical evaluation of epilepsy. *Brain.* (2001) 124:1683–700. doi: 10.1093/brain/124.9.1683
37. Kahane P, Landré E, Minotti L, Francione S, Ryvlin P. The Bancaud and Talairach view on the epileptogenic zone: a working hypothesis. *Epileptic Disord.* (2006) 8(Suppl. 2):S16–26.
38. Luders H, Najim I, Nair D. The epileptogenic zone: general principles. *Epileptic Discord.* (2008) 8:S1–9.
39. Lüders HO, Najm I, Nair D, Widdess-Walsh P, Bingman W. Definition and localization of the epileptogenic zone the epileptogenic zone: general principles. *Epileptic Disord.* (2006) 18:12–6. doi: 10.5698/1535-7597.18.1.12
40. Jin P, Wu D, Li X, Ren L, Wang Y. Towards precision medicine in epilepsy surgery. *Ann Transl Med.* (2016) 4:24. doi: 10.3978/j.issn.2305-5839.2015.12.65
41. Andrzejak RG, David O, Gnatkovsky V, Wendling F, Bartolomei F, Francione S, et al. Localization of epileptogenic zone on pre-surgical intracranial EEG recordings: toward a validation of quantitative signal analysis approaches. *Brain Topogr.* (2015) 28:832–7. doi: 10.1007/s10548-014-0380-8
42. Li YH, Ye XL, Liu QQ, Mao JW, Liang PJ, Xu JW, et al. Localization of epileptogenic zone based on graph analysis of stereo-EEG. *Epilepsy Res.* (2016) 128:149–57. doi: 10.1016/j.eplepsyres.2016.10.021
43. Chabardes S, Abel TJ, Cardinale F, Kahane P. Commentary: understanding stereoelectroencephalography: what's next? *Neurosurgery.* (2018) 82:E15–6. doi: 10.1093/neuros/nyx499
44. Reif PS, Strzelczyk A, Rosenow F. The history of invasive EEG evaluation in epilepsy patients. *Seizure.* (2016) 41:191–5. doi: 10.1016/j.seizure.2016.04.006
45. Talairach J, Bancaud J, Bonis A, Szikla G, Tournous P. Functional stereotaxic exploration of epilepsy. *Confin Neurol.* (1962) 22:328–31. doi: 10.1159/000104378
46. Talairach J, Szikla G. *Atlas of Stereotaxic Anatomy of the Telencephalon.* 1st ed. Paris: Masson (1976).
47. Talairach J, Tournoux P. *Co-Planar Sterotaxic Atlas of the Human Brain.* 1st ed. New York, NY: Thieme (1988).
48. Abel TJ, Osorio RV, Amorim-Leite R, Mathieu F, Kahane P, Minotti L, et al. Frameless robot-assisted stereoelectroencephalography in children: technical aspects and comparison with Talairach frame technique. *J Neurosurg Pediatr.* (2018) 22:37–46. doi: 10.3171/2018.1.PEDS17435
49. Bourdillon P, Châtillon CE, Moles A, Rheims S, Catenoix H, Montavont A, et al. Effective accuracy of stereoelectroencephalography: robotic 3D versus Talairach orthogonal approaches. *J Neurosurg.* (2019) 131:1938–46. doi: 10.3171/2018.7.JNS181164
50. Joswig H, Lau JC, Abdallat M, Parrent AG, MacDougall KW, McLachlan RS, et al. Stereoelectroencephalography versus subdural strip electrode implantations: feasibility, complications, and outcomes in 500 intracranial monitoring cases for drug-resistant epilepsy. *Neurosurgery.* (2020) 87:E23–30. doi: 10.1093/neuros/nyaa112
51. Gonzalez-Martinez J. The stereo-electroencephalography: the epileptogenic zone. *J Clin Neurophysiol.* (2016) 33:522–9. doi: 10.1097/WNP.0000000000000327
52. Baydin S, Gungor A, Holanda VM, Tanriover N, Danish SF. Microneuroanatomy of the anterior frontal laser trajectory to the insula. *World Neurosurg.* (2019) 132:e909–21. doi: 10.1016/j.wneu.2019.07.130
53. Camara D, Panov F, Oemke H, Ghatan S, Costa A. Robotic surgical rehearsal on patient-specific 3D-printed skull models for stereoelectroencephalography (SEEG). *Int J Comput Assist Radiol Surg.* (2019) 14:139–45.doi: 10.1007/s11548-018-1885-5
54. Bottan JS, Rubino PA, Lau JC, Macdougall KW, Parrent AG, Burneo JG, et al. Robot-assisted insular depth electrode implantation through oblique trajectories: 3-dimensional anatomical nuances, technique, accuracy, and safety. *Oper Neurosurg.* (2020) 18:278–83. doi: 10.1093/ons/opz154
55. Gil Robles S, Gelisse P, El Fertit H, Tancu C, Duffau H, Crespel A, et al. Parasagittal transinsular electrodes for stereo-EEG in temporal and insular lobe epilepsies. *Stereotact Funct Neurosurg.* (2009) 87:368–78. doi: 10.1159/000249818
56. Alomar S, Mullin JP, Smithason S, Gonzalez-Martinez J. Indications, technique, and safety profile of insular stereoelectroencephalography electrode implantation in medically intractable epilepsy. *J Neurosurg.* (2018) 128:1147–57. doi: 10.3171/2017.1.JNS161070
57. Tóth M, Janszky J. Intracranial EEG monitoring methods. *Ideggyogy Sz.* (2020) 73:79–83. doi: 10.18071/isz.73.0079
58. Serletis D, Bulacio J, Bingaman W, Najm I, González-Martínez J. The stereotactic approach for mapping epileptic networks: a prospective study of 200 patients. *J Neurosurg.* (2014) 121:1239–46. doi: 10.3171/2014.7.JNS132306
59. Yan H, Katz JS, Anderson M, Mansouri A, Remick M, Ibrahim GM, et al. Method of invasive monitoring in epilepsy surgery and seizure freedom and morbidity: a systematic review. *Epilepsia.* (2019) 60:1960–72. doi: 10.1111/epi.16315
60. Katz JS, Abel TJ. Stereoelectroencephalography versus subdural electrodes for localization of the epileptogenic zone: what is the evidence? *Neurotherapeutics.* (2019) 16:59–66. doi: 10.1007/s13311-018-0 0703-2
61. Arya R, Mangano FT, Horn PS, Holland KD, Rose DF, Glauser TA. Adverse events related to extraoperative invasive EEG monitoring with subdural grid electrodes: a systematic review and meta-analysis. *Epilepsia.* (2013) 54:828–39. doi: 10.1111/epi.12073
62. Mullin JP, Shriver M, Alomar S, Najm I, Bulacio J, Chauvel P, et al. Is SEEG safe? A systematic review and meta-analysis of stereo-electroencephalography-related complications. *Epilepsia.* (2016) 57:386–401. doi: 10.1111/epi.13298
63. Remick M, Ibrahim GM, Mansouri A, Abel TJ. Patient phenotypes and clinical outcomes in invasive monitoring for epilepsy: an individual patient data meta-analysis. *Epilepsy Behav.* (2019) 102:106652 doi: 10.1016/j.yebeh.2019.106652
64. Raftopoulos C, Vaz G, Tassigny D, van Rijckevorsel K. Invasive EEG in refractory epilepsy: insertion of subdural grids through linear craniectomy reduces complications and remains effective. *Neurochirurgie.* (2015) 61:16–21. doi: 10.1016/j.neuchi.2014.09.005
65. Abou-Al-Shaar H, Brock AA, Kundu B, Englot DJ, Rolston JD. Increased nationwide use of stereoelectroencephalography for intracranial epilepsy electroencephalography recordings. *J Clin Neurosci.* (2018) 53:132–4. doi: 10.1016/j.jocn.2018.04.064

66. Cardinale F, Rizzi M, Vignati E, Cossu M, Castana L, d'Orio P, et al. Stereoelectroencephalography: retrospective analysis of 742 procedures in a single centre. *Brain*. (2019) 142:2688–704. doi: 10.1093/brain/awz196
67. Dylgjeri S, Taussig D, Chipaux M, Lebas A, Fohlen M, Bulteau C, et al. Insular and insulo-opercular epilepsy in childhood: an SEEG study. *Seizure*. (2014) 23:300–8. doi: 10.1016/j.seizure.2014.01.008
68. Dorfmüller G, Ferrand-Sorbets S, Fohlen M, Bulteau C, Archambaud F, Delalande O, et al. Outcome of surgery in children with focal cortical dysplasia younger than 5 years explored by stereo-electroencephalography. *Child's Nerv Syst*. (2014) 30:1875–83. doi: 10.1007/s00381-014-2464-x
69. Gonzalez-Martinez J, Mullin J, Bulacio J, Gupta A, Enatsu R, Najm I, et al. Stereoelectroencephalography in children and adolescents with difficult-to-localize refractory focal epilepsy. *Neurosurgery*. (2014) 75:258–68; discussion: 267–8. doi: 10.1227/NEU.0000000000000453
70. Taussig D, Chipaux M, Lebas A, Fohlen M, Bulteau C, Ternier J, et al. Stereo-electroencephalography (SEEG) in 65 children: an effective and safe diagnostic method for pre-surgical diagnosis, independent of age. *Epileptic Disord*. (2014) 16:280–95. doi: 10.1684/epd.2014.0679
71. Taussig D, Dorfmüller G, Fohlen M, Jalin C, Bulteau C, Ferrand-Sorbets S, et al. Invasive explorations in children younger than 3 years. *Seizure*. (2012) 21:631–8. doi: 10.1016/j.seizure.2012.07.004
72. van Roost D, Solymosi L, Schramm J, Van Oosterwyck B, Elger CE. Depth electrode implantation in the length axis of the hippocampus for the presurgical evaluation of medial temporal lobe epilepsy: a computed tomography-based stereotactic insertion technique and its accuracy. *Neurosurgery*. (1998) 43:819–26; discussion: 826–7.doi: 10.1097/00006123-199810000-00058
73. Budke M, Avecillas-Chasin JM, Villarejo F. Implantation of depth electrodes in children using varioguider frameless navigation system: technical note. *Oper Neurosurg*. (2018) 15:302–9. doi: 10.1093/ons/opx192
74. Cossu M, Cardinale F, Colombo N, Mai R, Nobili L, Sartori I, et al. Stereoelectroencephalography in the presurgical evaluation of children with drug-resistant focal epilepsy. *J Neurosurg*. (2005) 103(4 Suppl.):333–43. doi: 10.3171/ped.2005.103.4.0333
75. Kassiri J, Pugh J, Carline S, Jurasek L, Snyder T, Wheatley M, et al. Depth electrodes in pediatric epilepsy surgery. *Can J Neurol Sci*. (2013) 40:48–55. doi: 10.1017/S0317167100012944
76. Park YS, Lee YH, Shim KW, Lee YJ, Kim HD, Lee JS, et al. Insular epilepsy surgery under neuronavigation guidance using depth electrode. *Child's Nerv Syst*. (2009) 25:591–7. doi: 10.1007/s00381-008-0764-8

16

Distinguishing Focal Cortical Dysplasia from Glioneuronal Tumors in Patients with Epilepsy by Machine Learning

Yi Guo [1,2], Yushan Liu [3], Wenjie Ming [2,4], Zhongjin Wang [2,4], Junming Zhu [2,5], Yang Chen [3], Lijun Yao [6], Meiping Ding [2,4] and Chunhong Shen [2,4*]*

[1] Department of General Practice, School of Medicine, Second Affiliated Hospital, Zhejiang University, Hangzhou, China, [2] Epilepsy Center, School of Medicine, Second Affiliated Hospital, Zhejiang University, Hangzhou, China, [3] School of Computer Science, Fudan University, Shanghai, China, [4] Department of Neurology, School of Medicine, Second Affiliated Hospital, Zhejiang University, Hangzhou, China, [5] Department of Neurosurgery, School of Medicine, Second Affiliated Hospital, Zhejiang University, Hangzhou, China, [6] Shanghai Pudong New Area Mental Health Center, Tongji University School of Medicine, Shanghai, China

***Correspondence:**
Chunhong Shen
2513109@zju.edu.cn
Lijun Yao
lyao@tongji.edu.cn

Purpose: We are aiming to build a supervised machine learning-based classifier, in order to preoperatively distinguish focal cortical dysplasia (FCD) from glioneuronal tumors (GNTs) in patients with epilepsy.

Methods: This retrospective study was comprised of 96 patients who underwent epilepsy surgery, with the final neuropathologic diagnosis of either an FCD or GNTs. Seven classical machine learning algorithms (i.e., Random Forest, SVM, Decision Tree, Logistic Regression, XGBoost, LightGBM, and CatBoost) were employed and trained by our dataset to get the classification model. Ten features [i.e., Gender, Past history, Age at seizure onset, Course of disease, Seizure type, Seizure frequency, Scalp EEG biomarkers, MRI features, Lesion location, Number of antiepileptic drug (AEDs)] were analyzed in our study.

Results: We enrolled 56 patients with FCD and 40 patients with GNTs, which included 29 with gangliogliomas (GGs) and 11 with dysembryoplasic neuroepithelial tumors (DNTs). Our study demonstrated that the Random Forest-based machine learning model offered the best predictive performance on distinguishing the diagnosis of FCD from GNTs, with an F1-score of 0.9180 and AUC value of 0.9340. Furthermore, the most discriminative factor between FCD and GNTs was the feature "age at seizure onset" with the Chi-square value of 1,213.0, suggesting that patients who had a younger age at seizure onset were more likely to be diagnosed as FCD.

Conclusion: The Random Forest-based machine learning classifier can accurately differentiate FCD from GNTs in patients with epilepsy before surgery. This might lead to improved clinician confidence in appropriate surgical planning and treatment outcomes.

Keywords: machine learning, epilepsy, focal cortical dysplasia, glioneuronal tumors, distinguish

INTRODUCTION

Focal cortical dysplasia (FCD) is a distinctive malformation of cortical development that is highly associated with refractory epilepsy. Around 12–40% of patients with FCD were submitted to surgery for refractory epilepsy (1). Neuropathological findings have also reported glioneuronal tumors (GNTs) are another important cause of refractory epilepsy in children and young adults, including gangliogliomas (GGs) and dysembryoplastic neuroepithelial tumors (DNTs) (2). Previous studies have demonstrated that patients with FCD and GNTs have different postoperative seizure outcomes. Up to 80% patients with GNTs could achieve seizure-free during the follow-up. However, only 40–50% patients with FCD experienced no seizures after surgery (3, 4). As for the surgical protocol in many patients with FCD, wide cortical resection over the MRI-delineated lesion with invasive electroencephalography is frequently recommended, due to obscure histologic boundary and poor prognosis (5). In contrast, recent studies on tumor-associated epilepsy have emphasized that total surgical resection of the tumor is sufficient and effective for seizure control in most patients with GNTs (6). Thus, it is crucial to make the differential diagnosis of FCD and GNTs preoperatively. However, their clinical manifestation and imaging findings could be similar, especially in cases of mass-like FCD (7). What' more, type III FCD was accompanied by an additional brain lesion as noted in the classification system by the International League Against Epilepsy (ILAE) (8).

Some factors have been reported to differentiate FCD from GNTs before surgery. Rácz's et al. study indicated that age at epilepsy onset was younger in patients with FCD compared to those with GNTs (9). Though ^{18}F-FDG PET can't contribute to the differentiation of FCD and GNTs, ^{11}C-methionine PET identified a significant difference between them (10). But, up to now, ^{11}C-methionine PET was unavailable in most hospitals worldwide. Several surface EEG biomarkers were also revealed to be significantly correlated with an underlying cortical dysplasia (11). Despite these factors, it remained a challenge to effectively differentiate FCD from GNTs preoperatively.

Machine learning, as an important branch of artificial intelligence, has been applied to automated seizure detection (12), prediction of antiepileptic drugs (AEDs) response (13), pre-surgical planning and surgical outcome prediction (14). In the present study, we adopted supervised machine learning-based algorithms to train the classifier to differentiate FCD from GNTs, using seven representative classification algorithms, i.e., Decision Tree (15), Random Forest (16), Logistic Regression (17), Support Vector Machine (SVM) (18), XGBoost (19), Catboost (20), and LightGBM (21). In addition, we included several features to predict different pathological results, attempting to identify the most valuable feature. Based on our results, one can use the trained classifier to make a diagnosis prediction of FCD or GNTs before surgery, hence helping clinicians to make better surgical planning.

METHODS

Patients and Definitions

The study was retrospectively conducted from January 2013 to December 2018 in the Second Affiliated Hospital of Zhejiang University, a tertiary referral hospital in Zhejiang, China. All the patients underwent epilepsy surgery at the Epilepsy Center. Inclusion criteria were as follows: (1) patients were diagnosed as epilepsy according to the guidelines for the Classification and Diagnosis of Epilepsy of ILAE (22). (2) the neuropathologic diagnosis of either FCD or GNTs was established by two senior neuropathologists (8, 23), discrepancies were discussed and resolved by verification from a third senior neuropathologist. (3) all the patients underwent a non-invasive pre-surgical evaluation, including long-term video-EEG monitoring, high-resolution MRI with epilepsy sequence and PET-CT for some of them; for patients whose surgical protocols were with difficulties, invasive evaluation with the stereo-electroencephalography was carried out. Among 308 patients who underwent epilepsy surgery from January 2013 to December 2018 in our center, 98 patients met inclusion criteria, 2 patients did not obtain informed consent, and 96 patients were included in the final analysis. Informed consents were obtained from all the participants, and the study was approved by the Second Affiliated hospital of Zhejiang University School of Medicine Ethics Committee.

The information of ten features (i.e., Gender, Past history, Age at seizure onset, Course of disease, Seizure type, Seizure frequency, Scalp EEG biomarkers, MRI features, Lesion location, Number of AEDs) were recorded. Past history included encephalitis, perinatal brain injury, febrile convulsion, traumatic brain injuries and other known secondary causes. Seizure type was classified according to the new operational classification by ILAE (24), and seizure frequency was grouped into four categories: every few years, once a year, once few months and several times a month (25). Video EEG (VEEG) was performed using digital VEEG systems (Nicolet, VIASYS, United States and Biologic, NATUS, United States), with scalp electrodes placed according to the international 10–20 system. All the patients were monitored for at least 24 h. For the patients with long-term monitoring, the first 24 h recordings were chosen without AEDs tapering. Two EEG experts were blind to the MRI results and underlying histopathology. EEG recordings were evaluated in both referential and bipolar montages, and positive biomarkers were considered to be present when consensus between two independent EEG experts was achieved. The positive biomarkers of FCD were defined as the presence of continuous epileptiform discharges, two types of rhythmic epileptiform discharges, polyspikes, repetitive activity and polyspikes, frequent rhythmic bursting epileptiform activity, or repetitive discharges according to Epitashvili's et al. study (11). Examples of positive EEG biomarkers were shown in (**Supplementary Figure 1**). As for MRI protocols, patients were conducted on a 3.0T scanner (MR750, GE Healthcare, United States) with an 8-channel brain phased array coil. High resolution coronal T2-weighted images perpendicular to the long axis of the hippocampus were acquired using spoiled gradient echo sequence with

TR/TE = 5,518/176 ms, flip angle = 110°, slice thickness = 2 mm, matrix = 512 × 512. Sagittal 3D T1-weighted images were acquired using brain volume imaging (BRAVO) sequence with TR/TE = 8.2/3.2 ms, TI = 450 ms, flip angle = 12°, slice thickness = 1 mm, matrix = 256 × 256. High resolution axial T2-weighted images and fluid-attenuated inversion-recovery (FLAIR) sequence were also obtained. Contrast-enhanced images T1-and T2-weighted images were obtained, if necessary. Typical MRI characteristics of FCD type I included subtle white matter signal changes and regional reduction of the white matter volume. Typical MRI characteristics of FCD type II included focal cortical thickening, blurring of the gray-white matter interface, focally increased signal on T2-weighted imaging, and a tail of increased signal from the cortex to an underlying ventricle on T2-weighted imaging (transmantle sign) (26, 27). GGs usually presents as a cyst with an enhancing mural nodule, with minimal to no surrounding edema and no significant mass effect. Foci of calcification are frequent (40–50%) in GGs and areas of cortical dysplasia can be seen adjacent to the tumor (28, 29). On MRI, DNTs appear well-demarcated and frequently wedge shaped, hypointense on T1WI, and hyperintense on T2WI, lack of edema and mass effect. Calcifications can be seen in 20% DNTs, and 20% DNTs have nodular or ring-like enhancement (28, 29). Typical characteristics of GGs and DNTs on MRI imaging were considered as typical characteristics of GNTs (28, 29). Typical MRI characteristics of FCD or GNTs were considered when consensus between two independent neuroradiologists was achieved. Examples of MRI for FCD and GNTs were shown in (**Supplementary Figure 2**).

Machine Learning

Our work was aiming to build a binary classification model capable of distinguishing FCD from GNTs. The process of the supervised machine learning-based analysis included the following steps, i.e., data preprocessing, feature selection, algorithm selection, parameter tuning, and performance evaluation. The method was as the same as our previous study (13). The workflow of data preparation and machine-learning based modeling was shown in the (**Supplementary Figure 3**).

Data Preprocessing

In our analysis, 56 patients with FCD and 40 with GNTs were recruited. To solve the unbalanced sample problem, we over-sampled the minority type to 56 by using the SMOTE technique (30). (https://www.jair.org/index.php/jair/article/view/10302). Then we randomly split the entire dataset into a training and validation dataset and a test dataset. The training and validation dataset were used to train and validate the prediction model, while the test dataset was applied to evaluate the prediction performance of the trained model. We used 50% of patients for training and validation, the rest for test. The aim of the training and validation stage is to find an optimal set of parameters that can achieve the highest prediction performance. We further applied the 5-fold cross-validation method by randomly dividing the training and validation dataset into 5 subsets with equal sample sizes. The cross-validation process was repeated for 5 rounds. For each round, one of the 5 subsets were retained as the validation data to evaluate the model, and the remaining 4 subsets were used for training. We have made our dataset available to the public via Harvard Dataverse (https://dataverse.harvard.edu/dataset.xhtml?persistentId=doi:10.7910/DVN/6F7QPP).

Algorithm Selection and Parameter Tuning

For machine learning algorithm selection, we included classical algorithms such as Random Forest, SVM, Decision Tree and Logistic Regression, as well as new algorithms, i.e., XGBoost, LightGBM, and CatBoost. For each algorithm, we should determine an optimal set of parameters. Based on the training and validation dataset, we applied grid search to go through the parameter space, which covers a finite set of parameter combinations. For each parameter combination, we evaluated the model's prediction performance using the training and validation dataset. We record the parameters leading to the highest F1-score. To train and evaluate the classification model (31), we used the scikit-learn library, a representative open source machine learning toolkit, written in the Python programming language. This library supports a number of supervised machine learning algorithms, including Decision Tree, Random Forest, Logistic Regression, Support Vector Machine (SVM), XGBoost, Catboost, and LightGBM. After selecting a specified algorithm, the scikit-learn library is able to process the training and validation dataset to obtain a classification model. Then this model can be further applied to the test dataset.

Performance Evaluation

Based on the test dataset, we used precision, recall, F1-score, and the AUC (Area Under the ROC Curve) value to evaluate the predictive performance of our trained model (32). Precision was the fraction of patients with FCD who were finally diagnosed with FCD. Recall was the fraction of patients with FCD who have been adequately identified by the model. F1-score was the harmonic mean of precision and recall, with its best value at 1 and worst value at 0. F1-score was calculated as follows:

$$F1 = \frac{2 \cdot precision \cdot recall}{precision + recall}$$

From the perspective of clinicians, high precision means that our prediction rarely over-reports or over-represents the fraction of patients with predicted FCD who are in fact diagnosed with FCD. Meanwhile, high recall means the fraction of patients with FCD who are uncovered accurately. A higher value of F1-score indicates a better overall predictive performance of a classifier. AUC is another important metric for evaluating a classification model's performance, which denotes the probability that a machine learning algorithm will rank higher of a random positive instance than a randomly chosen negative instance. The value of AUC is between 0 and 1. For a perfect classifier, the AUC value will be 1. For a completely random classifier, the AUC value will be 0.5. If the AUC value is smaller than 0.5, we could invert all the outputs of the classifier and obtain a new AUC value larger than 0.5. An AUC value close to 1 indicates that the model is good at distinguishing FCD from GNTs.

Statistical Analysis

Statistical analysis was performed using python. Continuous variable (course of disease) with normal distribution was represented as mean ± standard deviation (SD), non-normal variable (age at seizure onset) was reported as median [interquartile range (IQR)]. Categorical variables were described in the form of frequency and percentage. Independent student's *t*-test were conducted to compare the means of the continuous variables with normal distribution while Welch's *t*-test was used if the data was not normally distributed. Chi-Squared (χ^2) Statistics was used to compare the frequencies of categorical variables between FCD and GNTs Groups. And we calculated the Chi-Square (χ^2) Statistics to evaluate the dependence of each selected feature on different pathological results (33). A larger χ^2 value indicated a better discriminative power of the feature. A value of $p < 0.05$ was considered significant. All the tests were two tailed.

RESULTS

Patient Characteristics

A total of 96 patients who underwent epilepsy surgery were analyzed in our study, including 56 patients with FCD (FCD I: $n = 16$; FCD II: $n = 40$) and 40 patients with GNTs (GG: $n = 29$; DNTs = 11). Ten features were reviewed and recorded; the details were shown in **Table 1**. The median age at seizure onset (months) in FCD group was much lower than that in GNTs group (77 vs. 155, $P = 0.002$, also see **Figure 1**); Course of disease (months) in FCD group was longer than that in GNTs group, but not statistically significant (105 vs. 69, $P = 0.12$, also see **Figure 1**). Thirty-five (62.5%) patients with FCD showed scalp EEG biomarkers of FCD, whereas only 13 (32.5%) patients with GNTs had the positive biomarkers ($p = 0.04$, also see **Figure 1**). Thirty six (64.3%) patients with FCD had typical MRI characteristics of FCD, and 29 (72.5%) patients in GNTs group had typical MRI characteristics of GNTs ($p < 0.001$, also see **Figure 1**). As for AEDs, 37 (66.0%) patients in FCD group were taking more than 3 kinds of AEDs, while only 6 (15.0%) patients in GNTs group were taking 3 or more kinds of AEDs ($p < 0.001$, also see **Figure 1**). However, there were no significant differences in gender, past history, seizure type, seizure frequency, and lesion location between two groups with FCD and GNTs.

Machine Learning Algorithms Used to Distinguish FCD From GNTs

With the current dataset, we adopted supervised machine learning algorithms to preoperatively predict pathological diagnosis of patients with epilepsy. A wide variety of machine learning algorithms were selected to build classification models, including Random Forest, Catboost, SVM, XGBoost, LightGBM, Logistic Regression, and Decision Tree. As shown in **Table 2**, the F1-scores of these seven models (Random Forest, Catboost, SVM, XGBoost, LightGBM, Logistic Regression, and Decision Tree) were 0.9180, 0.9000, 0.8621, 0.8667, 0.8750, 0.8889, and 0.8000, and the AUC values were 0.9340, 0.9515, 0.9055, 0.9630, 0.8531, 0.9132, and 0.7873, respectively. The precision/positive predictive value and recall/sensitivity for each model were also described in **Table 2**. Overall, our data revealed that Random Forest and Catboost were most effective in distinguishing patients with FCDs from those with GNTs. Furthermore, Random Forest-based classifier achieved the highest F1-score of 0.9180 and an AUC value of 0.9340, providing the best discriminatory ability in the prediction of pathological diagnosis.

The Features Used to Distinguish FCD From GNTs

Next, the Chi-Square analysis was employed to identify the discriminative power of each feature to preoperatively make the diagnosis of FCD or GNTs. The top 5 ranked features that effectively contributed to distinguishing FCD from GNTs were Age at seizure onset, Course of disease, MRI features, Number of AEDs, and Scalp EEG biomarkers, with the Chi-square values of 1,213.000, 334.800, 19.969, 13.946, and 4.200, respectively (**Table 3**).

To visualize the difference between patients with FCD and GNTs, we analyzed in terms of Age at seizure onset, Course of disease, MRI features, Number of AEDs and Scalp EEG biomarkers as shown in **Figure 1**. Age at seizure onset was revealed to be the most discriminative feature to distinguish between patients with FCD and GNTs, meaning that younger age at seizure onset would increase the probability of the diagnosis of FCD.

DISCUSSION

In the present study, we demonstrated that the Random Forest-based machine learning model provided the best predictive performance on distinguishing FCD from GNTs, with an F1-score of 0.9180 and AUC value of 0.9340. Of ten included features, "Age at seizure onset" was revealed to be the most discriminative feature. With this supervised machine learning-based approach, one would accurately differentiate FCD from GNTs in patients with epilepsy before surgery, allowing clinicians to make the surgical planning properly and individually.

For all the patients who underwent epilepsy surgery, the ultimate desired outcomes were complete seizure freedom without further AEDs. Therefore, accurate preoperative diagnosis of FCD or GNTs based upon clinical features was of great importance, when planning the extent of resection and choosing the invasive evaluation as noted above. With widespread use in image recognition, language processing, and data mining, machine learning-based techniques have received increasing attention in medical applications, including the use of epilepsy (14). One challenge is that there are a series of potential supervised ML algorithms which could be selected. To our knowledge, which algorithm is the most suitable one for our problem is unknown. Our study focused on the differential diagnosis of FCD and GNTs before surgery, indicating that two classification algorithms (Random Forest and Catboost) were quite effective to predict between FCD and GNTs. Particularly, the Random Forest-based model performed best in prediction. Logistic regression was a widely used statistical method with an F1-score of 0.8889 in our study, which was much lower

TABLE 1 | Clinical characteristics of included patients with FCD and GNTs.

Variable	FCD ($n = 56$)	GNTs ($n = 40$)	Overall ($n = 96$)	*P*-value
Gender, *n* (%)				0.593
Female	27 (48.2%)	16 (40%)	43 (44.8%)	
Male	29 (51.8%)	24 (60%)	53 (55.2%)	
Past History, *n* (%)				0.949
Negative	52 (92.9%)	37 (92.5%)	89 (92.7%)	
Positive	4 (7.1%)	3 (7.5%)	7 (7.3%)	
Age at seizure onset (months), median (IQR)	77 (31, 125)	155 (70, 270)	108 (36, 228)	0.002*
Course of disease (months), Mean ± SD	105 ± 113	69 ± 107	90 ± 111	0.12
Seizure type, *n* (%)				0.978
FAS	14 (17.5%)	10 (18.2%)	24 (17.7%)	
FIAS	40 (50%)	22 (40%)	62 (45.9%)	
FBTCS	26 (32.5%)	23 (41.8%)	49 (36.4%)	
Seizure frequency, *n* (%)				0.184
Every few years	2 (3.6%)	7 (17.5%)	9 (9.4%)	
Once a year	0 (0%)	1 (2.5%)	1 (1.0%)	
Once few months	4 (7.1%)	5 (12.5%)	9 (9.4%)	
Several times a month	50 (89.3%)	27 (67.5%)	77 (80.2%)	
Scalp EEG biomarkers of FCD, *n* (%)				0.040*
Negative	21 (37.5%)	27 (67.5%)	48 (50.0%)	
Positive	35 (62.5%)	13 (32.5%)	48 (50.0%)	
MRI features, *n* (%)				<0.001*
Typical characteristics of GNTs	2 (3.6%)	29 (72.5%)	31 (32.3%)	
Typical characteristics of FCD	36 (64.3%)	6 (15%)	42 (43.8%)	
None	18 (32.1%)	5 (12.5%)	23 (23.9%)	
Lesion location, *n* (%)				0.130
Frontal lobe	31 (55.4%)	3 (7.5%)	34 (35.4%)	
Temporal lobe	19 (33.9%)	34 (85%)	53 (55.2%)	
Parietal lobe	4 (7.1%)	2 (5%)	6 (6.3%)	
Occipital lobe	1 (1.8%)	1 (2.5%)	2 (2.1%)	
Insular lobe	1 (1.8%)	0 (0%)	1(1.0%)	
Number of AEDs, *n* (%)				<0.001*
None	1 (1.8%)	8 (20%)	9 (9.4%)	
1 drug	3 (5.4%)	13 (32.5%)	16 (16.7%)	
2 drugs	15 (26.8%)	13 (32.5%)	28 (29.1%)	
≥3 drugs	37 (66.0%)	6 (15.0%)	43 (44.8%)	

*FCD, focal cortical dysplasia; GNTs, glioneuronal tumors; FAS, focal aware seizure; FIAS, focal impaired awareness seizure; FBTCS, focal to bilateral tonic-clonic seizure; AEDs, antiepileptic drugs; IQR, interquartile range; SD, standard deviation; *$P < 0.05$ was considered statistically significant.*

compared to that of Random Forest. Consequently, our Random Forest-based model would be considered as a potential and powerful classifier to predict the preoperative pathological diagnosis for patients with epilepsy. Consistent with our result, Paldino et al. have indicated that the Random Forest classifier achieved 100% sensitivity and 95.4% specificity in predicting language impairment with DTI-based whole-brain tractography data from pediatric patients with malformations of cortical development (34). A later study conducted by Grinspan et al. has also demonstrated that the Random Forest classifier achieved AUCs of 84.1 and 73.4% at each center in predicting emergency department visit rates for the following year, using a combination of demographic characteristics, insurance, comorbidity, and medication data in medical records at two pediatric referral centers (35). In our study, the consistent rate between conventional preoperative diagnosis and postoperative pathology was 76%, while the consistent rate was 89.6% when preoperative Random Forest algorithm was used to predict postoperative pathology, showing a statistically significant difference (**Supplementary Table 1**, $\chi^2 = 6.184$, $p = 0.013$). As far as we know, this was the first study reporting that machine learning-based algorithms could be used to differentiate FCD

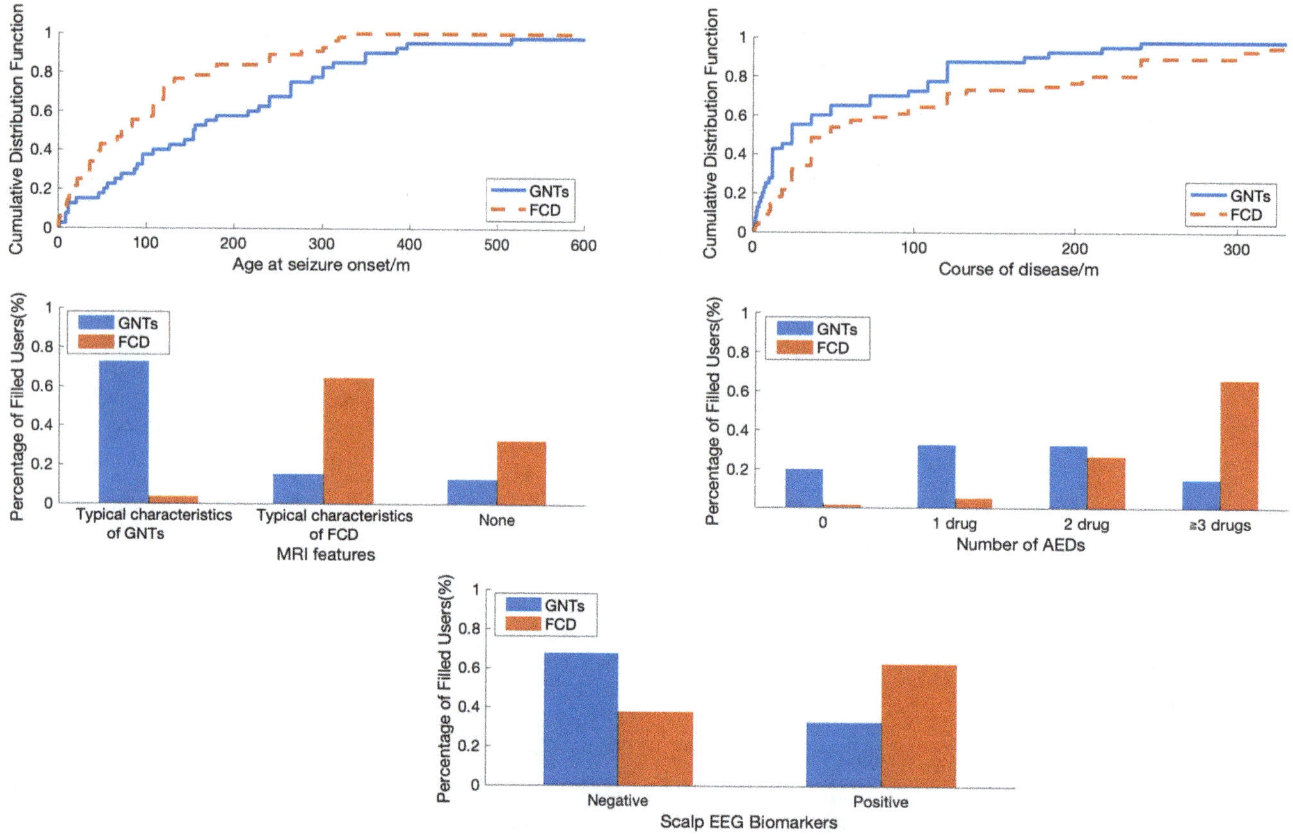

FIGURE 1 | The comparison of patients with FCD and GNTs in terms of different features. FCD, focal cortical dysplasia; GNTs, glioneuronal tumors; AEDs, antiepileptic drugs.

TABLE 2 | The performance of different algorithms to distinguish FCD from GNTs.

Algorithm	Precision/ Positive predictive value	Recall/ Sensitivity	F1-Score	AUC
Random forest	0.8750	0.9655	0.9180	0.9340
Catboost	0.8710	0.9310	0.9000	0.9515
Logistic regression	0.9600	0.8276	0.8889	0.9132
LightGBM	0.8000	0.9655	0.8750	0.8531
XGBoost	0.8387	0.8966	0.8667	0.9630
SVM	0.8621	0.8621	0.8621	0.9055
Decision tree	0.7742	0.8276	0.8000	0.7873

FCD, focal cortical dysplasia; GNTs, glioneuronal tumors.

from GNTs in patients with epilepsy. For the next step, we will use a larger sample to train our algorithm. One practical challenge is that different hospitals might host their patient databases on computers with different operating systems, including Windows, Linux and MacOSX. Our algorithm is implemented using the scikit-learn library (https://scikit-learn.org/stable/), which is an open source library written in the Python programming language. Thanks to the cross-platform nature of Python, our algorithm can be directly deployed on computers with any mainstream operating system without modification. Our algorithm could directly access a hospital's database of patient records, and read the patient information automatically to provide the predicted diagnosis of FCD or GNTs. In short, our algorithm has no special requirement for either the operating system or the computer hardware. It is convenient to be employed in clinical applications. If the diagnosis given by the classifier is FCD, wider cortical resection over the MRI-delineated lesion may be taken into consideration by neurosurgeons, in order to achieve favorable seizure outcomes. Furthermore, having a good knowledge of

TABLE 3 | The discriminative power of different features to distinguish FCD from GNTs.

Rank	Feature	Chi-square value
1	Age at seizure onset	1,213.000
2	Course of disease	334.800
3	MRI features	19.969
4	Number of AEDs	13.946
5	Scalp EEG biomarkers	4.200
6	Lesion location	2.287
7	Seizure frequency	1.760
8	Gender	0.285
9	Past history	0.004
10	Seizure type	0.001

FCD, focal cortical dysplasia; GNTs, glioneuronal tumors; AEDs, antiepileptic drugs.

the potential postsurgical outcome may improve clinicians' and patients' confidence in epilepsy surgery.

As for the top 5 ranked features which contributed most to distinguishing FCD from GNTs in patients with epilepsy, the feature "Age at seizure onset" had the highest Chi-square value at 1,213.000, suggesting patients who have the younger age at seizure onset were more likely to be diagnosed as FCD finally. This result was consistent with the study from Rácz et al. which indicated that age at epilepsy onset was significantly earlier in patients with FCD than that in GNTs (9). The second feature "Course of disease" had the Chi-square value at 334.800, suggesting that epileptic patients with FCD had a longer course of disease compared to patients with GNTs. A possible explanation could be that GNTs group had a higher proportion (72.5%) of patients with typical characteristics of GNTs and consequently underwent surgical treatment earlier, which was also a reason for the number difference of AEDs between two groups. As the commonly used method to distinguish FCD from GNTs, "MRI" was the third feature with the Chi-square value at 19.969, which was however obviously lower than the former. Epitashvili et al. have demonstrated that six surface EEG biomarkers (continuous epileptiform discharges, two types of rhythmic epileptiform discharges, polyspikes, repetitive activity, and polyspikes, frequent rhythmic bursting epileptiform activity or repetitive discharges) were significantly associated with an underlying cortical dysplasia (11). However, the single feature "Scalp EEG biomarkers" was also shown with less significance in our study, meaning the requirement of machine learning-based comprehensive evaluation progressed from signal processing analyses.

The predictive performance of a model depends on the large scale of dataset, the number and quality of features, and the design of the algorithms. Our study had some limitations. First, the current dataset was collected at a local tertiary hospital, and the sample may not be representative of all the regions in China and other countries. In the future, a prospective multicenter study with a larger sample size should be required. Second, ten features were included in our study, however the weight of each feature in the final model differed, which possibly increased the risk of overfitting or bias. Finally, some features were not included in this work, such as multiple seizure types, other MRI sequences (DTI) and PET-CT finding. The diagnostic validity of machine learning-based approach was associated with comprehensive parameters, thereby more features were considered, the higher level of performance we would achieve.

CONCLUSION

Taken together, this study highlighted the potential of a supervised machine learning-based model to differentiate FCD from GNTs in patients with epilepsy before surgery, contributing to appropriate surgical planning. With the availability and convenience of this model, clinicians will benefit from the novel approach in clinical applications.

AUTHOR CONTRIBUTIONS

YG and CHS: conceptualization and writing. YSL, LJY, and YC: methodology. WJM, ZJW, and JMZ: data collecting and confirmation. MPD and CHS: project administration and supervision. All authors contributed to the article and approved the submitted version.

REFERENCES

1. Guerrini R, Dobyns WB. Malformations of cortical development: clinical features and genetic causes. *Lancet Neurol.* (2014) 13:710–26. doi: 10.1016/S1474-4422(14)70040-7
2. Piao YS, Lu DH, Chen L, Liu J, Wang W, Liu L, et al. Neuropathological findings in intractable epilepsy: 435 Chinese cases. *Brain Pathol.* (2010) 20:902–8. doi: 10.1111/j.1750-3639.2010.00386.x
3. Kim DW, Lee SK, Chu K, Park KI, Lee SY, Lee CH, et al. Predictors of surgical outcome and pathologic considerations in focal cortical dysplasia. *Neurology.* (2009) 72:211–6. doi: 10.1212/01.wnl.0000327825.48731.c3
4. Englot DJ, Berger MS, Barbaro NM, Chang EF. Factors associated with seizure freedom in the surgical resection of glioneuronal tumors. *Epilepsia.* (2012) 53:51–7. doi: 10.1111/j.1528-1167.2011.03269.x
5. Krsek P, Maton B, Jayakar P, Dean P, Korman B, Rey G, et al. Incomplete resection of focal corticaldysplasia is the main predictor of poor postsurgical outcome. *Neurology.* (2009) 72:217–23. doi: 10.1212/01.wnl.0000334365.22854.d3
6. Zaatreh MM, Firlik KS, Spencer DD, Spencer SS. Temporal lobe tumoral epilepsy: characteristics and predictors of surgical outcome. *Neurology.* (2003) 61:636–41. doi: 10.1212/01.WNL.0000079374.78589.1B
7. Raybaud C, Shroff M, Rutka JT, Chuang SH. Imaging surgical epilepsy in children. *Childs Nerv Syst.* (2006) 22:786–809. doi: 10.1007/s00381-006-0132-5
8. Blumcke I, Thom M, Aronica E, Armstrong DD, Vinters HV, Palmini A, et al. The clinicopathologic spectrum of focal cortical dysplasias: a consensus classification proposed by anad hoc task force of the ILAE diagnostic methods commission. *Epilepsia.* (2011) 52:158–74. doi: 10.1111/j.1528-1167.2010.02777.x
9. Rácz A, Müller AM, Schwerdt J, Becker A, Vatter H, Elger CE. Age at epilepsy onset in patients with focal cortical dysplasias, gangliogliomas and dysembryoplastic neuroepithelial tumours. *Seizure.* (2018) 58:82–9. doi: 10.1016/j.seizure.2018.04.002

10. Phi JH, Paeng JC, Lee HS, Wang KC, Cho Bk, Lee JY, et al. Evaluation of focal cortical dysplasia and mixed neuronal and glial tumors in pediatric epilepsy patients using ^{18}F-FDG and ^{11}C-methionine pet. *J Nucl Med.* (2010) 51:728–34. doi: 10.2967/jnumed.109.070920
11. Epitashvili N, San Antonio-Arce V, Brandt A, Schulze-Bonhage A. Scalp electroencephalographic biomarkers in epilepsy patients with focal cortical dysplasia. *Ann Neurol.* (2018) 84:564–75. doi: 10.1002/ana.25322
12. Temko A, Thomas E, Marnane W, Lightbody G, Boylan GB. Performance assessment for EEG-based neonatal seizure detectors. *Clin Neurophysiol.* (2011) 122:474–82. doi: 10.1016/j.clinph.2010.06.035
13. Yao L, Cai M, Chen Y, Shen C, Shi L, Guo Y. Prediction of antiepileptic drug treatment outcomes of patients with newly diagnosed epilepsy by machine learning. *Epilepsy Behav.* (2019) 96:92–7. doi: 10.1016/j.yebeh.2019.04.006
14. Abbasi B, Goldenholz DM. Machine learning applications in epilepsy. *Epilepsia.* (2019) 60:2037–47. doi: 10.1111/epi.16333
15. Quinlan JR. *C4.5: Programs for Machine Learning.* Burlington, MA: Morgan Kaufmann Publishers Inc. (1993). 302p.
16. Breiman L. Random forests. *Mach Learn.* (2001) 45:5–32. doi: 10.1023/A:1010933404324
17. Cox DR. The regression analysis of binary sequences. *J Roy Stat Soc B.* (1958) 20:215–42. doi: 10.1111/j.2517-6161.1958.tb00292.x
18. Hearst MA, Dumais ST, Osuna E, Platt J, Scholkopf B. Support vector machines. *IEEE Intell Syst Appl.* (1998) 13:18–28. doi: 10.1109/5254.708428
19. Chen T, Guestrin C. XGBoost: a scalable tree boosting system. In: *Proceedings of the 22nd ACM SIGKDD International Conference on Knowledge Discovery and Data Mining.* San Francisco, CA: ACM (2016). p. 785–94.
20. Prokhorenkova LO, Gusev G, Vorobev A, Dorogush AV, Gulin A. CatBoost: unbiased boosting with categorical features. In: *Proceedings of the Advances in Neural Information Processing System.* Montreal (2018). p. 6639–9.
21. Ke G, Meng Q, Finley T, Wang TF, Chen W, Ma WD, et al. LightGBM: a highly efficient gradient boosting decision tree. In: *Proceeding of the Advances in Neural Information Processing Systems.* Long Beach, CA (2017). p. 3149–57.
22. Berg AT, Berkovic SF, Brodie MJ, Buchhalter J, Cross JH, van Emde Boas, et al. Revised terminology and concepts for organization of seizures and epilepsies: report of the ILAE commission on classification and terminology, 2005-2009. *Epilepsia.* (2010) 51:676–85. doi: 10.1111/j.1528-1167.2010.02522.x
23. Louis DN, Ohgaki H, Wiestler OD, Cavenee WK, Burger PC, Jouvet A, et al. The 2007 WHO classification of tumours of the central nervous system. *Acta Neuropathol.* (2007) 114:97–109. doi: 10.1007/s00401-007-0243-4
24. Fisher RS, Cross JH, French JA, Higurashi N, Hirsch E, Jansen FE, et al. Operational classification of seizure types by the international league against epilepsy: position paper of the ILAE commission for classification and terminology. *Epilepsia.* (2017) 58:522–30. doi: 10.1111/epi.13670
25. Choi H, Hamberger MJ, Munger Clary H, Leob R, Onchiri FM, Baker G, et al. Seizure frequency and patient-centered outcome assessment in epilepsy. *Epilepsia.* (2014) 55:1205–12. doi: 10.1111/epi.12672
26. Hong SJ, Bernhardt BC, Caldairou B, Hall JA, Guiot MC, Schrader D, et al. Multimodal MRI profiling of focal cortical dysplasia type II. *Neurology.* (2017) 88:734–42. doi: 10.1212/WNL.0000000000003632
27. Krsek P, Pieper T, Karlmeier A, Hildebrandt M, Kolodziejczyk D, Winkler P, et al. Different presurgical characteristics and seizure outcomes in children with focal cortical dysplasia type I or II. *Epilepsia.* (2009) 50:125–37. doi: 10.1111/j.1528-1167.2008.01682.x
28. Demir MK, Yapicier O, Yilmaz B, Kiliç T. Magnetic resonance imaging findings of mixed neuronal-glial tumors with pathologic correlation: a review. *Acta Neurol Belg.* (2018) 118:379–86. doi: 10.1007/s13760-018-0981-1
29. Abdel Razek AAK, Elsebaie NA, Zamora C, Castillo M. Imaging of neuronal and mixed glioneuronal tumors. *J Comput Assist Tomogr.* (2020) 44:356–69. doi: 10.1097/RCT.0000000000001010
30. Chawla NV, Bowyer KW, Hall LO Kegelmeyer WP. SMOTE: synthetic minority over-sampling technique. *J Artif Intrll Res.* (2002) 16:321–57. doi: 10.1613/jair.953
31. Pedregosa F, Varoquaux G, Gramfort A, Michel V, Thirion B, Grisel O, et al. Scikit-learn: machine learning in python. *J Mach Learn Res.* (2011) 12:2825–30. doi: 10.5555/1953048.2078195
32. Fawcett T. An introduction to ROC analysis. *Pattern Recogn Lett.* (2006) 27:861–74. doi: 10.1016/j.patrec.2005.10.010
33. Yang Y, Pedersen JO. A comparative study on feature selection in text categorization. In: *Proceedings of the Fourteenth International Conference on Machine Learning.* Burlington, MA: Morgan Kaufmann Publishers Inc. (1997). p. 412–20
34. Paldino MJ, Hedges K, Zhang W. Independent contribution of individual white matter pathways to language function in pediatric epilepsy patients. *Neuroimage Clin.* (2014) 6:327–32. doi: 10.1016/j.nicl.2014.09.017
35. Grinspan ZM, Patel AD, Hafeez B, Abramson EL, Kern LM. Predicting frequent emergency department use among children with epilepsy: a retrospective cohort study using electronic health data from 2 centers. *Epilepsia.* (2018) 59:155–69. doi: 10.1111/epi.13948

17

Semi-Automatic Extraction of Functional Dynamic Networks Describing Patient's Epileptic Seizures

Gaëtan Frusque [1], Pierre Borgnat [2], Paulo Gonçalves [1] and Julien Jung [3,4]*

[1] Univ Lyon, Inria, CNRS, ENS de Lyon, UCB Lyon 1, LIP UMR 5668, Lyon, France, [2] Univ Lyon, CNRS, ENS de Lyon, UCB Lyon 1, Laboratoire de Physique, UMR 5672, Lyon, France, [3] National Institute of Health and Medical Research U1028/National Center for Scientific Research, Mixed Unit of Research 5292, Lyon Neuroscience Research Center, Lyon, France, [4] Department of Functional Neurology and Epileptology, Member of the ERN EpiCARE Lyon University Hospital and Lyon 1 University, Lyon, France

***Correspondence:**
Gaëtan Frusque
gaetan.frusque@ens-lyon.fr

Intracranial electroencephalography (EEG) studies using stereotactic EEG (SEEG) have shown that during seizures, epileptic activity spreads across several anatomical regions from the seizure onset zone toward remote brain areas. A full and objective characterization of this patient-specific time-varying network is crucial for optimal surgical treatment. Functional connectivity (FC) analysis of SEEG signals recorded during seizures enables to describe the statistical relations between all pairs of recorded signals. However, extracting meaningful information from those large datasets is time consuming and requires high expertise. In the present study, we first propose a novel method named Brain-wide Time-varying Network Decomposition (BTND) to characterize the dynamic epileptogenic networks activated during seizures in individual patients recorded with SEEG electrodes. The method provides a number of pathological FC subgraphs with their temporal course of activation. The method can be applied to several seizures of the patient to extract reproducible subgraphs. Second, we compare the activated subgraphs obtained by the BTND method with visual interpretation of SEEG signals recorded in 27 seizures from nine different patients. As a whole, we found that activated subgraphs corresponded to brain regions involved during the course of the seizures and their time course was highly consistent with classical visual interpretation. We believe that the proposed method can complement the visual analysis of SEEG signals recorded during seizures by highlighting and characterizing the most significant parts of epileptic networks with their activation dynamics.

Keywords: epilepsy, functional connectivity, SEEG, epileptogenic networks, dynamical graph, subgraphs extraction

1. INTRODUCTION

About 30–40% of epileptic patients are drug resistant (1). For those patients, surgical resection of the epileptogenic brain structures is considered to promote seizure freedom (1). Intracranial EEG using depth EEG recordings or the stereoencephalography (SEEG) method is often required to guide tailored-surgical resection (2, 3).

The primary aim of SEEG is to delineate precisely the epileptogenic regions. However, since the pioneering works in SEEG, it has been shown that seizures cannot be considered as static phenomena with a single focus activation leading to clinical manifestations (4). SEEG recordings of focal seizures typically show that the epileptic activity spreads during seizures across several anatomical regions. It begins at the seizure onset zone and spreads toward remote brain areas. This dynamical pathological process can be described by several brain states characterized by transient and abnormal connectivity profiles within the epileptogenic network (5). A full and objective characterization of this patient-specific dynamic network is crucial for optimal surgical treatment.

Understanding brain network modifications operating at different time scales in the interictal state and during seizures is a very active stream of research. This is in line with computational neuroscience studies modeling neurological diseases as brain network disease (6–11).

In the field of epileptology, the structure of epileptic (or ictal) networks has been explored using connectivity analysis (functional or effective connectivity) and more recently, graph-theory analysis, (5). Functional connectivity (FC) approaches, based on linear or non-linear measures, quantify the statistical relations between any pair of recorded SEEG signals and their evolution across time. In most of the studies, pairwise correlations between remote sites are computed at specific time points [for a review, see (5)]. Those approaches unveil the organizational interactions of different regions of interest in the brains. They have proved very fruitful to investigate the neurophysiological correlations of symptoms during seizures, or to describe several subtypes of focal epilepsy involving specific networks (12–14). Graph theory is the study of graphs, which are mathematical structures used to model networks, and specifically pairwise relations between objects (8, 15). A graph is made up of vertices (also called nodes) that are connected by edges. Graph theory approaches allow the description of both local and global characteristics (16). For epilepsy, the nodes usually represent electrode contacts and the edges represent the FC measures. The resulting graph structure is known to contain relevant fingerprints of the seizure dynamic. Studying network structures with graph theory provides mathematical tools to investigate different subtypes of epilepsy (17). For example, it has been shown that the properties of networks' topology are different for temporal lobe, mesial temporal lobe, and neocortical epilepsy (18). Moreover, some studies suggest that investigating local properties of the network structure through graph theory concepts provides biomarkers for epileptogenic focus localization (19–21). Lastly, dynamic graph theory can also provide step-by-step modeling of the propagation of the seizure in the brain (19, 22).

A major challenge for the study of ictal networks is that seizures are a highly dynamical process with rapid transitions between network states (5, 23). To track network changes during the seizures, the network organization has to be described at short time scales. In the most straightforward approach, FC approaches forming the backbone of the network are estimated at different time steps of the seizure. Therefore, they are prone to create spurious connections and constitute a noisy estimation of the pathologic dynamic network. Moreover, as the brain activity is commonly monitored with more than 100 electrode contacts distributed along the stereotactic rods, the number of FC scales quadratically (100 electrode contacts providing around 5000 FC measures), making the study of FC over time a resources consuming task that requires high expertise.

One advantage of SEEG monitoring is to allow the recording of several seizures from the same patient, with the same measurement points (or nodes), yielding thus as many realizations of identically distributed dynamical networks of FC. Hence, several seizures from the same patient can be investigated that may share some connectivity features but with different dynamics. Methodological tools have to be proposed to extract relevant information from those large datasets. Ideally, such methods should summarize the dynamics of the seizures by providing several epileptogenic networks, with stable network structures, that characterize the different steps of the seizures and that are involved in the production and the propagation of the ictal events. Those network states may be common to the different seizures of the patient, but the timeline activation should follow a pattern that remains specific to each seizure (22).

Along these lines, we propose a novel semi-automatic method to characterize the dynamic epileptogenic network quantitatively and across time using SEEG signals. We propose to perform the joint analysis of all seizures of the same patient, first to reduce the measurement uncertainty in the calculation of FC indices, and second to make robust the identification of a time-functional pattern, systematic in all seizures and characteristic of a patient's pathology. First, the full FC matrix is computed for each time step using a classical FC measure, namely the Phase Locking Value (PLV) (24, 25). Then, the method extracts several pathological subgraphs with their own activation score during seizures. We expect each subgraph to comprise several brain nodes with high connectivity values. The paper is organized as follows: We extend our previous work (26) to seizures with different durations, we call this method the Brain-wide Time-varying Network Decomposition (BTND). On the application side, we validate the clinical use of the method on a larger clinical dataset.

2. MATERIALS AND METHODS

2.1. Description of the Brain-Wide Time-Varying Network Decomposition Method

For each patient, the dataset is composed of several SEEG recordings for different seizures. Seizures can have different durations. The proposed strategy can be summarized in four steps: (a) We chop each recording into short segments; (b) for each segment, we estimate via FC measures the connectivity for each pair of electrode contacts; (c) we rearrange the FC measures into a list of matrices representing the time evolution of FC for each seizure of a patient; (d) the list of matrices representing the multi-seizures brain-wide time-varying network is decomposed into FC subgraphs characteristic of one patient but common to

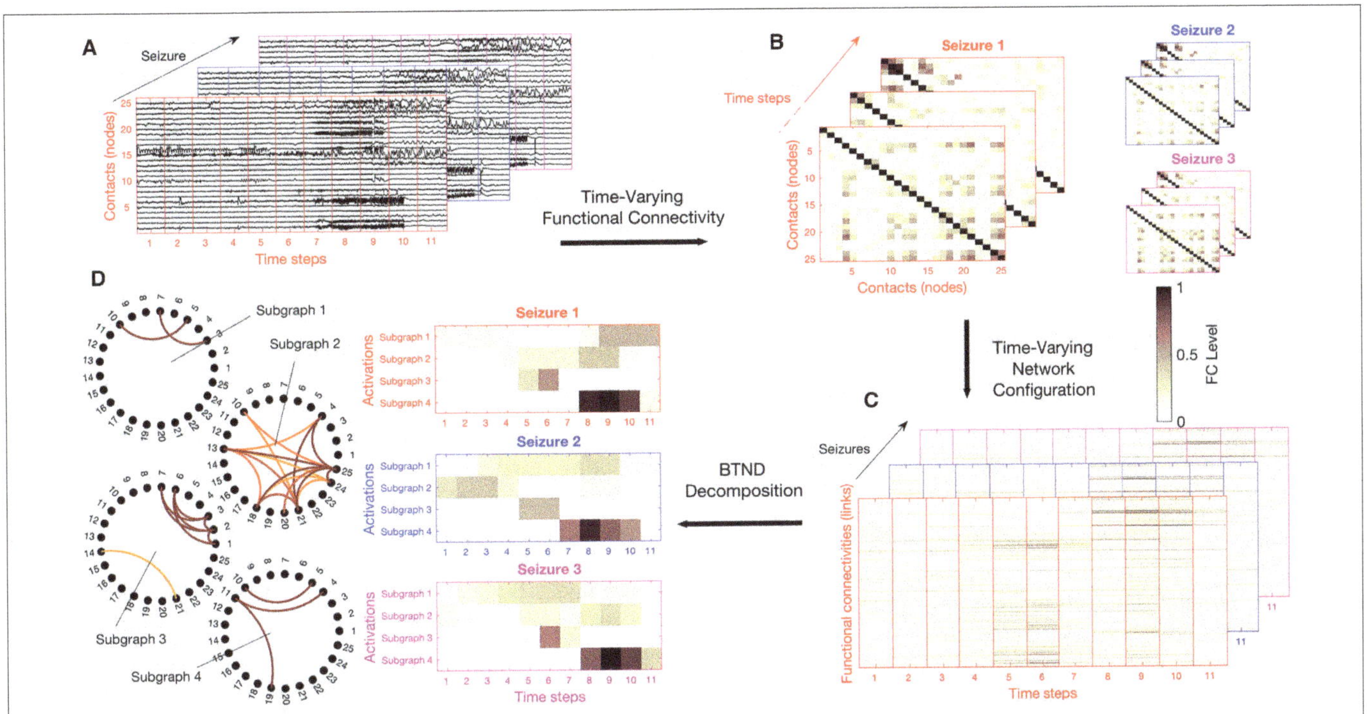

FIGURE 1 | Overview of the strategy: **(A)** We chop each recording in time segment, potentially with some overlapping. **(B)** For each segment, we compute the connectivity level of each pair of electrode contacts with a Functional connectivity (FC) measure. **(C)** We rearrange the FC measures in a vector, stacked in time they form for each seizure an FC matrix. **(D)** The list of FC matrix is decomposed into a set of FC graphs with their activation profiles respective to each seizure. Here, the number of subgraph is $K = 4$, and the activation profiles of each subgraph are represented for the 3 available seizures of this patient.

all his seizures, along with their activation profile specific to each seizure. The main steps of the method are illustrated in **Figure 1**.

2.2. Representation of the Multi-Seizure Brain-Wide Time-Varying Network

Practically, FC measurements are stored in a three-dimensional structure $\mathbf{X}_{lt}\{s\}$ corresponding to the FC of index l at time segment t and for the seizure s. The list of matrix $\mathbf{X}\{s\} \in \mathbb{R}^{L\times T(s)}$ $\forall s\,(1,\ldots,S)$ is the mathematical representation of the multi-seizures brain-wide time-varying network. Here, S is the total number of seizures recorded for the same patient. We remind that the number of time steps $T(s)$ can vary for each seizure. **Figure 1C** illustrates an example of list of matrices $\mathbf{X}\{s\}$.

2.3. The Optimization Problem Related to the BTND Method

The core of the BTND method is then to seek, for each seizure, for the following decomposition:

$$\mathbf{X}\{s\} \approx \mathbf{F}\mathbf{V}^t\{s\} \tag{1}$$

where $\mathbf{F} \in \mathbb{R}^{L\times K}$ contains the K FC subgraphs and $\mathbf{V}\{s\} \in \mathbb{R}^{T(s)\times K}$ are their respective temporal activations corresponding to the specific seizure s. This approach directly entails the requested decomposition since the columns of the matrix **F** contains the weights of the edges in the sub-graphs, as it can be seen in **Figure 1D** and matrices $\mathbf{V}\{s\}$ directly correspond to the activation profiles of each seizure depicted in **Figure 1D**.

However, the solution for the decomposition (1) is not unique, and to favor handily interpretability from the medical viewpoint, we impose several constraints on the components **F** and $\mathbf{V}\{s\}$:

a) because most of the functional connectivity measures and activation indices are naturally positive values, we impose **F** and **V** to be **non-negative** matrices;
b) to limit the complexity of the inferred subgraphs, we restrict the number of non-zero significant FC values, yielding a sparse matrix **F**. The **sparsity** constraint is meaningful in the context of epilepsy, where a large number of functional connectivities can be passively implied in the neurological process;
c) to promote FC subgraphs that are continuously activated over specific periods, we impose **sparsity** and **compactness** on $\mathbf{V}\{s\}$. These two constraints drastically improve the interpretability of the solution, as they prompt sparse and piecewise continuous activation periods that are close to cluster-like solutions. Formally, they correspond to the fused lasso constraint that reads:

$$C(\mathbf{v},\gamma,\eta)\ :\ \gamma\sum_{t=1}^{T}|\,v_t\,| + \eta\sum_{t=1}^{T-1}|\,v_{t+1}-v_t\,| + \sum_{t=1}^{T}v_t^2 \leq 1, \tag{2}$$

where the parameter γ and the parameter η compel each activation profile $\mathbf{v} = \mathbf{V}_{:k}\{s\}$, to be sparse and compact, respectively. As for the third term in expression (2), it prevents incoherent solutions due to scaling indeterminacy (27).

Finally, the BTND boils down to an instance of joint non-negative matrix factorization (28–31) that takes on the following form:

$$\begin{aligned} \underset{\mathbf{F},\mathbf{V}\{1\},\ldots,\mathbf{V}\{S\}}{\operatorname{argmin}} \quad & \sum_{s=1}^{S} \zeta_s \parallel \mathbf{X}\{s\} - \mathbf{F}\mathbf{V}\{s\}^t \parallel_F^2 + \lambda S \sum_{k=1}^{K} \sum_{l=1}^{L} \mid F_{lk} \mid, \\ s.t. \quad & C(\mathbf{V}_{:k}\{s\}, \gamma_s, \eta_s) \quad \forall k \in \{1,\ldots,K\}, \quad \forall s \in \{1,\ldots,S\}, \\ s.t. \quad & \mathbf{F} \geq 0, \qquad \mathbf{V}\{s\} \geq 0 \quad \forall s \in \{1,\ldots,S\}. \end{aligned} \tag{3}$$

The ζ_s are free parameters to balance the relative importance of each seizure (in our study, we consider all seizures evenly and select the ζ_s parameter according to the energy of each seizure, see the **Supplementary Materials** for more precision). The sparsity factor γ_s and the compactness factor η_s are chosen to adapt to the particular duration of each seizure s.

Then, the method is associated with three hyperparameters: λ and γ, respectively, controlling the **sparsity** level of the FC subgraphs and the activation profiles, and η regulating the temporal **compactness** of the activation profiles.

2.4. Additional Comments on BTND

Let us stress that the optimization problem of Equation (3) is non-convex, and therefore, different initial conditions yield different solutions corresponding to local maxima. As it is common practice for non-convex methods in machine learning [e.g., k-means for data clustering, (32)], we repeatedly solve (3) with a different initialization and retain the one that reached the smaller minimum cost function. In practice, we empirically chose 20 trials. As for the other hyper-parameters, we observed that $\eta = 0.2$ produces coherent activation profiles. Also, fixing $\lambda = \gamma$ simplifies the procedure without altering the results significantly. Then, λ is tuned so as to identify the 20% most resilient activated FC. To select the most pertinent number of subgraphs, we successively compute the decomposition for K ranging from 3 to 10. Based on an Elbow criterion and on visual inspection, we compare the quality of the resulting temporal activation and subgraphs, identifying thus the best value for K. Finally, we normalize each subgraph such that their connectivity strengths are between 0 and 1. We only retain connections above some threshold (empirically set to 0.2 in our experiments) to eliminate non-significant interactions.

For more details on the practical use of the method, see the **Supplementary Materials.** We provide the URL[1] for a Github repository with Matlab implementation of the proposed BTND method.

3. APPLICATION ON A REAL DATASET OF EPILEPTIC PATIENTS

3.1. Patients

To illustrate the clinical relevance of the BTND method, we applied the method on seizures recorded with intracranial EEG in 9 epileptic patients.

We included 9 adult patients suffering from drug-resistant focal epilepsy, followed in the Department of Functional Neurology and Epileptology at Lyon's University Hospital, who underwent intracranial EEG with SEEG according to the following criteria: (i) at least 1 seizure recorded during long-term monitoring; and (ii) conventional visual analysis of the SEEG signals identified clearly the seizure-onset zone.

Clinical details of all the patient included are listed in **Table 1**.

Among them, 8 patients presented seizures suggesting a temporal lobe involvement but with clinical features or morphological alterations on brain magnetic resonance imaging (MRI) not typical for medial temporal epilepsy requiring intracranial EEG. For one patient, clinical semiology suggested an involvement of operculo-insular cortex. Three patients underwent surgical resection of the epileptogenic cortex and all had a good surgical outcome (Engel class Ia for all patients with a follow-up duration between 4 and 48 months). For 2 patients, a focal thermolesion using SEEG electrodes was performed, resulting in a dramatic improvement of epilepsy (Engel Ia for both patients with 4 and 5 months of follow-up). For 2 patients, surgery was contraindicated because of the involvement of both temporal lobes during seizures. For 2 patients, surgical resection is planned based on SEEG findings but has not been performed at the time of the present study.

This study, involving human participants, was reviewed and approved by Ethics Committee CPP Lyon Sud EST IV (24/05/2012 N2012-A00516-37). The patients/participants provided their written informed consent to participate in this study.

3.2. SEEG Recordings

Intracerebral multi-contact electrodes (5–15 contacts, diameter 0.8 mm, length 2 mm, and 1.5 mm apart) were implanted according to Talairach's stereotactic method (3). Electrode location was verified with post-implantation MRI. Prolonged extra-operative recordings were performed to capture each patient's habitual seizures.

SEEG data were acquired with a 256 channel video EEG monitoring system, Micromed video EEG acquisition system (SD LTM express, Micromed, Treviso, Italy), using the following parameters: sampling rate 256 Hz, high-pass filter 0.15 Hz, low-pass filter 200 Hz, notch filter at 50 Hz.

The median number of bipolar contacts recorded per patient was 101 (range 64–130). The main cerebral structures targeted by intracranial electrodes for each patient are listed in the **Supplementary Table 1**. As a whole, for all patients, the medial temporal lobe (anterior hippocampus, posterior hippocampus, amygdala, entorhinal cortex), the temporal lateral neocortex and the insular cortex were always targeted. Depending on the

[1] https://github.com/FrusqueGaetan/BTND

TABLE 1 | Clinical details of each patient.

Patient	Brain MRI	Interictal EEG	Ictal EEG	FDG PET	Ictal semiology	Surgery	Surgical outcome
1	LT pole atrophy	LT slow wave activity and temporal spikes	LT ictal activity	left medial temporal hypoM + left anterior temporal neocortical hypoM	Oro alimentary automatisms + right hand dystonia + loss of consciousness	Left ALT	Ia (24 m)
2	LT post surgical sequelae	LT&RT spikes with left predominance	LT ictal activity	Left medial temporal hypoM + right medial temporal hypoM	Loss of consciousness + speech arrest	NA	NA
3	Right HS	Temporal spikes + temporal background slowing	RT basal ictal activity	Right medial temporal + RT pole hypo M + RT lateral neocortical hypoM	Left hand paresthesias + Ascending visceral sensation + tachycardia + loss of consciousness post icttal confusion	Right ATL	Ia (16 m)
4	Left HS, LT pole atrophy	LT&RT spikes with left predominance	LT ictal activity	LT pole + LT lateral neocortical hypo M	Oro alimentary automatismes + mental slowing with preserved consciousness	left ATL	Ia (48 m)
5	Post surgical right temporal lesion	RT spikes	RT ictal activity	RT pole hypoM	Loss of consciousness + bilateral dystonic arm posturing + oral automatisms	NA	NA
6	Normal	Normal	Left central activity	Left perisylvian Hypo M including anterior temporal gyrus + temporal pole + insula	Bilateral tonic posturing of arms + right head deviation + right arm paresthesias	Left operculo insular thermolesion	Ia (4 m)
7	Left amygdalar hyperintensity	LT spikes	LT ictal activity	LT pole hypoM + left medial temporal lobe hypoM	Cephalic sensation + dreamy state + language disturbance	Left medial temporal thermolesion	Ia (5 m)
8	Right HS	RT slow wave activity	RT ictal activity	Right medial temporal hypoM + right anterior temporal neocortical hypoM	Oro alimentary automat. + preserved consciousness + left facial clonus	NA	NA
9	Right HS	RT spikes	RT ictal activity	Right medial temporal hypoM	Verbal automatisms + dysgeusia + loss of consciousness	NA	NA

HS, hippocampal sclerosis; LT, left temporal; RT, right temporal; hypoM, hypometabolism; ATL, anterior temporal lobectomy; NA, not performed/surgical outcome is expressed as Engel Class.

electroclinical findings of each patient, frontal lobe, parietal lobe, and occipital cortex were targeted.

For 9 patients, all available seizures were extracted, forming a dataset composed of a total of 27 seizures. For 6 patients, 3 seizures were analyzed. For 2 patients, 4 seizures were analyzed and for 1 patient, a single seizure was available for analysis. For each seizure, we extracted signals for at least 1 min before the onset of the seizure and the whole course of the seizure.

The duration of the seizure was largely heterogeneous both at the inter-individual and intra-individual level. The median length of the seizures across patients was 96 s (range 18–337).

3.3. SEEG Signal Analysis

SEEG signals are considered in bipolar derivations; hence each signal is referenced to its closest neighbor. A high-pass filter, with a cut-off frequency equal to 20 Hz at -3 dB was applied on SEEG signals in order to highlight the high-frequency activity typical of seizure activity, particularly at seizure onset (33).

For each seizure, we computed the FC matrices during the pre-seizure period and the course of the whole seizure using a classical connectivity measure, the PLV (24, 25). Briefly, the PLV quantifies the synchronization in phase between two signal. The phase of each signal is computed by the Hilbert transform. The PLV is the time average of the relative phase difference. To compute the FC matrices, the SEEG signals were windowed with 4 s sliding windows moving by steps of 1 s. For each 4 s window, the PLV between all pairs of bipolar contacts was computed to produce the overall network at each time step.

Finally, the BTND method is applied to the set of several seizures for each patient, to decompose all seizures in several subgraphs, activating through time.

3.4. Comparison of Network Dynamics Estimated Through Conventional Visual Analysis and the BTND Method

Each seizure was pragmatically segmented in three main periods defined by visual analysis: seizure-onset, seizure propagation, and seizure ending. Visual analysis of the seizures was performed by an expert in clinical SEEG interpretation (JJ). Seizure onset corresponded to the time period with a dramatic change of SEEG signals with either low-voltage fast activity (typically above 20 Hz) or rhythmic spikes in a subset of electrode contacts. Seizure propagation corresponded to an extended time period where ictal SEEG discharge spread to several brain structures either locally or remotely from the seizure onset zone. The recruitment of these regions in the propagation zone can happen either by independent activation of the single areas or by activating multiple areas at the same time. Lastly, a seizure was supposed to have ended when the activation across brain structures was mostly synchronous (typically synchronous spikes) and stable in time and resolved ultimately.

For each time period, we determined the electrode contacts that were involved in the ictal wave with a conventional visual inspection. The electrode contacts were then pooled in several anatomical predefined subregions.

For each patient, the output of the BTND method provided the temporal profile of activation of several common subgraphs of the whole network during each seizure. The list of activated subgraphs at each time period of the seizure was then collected. Each subgraph included several contacts with strong functional connectivity. At each time period, we determined which anatomical subregions were connected based on the activated subgraphs.

Lastly, a qualitative comparison between the set of activated structures determined by visual analysis and the BTND method was performed for each seizure.

3.5. Results for the Real Dataset of Epileptic Patients

The overall functional connectivity organization was extracted in all 27 seizures using the BTND method. This means that the seizures (from 1 to 4) of one patient are processed together according to BTND. **Table 2** provides the qualitative comparison between the set of activated structures between visual analysis and the BTND method for patients 1 and 2. Also, **Tables 3, 4** show the same qualitative comparison for, respectively, patients 2–4 and patients 5–9.

Using this method, we found, in the case of 6 patients, that 6 distinct functional subgraphs characterized the organization of seizures; 7 subgraphs for 1 patient; 5 subgraphs for another one; and only 4 subgraphs characterized seizures for the last patient. However, for each patient, some subgraphs were more strongly activated before seizure onset or were continuously activated before seizure onset and remained active during the course of the seizures. Those subgraphs were considered as non-specific subgraphs for the ictal events. For 5 patients, 2 subgraphs were non-specific while for 4 patients a single subgraph was non-specific.

At seizure onset, a single subgraph was activated for 1 patient, two subgraphs were activated for 4 patients, three subgraphs were activated for 3 patients, and 5 subgraphs were activated for 1 patient. For 24 seizures in 6 patients, the seizure onset determined by visual analysis overlapped closely with the network disclosed by the BTND method. For those patients, the cortical regions underlying the seizure-onset zone determined through visual analysis were included in the seizure-onset subgraphs. However, the seizure-onset subgraph also included other regions with strong functional connectivity not directly outside of the seizure-onset zone. For one of those 6 patients (Pt 2), the seizure involved either the left or the right medial temporal lobe at seizure onset. The seizure-onset subgraph was different for each seizure, and the lateralization of the activated structures was concordant with visual analysis. For 3 seizures in one patient (Pt 9), the seizure-onset subgraph was discordant from the seizure onset-zone. For this patient, the seizure-onset zone involved either right or left medial temporal lobe depending on the seizure. The seizure-onset subgraph for this patient was wrongly lateralized to the right or the left temporal lobe.

During seizure propagation, there was always a close spatial overlap between the activated subgraphs and the brain regions involved at each part of the seizure in all patients. For the 27 seizures in the 9 patients, the brain regions involved during seizure propagation were included in activated subgraphs. However, the congruence between activated subgraphs and regions disclosed by visual analysis was not perfect: a minority of regions were revealed by the BTND method but was not detected by visual analysis.

During seizure ending, a tight spatial overlap was also observed between activated subgraphs and brain regions determined by visual analysis. For 23 seizures, the brain regions involved at seizure ending were included in activated subgraphs. For 4 seizures in 1 patient, visual analysis disclosed more activated regions than the BTND method (Pt 4).

The detailed results are now presented for two cases (Pt 1 and Pt 2).

CASE 1:

Pt 1 is a 49 years old male patient. Presurgical non-invasive investigations suggested left temporal lobe epilepsy but some radiological features were considered as atypical for mesial temporal lobe epilepsy syndrome and prompted invasive EEG with SEEG. SEEG targeted several regions within left temporal lobe (anterior hippocampus, posterior hippocampus, amygdala, temporal pole, anterior temporal neocortex, posterior temporal lobe), left orbito frontal cortex, and right temporal lobe (right amygdala, right anterior temporal neocortex).

Three seizures were recorded during SEEG. During the 3 seizures, the initial seizure-onset activity developed in left anterior and posterior hippocampus with secondary involvement of the temporal pole, amygdalar nucleus, and left anterior temporal neocortex at the end of the seizures.

The BTND method applied to the three seizures decomposed the connectivity pattern in 6 subgraphs. **Figure 2** shows the recording of two seizures (seizure 1 and 2) of the patient 1 for selected electrode contacts. Below each recording, we provide the activation profiles of all subgraphs obtained by the BTND for this specific seizure. On top is represented the main cerebral structures targeted by intracranial electrodes for this patient. **Figure 3** shows the 6 FC subgraphs revealed by the BTND.

One subgraph was active before the seizure and during the whole course of the seizures. This subgraph was mostly composed of local connections within temporal lobe (mostly within anterior hippocampus, posterior hippocampus, amygdala). At the seizure onset, during the first seconds of the seizure, there was a reproducible activation of one subgraph, that involved mostly connections between anterior hippocampus and amygdala, posterior hippocampus, and posterior temporal neocortex. A few seconds later, a strong activation of another subgraph was observed that involved mostly connections between medial temporal lobe and temporal pole. During the course of the seizures, there was a consistent activation of three other subgraphs, with a very similar pattern between seizures. Those

TABLE 2 | Qualitative comparison between the set of activated structures determined by visual analysis and the BTND method for the patient 1 and 2.

		Seizure onset	Seizure propagation	Seizure ending
Patient 1	Seiz. 1	**Clinical**:L ANT HIPPOC + L POST HIPPOC **Method**: subg3 + (subg1)	**Clinical**: L ANT HIPPOC + L POST HIPPOC + L TEMP POLE **Method**: subg3 + subg2 + (subg1)	**Clinical**: L ANT HIPPOC + L POST HIPPOC + L TEMP POLE + L ANT TEMP NEOCORTEX **Method**: subg4 + subg5 + subg6 + (subg1)
	Seiz. 2	**Clinical**:L ANT HIPPOC + L POST HIPPOC **Method**: subg3 + (subg1)	**Clinical**: L ANT HIPPOC + L POST HIPPOC + L TEMP POLE **Method**: subg3 + subg2 + (subg1)	**Clinical**: L ANT HIPPOC + L POST HIPPOC + L TEMP POLE + L ANT TEMP NEOCORTEX **Method**: subg4 + subg5 + subg6 + (subg1)
	Seiz. 3	**Clinical**:L ANT HIPPOC + L POST HIPPOC **Method**: subg3 + (subg1)	**Clinical**: L ANT HIPPOC + L POST HIPPOC + L TEMP POLE **Method**: subg3 + subg2 + (subg1)	**Clinical**: L ANT HIPPOC + L POST HIPPOC + L TEMP POLE + L ANT TEMP NEOCORTEX **Method**: subg4 + subg5 + subg6 + (subg1)
	subgraphs	**subg1**: L ANT HIPPOC + L AMYG, **subg2**: L ANT HIPPOC + L POST HIPPOC + L TEMPORAL POLE + L AMYG, **subg3**: L ANT HIPPOC + L POST HIPPOC + L POST TEMPORAL NEOCORTEX + L AMYG, **subg4**: L POST TEMPORAL NEOCORTEX + L TEMPORAL POLE + L ANT HIPPOC + L POST HIPPOC **subg5**: L ANT TEMPORAL NEOCORTEX + L TEMP POLE, **subg6**: L TEMPORAL POLE + L ANT TEMPORAL NEOCORTEX.		
Patient 2	Seiz. 1	**Clinical**: L ANT HIPPOC + L POST HIPPOC **Method**: subg1 + (subg7)	**Clinical**: L ANT HIPPOC + L POST HIPPOC + L ANT TEMPORAL NEOCORTEX + L ORBITO FRONTAL NEOCORTEX **Method**: subg2 + (subg7)	**Clinical**: R ANT HIPPOC + R POST HIPPOC + R AMYG **Method**:subg3 + subg4 + subg5 + subg6 + (subg7)
	Seiz. 2	**Clinical**: R ANT HIPPOC + R POST HIPPOC + R AMYG + R ENTORHINAL CORTEX **Method**: subg3 + subg4 + (subg7)	**Clinical**: R ANT HIPPOC + R POST HIPPOC + R AMYG + R ENTORHINAL CORTEX + R ANT TEMPORAL NEOCORTEX **Method**: subg5 + (subg7)	**Clinical**: L ANT HIPPOC + L POST HIPPOC **Method**: subg1 + subg2 + subg6 + (subg7)
	Seiz. 3	**Clinical**: R ANT HIPPOC + R POST HIPPOC + R AMYG + R ENTORHINAL CORTEX **Method**: subg3 + subg4 + (subg7)	**Clinical**: R ANT HIPPOC + R POST HIPPOC + R AMYG + R ENTORHINAL CORTEX + R ANT TEMPORAL NEOCORTEX **Method**: subg5 + (subg7)	**Clinical**: L ANT HIPPOC + L POST HIPPOC **Method**: subg1 + subg5 + subg6 + (subg7)
	subgraphs	**subg1**: L ANT HIPPOC + L POST HIPPOC, **subg2**: L ANT HIPPOC + L POST HIPPOC + L ENTORHINAL CORTEX + L ORBITO FRONTAL CORTEX, **subg3**: R ANT HIPPOC + R POST HIPOC + R AMYG + R ENTORHINAL CORTEX, **subg4**: R ANT HIPPOC + R POST HIPOC + R AMYG + R ENTORHINAL CORTEX, **subg5**: R ANT HIPPOC + R POST HIPPOC + R ENTORHINAL CORTEX + R ORBITO FRONTAL CORTEX + R ANT TEMPORAL NEORTEX, **subg6**: R ANT TEMPORAL NEOCORTEX + R POST TEMPORAL NEOCORTEX, **subg7**: L ANT TEMPORAL NEOCORTEX		

Legend; subg: subgraph, Seiz.: seizure, L: left, R: right, ANT HIPPOC: anterior hippocampus, POST HIPPOC: posterior hippocampus, ANT TEMPORAL NEOCORTEX: anterior temporal neocortex, POST TEMPORAL NEOCORTEX: posterior temporal neocortex, AMYG: amygdala.

TABLE 3 | Qualitative comparison between the set of activated structures determined by visual analysis and the Brain-wide Time-varying Network Decomposition (BTND) method for the patients 3, 4, and 5 (see legend **Table 2**).

		Seizure onset	Seizure propagation	Seizure ending
Patient 3	Seiz. 1	**Clinical**: R ANT HIPPOC **Method**: (subg2)	**Clinical**: R ANT HIPPOC + R POST HIPPOC + R ENT CX **Method**: subg1	**Clinical**: R ANT HIPPOC + R POST HIPPOC + R ENT CX + R TEMPORAL LATERAL + R OCCIPITAL CX + R PARIETAL CX + R POST CENTRAL OPERC **Method**: subg3 + subg4 + subg5 + subg6
	Seiz. 2	**Clinical**: R ANT HIPPOC + R POST HIPPOC **Method**: (subg2) + subg3 + subg5	**Clinical**: R ANT HIPPOC + R POST HIPPOC + R ENT CX **Method**: subg1	**Clinical**: R ANT HIPPOC + R POST HIPPOC + R ENT CX + R TEMPORAL LATERAL + R OCCIPITAL CX + R PARIETAL CX + R POST CENTRAL OPERC **Method**: subg3 + subg4 + subg5 + subg6
	Seiz. 3	**Clinical**: R ANT HIPPOC + R POST HIPPOC **Method**: (subg2) + subg3 + subg5	**Clinical**: R ANT HIPPOC + R POST HIPPOC + R ENT CX + R TEMPORAL LATERAL + R OCCIPITAL CX + R PARIETAL CX + R POST CENTRAL OPERC **Method**: subg1 + (subg2) + subg4 + subg6	**Clinical**: R ANT HIPPOC + R POST HIPPOC + R ENT CX + R TEMPORAL LATERAL + R OCCIPITAL CX + R PARIETAL CX + R POST CENTRAL OPERC **Method**: (subg2) + subg4
	subgraphs	**subg1**: R ANT HIPPOC + R POST HIPPOC + R AMYG + R ENT CX, **subg2**: R ANT HIPPOC, **subg3**: R PARIETAL CX + R OCCIPITAL CX, **subg4**: R TEMP LATERAL, **subg5**: R TEMP LATERAL + R POST CENTRAL OPERC, **subg6**: R TEMP LATERAL,		
Patient 4	Seiz. 1	**Clinical**: L ANT HIPPOC + L POST HIPPOC + L TEMP POLE **Method**: subg2 + (subg1)	**Clinical**: L ANT HIPPOC + L POST HIPPOC + L TEMP POLE + L POST TEMP NEOCORTEX + R AMYG + R ANT HIPPOC **Method**: subg3 + subg4 + subg5	**Clinical**:L ANT HIPPOC + L POST HIPPOC + L TEMP POLE + L POST TEMP NEOCORTEX + R AMYG + R ANT HIPPOC **Method**: subg4 + subg5 + (subg6)
	Seiz. 2	**Clinical**: L ANT HIPPOC + L POST HIPPOC + L TEMP POLE **Method**: subg2 + (subg1)	**Clinical**: L ANT HIPPOC + L POST HIPPOC + L TEMP POLE + L POST TEMP NEOCORTEX + R AMYG + R ANT HIPPOC **Method**: subg3 + subg4 + subg5	**Clinical**: L ANT HIPPOC + L POST HIPPOC + L TEMP POLE + L POST TEMP NEOCORTEX + R AMYG + R ANT HIPPOC **Method**: subg4 + subg5 + (subg6)
	Seiz. 3	**Clinical**: L ANT HIPPOC + L POST HIPPOC + L TEMP POLE **Method**: subg2 + (subg1)	**Clinical**: L ANT HIPPOC + L POST HIPPOC + L TEMP POLE + L POST TEMP NEOCORTEX + R AMYG + R ANT HIPPOC **Method**: subg3 + subg4 + subg5	**Clinical**: L ANT HIPPOC + L POST HIPPOC + L TEMP POLE + L POST TEMP NEOCORTEX + R AMYG + R ANT HIPPOC **Method**: subg4 + subg5 + (subg6)
	Seiz. 4	**Clinical**: L ANT HIPPOC + L POST HIPPOC + L TEMP POLE **Method**: subg2 + (subg1)	**Clinical**: L ANT HIPPOC + L POST HIPPOC + L TEMP POLE + L POST TEMP NEOCORTEX + R AMYG + R ANT HIPPOC **Method**: subg3 + subg4 + subg5	**Clinical**: L ANT HIPPOC + L POST HIPPOC + L TEMP POLE + L POST TEMP NEOCORTEX + R AMYG + R ANT HIPPOC **Method**: subg4 + subg5 + (subg6)
	subgraphs	**subg1**: L ANT TEMP NEOCORTEX + R ANT HIPPOC, **subg2**: L ANT HIPPOC + L POST HIPPOC, **subg3**: L POST TEMPORAL NEOCORTEX + L AMYGDALA + L ANTERIOR CINGULATE, **subg4**: R AMYGD + R ANT HIPPOC + L ANT HIPPOC + L AMYG, **subg5**: R AMYGD + R ANT HIPPOC **subg6**: L TEMP LATERAL + L TEMP POST		
Patient 5	Seiz. 1	**Clinical**: R ANT HIPPOC + R POST HIPPOC + R TEMP POLE + R AMYG **Method**: subg3 + (subg1)	**Clinical**: R ANT HIPPOC + R POST HIPPOC + R TEMP POLE + R AMYG **Method**: subg3 + subg2 + (subg1)	**Clinical**:R ANT HIPPOC + R POST HIPPOC + R TEMP POLE + R AMYG **Method**: subg3 + (subg4) + (subg1)
	Seiz. 2	**Clinical**: R ANT HIPPOC + R POST HIPPOC + R TEMP POLE + R AMYG **Method**: subg3 + (subg1)	**Clinical**:R ANT HIPPOC + R POST HIPPOC + R TEMP POLE + R AMYG + R POST TEMP NEOCORTEX **Method**: subg3 + subg2 + (subg1)	**Clinical**: R ANT HIPPOC + R POST HIPPOC + R TEMP POLE + R AMYG + R POST TEMP NEOCORTEX **Method**: subg3 + (subg4) + (subg1)
	Seiz. 3	**Clinical**: R ANT HIPPOC + R POST HIPPOC + R TEMP POLE + R AMYG **Method**: subg3 + (subg1)	**Clinical**: R ANT HIPPOC + R POST HIPPOC + R TEMP POLE + R AMYG + R POST TEMP NEOCORTEX + R ORBITO FRONTAL CX **Method**: subg3 + subg2 + (subg1)	**Clinical**: R ANT HIPPOC + R POST HIPPOC + R TEMP POLE + R AMYG + R POST TEMP NEOCORTEX R ORBITO FRONTAL CX **Method**: subg3 + (subg4) + (subg1)
	Seiz. 4	**Clinical**: R ANT HIPPOC + R POST HIPPOC + R TEMP POLE + R AMYG **Method**: subg3 + (subg1)	**Clinical**: R ANT HIPPOC + R POST HIPPOC + R TEMP POLE + R AMYG + R POST TEMP NEOCORTEX **Method**: subg3 + subg2+ (subg1)	**Clinical**: R ANT HIPPOC + R POST HIPPOC + R TEMP POLE + R AMYG + R POST TEMP NEOCORTEX **Method**: subg3 + (subg4) + (subg1)
	subgraphs	**subg1**: R LAT TEMP NEOCORTEX + R LAT FRONTAL CORTEX, **subg2**: R ANT HIPPOC + R POST HIPPOC + R AMY + R TEMPORAL POLE, **subg3**: R ANT HIPPOC + R POST HIPPOC **subg4**: R POST HIPPOC + R ORBITO FRONTAL CX + R TEMPORAL POST NEOCORTEX		

TABLE 4 | Qualitative comparison between the set of activated structures determined by visual analysis and the Brain-wide Time-varying Network Decomposition (BTND) method for the patients 6, 7, 8, and 9 (see legend **Table 2**).

		Seizure onset	Seizure propagation	Seizure ending
Patient 6	Seiz. 1	**Clinical**: L PRECENTRAL OPERCULUM + L POST CENTRAL OPERCULUM + L FRONTAL CORTEX **Method**: subg2 + subg3 + subg4 + (subg1) (subg5)	**Clinical**: L PRECENTRAL OPERCULUM + L POST CENTRAL OPERCULUM + L FRONTAL CORTEX **Method**: subg2 + subg3 + subg4 + (subg1) (subg5)	**Clinical**: L PRECENTRAL OPERCULUM + L POST CENTRAL OPERCULUM + L FRONTAL CORTEX **Method**: subg4 + (subg1) (subg5)
	Seiz. 2	**Clinical**: L PRECENTRAL OPERCULUM + L POST CENTRAL OPERCULUM + L FRONTAL CORTEX **Method**: subg2 + subg3 + subg4 + (subg1) (subg5)	**Clinical**: L PRECENTRAL OPERCULUM + L POST CENTRAL OPERCULUM + L FRONTAL CORTEX **Method**: subg2 + subg3 + subg4 + (subg1) (subg5)	**Clinical**: L PRECENTRAL OPERCULUM + L POST CENTRAL OPERCULUM + L FRONTAL CORTEX **Method**: subg4 + (subg1) (subg5)
	Seiz. 3	**Clinical**: L PRECENTRAL OPERCULUM + L POST CENTRAL OPERCULUM + L FRONTAL CORTEX **Method**: subg2 + subg3 + subg4 + (subg1) (subg5)	**Clinical**: L PRECENTRAL OPERCULUM + L POST CENTRAL OPERCULUM + L FRONTAL CORTEX **Method**: subg2 + subg3 + subg4 + (subg1) (subg5)	**Clinical**: L PRECENTRAL OPERCULUM + L POST CENTRAL OPERCULUM + L FRONTAL CORTEX **Method**: subg4 + (subg1) (subg5)
	subgraphs	**subg1**: L PRECENTRAL OPERCULUM + L POST CENTRAL OPERCULUM + L FRONTAL CORTEX, **subg2**: L PRECENTRAL OPERCULUM + L POST CENTRAL OPERCULUM + L FRONTAL CORTEX + L PARIETAL CORTEX, **subg3**: L POST CENTRAL OPERCULUM + L PARIETAL CORTEX, **subg4**: L TEMPORAL LOBE + L POST PARIETAL CORTEX		
Patient 7	Seiz. 1	**Clinical**: L ANT HIPPOC + L POST HIPPOC + L AMYGD **Method**: subg2 + (subg1)	**Clinical**: L ANT HIPPOC + L POST HIPPOC + L AMYGD + L ANT TEMPORAL NEOCORTEX **Method**: subg3 (+subg1)	**Clinical**: L ANT HIPPOC + L POST HIPPOC + L AMYGD + L ANT TEMPORAL NEOCORTEX **Method**: subg4 + subg5 + subg6 (+subg1)
	subgraphs	**subg1**: L ANT TEMPORAL NEOCORTEX, **subg2**: L ANT HIPPOC + L POST HIPPOC + L AMYGD, **subg3**: L ANT HIPPOC + L POST HIPPOC + L AMYGD, **subg4**: L ANT TEMPORAL NEOCORTEX, **subg5**: L ANT TEMPORAL NEOCORTEX, **subg6**: L ANT HIPPOC + L POST HIPPOC + L AMYGD.		
Patient 8	Seiz. 1	**Clinical**: R ANT HIPPOC + R POST HIPPOC + R AMYG + R ENTORINAL CORTEX + R TEMP POLE **Method**: subg3 + subg6 + (subg1) + (subg2)	**Clinical**: R ANT HIPPOC + R POST HIPPOC + R AMYG + R ENTORINAL CORTEX + R TEMP POLE **Method**: subg3 + subg4 + (subg1)	**Clinical**: R ANT HIPPOC + R POST HIPPOC + R AMYG + R ENTORINAL CORTEX + R TEMP POLE **Method**: subg1 + subg4 + subg5 + (subg2)
	Seiz. 2	**Clinical**: R ANT HIPPOC + R POST HIPPOC + R AMYG + R ENTORINAL CORTEX + R TEMP POLE **Method**: subg3 + subg6 + (subg2)	**Clinical**: R ANT HIPPOC + R POST HIPPOC + R AMYG + R ENTORINAL CORTEX + R TEMP POLE **Method**: subg5 + subg6 + (subg2)	**Clinical**: R ANT HIPPOC + R POST HIPPOC + R AMYG + R ENTORINAL CORTEX + R TEMP POLE + R ANT TEMPORAL NEOCORTEX **Method**: subg1 + subg4 + subg5 + (subg2)
	Seiz. 3	**Clinical**: R ANT HIPPOC + R POST HIPPOC + R AMYG + R ENTORINAL CORTEX + R TEMP POLE **Method**: subg3 + subg6 + (subg2)	**Clinical**: R ANT HIPPOC + R POST HIPPOC + R AMYG + R ENTORINAL CORTEX + R TEMP POLE **Method**: subg5 + subg6 + (subg2)	**Clinical**: R ANT HIPPOC + R POST HIPPOC + R AMYG + R ENTORINAL CORTEX + R TEMP POLE + R ANT TEMPORAL NEOCORTEX **Method**: subg3 + subg6 + (subg1) + (subg2)
	subgraphs	**subg1**: R ANT TEMPORAL NEOCORTEX + R POST TEMPORAL NEOCORTEX, **subg2**: R POST HIPPOC + R ANT TEMPORAL NEOCORTEX + R POST TEMPORAL NEOCORTEX, **subg3**: R ANT HIPPOC + R AMYG, **subg4**: R ENTORHINAL CORTEX + R TEMPORAL POLE + R ANT TEMPORAL NEOCORTEX, **subg5**: R ANT HIPPOC + R POST HIPPOC + R AMYG, **subg6**: R ANT HIPPOC + R AMYG		
Patient 9	Seiz. 1	**Clinical**: R ANT HIPPOC + R POST HIPPOC + R AMYG + R ENTORINAL CORTEX + R TEMP POLE **Method**: subg2 + (subg1)	**Clinical**: L ANT HIPPOC + L TEMP POLE **Method**: subg2 + subg3 + (subg1)	**Clinical**: R ANT HIPPOC + R POST HIPPOC + R AMYG + R ENTORINAL CORTEX + R TEMP POLE + L TEMP POLE + R ANT TEMPORAL NEOCORTEX L ANT HIPPOC **Method**: subg3 + subg4 + subg5 + subg6
	Seiz. 2	**Clinical**: L ANT HIPPOC + L TEMP POLE **Method**: subg3 + (subg5) + (subg1)	**Clinical**: R ANT HIPPOC + R POST HIPPOC + R AMYG + R ENTORINAL CORTEX + R TEMP POLE **Method**: subg2 + subg3 + (subg5) + (subg1)	**Clinical**: R ANT HIPPOC + R POST HIPPOC + R AMYG + R ENTORINAL CORTEX + R TEMP POLE + L TEMP POLE + R ANT TEMPORAL NEOCORTEX L ANT HIPPOC **Method**: subg4 + subg5 + (subg1)
	Seiz. 2	**Clinical**: L ANT HIPPOC + L TEMP POLE **Method**: subg3 + (subg5) + (subg1)	**Clinical**: R ANT HIPPOC + R POST HIPPOC + R AMYG + R ENTORINAL CORTEX + R TEMP POLE **Method**: subg2 + subg3 + (subg5) + (subg1)	**Clinical**: R ANT HIPPOC + R POST HIPPOC + R AMYG + R ENTORINAL CORTEX + R TEMP POLE + L TEMP POLE + R ANT TEMPORAL NEOCORTEX L ANT HIPPOC **Method**: subg4 + subg5 + (subg6)
	subgraphs	**subg1**: L POST TEMPORAL NEOCORTEX + L ANT TEMP NEOCORTEX + R ANT HIPPOC + R LAT TEMPORAL NEOCORTEX, **subg2**: L ANT HIPPOC + L ANT TEMPORAL NEOCORTEX + L POST TEMPORAL NEOCORTEX, **subg3**: R ANT HIPPOC + R POST HIPPOC + R ENTORHINAL CX + R AMYG, **subg4**: L ANT HIPPOC + L ANT TEMPORAL NEOCORTEX, **subg5**: + L POST TEMPORAL NEOCORTEX + L ANT TEMP NEOCORTEX + R ANT HIPPOC + R LAT TEMPORAL NEOCORTEX, **subg6**: R ANT TEMPORAL NEOCORTEX + R POST TEMPORAL NEOCORTEX		

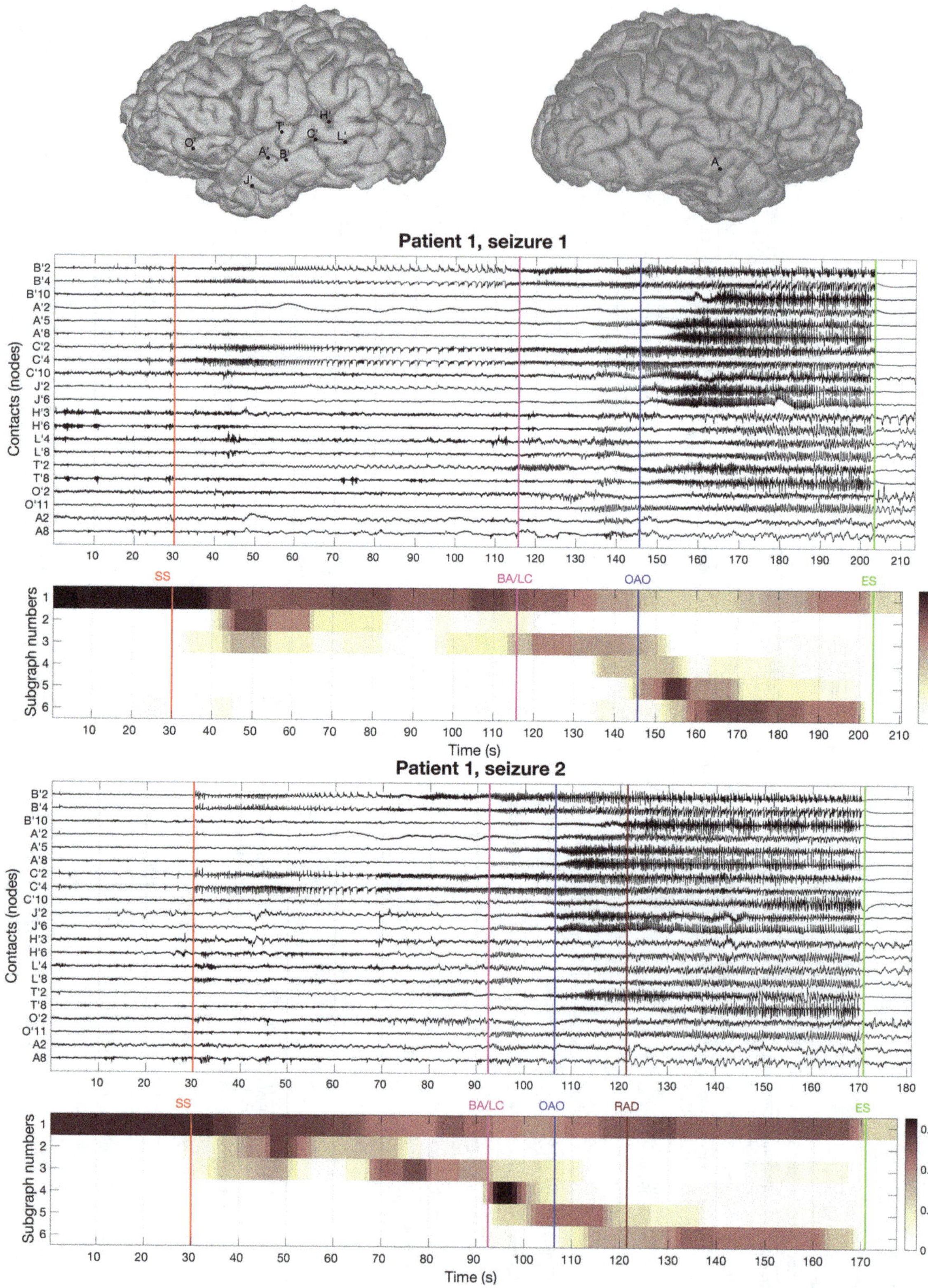

FIGURE 2 | On top is represented the main cerebral structures targeted by intracranial electrodes for the patient 1. Then we picture the recording of two seizures of the patient 1 for selected electrode contacts. Under each seizure, we show the activation level of each subgraph obtained by the BTND decomposition. A subgraph is composed of pairs of contacts with high FC values. The activation level shows the FC dynamic of a subgraph. The main features of ictal semiology are represented by vertical lines, SS, start of the seizure; BA/LC, clinical onset with behavioral arrest and loss of consciousness; OAO, oro alimentary automatisms; RAD, right arm dystonia; SE, end of the seizure.

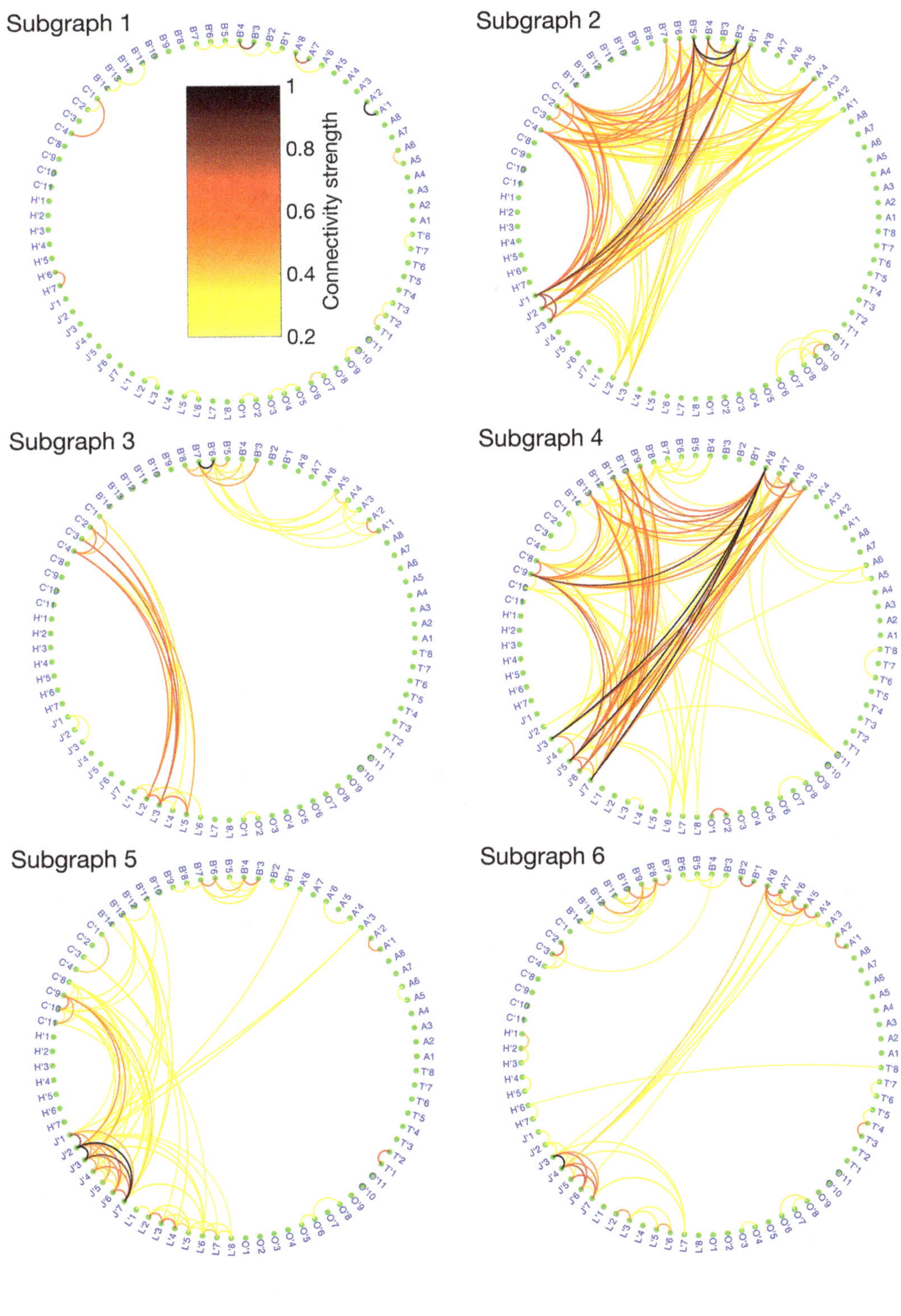

Legend ; B'2 : Left hippocampus B'4 : Left hippocampus B'10 : middle temporal gyrus A'2 : left amygdala A'5 : left amygdala A'8 : left middle temporal gyrus C'2 : left posterior hippocampus C'4 :left posterior hippocampus C'10 : left anterior temporal gyrus J'2 : left temporal pole J'6 : left temporal pole H'3 : left posterior insula H'6 : left temporal operculum L'4 : left posterior temporal neocortex L'8 : left posterior temporal neocortex T'2 : left anterior insula T'8 : left superior temporal gyrus O'2 : left orbitofrontal cortex O'11 : left orbito frontal cortex A2 : right amygdala A8 : right middle temporal gyrus.

FIGURE 3 | Six functional connectivity (FC) subgraphs revealed by the Brain-wide Time-varying Network Decomposition (BTND) decomposition for the patient 1. The colorbar is the same for each graph. Only the electrode contacts that show one or several connections in at least one subgraph are represented.

subgraphs contained mostly connections between anterior lateral temporal neocortex, temporal posterior neocortex, and temporal pole. As a whole, the pattern of activations was very similar for the three seizures and was very consistent with visual analysis of the seizures.

From a clinical point of view, at seizure onset, the patient was asymptomatic and the seizure remained clinically silent for almost 80 s. First clinical symptoms (behavioral arrest and loss of consciousness) occurred more than 1 min after seizure onset during the course propagation. Secondary clinical manifestations included oro alimentary automatisms (seizure 1) and right arm dystonia (seizure 2). Those symptoms occurred while several modules were simultaneously activated.

The patient underwent left anterior lobectomy that resulted in seizure freedom with more than 24 months of follow-up.

CASE 2:

Pt 2 is a 37 years old female patient. Presurgical non-invasive investigations suggested that both temporal lobes could trigger habitual epileptic seizures of the patient. Intracranial EEG using SEEG was thus required to evaluate the intrinsic epileptogenicity of each temporal lobe. Intracranial SEEG electrodes targeted mostly both medial and lateral temporal lobes (left and right anterior hippocampus, left and right temporal pole, right amygdala, left and right anterior temporal neocortex, left and right posterior temporal neocortex, left and right insula), but also left and right orbitofrontal cortex.

Three seizures were recorded during SEEG. For the seizure 1, seizure-onset was characterized by a rapid discharge in the left anterior and posterior hippocampus with secondary spread to left anterior lateral temporal and left orbito frontal cortex fast activity and at the end of the seizure propagation to right temporal lobe (right hippocampus and right amygdala). For two seizures (seizures 2 and 3), the initial seizure-onset activity developed in right hippocampus, right amygdala, and right entorhinal cortex with a secondary ictal spread to right anterior temporal cortex and with a propagation to left temporal lobe at seizure ending.

The BTND method applied to the three seizures decomposed the connectivity pattern in 7 subgraphs. **Figure 4** shows the recording of two seizures (seizures 1 and 2) of the Patient 2 for selected electrode contacts. Below each recording, we provide the activation profiles of all subgraphs obtained by the BTND for this specific seizure. On top is represented the main cerebral structures targeted by intracranial electrodes for this patient. **Figure 5** shows the 7 FC subgraphs revealed by the BTND.

One subgraph was mostly composed of connections within left medial temporal lobe and left orbitofrontal cortex. Another subgraph was mostly composed of connections within left anterior temporal neocortex. The remaining five subgraphs consisted of regions connecting mostly right medial temporal structures (hippocampus, amygdala, entorhinal cortex) and/or right lateral temporal neocortex. The time course of activation of those subgraphs was closely related to the ictal involvement of both temporal lobes revealed by visual analysis of the seizures: involvement of the left (right) medial temporal lobe was paralleled by an activation of the left (right) subgraphs in a timely fashion, depending on the seizure.

Clinically, ictal semiology for seizure 1 consisted of nausea and olfactory hallucinations with preserved consciousness reported consciously by the patient 30 s after EEG onset followed by behavioral arrest with loss of consciousness more 60 seconds later. Loss of consciousness occurred lately during the course of the seizure when both temporal lobes were involved. At that time, the BTND method showed activation of modules in both temporal lobes. Seizure 2 was a nocturnal seizure with mild clinical semiology, mostly consisting of nocturnal arousal and confusion.

Since SEEG revealed an intrinsic epileptogenicity of both temporal lobes, surgical resection was contraindicated.

4. DISCUSSION

This study investigated a new method named BTND to decompose the multi-seizure brain-wide time-varying network obtained by means of FC. The dataset is visualized as FC subgraphs characterizing the dynamic of all seizures from the same patient. The FC measure used was the PLV, estimated at different time steps of the seizure and applied on large band signal (20–100 Hz). We compared the obtained decomposition of ictal events from 9 patients who have drug-resistant focal epilepsy (observation of a total of 27 seizures) to the visual interpretation from the clinician. Overall, for every patient, results consisting of spatially localized FC subgraphs with stepwise activation were easily interpretable. For 8 of the 9 patients, the decomposition matched with the clinical observation entailing the BTND method as a relevant tool to visualize the multi-seizure brain-wide time-varying network.

4.1. Investigating Seizure Dynamics With Brain-Wide Time-Varying Network

It is well-established that the brain is a complex network, with a sophisticated structural connectivity architecture and specific anatomical networks shaping sensory and cognitive processes (34, 35). Functional connectivity measures are a statistical way to investigate the interrelations between brain regions, forming a physiological or pathological brain network (36). When applied on static processes, FC network analysis can provide an instantaneous picture of a stable network. In the field of clinical neuroscience, this proved to be useful for studying stable disease traits like the effects of specific lesions (10) or the effects of drugs on the brain (6, 11, 37). Graph theory-based measures can then provide quantitative tools to explore the overall topology of the network (35). Thus, specific metrics such as modularity, clustering coefficients, or efficiency originating from graph theory (16) were proposed as a useful strategy, for example, to classify patients with Alzheimer disease from standard patients (9) or to explain the effect of physical activity on relations between brain regions (38).

However, static network analysis does not capture one fundamental property of epileptic seizures, the dynamic propagation of the ictal wave. Analysis of time-varying network inferred by dynamic FC measures is a recent topic. Newly

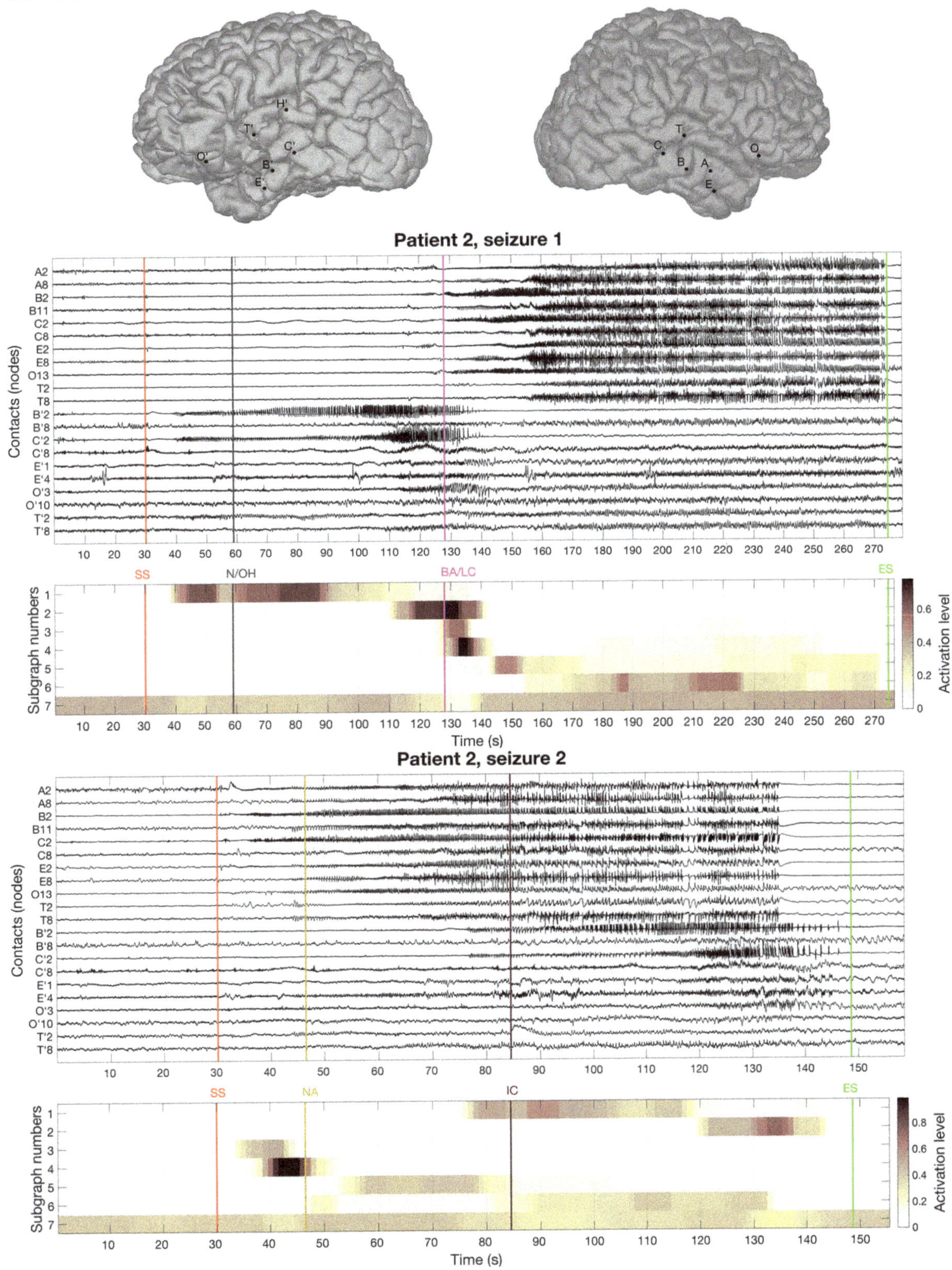

FIGURE 4 | On top is represented the main cerebral structures targeted by intracranial electrodes for patient 2. Then we picture the recording of two seizures of the patient 2 for selected electrode contacts. Under each seizure, we show the activation level of each subgraph obtained by the Brain-wide Time-varying Network Decomposition (BTND) decomposition. A subgraph is composed of pairs of contacts with high functional connectivity (FC) values. The activation level shows the FC dynamic of a subgraph. The main features of ictal semiology are represented by vertical lines, BA/LC, behavioral arrest and loss of consciousness; N/OH, clinical onset with nausea and olfactory hallucinations; NA, nocturnal arousal; IC, ictal confusion.

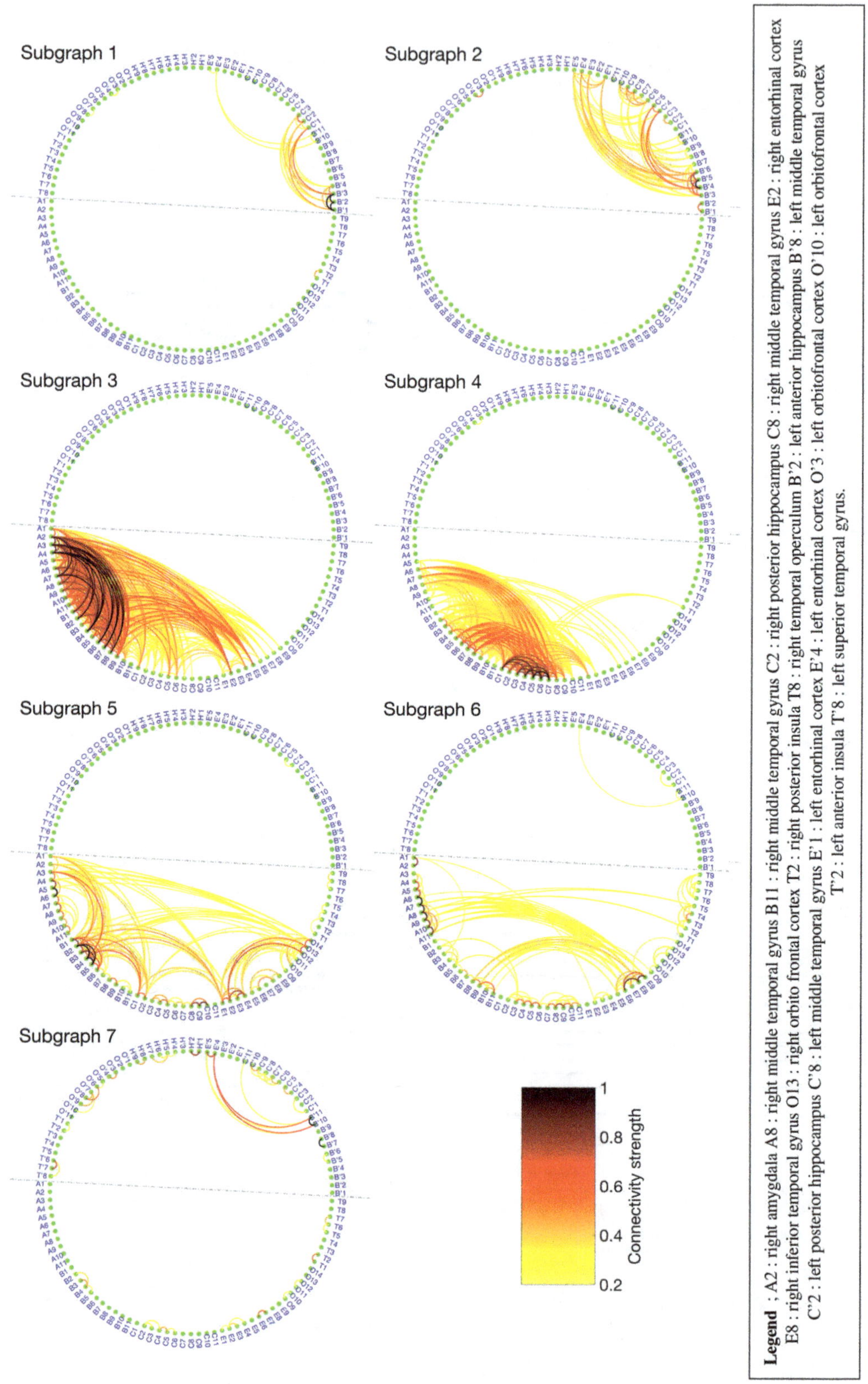

FIGURE 5 | Seven functional connectivity (FC) subgraphs revealed by the Brain-wide Time-varying Network Decomposition (BTND) decomposition for the patient 2. Only the electrode contacts that show one or several connections in at least one subgraph are represented. The dotted line separates the electrode contacts located in the right hemisphere from those located in the left hemisphere.

emerging dynamic measures that quantify how community organization evolved in time have been proposed in recent years (39). In this context, Kerr et al. (40) shows that simple metrics using the first eigenvector of each FC network lead to the separation of ictal, pre-ictal, or non-ictal events of a recording. A similar metric demonstrated in (22) used to describe the seizure as a succession of states. The strategy can be used to decompose the time axes in states, and then to extract the major FC network of each state (41). Despite producing intelligible results, this strategy hampers the identification of FC subgraphs with interconnected temporal activation, and prevents highlighting some complex relations between brain regions. A complementary approach has been proposed in (23): the authors identify first the main subgraphs of the seizures by modularity optimization (42), and the evolution in time of the main subgraphs leads to a decomposition of the seizure in time states. It should be noticed that this approach is not fundamentally different from the study of static graphs since the subgraphs and their time evolution are determined independently. However, in addition to finding a measure characterizing each FC graph, one must know how to analyze the temporal evolution of the proposed scores. It becomes even more complicated when several modalities are used, as in (43), where several seizures are analyzed for different frequency bands over time.

The present study proposes another strategy, consisting of decomposing all modalities characterizing the dataset simultaneously. Thus, the main advantages of the proposed method are that the analysis pipeline provides both the subgraphs and their temporal activations. The output of the process highlights the main components of the connectivity structure and summarizes a large amount of data with an automatic approach. A similar approach has already been employed in the context of epilepsy in (44) to decompose FC matrices from seizures into FC subgraphs with their respective activation profile. Khambhati et al. (44) demonstrate that inferred FC subgraphs during interictal periods can predict brain regions that generate seizures, and that those subgraphs undergo slower and more coordinated fluctuations during the ictal events compared to interictal states. However, this kind of simultaneous decompositions can produce results that are difficult to interpret. Therefore, for an application different from epilepsy, a sparsity constraint applied on activation profile was shown to enforce intelligibility of the results (45), providing FC subgraphs discriminating the brain network's dynamic in neurodevelopment. Moreover, contrary to our study, the decomposition from (44) does not integrate the different seizures of the same patient to obtain more reproducible FC subgraphs. Tools to decompose several modalities, like tensor decomposition (46–48), were already applied in neuroscience (41, 49, 50) and recently in the context of epilepsy (26). In (26), we proposed a specific tensor decomposition with relevant constraints to encourage the inference of interpretable clusters of FC common to several seizures of the same patient. However, this method is only applicable if all seizures from the same patient have similar durations. In the present study, we developed a new method offering the possibility of decomposing several seizures with different durations from the same patient, which is a more realistic situation in a clinical setting.

4.2. Limitations

The BTND method can produce relevant FC, but several limitations have to be addressed. First, the method requires 3 parameters that are directly related to the obtained FC results. We expose a simple procedure to choose each parameter that produces relevant results for each of the 27 seizures. However, the optimal selection of these parameters may be dependent on the FC measure and might be adapted for other clinical applications. Second, for one patient, the BTND method identified a seizure-onset subgraph that was discordant from the seizure onset-zone. For that patient, at seizure-onset, there was a rapid discharge within the seizure-onset zone (without any focal change of synchrony) and a spiking activity within the contralateral hemisphere (accompanied with an increase in synchrony). The increase of FC evaluated by the phase-locking value was wrongly lateralized, emphasizing that the BTND method is dependent on the FC measure used to infer the brain-wide time-varying network. Thus, using another FC measure could be envisaged for this patient. In addition, several studies have already shown that seizure-onset is often marked by a dramatic decrease in seizure connectivity among recorded brain structures. At the same time, synchrony increases progressively during the seizure (51, 52). It might be thus expected that seizure-onset should be characterized by a decrease of activation of subgraphs located within the seizure-onset zone with the BTND method in some patients. It is important to consider that our procedure only highlights functional subgraphs associated with high values of functional connectivity. Thus, it is ideal for showing activations of synchrony in different areas of the brain. However, it is not able to explicitly demonstrate the deactivations that may occur in the brain at the early start of the seizure when SEEG activities in different areas of the brain are suddenly decorrelated. Lastly, direct validation of the method is out of reach since there is no perfect gold standard for the estimation of the connectivity pattern in epileptic patients. We chose to make a correspondence between the propagation patterns disclosed by classical visual interpretation of SEEG signals and the BTND method. Simulation studies generating neural models of epileptic activity with a known connectivity pattern could represent an alternative in future studies.

4.3. Clinical Application of the Method

In the present study, we presented an automatic method to describe the connectivity structures of epileptic seizures using an original algorithm with several constraints optimized for that clinical context.

As a whole, we found that the method produces several subgraphs of connections with their activation time course that parallel the patterns of propagation of the seizures closely. In 24/27 seizures, one or two subgraphs overlapped clearly with the seizure onset zone. This suggests that the method can help to localize the seizure-onset zone if there is an increase in synchrony at seizure-onset revealed by FC. This finding confirms several studies evidencing that focal modulations of synchrony help to localize the seizure-onset zone to be surgically resected (5, 53). Moreover, thanks to the sparsity and temporal coherence constraints, the method effortlessly reveals how FC synchrony propagates to the different regions of the brain. As a whole, the method summarizes a vast amount of complex interactions with high readability. We believe that the method is thus highly valuable in clinical studies focusing on connectivity in epileptic patients. For example, this may help to unravel the neural bases of clinical semiology of seizures, which are often related to ictal dysfunction of widespread brain networks involving cortical or subcortical structures. The BTND method provides an exhaustive view of the structure of functional networks at each period of the seizure enabling a fine-grained correlation ictal semiology and network analysis. Lastly, clinical interpretation of SEEG signals is mostly focused on changes of power in large frequency bands (typically high-frequency above 20 Hz at seizure-onset and low band or large band frequency during propagation) revealed by visual inspection. The BTND method enables the detection of changes of synchrony revealed by functional connectivity measures, which are not necessarily paralleled by changes of power. In that respect, we believe that the method may thus contribute to bringing into clinical practice computational measures complementary to a visual interpretation of seizures.

5. CONCLUSION

We present here a novel approach to decompose epileptic seizures in several time-varying subgraphs with high and reproducible functional connectivity values. The method extracts the most significant subgraphs and their corresponding time course of activation. We suggest that this represents a first step to simplify the interpretation of large datasets of functional connectivity for clinical practice. We believe that this will enable further studies investigating the clinical relevance of networks identification for epilepsy surgery.

ETHICS STATEMENT

The studies involving human participants were reviewed and approved by CPP Lyon Sud EST IV (24/05/2012 N2012-A00516-37). The patients/participants provided their written informed consent to participate in this study. Written informed consent was obtained from the individual(s) for the publication of any potentially identifiable images or data included in this article.

AUTHOR CONTRIBUTIONS

GF: concept, method design, data analysis, bibliographic review, writing contributions to the manuscript introduction, materials and methods and discussion, and submission. PB and PG: critical review of the manuscript and scientific supervision (data analysis). JJ: concept, experiment design, scientific supervision (clinic), bibliographic review, writing contributions to the manuscript introduction, application, and discussion. All authors contributed to the article and approved the submitted version.

REFERENCES

1. Ryvlin P, Cross JH, Rheims S. Epilepsy surgery in children and adults. *Lancet Neurol.* (2014) 13:1114–26. doi: 10.1016/S1474-4422(14)70156-5
2. Guenot M, Isnard J, Ryvlin P, Fischer C, Ostrowsky K, Mauguiere F, et al. Neurophysiological monitoring for epilepsy surgery: the Talairach SEEG method. *Stereotact Funct Neurosurg.* (2001) 77:29–32. doi: 10.1159/000064595
3. Isnard J, Taussig D, Bartolomei F, Bourdillon P, Catenoix H, Chassoux F, et al. French guidelines on stereoelectroencephalography (SEEG). *Neurophysiol Clin.* (2018) 48:5–13. doi: 10.1016/j.neucli.2017.11.005
4. Chauvel P, Gonzalez-Martinez J, Bulacio J. Presurgical intracranial investigations in epilepsy surgery. *Handb Clin Neurol.* (2019) 161:45–71. doi: 10.1016/B978-0-444-64142-7.00040-0
5. Bartolomei F, Lagarde S, Wendling F, McGonigal A, Jirsa V, Guye M, et al. Defining epileptogenic networks: contribution of SEEG and signal analysis. *Epilepsia.* (2017) 58:1131–47. doi: 10.1111/epi.13791
6. Hallett M, de Haan W, Deco G, Dengler R, Di Iorio R, Gallea C, et al. Human brain connectivity: Clinical applications for clinical neurophysiology. *Clin Neurophysiol.* (2020) 131:1621–51. doi: 10.1016/j.clinph.2020.03.031
7. van Mierlo P, Höller Y, Focke NK, Vulliemoz S. Network perspectives on epilepsy using EEG/MEG source connectivity. *Front Neurol.* (2019) 10:721. doi: 10.3389/fneur.2019.00721
8. van den Heuvel MP, Sporns O. A cross-disorder connectome landscape of brain dysconnectivity. *Nat Rev Neurosci.* (2019) 20:435–46. doi: 10.1038/s41583-019-0177-6
9. Rubinov M, Knock SA, Stam CJ, Micheloyannis S, Harris AW, Williams LM, et al. Small-world properties of nonlinear brain activity in schizophrenia. *Hum Brain Mapp.* (2009) 30:403–16. doi: 10.1002/hbm.20517
10. Sponheim SR, McGuire KA, Kang SS, Davenport ND, Aviyente S, Bernat EM, et al. Evidence of disrupted functional connectivity in the brain after combat-related blast injury. *Neuroimage.* (2011) 54:S21–9. doi: 10.1016/j.neuroimage.2010.09.007
11. Alonso JF, Mananas MA, Romero S, Hoyer D, Riba J, Barbanoj MJ. Drug effect on EEG connectivity assessed by linear and nonlinear couplings. *Hum Brain Mapp.* (2010) 31:487–97. doi: 10.1002/hbm.20881
12. Bartolomei F, Trebuchon A, Gavaret M, Regis J, Wendling F, Chauvel P. Acute alteration of emotional behaviour in epileptic seizures is related to transient desynchrony in emotion-regulation networks. *Clin. Neurophysiol.* (2005) 116:2473–9. doi: 10.1016/j.clinph.2005.05.013
13. Bartolomei F, Gavaret M, Hewett R, Valton L, Aubert S, Regis J, et al. Neural networks underlying parietal lobe seizures: a quantified study from intracerebral recordings. *Epilepsy Res.* (2011) 93:164–76. doi: 10.1016/j.eplepsyres.2010.12.005
14. Bartolomei F, Barbeau EJ, Nguyen T, McGonigal A, Regis J, Chauvel P, et al. Rhinal-hippocampal interactions during déjà vu. *Clin. Neurophysiol.* (2012) 123:489–95. doi: 10.1016/j.clinph.2011.08.012
15. Stacey W, Kramer M, Gunnarsdottir K, Gonzalez-Martinez J, Zaghloul K, Inati S, et al. Emerging roles of network analysis for epilepsy. *Epilepsy Res.* (2020) 159:106255. doi: 10.1016/j.eplepsyres.2019.106255
16. Bullmore E, Sporns O. Complex brain networks: graph theoretical analysis of structural and functional systems. *Nat. Rev. Neurosci.* (2009) 10:186–98. doi: 10.1038/nrn2575
17. Hong SJ, Bernhardt BC, Gill RS, Bernasconi N, Bernasconi A. The spectrum of structural and functional network alterations in malformations of cortical development. *Brain.* (2017) 140:2133–43. doi: 10.1093/brain/awx145
18. Bartolomei F, Bettus G, Stam CJ, Guye M. Interictal network properties in mesial temporal lobe epilepsy: a graph theoretical study from intracerebral recordings. *Clin. Neurophysiol.* (2013) 124:2345–53. doi: 10.1016/j.clinph.2013.06.003
19. Van Mierlo P, Carrette E, Hallez H, Raedt R, Meurs A, Vandenberghe S, et al. Ictal-onset localization through connectivity analysis of intracranial EEG signals in patients with refractory epilepsy. *Epilepsia.* (2013) 54:1409–18. doi: 10.1111/epi.12206
20. Wang My, Wang J, Zhou J, Guan Yg, Zhai F, Liu Cq, et al. Identification of the epileptogenic zone of temporal lobe epilepsy from stereo-electroencephalography signals: a phase transfer entropy and graph theory approach. *Neuroimage Clin.* (2017) 16:184–95. doi: 10.1016/j.nicl.2017.07.022
21. Wilke C, Van Drongelen W, Kohrman M, He B. Neocortical seizure foci

localization by means of a directed transfer function method. *Epilepsia*. (2010) 51:564–72. doi: 10.1111/j.1528-1167.2009.02329.x

22. Burns SP, Santaniello S, Yaffe RB, Jouny CC, Crone NE, Bergey GK, et al. Network dynamics of the brain and influence of the epileptic seizure onset zone. *Proc Natl Acad Sci USA*. (2014) 111:E5321–30. doi: 10.1073/pnas.1401752111
23. Khambhati AN, Davis KA, Oommen BS, Chen SH, Lucas TH, Litt B, et al. Dynamic network drivers of seizure generation, propagation and termination in human neocortical epilepsy. *PLoS Comput Biol.* (2015) 11: e1004608. doi: 10.1371/journal.pcbi.1004608
24. Lachaux JP, Rodriguez E, Martinerie J, Varela FJ. Measuring phase synchrony in brain signals. *Hum Brain Mapp*. (1999) 8:194–208. doi: 10.1002/(sici)1097-0193(1999)8:4<194::aid-hbm4>3.0.co;2-c
25. Aydore S, Pantazis D, Leahy RM. A note on the phase locking value and its properties. *Neuroimage*. (2013) 74:231–44. doi: 10.1016/j.neuroimage.2013.02.008
26. Frusque GM, Jung J, Borgnat P, Goncalves P. Multiplex network inference with sparse tensor decomposition for functional connectivity. *IEEE Trans Signal Inform Process Netw*. (2020) 6:316–28. doi: 10.1109/TSIPN.2020.2984853
27. Mairal J, Bach F, Ponce J, Sapiro G. Online learning for matrix factorization and sparse coding. *J Mach Learn Res*. (2010) 11:19–60. doi: 10.1145/1553374.1553463
28. Wang HQ, Zheng CH, Zhao XM. j NMFMA: a joint non-negative matrix factorization meta-analysis of transcriptomics data. *Bioinformatics*. (2015) 31:572–80. doi: 10.1093/bioinformatics/btu679
29. Lahoti P, Garimella K, Gionis A. Joint non-negative matrix factorization for learning ideological leaning on twitter. In: *Proceedings of the Eleventh ACM International Conference on Web Search and Data Mining*. Marina Del Rey, CA (2018). p. 351–9. doi: 10.1145/3159652.3159669
30. Kim H, Choo J, Kim J, Reddy CK, Park H. Simultaneous discovery of common and discriminative topics via joint nonnegative matrix factorization. In: *Proceedings of the 21th ACM SIGKDD International Conference on Knowledge Discovery and Data Mining*. Sydney, NSW (2015). p. 567–76. doi: 10.1145/2783258.2783338
31. Jiang X, Hu X, Xu W. Microbiome data representation by joint nonnegative matrix factorization with Laplacian regularization. *IEEE/ACM Trans Comput Biol Bioinform*. (2015) 14:353–9. doi: 10.1109/TCBB.2015.2440261
32. Jain AK. Data clustering: 50 years beyond K-means. *Pattern Recogn Lett*. (2010) 31:651–66. doi: 10.1016/j.patrec.2009.09.011
33. Bartolomei F, Chauvel P, Wendling F. Epileptogenicity of brain structures in human temporal lobe epilepsy: a quantified study from intracerebral EEG. *Brain*. (2008) 131(Pt 7):1818–30. doi: 10.1093/brain/awn111
34. Bassett DS, Sporns O. Network neuroscience. *Nat Neurosci*. (2017) 20:353–64. Number:3. doi: 10.1038/nn.4502
35. Stam CJ. Modern network science of neurological disorders. *Nat Rev Neurosci*. (2014) 15:683–95. doi: 10.1038/nrn3801
36. He B, Astolfi L, Valdes-Sosa PA, Marinazzo D, Palva S, Benar CG, et al. Electrophysiological brain connectivity: theory and implementation. *IEEE Trans Biomed Eng*. (2019) 66:2115–37. doi: 10.1109/TBME.2019.2913928
37. Douw L, van Dellen E, Gouw AA, Griffa A, de Haan W, van den Heuvel M, et al. The road ahead in clinical network neuroscience. *Netw Neurosci*. (2019) 3:969–93. doi: 10.1162/netn_a_00103
38. Kamijo K, Takeda Y, Hillman CH. The relation of physical activity to functional connectivity between brain regions. *Clin Neurophysiol*. (2011) 122:81–9. doi: 10.1016/j.clinph.2010.06.007
39. Khambhati AN, Sizemore AE, Betzel RF, Bassett DS. Modeling and interpreting mesoscale network dynamics. *Neuroimage*. (2018) 180:337–49. doi: 10.1016/j.neuroimage.2017.06.029
40. Kerr MS, Burns SP, Gale J, Gonzalez-Martinez J, Bulacio J, Sarma SV. Multivariate analysis of SEEG signals during seizure. In: 2011 Annual International Conference of the IEEE Engineering in Medicine and Biology Society. Boston, MA: IEEE (2011). p. 8279–82. doi: 10.1109/IEMBS.2011.6092041
41. Mahyari AG, Zoltowski DM, Bernat EM, Aviyente S. A tensor decomposition-based approach for detecting dynamic network states from EEG. *IEEE Trans Biomed Eng*. (2017) 64:225–37. doi: 10.1109/TBME.2016.2553960
42. Newman M. *Networks*. Oxford University Press (2018). doi: 10.1093/oso/9780198805090.001.0001
43. Le Van Quyen M, Soss J, Navarro V, Robertson R, Chavez M, Baulac M, et al. Preictal state identification by synchronization changes in long-term intracranial EEG recordings. *Clin Neurophysiol*. (2005) 116:559–68. doi: 10.1016/j.clinph.2004.10.014
44. Khambhati AN, Bassett DS, Oommen BS, Chen SH, Lucas TH, Davis KA, et al. Recurring functional interactions predict network architecture of interictal and ictal states in neocortical epilepsy. *eNeuro*. (2017) 4:ENEURO.0091-16.2017. doi: 10.1523/ENEURO.0091-16.2017
45. Chai LR, Khambhati AN, Ciric R, Moore TM, Gur RC, Gur RE, et al. Evolution of brain network dynamics in neurodevelopment. *Netw Neurosci*. (2017) 1:14–30. doi: 10.1162/NETN_a_00001
46. Cichocki A. Tensor decompositions: a new concept in brain data analysis? *arXiv preprint arXiv:*13050395. (2013).
47. Kolda T, Bader B. Tensor decompositions and applications. *SIAM Rev*. (2009) 51:455–500. doi: 10.1137/07070111X
48. Comon P. Tensors: a brief introduction. *IEEE Signal Process Mag*. (2014) 31:44–53. doi: 10.1109/MSP.2014.2298533
49. Leonardi N, Van De Ville D. Identifying network correlates of brain states using tensor decompositions of whole-brain dynamic functional connectivity. In: 2013 International Workshop on Pattern Recognition in Neuroimaging (PRNI). IEEE (2013). p. 74–7. doi: 10.1109/PRNI.2013.28
50. Ozdemir A, Bernat EM, Aviyente S. Recursive tensor subspace tracking for dynamic brain network analysis. *IEEE Trans Signal Inform Process Netw*. (2017) 3:669–82. doi: 10.1109/TSIPN.2017.2668146
51. Wendling F, Bartolomei F, Bellanger JJ, Bourien J, Chauvel P. Epileptic fast intracerebral EEG activity: evidence for spatial decorrelation at seizure onset. Brain. (2003) 126:1449–59. doi: 10.1093/brain/awg144
52. Jiruska P, de Curtis M, Jefferys JGR, Schevon CA, Schiff SJ, Schindler K. Synchronization and desynchronization in epilepsy: controversies and hypotheses. *J Physiol*. (2013) 591:787–97. Number:4. doi: 10.1113/jphysiol.2012.239590
53. van Mierlo P, Papadopoulou M, Carrette E, Boon P, Vandenberghe S, Vonck K, et al. Functional brain connectivity from EEG in epilepsy: seizure prediction and epileptogenic focus localization. *Prog Neurobiol*. (2014) 121:19–35. doi: 10.1016/j.pneurobio.2014.06.004

18

Expert-Level Intracranial Electroencephalogram Ictal Pattern Detection by a Deep Learning Neural Network

Alexander C. Constantino [1†], Nathaniel D. Sisterson [2†], Naoir Zaher [3,4], Alexandra Urban [3,4], R. Mark Richardson [2,5] and Vasileios Kokkinos [2,5]*

[1] Brain Modulation Lab, Department of Neurological Surgery, University of Pittsburgh School of Medicine, Pittsburgh, PA, United States, [2] Department of Neurosurgery, Massachusetts General Hospital, Boston, MA, United States, [3] Department of Neurology, University of Pittsburgh School of Medicine, Pittsburgh, PA, United States, [4] University of Pittsburgh Comprehensive Epilepsy Center, Pittsburgh, PA, United States, [5] Harvard Medical School, Boston, MA, United States

***Correspondence:**
R. Mark Richardson
mark.richardson@mgh.harvard.edu

Background: Decision-making in epilepsy surgery is strongly connected to the interpretation of the intracranial EEG (iEEG). Although deep learning approaches have demonstrated efficiency in processing extracranial EEG, few studies have addressed iEEG seizure detection, in part due to the small number of seizures per patient typically available from intracranial investigations. This study aims to evaluate the efficiency of deep learning methodology in detecting iEEG seizures using a large dataset of ictal patterns collected from epilepsy patients implanted with a responsive neurostimulation system (RNS).

Methods: Five thousand two hundred and twenty-six ictal events were collected from 22 patients implanted with RNS. A convolutional neural network (CNN) architecture was created to provide personalized seizure annotations for each patient. Accuracy of seizure identification was tested in two scenarios: patients with seizures occurring following a period of chronic recording (scenario 1) and patients with seizures occurring immediately following implantation (scenario 2). The accuracy of the CNN in identifying RNS-recorded iEEG ictal patterns was evaluated against human neurophysiology expertise. Statistical performance was assessed *via* the area-under-precision-recall curve (AUPRC).

Results: In scenario 1, the CNN achieved a maximum mean binary classification AUPRC of 0.84 ± 0.19 (95%CI, 0.72–0.93) and mean regression accuracy of 6.3 ± 1.0 s (95%CI, 4.3–8.5 s) at 30 seed samples. In scenario 2, maximum mean AUPRC was 0.80 ± 0.19 (95%CI, 0.68–0.91) and mean regression accuracy was 6.3 ± 0.9 s (95%CI, 4.8–8.3 s) at 20 seed samples. We obtained near-maximum accuracies at seed size of 10 in both scenarios. CNN classification failures can be explained by ictal electro-decrements, brief seizures, single-channel ictal patterns, highly concentrated interictal activity, changes in the sleep-wake cycle, and progressive modulation of electrographic ictal features.

Conclusions: We developed a deep learning neural network that performs personalized detection of RNS-derived ictal patterns with expert-level accuracy. These results suggest the potential for automated techniques to significantly improve the management of closed-loop brain stimulation, including during the initial period of recording when the device is otherwise naïve to a given patient's seizures.

Keywords: epilepsy, responsive neurostimulation, seizure detection, ictal pattern, deep learning

INTRODUCTION

Since its clinical establishment in the early twentieth century, intracranial electroencephalography (iEEG) has become the fundamental modality for evaluation and subsequent management in epilepsy surgery (1–4). Recorded either with the use of subdural electrodes (5) or stereotactic electroencephalography (sEEG) (6), the iEEG allows for localization of the epileptogenic zone or the epileptogenic network giving rise to seizures (7, 8). Computer-assisted signal processing methodologies became popular in the field to support the tedious task of seizure onset localization (9–11).

Deep learning methodologies have been successful in the medical field due to their efficiency in information extraction from raw data (12). One of the most recently established approaches to machine-learning is the convolutional neural network (CNN) model. CNNs are artificial neural networks with multiple consecutive layers that perform convolutions in a hierarchical fashion (13, 14). They are considered to be the deep learning model of choice in applications that require processing of multiple array data, as they can successfully identify local conjunctions in data and build high-level features from low-level ones (15). In the brain-related sciences and clinical fields, neural networks have become a core entity of brain-computer interfaces (16–23), assisted diagnosis and rehabilitation for brain disorders (24–27), and allowed methodological improvements in neuroscience (28–31). For electroencephalographic (EEG) data analysis specifically, deep learning by means of CNNs has been applied for feature extraction purposes (32–34), prediction of cognitive performance (35, 36), and identification of evoked potentials (37).

In recent years, deep learning has been applied in extracranial EEG data to facilitate seizure detection in adult (38–41), children (42), and neonatal populations (43), as well as to identify interictal EEG features (44, 45). Fewer studies, have used deep learning to detect seizures from iEEG data (46). Machine learning approaches have also been used to link extracranial EEG with ECoG discharges (47), predict epileptic seizures (41, 48), and design seizure-detection embedded systems (49). The studies aiming at developing deep learning approaches using intracranial seizure data derived from pre-surgical evaluations for epilepsy are highly limited by the small number of recorded seizures available per patient.

More recently, neuromodulation by the Food and Drug Administration (FDA)-approved RNS System has been used in the U.S.A. as an alternative minimally invasive and personalized therapy for patients with pharmacoresistant focal epilepsy (50). The RNS system is an implantable closed-loop electrical stimulation device that applies electrical stimulation to epileptogenic tissue upon detection of ictal patterns (51–54). The electric current applied locally over the seizure onset areas affects the progress of the detected ongoing ictal patterns by acutely causing their attenuation (55) or by chronically inducing changes in the epileptic synchronization and neuronal recruitment properties of the underlying epileptogenic tissue (56). For the first time in the history of iEEG, RNS allows the recording of iEEG epochs over long periods of time, resulting in the accumulation of hundreds and often thousands of iEEG epochs per patient per year. However, a study to evaluate the efficiency of CNNs in large intracranial RNS-derived seizure datasets remains lacking. As a consequence, the development of reliable automated seizure detection methods is urgently needed to support routine clinical evaluation of RNS patients, as well as to facilitate analytics for personalized treatment (57). Our study addresses this need and evaluates the efficiency of deep learning methodology in detecting iEEG ictal patterns using a large RNS-derived dataset of ictal patterns.

METHOD

Patients

Patients included in this study suffered from focal epilepsy, diagnosed according to current ILAE criteria (58, 59). Patients underwent investigative intracranial recording procedures, either by subdural electrodes, or by robotic-assisted stereotactic EEG, to identify the focus and extent of their epileptogenic zone. After a review of all available patient data during weekly multidisciplinary epilepsy conferences and consideration of available therapeutic options, closed-loop neurostimulation therapy (RNS, NeuroPace, Mountain View, CA, USA) was recommended. Our patients were implanted with the RNS system between January 2015 and June 2018, and the use of their data for this study was approved by the University of Pittsburgh Institutional Review Board (IRB).

RNS Implantation

RNS leads were implanted as closely as possible to the recorded and/or hypothesis-derived epileptogenic regions (**Supplementary Figure 1**). Patients with a diagnosis of neocortical epilepsy onset were implanted either with strips placed over the focus, or depth leads placed through the focus, or a combination of both. Patients with a diagnosis of malformations of cortical development were implanted with depth leads across the posterior-anterior direction of the lesion. Patients with a diagnosis of mesio-temporal epilepsy were implanted with depth electrodes placed across the posterior-anterior axis of the hippocampus. Patients with a diagnosis of idiopathic generalized epilepsy were implanted in the thalamus by oblique depth electrodes targeting the centro-median nucleus.

Assessment of electrode locations was performed by fusion of the post-surgical CT with the pre-surgical MRI.

Data Acquisition

iEEG data recorded from the RNS system were obtained from NeuroPace. Additional RNS-related metadata, including recording, detection and stimulation settings, were collected directly from the NeuroPace Patient Data Management System (PDMS) using purpose-built software. Recordings consisted exclusively of 90 s duration, 4-channel ECoGs, online band-pass filtered at 4–125 Hz, sampled at 250 Hz and digitized by a 10-bit ADC. iEEG channel derivations were bipolar between neighboring electrode contacts (**Supplementary Figure 1**), grounded to the case of the RNS pulse generator. All electrode impedances measured below 1 kOhm for all recordings. Both scheduled and detection-triggered iEEG recordings were obtained and used in this study. Scheduled recordings were triggered by the RNS device's onboard clock to occur either every 12 or 24 h and offered a continuous sampling of spontaneous neurophysiologic activity. Detection triggered recordings were initiated by one of the onboard closed-loop algorithms. Patients were instructed to download their raw iEEG data daily to a local computer, through a transcutaneous telemetry wand, which was in turn uploading the recordings to the NeuroPace PDMS on a weekly basis. Immediately post-implantation, the device was set to passive recording mode for ~1 month, during which no stimulation was delivered in order to record baseline activity (baseline epoch). Once baseline activity was reviewed, stimulation parameters were configured and activated. During the rest of the post-implantation period the device delivered detection-triggered stimulation therapy and parameters were periodically modified in subsequent clinic visits based on evaluation of seizure control status. The time interval during which RNS parameters remain unchanged is referred to as programming epoch.

Data Labeling

In accordance with established clinical practice, iEEG ictal patterns were visually identified by an experienced epilepsy surgery neurophysiologist (V.K.) and in turn confirmed by a board-certified epileptologist (N.Z.). The evaluation process was not influenced by and did not take into account the "long-episode" detections of the RNS system. The onset of ictal patterns was annotated by a cursor marker. The term "ictal pattern" is used instead of the term "seizure," as the device provides no information regarding the clinical manifestation of the electrographic events. The iEEG ictal pattern onset was defined as the point in time after which the iEEG recording background was no longer interictal and was followed by a paroxysmal discharge of ictal features with evolution in frequency and morphology over time. Interictal background was evaluated from scheduled recordings that did not contain iEEG ictal patterns.

Data Augmentation

To reduce overfitting of the model to the training data, we applied label-preserving transformations to iEEGs in the training set (60). We padded the iEEGs with 30 s of zero-voltage measurements before and after the recording, and then chose a 90-s crop uniformly at random. We also rescaled the data by multiplying each signal by a factor between 0.8 and 1.2, chosen uniformly at random for each iEEG. The network was evaluated on untransformed iEEGs from separate validation sets.

Model Architecture and Training

We used a convolutional neural network with high-level architecture shown in **Figure 1**. The network contains 23 convolutional layers with residual connections to make optimization of such a deep network tractable (61). The network takes as input a time-series of intracranial voltage measurements and a patient identifier. The patient identifier facilitates personalized ictal pattern prediction by allowing the network to make predictions conditioned to a particular patient. The network outputs two predictions: a probability that the recording contains an ictal pattern, and the onset time of the ictal pattern in seconds. We jointly optimize both losses using a hybrid loss function. Defining $s \in \{0, 1\}$ as ictal pattern label, $\hat{s}$ as predicted ictal pattern probability, t as ictal pattern onset time, and $\hat{t}$ as predicted ictal pattern onset time, the loss for one example is:

$$L\left(s, \hat{s}, t, \hat{t}\right) = crossentropy\left(s, \hat{s}\right) + 0.1\ huber\left(t, \hat{t}\right)$$

where

$$crossentropy\left(s, \hat{s}\right) = -s \log\left(\hat{s}\right) - (1 - s) \log\left(1 - \hat{s}\right)$$

and

$$\text{huber}\left(t, \hat{t}\right) = \begin{cases} \frac{1}{2}\left(t - \hat{t}\right)^2 & \text{for } \left|t - \hat{t}\right| \le 1 \\ \left|t - \hat{t}\right| - \frac{1}{2} & \text{otherwise} \end{cases}$$

The network contains 11 residual blocks with 2 one-dimensional convolutional layers per block. The convolutional kernel size is 16. The number of filters is 16 in the first layer and increases linearly to 116 in the penultimate residual block. At that point, the filters are concatenated with one-hot encoded patient IDs followed by the final residual block. At the first convolutional layer and at the start of every other residual block, the stride is 2, which down samples the data by a factor of 2 every other residual block. Alternating residual connections also use a stride of 2 in their convolution.

Before each convolutional layer, we apply batch normalization (62) followed by rectified linear activations (63). We initialize the weights (64) and train the network using stochastic gradient descent for 20 epochs with a batch size of 128. We use cyclical learning rates (65) by cycling the learning rate from 0.1 to 0.025 every 4 epochs. For the final two epochs, the learning rate is held at 0.025. Experiments were conducted on Nvidia Tesla K80 accelerators using TensorFlow 1.13.

Accuracy is evaluated by concordance with expert identification, as well as the empirical time constraint for detecting the ictal pattern onset at an interval of less than ±5 s from the expert onset marking, corresponding to half the 20 s EEG review page typically used in clinical routine.

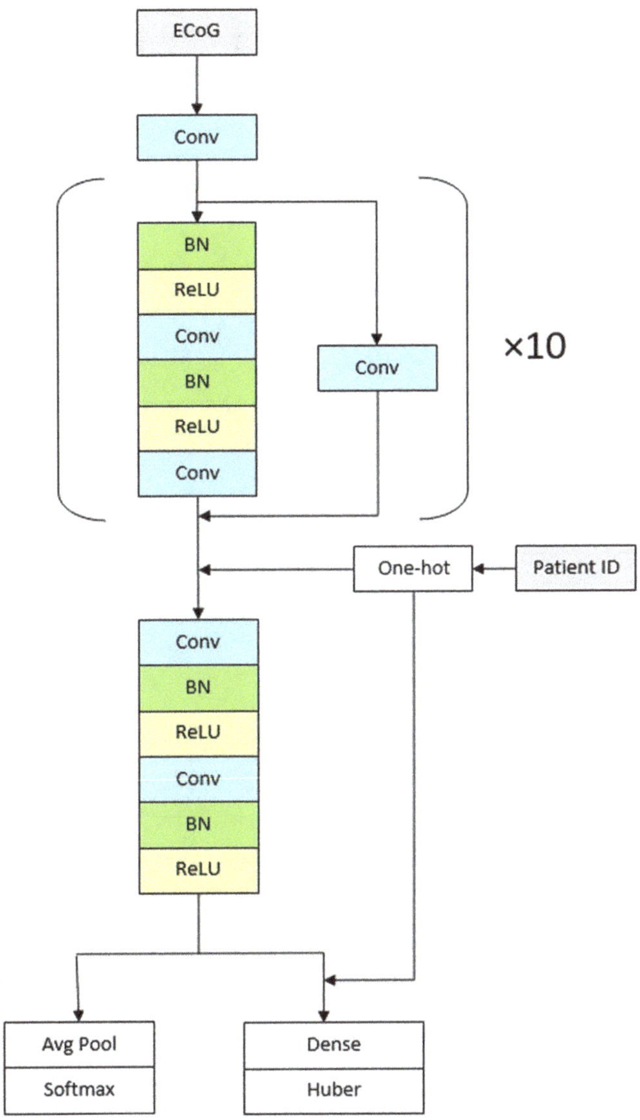

FIGURE 1 | Architecture of the network. The CNN contains 23 convolutional layers with residual connections. The network takes as input a time-series of intracranial voltage measurements and a patient identifier. Before each convolutional layer, batch normalization is applied followed by rectified linear activations. The network contains 11 residual blocks with 2 one-dimensional convolutional layers per block. The convolutional kernel size is 16. The number of filters is 16 in the first layer and increases linearly to 116 in the penultimate residual block. The network outputs two predictions: a probability that the recording contains an ictal pattern, and the onset time of the ictal pattern in seconds (Conv, convolutional layer; BN, batch normalization; ReLU, rectified linear activations).

Annotated iEEG ictal patterns from the dataset were partitioned into training and testing sets; the training set was used to introduce data and the testing set to measure algorithm performance. We decided to create the following two experimental scenarios that correspond to actual clinical situations: (1) when a patient already implanted with RNS moves his epilepsy care to a new center, and the new center receives all prior RNS recordings for analysis, or when an RNS clinic physician moves to a new center, where a list of RNS patients is already registered for care (scenario 1) and, (2) the situation when a new patient is implanted (scenario 2). To test the 1st scenario on previously unseen data of patients that have already been recorded for some time (scenario 1), cross-validation was performed using leave-one-out methodology. This was done by training and evaluating the network on all ictal patterns obtained from all except one patient. Ictal patterns from this "hold-one-out" patient were randomly selected to form a seed set that was then used to train the CNN. The size of seed set was increased from $n = 0$ to $n = 30$ at increments of 5. In addition, each seed set was paired with an equal number of interictal epochs free from ictal patterns; for this purpose, non-ictal scheduled recordings from the "hold-one-out" patient were used to pair seed set recordings containing ictal patterns from the same patient. We then evaluated CNN accuracy on the held-out data, i.e., ictal patterns of the "hold-one-out" patient not used in the seed set. This experiment was repeated in separate iterations for all patients. To test the 2nd scenario on data of newly implanted patients (scenario 2), we used the "hold-one-out" patient's earliest available consecutive ictal patterns as seed set, corresponding to the baseline and early stimulation programming epochs, and then trained and evaluated the network as in scenario 1. Testing in both scenarios was performed in 12/22 patients for which at least $n + 5$ iEEG ictal patterns (i.e., # of ictal patterns > 35) were available (**Table 1**). The data of the rest of the patients were not used for testing. We trained our CNN to classify each iEEG epoch as containing an ictal pattern vs. no ictal pattern. Binary classification or detection accuracy was evaluated using area under precision-recall curve (AUPRC), which incorporates positive-predictive value to adjust for the significant class imbalance in our data set. For regression accuracy (predicting the time at which an ictal pattern begins), we used mean absolute error.

Statistical Analyses

Kruskal-Wallis-tests were used to compare AUPRC results between implant location groups, with an a priori level of significance set to 0.05. All analyses were performed using R 3.1.6 (R Foundation for Statistical Computing, Vienna, Austria) and all data was stored on Microsoft SQL Server 2012 R2 (Microsoft Corporation, Redmond, Washington, USA).

RESULTS

In this study we used a large RNS-derived intracranial dataset comprised of 5,226 ictal pattern events, marked and verified by consensus by two epilepsy experts (agreement on 99.8% of markings), in 18,368 epochs of ~90 s duration from 22 epilepsy patients implanted with RNS, corresponding to a total of 7,346 days of intracranial recording. The mean total post-implantation recording period was 47.7 ± 7.5 weeks (minimum 2.4 weeks, maximum 111.9 weeks). The mean patient age was 33.9 ± 2.5 years and 13 (59.1%) were women (**Table 1**).

In scenario 1, the CNN achieved a maximum mean binary classification AUPRC of 0.84 ± 0.19 (95%CI, 0.72–0.93) (**Figure 2A**) and mean regression accuracy of 6.3 ± 1.0 s

TABLE 1 | Patient demographics and RNS data features.

Patient	Age	Gender	Implantation site	# of days with RNS	# of iEEG files	# of ictal patterns
1	21	F	Thalamus	95	349	11
2	22	M	Developmental malformation	166	333	13
3*	42	F	Neocortex	677	1,682	430
4*	22	F	Hippocampus	393	1,316	452
5*	39	F	Hippocampus	314	716	73
6	29	M	Developmental malformation	152	294	9
7*	22	F	Hippocampus	461	1,396	567
8*	34	F	Neocortex	600	1,172	113
9*	24	M	Neocortex	425	1,304	258
10	19	F	Thalamus	355	16	5
11*	39	F	Developmental malformation	297	834	720
12*	31	M	Hippocampus	261	443	47
13	46	M	Hippocampus	17	46	4
14	53	M	Neocortex	42	90	1
15	22	M	Thalamus	171	529	13
16*	63	F	Neocortex	732	4,110	2,057
17	35	F	Neocortex	19	95	4
18	37	M	Neocortex	735	508	20
19	31	F	Thalamus	73	299	9
20*	38	F	Hippocampus	202	522	93
21*	30	M	Hippocampus	376	796	159
22*	47	F	Developmental malformation	783	1,518	168
			Total	7,346	18,368	5,226

**Patients with > 35 iEEG ictal patterns used in the testing dataset.*

(95%CI, 4.3–8.5 s) at 30 seed samples (**Figure 2B**). In scenario 2, maximum mean AUPRC was 0.80 ± 0.19 (95%CI, 0.68–0.91) (**Figure 2C**) and mean regression accuracy of 6.3 ± 0.9 s (95%CI, 4.8–8.3 s) at 20 seed samples (**Figure 2D**). However, we obtained near-maximum accuracies at seed size of 10 in both scenarios (**Figure 2**), suggesting significant transference between patients at a small seed size.

Sub-analysis by brain region implanted in scenario 1 showed an AUPRC of 0.88 ± 0.08 (95%CI, 0.83–0.93) for the hippocampus, 0.92 ± 0.09 (95%CI, 0.88–0.96) for developmental anomalies, and 0.73 ± 0.24 (95%CI, 0.60–0.86) for the neocortex ($p = 0.35$). In scenario 2, the AUPRC was 0.89 ± 0.09 (95%CI, 0.85–0.94) for the hippocampus, 0.93 ± <0.01 (95%CI, 0.93–0.93) for developmental anomalies, and 0.59 ± 0.29 (95%CI, 0.44–0.75) for the neocortex ($p = 0.15$).

Examples of successful detections are presented in **Figure 3A**. In order to appreciate confounds that influenced accuracy and resulted in suboptimal detections, we performed manual review of failed detection items and identified 7 main categories of CNN pitfall conditions: (1) Ictal electro-decrements that reduce the signal amplitude to baseline levels (**Figure 3B$_1$**). (2) Brief ictal patterns that can be confused for interictal bursts (**Figure 3B$_2$**). (3) Ictal patterns isolated to a single channel (**Figure 3B$_3$**). (4) Highly concentrated interictal activity (**Figure 3B$_4$**). (5) Changes in the brain state in the context of the sleep-wake cycle (**Figure 3B$_5$**). (6) Progressive modulation of electrographic ictal features [not shown, see (56)]. (7) Undetermined reasons (**Figure 3B$_6$**).

DISCUSSION

This study describes a deep neural network that achieved high accuracy in seizure detection using a large dataset of expert-validated ictal patterns from the iEEG recordings of RNS-implanted epilepsy patients. The large size of our dataset allowed us to test two scenarios: (1) to evaluate seizure detection in an existing collection of recordings (including a random selection of the patient's ictal patterns in the training dataset) (scenario 1), and (2) to evaluate seizure detection on a prospective basis for new patients (including the earliest consecutive recorded ictal patterns of the patient in the training dataset) (scenario 2). We performed our evaluations using hold-one-patient-out cross validation. Specifically, the model was trained on 22 patients and evaluated in 12/22 patients for which at least > 35 ictal patterns were available, in a hold-one-patient-out cross validation fashion. For the "chronic recording scenario" (scenario 1), the model was trained on 22 patients, 0–30 seed examples from the test patient chosen uniformly at random, and it was evaluated on the remaining examples for the test "hold-one-out" patient. For the "recent recording scenario" (scenario 2), the model was also trained on 22 patients and the 0–30 seed examples were chosen to be the earliest possible recordings for the test patient, to evaluate the ability of the model to predict future examples for that patient. In turn, we report average results over all possible "hold-one-out" patients (12 total, after excluding patients with fewer than 35 ictal events). Our deep learning architecture achieved accuracy comparable to experts in both clinically

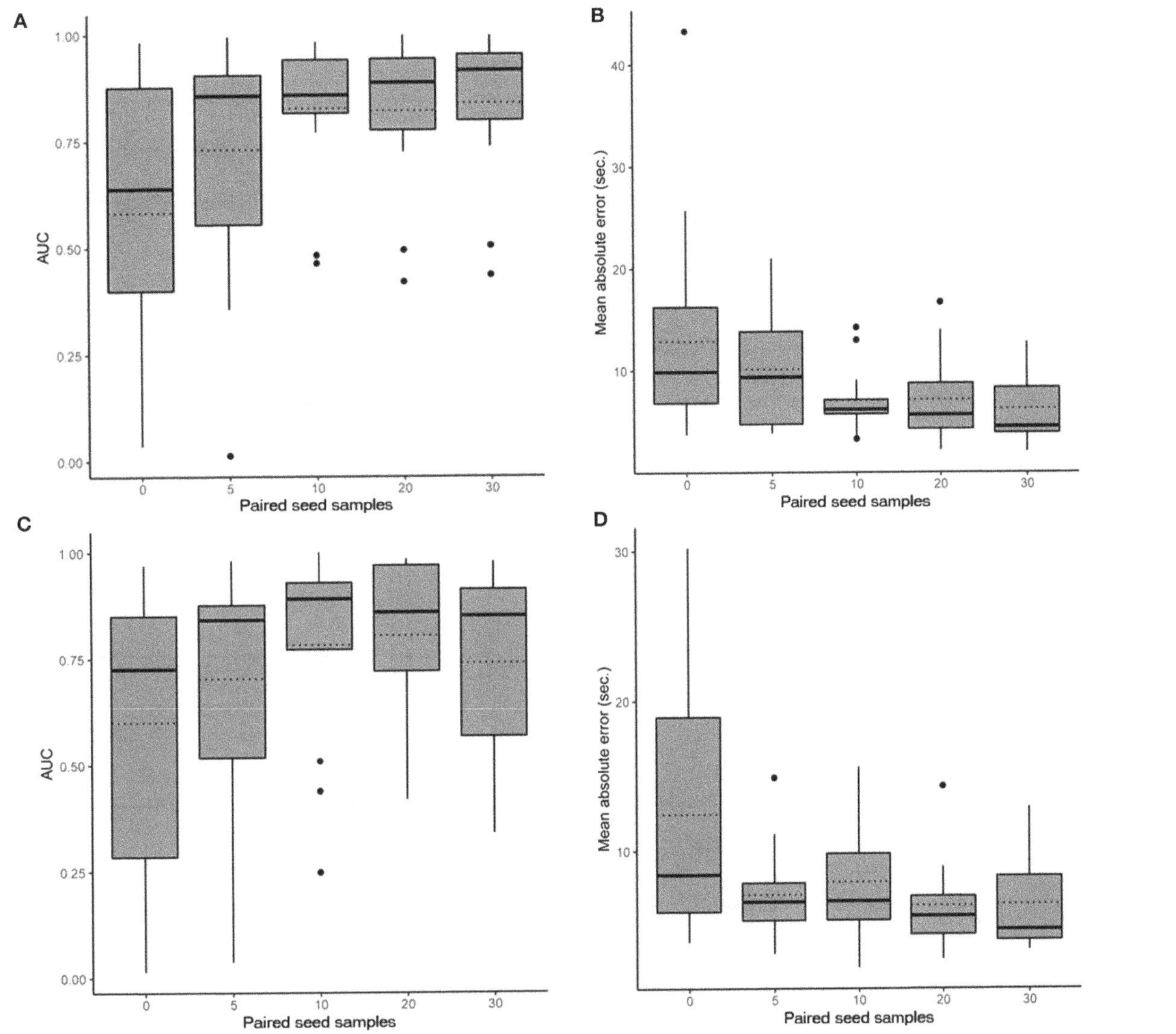

FIGURE 2 | Performance evaluation of the CNN. Box plots show the 25th and 75th percentiles, median (solid), mean (dotted), minimum, and maximum values with outliers shown as dots. **(A)** AUPRC results (accounting for all past patients) for different numbers of paired seed data for our CNN in scenario 1 when detecting iEEG ictal patterns vs. non-ictal patterns. **(B)** Absolute mean regression error results for our CNN in scenario 1. **(C)** AUPRC results (accounting for all past patients) for different numbers of paired seed data for our CNN in scenario 2 when detecting iEEG ictal patterns vs. non-ictal patterns. **(D)** Absolute mean regression error results for our CNN in scenario 2.

relevant scenarios (0.84 and 0.80, respectively) using limited seed datasets containing 30 random and 20 consecutive ictal patterns, respectively. In the only previous report investigating the inter-rater reliability of RNS-derived intracranial seizure detection by experts (66), a manual review of 7,221 RNS-recorded electrographic epileptic events from 22 patients, experts reached an overall 0.79 agreement.

We also observed that AUPRC accuracy between just 5 vs. 10 seeds increased significantly, and although we obtained maxima at 20 and 30 seeds, the difference between 10, 20, and 30 seeds was not clinically meaningful. The standard procedure following RNS implantation requires 3–4 weeks of recording without therapeutic stimulation (baseline period) in order to collect ictal events and manually tune the on-board RNS detectors (51–54). Our model's training data requirements fit nicely with the RNS procedure, and the CNN could be used to improve the device's event detection capabilities in real-time. Specifically, it could use the baseline seizure data for training to improve the overall detection accuracy, and greatly reduce the need for the current practice of repeated heuristic manual adjustments of detection parameters (67).

Finally, we observed that although there was no statistically significant difference in ictal pattern identification between implanted anatomy groups, ictal patterns in developmental

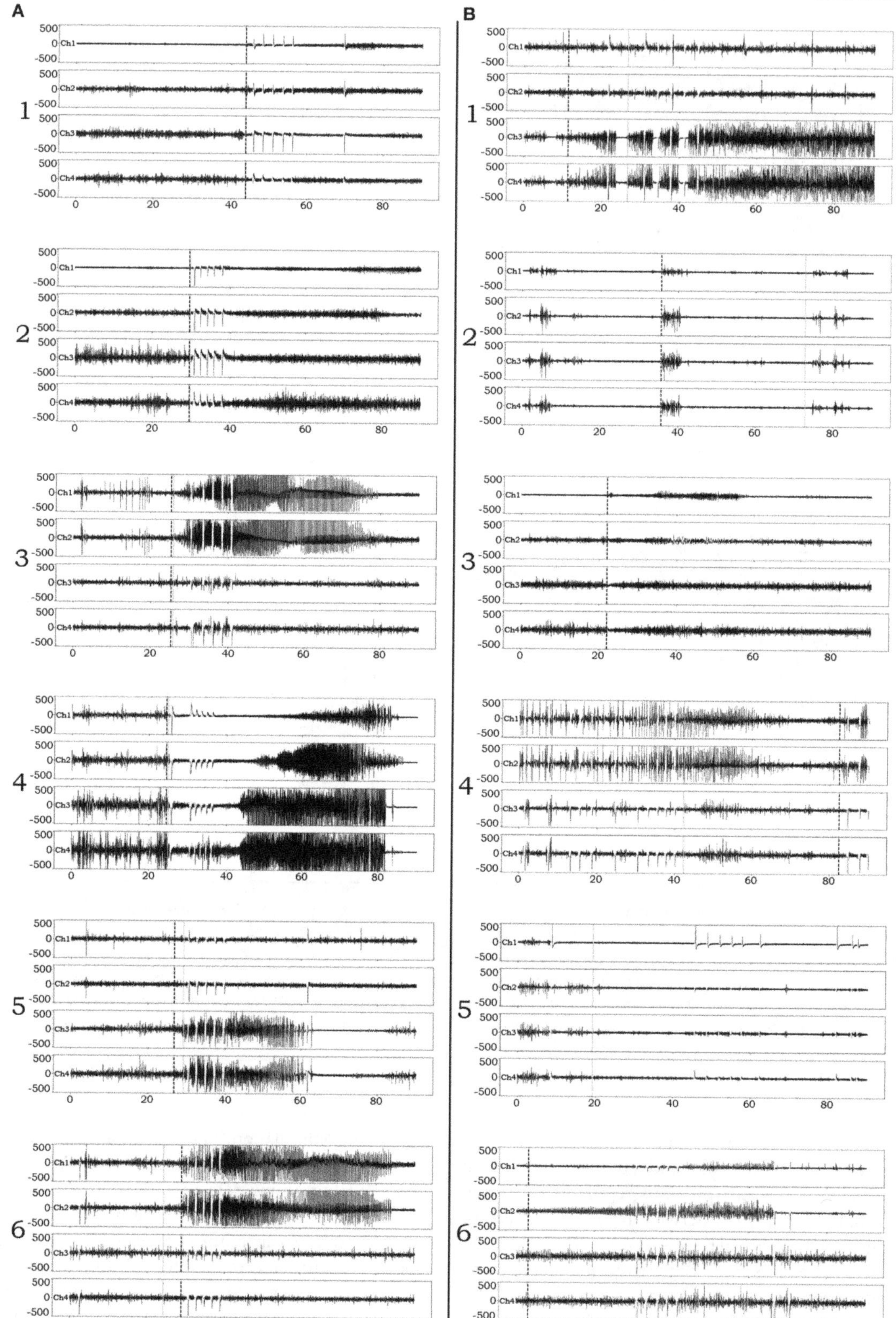

FIGURE 3 | Examples of iEEG ictal pattern detection by the deep-learning neural network. Black dotted vertical lines represent the ictal pattern onset marking set by expert neurophysiologists. Green dotted vertical lines represent the CNN's annotation. **(A)** Examples of successful identifications of RNS ictal patterns with variable

(Continued)

FIGURE 3 | degrees of onset accuracy (1–6). **(B)** Examples of unsuccessful identifications. 1. Although the CNN classifies an ictal pattern in the epoch file, the actual onset is missed due to the presence of semi-regular brief diffuse electro-decrements at the beginning of the ictal pattern. 2. Although the CNN classifies an ictal pattern in the epoch file, the marker is placed at the onset of brief interictal activity that resembles the actual, also brief, ictal pattern. 3. Ictal pattern taking place in a single channel, in a patient with distant electrode implantation, is not acknowledged by the CNN (false negative). 4. Highly concentrated interictal activity is annotated by the CNN as ictal pattern (most of the times resulting in a false positive, unless an ictal pattern co-existed in the epoch file as in this example). 5. The recording occurred during the transition from sleep to wakefulness (arousal) and the CNN annotated the sudden introduction of normal background high frequencies as ictal pattern onset (false positive). 6. The CNN missed the ictal pattern for no apparent reason.

malformations and the hippocampus were more reliably classified than neocortical patterns. For that reason, we performed manual review of failed classifications and determined several systematic causes that turned out to have negatively affected the ictal pattern onset accuracy, although the mean values were well within the pre-determined tolerance window. Most failures and misses that we identified and hereby report have a neurophysiological rather than a computational background, comprised of a constellation of patterns that have often raised concerns within the epilepsy community (68, 69): patterns of interictal activity (70, 71), ictal electrodecrement patterns (72), iEEG patterns during the shift from sleep to wakefulness (73) and vice-versa (74), brief and regionally isolated ictal patterns (75), as well as the recently highlighted effect of ictal pattern modulation due to prolonged stimulation (56, 76). The overall lack of major confounds related to RNS anatomical substrates, suggests that the variety introduced by the anatomical origin of ictal patterns is unlikely to interfere with deep learning and performance.

We took several measures to quantify and reduce model overfitting. First, we report cross-validated results wherein the model is evaluated on different recordings than which it is trained on. Also, we did not extensively or automatically tune hyperparameters. For example, our learning rate varies from 0.1 to 0.025 and we train for exactly 20 epochs. Finally, we trained with both batch normalization (62) and dropout (77) that have experimentally been shown to act as regularizers.

The use of this CNN as an off-line tool can have an important impact in the routine clinical evaluation of epileptic patients implanted with RNS. Due to its high reliability in detecting ictal patterns, our tool can reflect an accurate overview of the patient's progress with neurostimulation therapy and support further quantitative assessments (57). Improvements in accuracy of seizure detection can also identify potential breakthrough seizures early enough for the physician to adjust and adapt the treatment strategy and achieve better seizure control, reducing thereby the risk of life-threatening emergencies such as status epilepticus and sudden unexpected death in epilepsy (54, 78).

We developed and presented a deep learning neural network that performs detection of RNS-derived ictal patterns with the highest published accuracy to date. The key to its performance is the large training dataset that allows the network to develop expertise; a pool of data that only the RNS device can provide due to its ability to sample and record neural activity over long periods of time. We are confident that this technology will improve the management of RNS patients and become pivotal for applications requiring high accuracy in intracranial seizure detection.

AUTHOR CONTRIBUTIONS

AC, NS, RMR, and VK designed the study and interpreted data. AC and NS organized the RNS data from the clinical system, created the figures, and result metrics. AC created the convolutional neural network and performed the experiments. NZ and VK reviewed and marked seizure patterns in the RNS-derived iEEG data. AU directed the RNS clinic and managed patient compliance with clinical data uploads. RMR performed the RNS implantations. All authors read and approved the submitted manuscript.

ACKNOWLEDGMENTS

We are grateful to the epilepsy patients who provided us the privileged opportunity to evaluate their brain recordings.

SUPPLEMENTARY MATERIAL

Supplementary Figure 1 | RNS iEEG data acquisition. a. Pre-operative MRI and post-implantation CT fused image aligned in the axial plane across the trajectory of the implanted RNS lead in the left hippocampus of patient 6. b. iEEG data from the baseline period. The two distal anterior hippocampal contacts make bipolar channel 1, and the two proximal posterior hippocampal ones make bipolar channel 2, that record a unilateral iEEG seizure pattern in the left hippocampus during the baseline period starting in channel 2 (onset at red line). c. Respective iEEG data from the 1st programming epoch where stimulation was activated. During stimulation the amplifier is disconnected, thereby generating a rectangular pulse artifact in the time domain. d, e, and f show the respective imaging and data for an independent right hippocampal electrographic seizure pattern starting in channel 3 of the same patient.

REFERENCES

1. Foerster O, Altenberger H. Elektrobiologische vorgänge an der menschlichen hirnrinde. *Dtsch Nervenheilkd.* (1935) 135:277–88. doi: 10.1007/BF01732786
2. Jasper HH. Electrocorticography. In: Penfield W, Erickson TC, editorss. *Epilepsy and Cerebral Localization*. Springfield, Il: Charles C Thomas Publisher (1941). p. 380–454.
3. Penfield W, Rasmussen T. *The Cerebral Cortex of Man: A Clinical Study of Localization of Function*. New York: Macmillan (1950). p. 248.
4. Penfield W, Jasper HH. *Epilepsy and the Functional Anatomy of the Human Brain*. Boston: Little, Brown and Company (1954). p. 896.
5. Lüders H, Lesser RP, Dinner DS, Morris HH, Hahn JF, Friedman L, et al. Commentary: chronic intracranial recording and stimulation with subdural electrodes. In: Engel J, Jr., editor. *Surgical Treatment of the Epilepsies*. New York, NY: Raven Press (1987). p. 297–321.
6. Bancaud J, Talairach J. *La Stéréo-électroencéphalographie dans l'épilepsie: informations neurophysiopathologiques apportées par l'investigation fonctionnelle stéréotaxique*. Paris: Masson (1965).

7. Lüders HO, Awad I. Conceptual considerations. In: Lüders H, editor. *Epilepsy Surgery*. New York, NY: Raven Press (1992). p. 51–62.
8. Palmini A, Gambardella A, Andermann F, Dubeau F, da Costa JC, Olivier A, et al. Intrinsic epileptogenicity of human dysplastic cortex as suggested by corticography and surgical results. *Ann Neurol.* (1995) 37:476–87. doi: 10.1002/ana.410370410
9. Bartolomei F, Chauvel P, Wendling F. Epileptogenicity of brain structures in human temporal lobe epilepsy: a quantified study from intracerebral EEG. *Brain.* (2008) 131:1818–30. doi: 10.1093/brain/awn111
10. David O, Blauwblomme T, Job AS, Chabardès S, Hoffmann D, Minotti L, et al. Imaging the seizure onset zone with stereo-electroencephalography. *Brain.* (2011) 134:2898–911. doi: 10.1093/brain/awr238
11. Grinenko O, Li J, Mosher JC, Wang IZ, Bulacio JC, Gonzalez-Martinez J, et al. A fingerprint of the epileptogenic zone in human epilepsies. *Brain.* (2018) 141:117–31. doi: 10.1093/brain/awx306
12. LeCun Y, Bengio Y, Hinton G. Deep learning. *Nature.* (2015) 521:436–44. doi: 10.1038/nature14539
13. LeCun Y, Boser B, Denker JS, Henderson D, Howard RE, Hubbard W, et al. Handwritten digit recognition with a back-propagation network. In: *Proc Advances in Neural Information Processing Systems.* (1990). p. 396–404.
14. LeCun Y, Bottou L, Bengio Y, Haffner P. Gradient-based learning applied to document recognition. *Proc IEEE.* (1998) 86:2278–324. doi: 10.1109/5.726791
15. Schmidhuber J. Deep learning in neural networks: an overview. *Neural Networks.* (2015) 61:85–117. doi: 10.1016/j.neunet.2014.09.003
16. Nijboer F, Sellers EW, Mellinger J, Jordan MA, Matuz T, Furdea A, et al. A P300-based brain-computer interface for people with amyotrophic lateral sclerosis. *Clin Neurophysiol.* (2008) 119:1909–16. doi: 10.1016/j.clinph.2008.03.034
17. Munbinger JI, Halder S, Kleih SC, Furdea A, Raco V, Hosle A, et al. Brain painting: first evaluation of a new brain-computer interface application with ALS-patients and healthy volunteers. *Front Neurosci.* (2010) 4:182. doi: 10.3389/fnins.2010.00182
18. Tonin L, Carlson T, Leeb R, Millan Jd R. Brain-controlled telepresence robot by motor-disabled people. In: *2011 Annual International Conference of the IEEE Engineering in Medicine and Biology Society.* (2011). p. 4227–30.
19. Wang Z, Lyu S, Schalk G, Ji Q. Deep feature learning using target priors with applications in ECoG signal decoding for BCI. In: *Proceedings of the Twenty-Third International Joint Conference on Artificial Intelligence, IJCAI.* Beijing: AAAI Press (2013). p. 1785–91.
20. Sakhavi S, Guan C, Yan S. Parallel convolutional-linear neural network for motor imagery classification. In: *23rd European Signal Processing Conference (EUSIPCO).* (2015). p. 2736–40.
21. Manor R, Mishali L, Geva AB. Multimodal neural network for rapid serial visual presentation brain computer interface. *Front Comput Neurosci.* (2016) 10:130. doi: 10.3389/fncom.2016.00130
22. Tabar YR, Halici U. A novel deep learning approach for classification of EEG motor imagery signals. *J Neural Eng.* (2017) 14:016003. doi: 10.1088/1741-2560/14/1/016003
23. Tang Z, Li C, Sun S. Single-trial EEG classification of motor imagery using deep convolutional neural networks. *Optik Int J Light Electron Opt.* (2017) 130:11–8. doi: 10.1016/j.ijleo.2016.10.117
24. Ramos-Murguialday A, Broetz D, Rea M, Laer L, Yilmaz O, Brasil FL, et al. Brain-machine interface in chronic stroke rehabilitation: a controlled study. *Ann Neurol.* (2013) 74:100–8. doi: 10.1002/ana.23879
25. Moghimi S, Kushki A, Guerguerian AM, Chau T. A review of EEG-based brain-computer interfaces as access pathways for individuals with severe disabilities. *Assist Technol.* (2013) 25:99–110. doi: 10.1080/10400435.2012.723298
26. Ortiz-Garcia A, Muruilla J, Gorriz JM, Ramirez J. Ensembles of deep learning architectures for the early diagnosis of Alzheimer's disease. *Int J Neural Syst.* (2016) 26:1650025. doi: 10.1142/S0129065716500258
27. Acharya UR, Oh SL, Hagiwara Y, Tan JH, Adeli H, Subha DP. Automated EEG-based screening of depression using deep convolutional network. *Comp Methods Program Biomed.* (2018) 161:103–13. doi: 10.1016/j.cmpb.2018.04.012
28. Das K, Giesbrecht B, Eckstein MP. Predicting variations ofperceptual performance across individuals from neural activity using pattern classifiers. *NeuroImage.* (2010) 51:1425–37. doi: 10.1016/j.neuroimage.2010.03.030
29. Knops A, Thirion B, Hubbard EM, Michel V, Dehaene S. Recruitment of an area involved in eye movements duringmental arithmetic. *Science.* (2009) 324:1583–5. doi: 10.1126/science.1171599
30. Kurth-Nelson Z, Economides M, Dolan RJ, Dayan P. Fastsequences of non-spatial state representations in humans. *Neuron.* (2016) 91:194–204. doi: 10.1016/j.neuron.2016.05.028
31. Stansbury DE, Naselaris T, Gallant JL. Natural scene statistics account for the representation of scene categories inhuman visual cortex. *Neuron.* (2013) 79:1025–34. doi: 10.1016/j.neuron.2013.06.034
32. Ren Y, Wu Y. Convolutional deep belief networks for feature extraction of EEG signal. In: *2014 International Joint Conference on Neural Networks (IJCNN).* (2014). p. 2850–3.
33. Stober S, Cameron DJ, Grahn JA. Using convolutional neural networks to recognize rhythm stimuli from electroencephalography recordings. In: *Proceedings of the 27th International Conference on Neural Information Processing Systems, NIPS.* Cambridge, MA: MIT Press (2014). p. 1449–57.
34. Schirrmeister RT, Springerberg JT, Fiederer LDJ, Glasstetter M, Eggensperger K, Tangerman M, et al. Deep learning with convolutional neural networks for EEG decoding and visualization. *Hum Brain Map.* (2017) 38:5391–420. doi: 10.1002/hbm.23730
35. Hajinoroozi M, Mao Z, Jung T-P, Lin C-T, Huang Y. EEG-based prediction of driver's cognitive performance by deep convolutional neural network. *Signal Process Image Commun.* (2016) 47:549–55. doi: 10.1016/j.image.2016.05.018
36. Sun X, Qian C, Chen Z, Wu Z, Luo B, Pan G. Remembered or forgotten?-An EEG-based computational prediction approach. *PLoS ONE.* (2016) 11:e0167497. doi: 10.1371/journal.pone.0167497
37. Cecotti H, Graser A. Convolutional neural networks for P300 detection with application to brain-computer interfaces. *IEEE Trans Pattern Anal Mach Intell.* (2011) 33:433–45. doi: 10.1109/TPAMI.2010.125
38. Page A, Shea C, Mohsenin T. Wearable seizure detection using convolutional neural networks with transfer learning. In: *2016 IEEE International Symposium on Circuits and Systems (ISCAS).* (2016). p. 1086–9.
39. Acharya UR, Oh SL, Hagiwara Y, Tan JH, Adeli H. Deep convolutional neural network for the automated detection and diagnosis of seizure using EEG signals. *Comput Biol Med.* (2018) 100:270–8. doi: 10.1016/j.compbiomed.2017.09.017
40. Wei X, Zhou L, Chen Z, Zhang L, Zhou Y. Automatic seizure detection using three-dimensional CNN based on multi-channel EEG. *BMC Med Inform Decis Mak.* (2018) 18(Suppl. 5):111. doi: 10.1186/s12911-018-0693-8
41. Zhang Y, Yang S, Liu Y, Zhang Y, Han B, Zhou F. Integration of 24 feature types to accurately detect and predict seizures using scalp EEG signals. *Sensors (Basel).* (2018) 18:E1372. doi: 10.3390/s18051372
42. Thodoroff P, Pineau J, Lim A. Learning robust features using deep learning for automatic seizure detection. In: *JMLR Workshop and Conference Proceedings* (2016).
43. Ansari AH, Cherian PJ, Caicedo A, Naulaers G, De Vos M, Van Huffel. S. Neonatal seizure detection using deep convolutional neural networks. *Int J Neural Syst.* (2018) 2:1850011. doi: 10.1142/S0129065718500119
44. Johansen AR, Jin J, Maszczyk T, Dauwels J, Cash SS, Westover MB. Epileptiform spike detection *via* convolutional neural networks. *Proc IEEE Int Conf Acoust Speech Signal Process.* (2016) 2016:754–8. doi: 10.1109/ICASSP.2016.7471776
45. Jing J, Sun H, Kim JA, Herlopian A, Karakis I, Ng M, et al. Development of expert-level automated detection of epileptiform discharges during electroencephalogram interpretation. *JAMA Neurol.* (2019) 77:103–8. doi: 10.1001/jamaneurol.2019.3485
46. Truong ND, Nguyen AD, Kuhlmann L, Bonyadi MR, Yang J, Ippolito S, et al. Convolutional neural networks for seizure prediction using intracranial and scalp electroencephalogram. *Neural Netw.* (2018) 105:104–11. doi: 10.1016/j.neunet.2018.04.018
47. Antoniades A, Spyrou L, Martin-Lopez D, Valentin A, Alarcon G, Sanei S, et al. Deep neural architectures for mapping scalp to intracranial EEG. *Int J Neural Syst.* (2018) 28:1850009. doi: 10.1142/S0129065718500090
48. Liang J, Lu R, Zhang C, Wang F. Predicting seizures from electroencephalography recordings: a knowledge transfer strategy. In: *2016 IEEE International Conference on Healthcare Informatics (ICHI).* (2016). p. 184–91.
49. Heller S, Hugle M, Nematollahi I, Manzouri F, Dumpelmann M, Schulze-Bonhage A, et al. Hardware implementation of a performance

and energy-optimized convolutional neural network for seizure detection. *Annu Int Conf IEEE Eng Med Biol Soc.* (2018) 2018:2268–71. doi: 10.1109/EMBC.2018.8512735

50. Sun FT, Morrell MJ. Closed-loop neurostimulation: the clinical experience. *Neurotherapeutics.* (2014) 11:553–63. doi: 10.1007/s13311-014-0280-3
51. Geller EB, Skarpaas TL, Gross RE, Goodman RR, Barkley GL, Bazil CW, et al. Brain-responsive neurostimulation in patients with medically intractable mesial temporal lobe epilepsy, *Epilepsia.* (2017) 58:994–1004. doi: 10.1111/epi.13740
52. Jobst BC, Kapur R, Barkley GL, Bazil CW, Berg MJ, Bergey GK, et al. Brain-responsive neurostimulation in patients with medically intractable seizures arising from eloquent and other neocortical areas. *Epilepsia.* (2017) 58:1005–14. doi: 10.1111/epi.13739
53. Razavi B, Rao VR, Lin C, Bujarski KA, Patra SE, Burdette DE, et al. Real-world experience with direct brain-responsive neurostimulation for focal onset seizures. *Epilepsia.* (2020) 61:1749–57. doi: 10.1111/epi.16593
54. Nair DR, Laxer KD, Weber PB, Murro AM, Park YD, Barkley GL, et al. Nine-year prospective efficacy and safety of brain-responsive neurostimulation for focal epilepsy. *Neurology.* (2020) 95:e1244–56. doi: 10.1212/WNL.0000000000010154
55. Kossoff EH, Ritzl EK, Politsky JM, Murro AM, Smith JR, Duckrow RB, et al. Effect of an external responsive neurostimulation on seizures and electrographic discharges during subdural electrode monitoring. *Epilepsia.* (2004) 45:1560–7. doi: 10.1111/j.0013-9580.2004.26104.x
56. Kokkinos V, Sisterson ND, Wozny TA, Richardson RM. Association of closed-loop brain stimulation neurophysiological features with seizure control among patients with focal epilepsy. *JAMA Neurol.* (2019) 76:800–8. doi: 10.1001/jamaneurol.2019.0658
57. Sisterson ND, Wosny TA, Kokkinos V, Constantino A, Richardson RM. Closed-loop brain stimulation for drug-resistant epilepsy: towards an evidence-based approach to personalized medicine. *Neurotherapeutics.* (2019) 16:119–27. doi: 10.1007/s13311-018-00682-4
58. Berg AT, Berkovic SF, Brodie MJ, Buchhalter J, Cross JH, van Emde Boas W, et al. Revised terminology and concepts for organization of seizures and epilepsies: report of the ILAE commission on classification and terminology, 2005-2009. *Epilepsia.* (2010) 51:676–85. doi: 10.1111/j.1528-1167.2010.02522.x
59. Fisher RS, Cross JH, French JA, Higurashi N, Hirsch E, Jansen FE, et al. Operational classification of seizure types by the international league against epilepsy: position paper of the ILAE commission for classification and terminology. *Epilepsia.* (2017) 58:522–30. doi: 10.1111/epi.13670
60. Krizhevsky A, Sutskever I, Hinton GE. Imagenet classification with deep convolutional neural networks. *Adv Neural Inform Process Syst.* (2012) 1097–105. doi: 10.1145/3065386
61. He K, Zhang X, Ren S, Sun J. Deep residual learning for image recognition. In: *Proceedings of the IEEE Conference on Computer Vision and Pattern Recognition.* (2016). p. 770–8.
62. Ioffe S, Szegedy C. Batch normalization: accelerating deep network training by reducing internal covariate shift. *ArXiv: 1502.03167.* (2015).
63. Nair V, Hinton GE. Rectified linear units improve restricted boltzmann machines. In: *Proceedings of the 27th International Conference on Machine Learning (ICML-10).* (2010). p. 807–14.
64. He K, Zhang X, Ren S, Sun J. Delving deep into rectifiers: surpassing human-level performance on imagenet classification. In: *Proceedings of the IEEE International Conference on Computer Vision.* (2015). p. 1026–34.
65. Smith LN. Cyclical learning rates for training neural networks. In: *IEEE Winter Conference on Applications of Computer Vision (WACV).* (2017). p. 464–72.
66. Quigg M, Sun F, Fountain NB, Jobst BC, Wong VS, Mirro E, et al. Interrater reliability in interpretation of electrocorticographic seizure detections of the responsive neurostimulator. *Epilepsia.* (2015) 56:968–71. doi: 10.1111/epi.12998
67. Sisterson ND, Wozny TA, Kokkinos V, Bagic A, Urban AP, Richardson RM. A rational approach to understanding and evaluating responsive neurostimulation. *Neuroinformatics.* (2020) 18:365–75. doi: 10.1007/s12021-019-09446-7
68. Nadler JV, Spencer DD. What is a seizure focus? *Adv Exp Med Biol.* (2014) 813:55–62. doi: 10.1007/978-94-017-8914-1_4
69. Alter AS, Dhamija R, McDonough TL, Shen S, McBrian DK, Mandel AM, et al. Ictal onset patterns of subdural intracranial electroencephalogram in children: how helpful for predicting epilepsy surgery outcome? *Epilepsy Res.* (2019) 149:44–52. doi: 10.1016/j.eplepsyres.2018.10.008
70. Fisher RS, Scharfman HE, deCurtis M. How can we identify ictal and interictal abnormal activity? *Adv Exp Med Biol.* (2014) 813:3–23. doi: 10.1007/978-94-017-8914-1_1
71. Krishnan B, Vlachos I, Faith A, Mullane S, Williams K, Alexopoulos A, et al. A novel spatiotemporal analysis of peri-ictal spiking to probe the relation of spikes and seizures in epilepsy. *Ann Biomed Eng.* (2014) 42:1606–17. doi: 10.1007/s10439-014-1004-x
72. Singh S, Sandy S, Wiebe S. Ictal onset on intracranial EEG: do we know it when we see it? State of the evidence. *Epilepsia.* (2015) 56:1629–38. doi: 10.1111/epi.13120
73. Malow A, Bowes RJ, Ross D. Relationship of temporal lobe seizures to sleep and arousal: a combined scalp-intracranial electrode study. *Sleep Mar.* (2000) 23:231–4. doi: 10.1093/sleep/23.2.1j
74. Klimes P, Cimbalnik J, Brazdil M, Hall J, Dubeau F, Gotman J, et al. NREM sleep is the state of vigilance that best identifies the epileptogenic zone in the interictal electroencephalogram. *Epilepsia.* (2019) 60:2404–15. doi: 10.1111/epi.16377
75. Perucca P, Dubeau F, Gotman J. Intracranial electroencephalographic seizure-onset patterns: effect of underlying pathology. *Brain.* (2014) 137:183–96. doi: 10.1093/brain/awt299
76. Sisterson ND, Kokkinos V. Neuromodulation of epilepsy networks. *Neurosurg Clin N Am.* (2020) 31:459–70. doi: 10.1016/j.nec.2020.03.009
77. Srivastava N, Hinton G, Krizhevsky A, Sutskever I, Salakhutdinov R. Dropout: a simple way to prevent neural networks from overfitting. *J Mach Learn. Res.* (2014) 15:1929–1958.
78. Bauer D, Quigg M. Optimizing management of medically responsive epilepsy. *Continuum (Minneap Minn).* (2019) 25:343–61. doi: 10.1212/CON.0000000000000709

19

Enhancing Safety in Epilepsy Surgery (EASINESS): Study Protocol for a Retrospective, Multicenter, Open Registry

Richard Drexler[1], Sharona Ben-Haim[2], Christian G. Bien[3], Valeri Borger[4], Francesco Cardinale[5], Alexandre Carpentier[6], Fernando Cendes[7], Sarat Chandra[8], Hans Clusmann[9], Albert Colon[10], Marco de Curtis[11], Daniel Delev[9], Giuseppe Didato[11], Lasse Dührsen[1], Jibril Osman Farah[12], Marc Guenot[13,14], Saadi Ghatan[15], Claire Haegelen[13,14], Hajo Hamer[16], Jason S. Hauptmann[17], Rosalind L. Jeffree[18,19], Thilo Kalbhenn[20], Josua Kegele[21], Niklaus Krayenbühl[22], Johannes Lang[16], Bertrand Mathon[6], Georgios Naros[21], Julia Onken[23], Fedor Panov[15], Christian Raftopoulos[24], Franz L. Ricklefs[1], Kim Rijkers[25], Michele Rizzi[26], Karl Rössler[27], Olaf Schijns[25,28], Ulf C. Schneider[23], Andrea Spyrantis[29], Adam Strzelczyk[29], Stefan Stodieck[30], Manjari Tripathi[8], Sumeet Vadera[31], Mario A. Alonso-Vanegas[32], José Géraldo Ribero Vaz[24], Jörg Wellmer[33], Tim Wehner[33], Manfred Westphal[1] and Thomas Sauvigny[1]*

Correspondence:
Richard Drexler
r.drexler@uke.de

[1] Department of Neurosurgery, University Medical Center Hamburg-Eppendorf, Hamburg, Germany, [2] Department of Neurosurgery, University of California San Diego, San Diego, CA, United States, [3] Epilepsy Centre Bethel, Krankenhaus Mara, Bielefeld, Germany, [4] Department of Neurosurgery, University Hospital Bonn, Bonn, Germany, [5] "C. Munari" Epilepsy Surgery Center, Niguarda Hospital, Milan, Italy, [6] Department of Neurosurgery, Pitié-Salpêtrière Hospital, Paris, France, [7] Department of Neurology, University of Campinas, Campinas, Brazil, [8] Department of Neurosurgery, AIIMS, New Delhi, India, [9] Department of Neurosurgery, University Hospital RWTH Aachen, Aachen, Germany, [10] School for Mental Health and Neuroscience (MHeNS), University Maastricht (UM), Maastricht, Netherlands, [11] Epilepsy Unit, IRCCS "C. Besta" Neurological Institute Foundation, Milan, Italy, [12] The Walton Centre NHS Foundation Trust, Liverpool, United Kingdom, [13] Department of Functional Neurosurgery, P. Wertheimer Hospital, Hospices Civils de Lyon, Lyon, France, [14] Department for Neurosurgery, University of Lyon, Lyon, France, [15] Department of Neurosurgery, Icahn School of Medicine at Mount Sinai, New York, NY, United States, [16] Epilepsy Center, Department of Neurology, University of Erlangen-Nürnberg, Erlangen, Germany, [17] Department of Neurosurgery, University of Washington, Seattle, WA, United States, [18] Department of Neurosurgery, Royal Brisbane and Womens Hospital, Brisbane, QLD, Australia, [19] Herston Clinical School, University of Queensland, Brisbane, QLD, Australia, [20] Department of Neurosurgery (Evangelisches Klinikum Bethel), Bielefeld University, Medical School, Bielefeld, Germany, [21] Department of Neurology and Epileptology, Hertie Institute of Clinical Brain Research, University of Tubingen, Tubingen, Germany, [22] Division of Pediatric Neurosurgery, University Children's Hospital Zurich, University of Zurich, Zurich, Switzerland, [23] Department of Neurosurgery, Universitätsmedizin Charité-Berlin, Berlin, Germany, [24] Department of Neurosurgery, University Hospital St-Luc, Université Catholique de Louvain (UCL), Brussels, Belgium, [25] Department of Neurosurgery, Academic Center for Epileptology UMC Maastricht, Maastricht, Netherlands, [26] Department of Neurosurgery, Fondazione IRCCS Istituto Neurologico Carlo Besta, Milan, Italy, [27] Department of Neurosurgery, Medical University Vienna, Vienna, Austria, [28] School for Mental Health and Neuroscience (MHeNS), University Maastricht (UM), Maastricht, Netherlands, [29] Department of Neurosurgery and Epilepsy Center Frankfurt Rhine-Main, Center of Neurology and Neurosurgery, Goethe-University Frankfurt, Frankfurt, Germany, [30] Hamburg Epilepsy Center, Protestant Hospital Alsterdorf, Department of Neurology and Epileptology, Hamburg, Germany, [31] Department of Neurological Surgery, University of California Irvine, Irvine, CA, United States, [32] National Institute of Neurology and Neurosurgery, Manuel Velasco Suarez, Mexico City, Mexico, [33] Ruhr - Epileptology, Department of Neurology, University Hospital Knappschafts-Krankenhaus, Ruhr - University Bochum, Bochum, Germany

Introduction: Optimizing patient safety and quality improvement is increasingly important in surgery. Benchmarks and clinical quality registries are being developed to assess the best achievable results for several surgical procedures and reduce unwarranted variation between different centers. However, there is no clinical database from international centers for establishing standardized reference values of patients undergoing surgery for mesial temporal lobe epilepsy.

Design: The Enhancing Safety in Epilepsy Surgery (EASINESS) study is a retrospectively conducted, multicenter, open registry. All patients undergoing mesial temporal lobe epilepsy surgery in participating centers between January 2015 and December 2019 are included in this study. The patient characteristics, preoperative diagnostic tools, surgical data, postoperative complications, and long-term seizure outcomes are recorded.

Outcomes: The collected data will be used for establishing standardized reference values ("benchmarks") for this type of surgical procedure. The primary endpoints include seizure outcomes according to the International League Against Epilepsy (ILAE) classification and defined postoperative complications.

Discussion: The EASINESS will define robust and standardized outcome references after amygdalohippocampectomy for temporal lobe epilepsy. After the successful definition of benchmarks from an international cohort of renowned centers, these data will serve as reference values for the evaluation of novel surgical techniques and comparisons among centers for future clinical trials.

Clinical Trial Registration: This study is indexed at clinicaltrials.gov (NT 04952298).

Keywords: epilepsy, epilepsy surgery, temporal lobe epilepsy, outcome, benchmark, seizure outcome, amygdalohippocampectomy, anteromedial resection

INTRODUCTION

Surgeons strive for the best possible outcome from their operations with the greatest possible chance for recovery and cure of the patients. To optimize the outcome, the continuous monitoring and measurement of key elements of surgical procedures are indispensable. To this end, the number of clinical registries has increased in recent years (1). To evaluate surgical quality, recent initiatives aim to assess the best achievable results for several surgical procedures and reduce unwarranted variation between different centers (2–4). A standardized methodology to describe optimal outcomes in neurosurgery is lacking. The most appealing concept in surgery is a combination of various clinical indicators with risk stratification and a focus on treatment efficacy and adverse events. This offers a more reliable analysis than single-outcome indicators, such as survival or readmission rate (5–10). Nevertheless, an establishment of clinical databases from international centers with an accurate collection of demographic, management, and outcome data for respective surgical procedures is needed. The importance of establishing benchmarks has been demonstrated for various surgical procedures in general and visceral surgery (11–15). As yet, there is very little published about acceptable neurosurgical benchmarks. A benchmark establishes standardized reference values which represent the acceptable common outcome of high-volume centers and can be used for comparison and improvement. Best results are obtained from patients at the lowest risk (10). Therefore, the cohort must be divided into low-risk and high-risk patients according to the defined benchmark criteria that predict a potentially worse postoperative outcome.

The aim of this international multicenter register [Enhancing Safety in Epilepsy Surgery (EASINESS)] is to define robust and standardized outcome references after amygdalohippocampectomy and anteromedial temporal lobectomy for temporal lobe epilepsy. After the successful determination of benchmarks from an international cohort of renowned centers, these data will serve as reference values for the evaluation of novel surgical techniques and comparisons among centers for future clinical trials. They will provide feedback to participating centers to enable deficiencies in care to be addressed, thereby enabling quality improvement. This registry will demonstrate the feasibility and utility of risk-stratified benchmarked data for neurosurgical practice.

MATERIALS AND METHODS

Study Design

The EASINESS is a retrospectively conducted, multicenter, open registry. The study is a procedure-specific registry, initiated by the Department of Neurosurgery, University Medical Center Hamburg-Eppendorf, Germany. The selected members of participating neurosurgical or epilepsy centers will be invited to form a Steering Committee, which will be responsible for the scientific goals and guarantee the reliability of the data analysis. Neurosurgical, neurological, and epilepsy units from all countries are invited to join the trial and to recruit patients if the center- and patient-specific inclusion criteria are met.

Study Setting and Type of Participants

All patients undergoing mesial temporal lobe epilepsy surgery between January 1, 2015 and December 31, 2019 are included in the study. The following surgical procedures are included: selective amygdalohippocampectomy including anterior parahippocampal gyrus/entorhinal cortex, anteromedial temporal lobe resection including amygdalohippocampectomy with approximately anterior third of the temporal neocortex,

TABLE 1 | Inclusion and exclusion criteria for centers and patients to participate in the Enhancing Safety in Epilepsy Surgery (EASINESS) registry.

Inclusion criteria	Exclusion criteria
Center-specific: 1. Centers with ≥30 seizure-specific resections (excluding vagus nerve stimulation) as an average per year during the study period	
Patient-specific: 1. Patients who went through mesial temporal lobe epilepsy surgery, including: a. Selective Amygdalohippocempectomy including anterior parahippocampal gyrus / entorhinal cortex b. Anteromedial temporal lobe resection including amygdalohippocampectomy c. Anterior temporal lobe resection	1. Patients who went through neocortical temporal resection only 2. Patients who went through recurrent resection

amygdala, uncus, hippocampus, anterior parahippocampal gyrus/entorhinal cortex, and anterior temporal lobe resection with two-thirds of the temporal neocortex, amygdala, uncus, hippocampus, and anterior parahippocampal gyrus/entorhinal cortex (16, 17). Patients who went through deep brain stimulation, vagus nerve stimulation, neocortical temporal resection only, or a recurrent resection are not included in this study.

Center-Specific Inclusion Criteria

The participating centers need to perform 30 or more seizure-specific resections as an average per year during the 5-year study period. This threshold is based on the recommendations of the German Society for Epileptology and the Austrian, German, and Swiss working group on presurgical epilepsy diagnosis and operative epilepsy treatment for certification as an epilepsy center performing epilepsy surgery (18, 19). International centers may be accepted on a case-by-case basis if they meet the alternative local guidelines for epilepsy center definition. The implantation of vagus nerve stimulators was not counted toward the number of seizure-specific procedures (**Table 1**).

Informed Consent

Written informed consent is not required in this retrospective study since all patient data are processed anonymously. The study was approved by the Institutional Ethics Committee centrally at University Medical Center Hamburg-Eppendorf and local governance approval was obtained by each site as necessary. The patients' data were extracted and analyzed following the declaration of Helsinki.

Data Collection

According to a standardized template for mesial temporal lobe epilepsy surgery, patient-specific data, surgical details, postoperative complications, and long-term seizure outcome including neuropsychological assessment will be recorded. The data acquisition will be electronic-based (case report form, CRF), and patient-specific data will be de-identified by the study center. The data will then be transferred into an electronic database and further analyses made at the Department of Neurosurgery, University Medical Center Hamburg-Eppendorf.

Case Report Form

The specially designed and developed Case Report Form (CRF) consists of four parts (**Figure 1**).

1. *Patient characteristics:* The first part of the CRF covers preoperative characteristics including patient demographic and baseline characteristics (sex, age, body mass index, educational status, neurological status), comorbidities (diabetes, congestive heart failure, coagulopathy, and COPD), and the American Society of Anesthesiologists (ASA) Physical Status Classification. In addition, seizure-specific features such as a history of neonatal seizure, febrile seizure, encephalitis or meningitis, age at epilepsy onset, type of seizure, average monthly frequency of seizures, and a number of anticonvulsive drugs at the time of surgery are registered. Furthermore, presurgical diagnostic tools (e.g., invasive monitoring, PET, SPECT, MEG) and possible lesions in MRI will be documented.
2. *Surgical data:* This part covers all aspects of mesial temporal lobe epilepsy surgery. Here, type of procedure, intraoperative navigation, resection of the dominant or non-dominant hemisphere, side of resection, and the operating duration are registered.
3. *Postoperative complications:* The fourth part addresses all questions of the outcome until discharge after index surgery. Postoperative complications such as stroke, surgical site infection, meningitis, reoperation, new neurological deficits, and in-hospital mortality will be recorded. In addition, the histological finding of the resected lesion is registered.
4. *Follow-up:* Long-term clinical and seizure outcome after 12 months and an optional later time will be recorded. Here, long-term complications such as reoperation, temporalis muscle atrophy, and neurological deficits are registered. To analyze the seizure-specific outcome after surgery, the International League Against Epilepsy (ILAE) outcome scale, neuropsychological assessment (verbal and figural memory, attention), and the number of antiseizure medications will be documented.

Data Management

Data collection will be performed locally at each site and de-identified in an independent database, then submitted to the Department of Neurosurgery at University Medical Center Hamburg-Eppendorf (Germany). All results, including patient-specific data, surgical techniques, complications, and long-term outcomes, will be submitted for publication in peer-reviewed journals and/or reported at professional scientific meetings. Every participating center can submit further scientific questions which will be evaluated by the steering committee for approval or rejection. The by-laws of the steering committee are accessible from the principal investigator upon request. This study is indexed at clinicaltrials.gov (NT 04952298).

Center-specific data:

- Number of yearly seizure-specific resections (excluding vagus nerve stimulation) during the study period
- Number of yearly mesial temporal lobe epilepsy surgery during the study period

↓

Preoperative patient characteristics:

- Basic features (sex, age, body mass index, education status, ASA physical status classification)
- Comorbidities (diabetes, congestive heart failure, coagulopathy, COPD)
- History of neonatal or febrile seizures, and meningitis or encephalitis
- Age at epilepsy onset
- Type of seizure
- Average monthly frequency of seizures impairing awareness in year before surgery
- Number of anticonvulsive drugs at time of surgery
- Neurological deficit
- Preoperative MRI (Identifiable lesion, post-processing conducted)
- Preoperative invasive monitoring (sEEG, subdural electrodes/ECoG)
- Preoperative diagnostic tool (PET, SPECT, MEG, Wada)

↓

Surgical data:

- Type of procedure
- Intraoperative navigation
- Dominant or non-dominant hemisphere
- Side of procedure
- Operating duration

↓

Postoperative complications:

- Complication of any severity (stroke, surgical site infection, meningitis)
- Reoperation rate
- Neurological deficit
- In-hospital mortality
- Reoperation
- Length of ICU and postoperative stay
- Histological finding (hippocampal sclerosis, focal cortical dysplasia, DNET, ganglioglioma, others)
- 3D-Volumetry of extent of resection on MRI >3months postoperatively if applicable

↓

Follow-up at 12 months and last seen:

- Reoperation rate
- Temporalis muscle atrophy
- Neurological deficit
- ILAE Outcome Scale
- Neuropsychological assessment (verbal memory, figural memory, attention)
- Number of anticonvulsive drugs

FIGURE 1 | Study protocol of the Enhancing Safety in Epilepsy Surgery (EASINESS) registry.

Statistics

The endpoints will be evaluated using descriptive statistics, and the key figures of the distributions will be presented in tables. Statistical analyses will be made as described in previous studies which established the concept of benchmarking for other surgical procedures (10, 11, 15). Hereby, the cohort is stratified into patients with a low-preoperative and high-preoperative risk profile according to comorbidities which are proven to negatively impact the postoperative course. Afterward, the benchmark cut-off for each outcome indicator is set at the 75th percentile of the median of all centers (10). Depending on the composition of the data, $\chi 2$, Mann-Whitney U, and *t*-tests, or Pearson or Spearman correlation coefficients, will be conducted. The relationships between multiple independent variables on the dependent variable(s) will be tested using multivariate regression analysis.

Registry Reports

The results of the EASINESS registry will be published by the Steering Committee and distributed to all participating centers following careful analysis by the principal investigators (R.D. and T.S.) at the Department of Neurosurgery, University Medical Center Hamburg-Eppendorf.

DISCUSSION

In recent years, quality monitoring and improvement have become more important in the field of healthcare, especially in surgery (20, 21). As a various single- and multiple-outcome indicators for evaluating the quality of surgical procedures were introduced, the concept of benchmarking as introduced by Staiger et al. seems to be the most reliable concept for establishing standardized outcome references and defining acceptable outcomes (10). Benchmarking offers an opportunity to present valid, internationally applicable reference values which originate from the daily routine of a large representative cohort. This will be the first internationally validated benchmark data for neurosurgery and as such will demonstrate that such data collection is both feasible and useful.

Unlike data from randomized controlled trials, which have stringent patient selection criteria and questionable generalizability, this study has only a few patient-specific inclusion criteria, and the results will therefore be generalizable to usual neurosurgical practice.

The EASINESS is a retrospectively conducted, multicenter, open registry with narrowly defined inclusion criteria for international centers. The objective is the application of the previously described benchmarking to define robust and standardized outcome references after temporal lobe epilepsy surgery. Afterward, these benchmarks from an international cohort of high-volume centers will serve as reference values for the evaluation of novel surgical techniques and comparisons among centers or future clinical trials. Furthermore, EASINESS has been established with an interdisciplinary approach collecting outcome data from both a neurosurgical and epileptogenic perspective and presenting novel valuable data compared with existing registries.

Limitations of This Study

The results of this registry should be interpreted considering the limitation that the study design is a retrospective, non-randomized design which could introduce some bias.

AUTHOR CONTRIBUTIONS

RD, LD, and TS contributed to conceptualization and design. All authors drafted the manuscript, critically revised it and collect the data.

REFERENCES

1. Stey AM, Russell MM, Ko CY, Sacks GD, Dawes AJ, Gibbons MM. Clinical registries and quality measurement in surgery: a systematic review. *Surgery.* (2015) 157:381–95. doi: 10.1016/j.surg.2014.08.097
2. Khuri SF, Daley J, Henderson W, Hur K, Demakis J, Aust JB, et al. The Department of Veterans Affairs' NSQIP: the first national, validated, outcome-based, risk-adjusted, and peer-controlled program for the measurement and enhancement of the quality of surgical care. National VA Surgical Quality Improvement Program. *Ann Surg.* (1998) 228:491–507. doi: 10.1097/00000658-199810000-00006
3. Rowell KS, Turrentine FE, Hutter MM, Khuri SF, Henderson WG. Use of national surgical quality improvement program data as a catalyst for quality improvement. *J Am Coll Surg.* (2007) 204:1293–300. doi: 10.1016/j.jamcollsurg.2007.03.024
4. Kao LS, Lally KP, Thomas EJ, Tyson JE. Improving quality improvement: a methodologic framework for evaluating effectiveness of surgical quality improvement. *J Am Coll Surg.* (2009) 208:621–6. doi: 10.1016/j.jamcollsurg.2009.01.021
5. Dimick JB, Welch HG, Birkmeyer JD. Surgical mortality as an indicator of hospital quality: the problem with small sample size. *JAMA.* (2004) 292:847–51. doi: 10.1001/jama.292.7.847
6. Porter ME. What is value in health care? *N Engl J Med.* (2010) 363:2477–81. doi: 10.1056/NEJMp1011024
7. Donabedian A. The quality of care. How can it be assessed? *JAMA J Am Med Assoc.* (1988) 260:1743–8. doi: 10.1001/jama.260.12.1743
8. Salet N, Bremmer RH, Verhagen MAMT, Ekkelenkamp VE, Hansen BE, de Jonge PJF, et al. Is Textbook Outcome a valuable composite measure for short-term outcomes of gastrointestinal treatments in the Netherlands using hospital information system data? A retrospective cohort study. *BMJ Open.* (2018) 8:e019405. doi: 10.1136/bmjopen-2017-019405
9. Mainz J. Defining and classifying clinical indicators for quality improvement. *Int J Qual Health Care J Int Soc Qual Health Care.* (2003) 15:523–30. doi: 10.1093/intqhc/mzg081
10. Staiger RD, Schwandt H, Puhan MA, Clavien P-A. Improving surgical outcomes through benchmarking. *Br J Surg.* (2019) 106:59–64. doi: 10.1002/bjs.10976
11. Muller X, Marcon F, Sapisochin G, Marquez M, Dondero F, Rayar M, et al. Defining benchmarks in liver transplantation: a multicenter outcome analysis determining best achievable results. *Ann Surg.* (2018) 267:419–25. doi: 10.1097/SLA.0000000000002477
12. Raptis DA, Sánchez-Velázquez P, Machairas N, Sauvanet A, Rueda de. Leon A, Oba A, et al. Defining benchmark outcomes for pancreatoduodenectomy with portomesenteric venous resection. *Ann Surg.* (2020) 272:731–7. doi: 10.1097/SLA.0000000000004267
13. Raptis DA, Linecker M, Kambakamba P, Tschuor C, Müller PC, Hadjittofi C, et al. Defining benchmark outcomes for ALPPS. *Ann Surg.* (2019) 270:835–41. doi: 10.1097/SLA.0000000000003539

14. Rössler F, Sapisochin G, Song G, Lin Y-H, Simpson MA, Hasegawa K, et al. Defining benchmarks for major liver surgery: a multicenter analysis of 5202 living liver donors. *Ann Surg.* (2016) 264:492–500. doi: 10.1097/SLA.0000000000001849
15. Sánchez-Velázquez P, Muller X, Malleo G, Park J-S, Hwang H-K, Napoli N, et al. Benchmarks in pancreatic surgery: a novel tool for unbiased outcome comparisons. *Ann Surg.* (2019) 270:211–8. doi: 10.1097/SLA.0000000000003223
16. Schramm J. Temporal lobe epilepsy surgery and the quest for optimal extent of resection: a review. *Epilepsia.* (2008) 49:1296–307. doi: 10.1111/j.1528-1167.2008.01604.x
17. Al-Otaibi F, Baeesa SS, Parrent AG, Girvin JP, Steven D. Surgical techniques for the treatment of temporal lobe epilepsy. *Epilepsy Res Treat.* (2012) 2012:1–13. doi: 10.1155/2012/374848
18. Schmitz B, Mayer T, Neubauer B, Rosenow F, Bast T. Definition von Epilepsiezentren [Internet]. (2010). Available online at: http://www.izepilepsie.de/cweb2/cgi-bin-noauth/cache/VAL_BLOB/4092/4092/1106/definitionepilepsiezentren.pdf
19. Rosenow F, Bast T, Czech T, Feucht M, Hans VH, Helmstaedter C, et al. Revised version of quality guidelines for presurgical epilepsy evaluation and surgical epilepsy therapy issued by the Austrian, German, and Swiss working group on presurgical epilepsy diagnosis and operative epilepsy treatment. *Epilepsia.* (2016) 57:1215–20. doi: 10.1111/epi.13449
20. Ettorchi-Tardy A, Levif M, Michel P. Benchmarking: a method for continuous quality improvement in health. *Healthc Policy Polit Sante.* (2012) 7:e101–119. doi: 10.12927/hcpol.2012.22872
21. von Eiff W. International benchmarking and best practice management: in search of health care and hospital excellence. *Adv Health Care Manag.* (2015) 17:223–52. doi: 10.1108/S1474-823120140000017014

20

Quantification and Selection of Ictogenic Zones in Epilepsy Surgery

Petroula Laiou[1,2,3], Eleftherios Avramidis[4], Marinho A. Lopes[1,2,3,5], Eugenio Abela[6], Michael Müller[7,8], Ozgur E. Akman[3], Mark P. Richardson[6], Christian Rummel[7], Kaspar Schindler[8] and Marc Goodfellow[1,2,3,5]*

[1] Living Systems Institute, University of Exeter, Exeter, United Kingdom, [2] EPSRC Centre for Predictive Modelling in Healthcare, University of Exeter, Exeter, United Kingdom, [3] College of Engineering, Mathematics and Physical Sciences, University of Exeter, Exeter, United Kingdom, [4] Research Computing Services, University of Cambridge, Cambridge, United Kingdom, [5] Wellcome Trust Centre for Biomedical Modelling and Analysis, University of Exeter, Exeter, United Kingdom, [6] Institute of Psychiatry, Psychology and Neuroscience, King's College London, London, United Kingdom, [7] Support Center for Advanced Neuroimaging, University Institute for Diagnostic and Interventional Neuroradiology, Inselspital, Bern University Hospital, University of Bern, Bern, Switzerland, [8] Department of Neurology, Inselspital, University Hospital Bern, Bern, Switzerland

***Correspondence:**
Petroula Laiou
p.laiou@exeter.ac.uk*

Network models of brain dynamics provide valuable insight into the healthy functioning of the brain and how this breaks down in disease. A pertinent example is the use of network models to understand seizure generation (ictogenesis) in epilepsy. Recently, computational models have emerged to aid our understanding of seizures and to predict the outcome of surgical perturbations to brain networks. Such approaches provide the opportunity to quantify the effect of removing regions of tissue from brain networks and thereby search for the optimal resection strategy. Here, we use computational models to elucidate how sets of nodes contribute to the ictogenicity of networks. In small networks we fully elucidate the ictogenicity of all possible sets of nodes and demonstrate that the distribution of ictogenicity across sets depends on network topology. However, the full elucidation is a combinatorial problem that becomes intractable for large networks. Therefore, we combine computational models with a genetic algorithm to search for minimal sets of nodes that contribute significantly to ictogenesis. We demonstrate the potential applicability of these methods in practice by identifying optimal sets of nodes to resect in networks derived from 20 individuals who underwent resective surgery for epilepsy. We show that they have the potential to aid epilepsy surgery by suggesting alternative resection sites as well as facilitating the avoidance of brain regions that should not be resected.

Keywords: epilepsy surgery, brain networks, ictogenesis, graph theory, optimization, genetic algorithm

INTRODUCTION

Approximately 30% of people with epilepsy have refractory seizures, i.e. their seizures cannot be controlled by medication (1, 2). In these cases, the surgical removal or disconnection of the putative "epileptogenic zone" (EZ), i.e. the region of brain tissue thought to be indispensable for the generation of seizures, is a potential therapeutic option that can alleviate seizures in many cases (3, 4). The epileptogenic zone is currently defined retrospectively: diverse information is integrated by clinical teams to define targets for resection, and if seizure freedom is achieved after surgery, the EZ is assumed to have been removed (3). Unfortunately, post-operative seizure freedom rates are currently sub-optimal and not everyone who could potentially benefit from surgery is identified as a candidate (5–9). In order to improve the success of epilepsy surgery and widen its potential usage, a better understanding of the mechanisms of seizure generation is required, and improved, quantitative methods to prospectively map the EZ need to be developed (10, 11).

Computational studies of seizure generation in large-scale brain networks with the aim to inform epilepsy surgery have recently begun to emerge (11–14). In an early such study we introduced a quantitative framework for prospectively evaluating the effect that surgical removal of tissue would have (11). The framework proceeds by first mapping an ictogenic network i.e. a set of brain regions, together with connections between them, that are important for the generation of seizures. A dynamic model is then applied to this network in order to simulate epileptiform dynamics and thereby quantify the seizure generating capability of the network. This is captured in a quantity called Brain Network Ictogenicity (*BNI*) that can be measured from simulations of the model (15). Crucially, measuring the *BNI* for a network provides a baseline against which the effect of perturbations, such as the removal of nodes (which is a proxy for surgery), can be quantified. We recently showed that our model could accurately delineate surgeries that resulted in seizure freedom from those that did not (11). Subsequent studies have added evidence for the potential use of models to guide epilepsy surgery (12, 13). Using models to quantify ictogenicity opens up avenues for the improvement of pre-surgical mapping. For example, putative resections can be quantitatively compared *in silico*, and resections providing large reductions in ictogenicity (i.e. substantial reduction in seizure occurrence) can be sought. This in itself leads to a re-imagining of the concept of the epileptogenic zone for pre-surgical planning: rather than searching for correlates of a region of tissue that should render a person seizure free, we can quantify the seizure reducing capabilities of removing many alternative sets of nodes in a network prospectively, *in silico*.

Here, we use a quantity called Set Ictogenicity (*SI*) [previously introduced as ΔBNI (11)] to represent the extent to which ictogenicity is reduced when a given set of nodes is removed from a network. *SI* can be quantified for any potential set of nodes in a resection using the framework described above. Once the effect of removing a set of nodes can be quantified, one can compare the effect of removing different sets, and choose the set with the minimal number of nodes that would yield the largest reduction in ictogenicity (i.e. find the set with largest *SI*, which would be designated as a putative EZ). However, to ensure an optimal solution is uncovered, one would have to evaluate the *SI* of all possible combinations of sets of nodes within a given network. Unfortunately, this is a combinatorial optimization problem in which the number of sets to search through quickly becomes intractable, even for moderately sized networks (16, 17). Though in practice constraints on the location of resections may exist, alternative strategies to exhaustive searches have to be explored. One could use heuristics that are quick but do not guarantee finding an optimum (18, 19). For example, previous approaches (11, 12, 20) applied heuristics to attempt to identify a set of nodes that optimally reduces the network ictogenicity. However, the selection of nodes of that set was solely based on the contribution of single nodes to seizure generation. In other application areas, combinatorial problems have previously been approached using global non-deterministic search strategies, like simulated annealing (21), evolution strategies (22), genetic algorithms (16, 17) and particle swarm optimization (23). The deployment of such approaches to brain networks would enable us to gain a deeper insight into the way that ictogenesis is distributed throughout networks and facilitate the development of optimal strategies for epilepsy surgery.

Here we use computational models to study the ictogenicity of sets of nodes within a network. We use artificial networks to explore how *SI* varies across sets of nodes within networks of different topologies and to characterize the relationship between common graph metrics and *SI*. To facilitate the search for optimal resections, we develop and validate a multi-objective genetic algorithm to uncover sets of nodes that optimally reduce the ictogenicity of a network. In addition, we apply the methodology to a cohort of 20 people who underwent epilepsy surgery. Finally, we discuss the potential benefits of these approaches to both enhance our understanding of epilepsy and advance pre-surgical planning in practice.

MATERIALS AND METHODS

Simulation of Brain Dynamics

We use a mathematical modeling framework to simulate and predict the outcome of epilepsy surgery (11). The framework uses intracranial electroencephalographic (iEEG) recordings (**Figure 1A**) to construct functional networks (**Figure 1B**), where nodes are associated with electrodes and edges denote interrelations between the recorded signals. We use a surrogate corrected version of mutual information (10, 24) that detects non-linear dependencies in excess of linear relationships to define weighted edges of the network (see **Supplementary Text S1** and **Supplementary Figure 1**). We then place a mathematical model on each node (**Figure 1C**). We use the canonical theta model (20, 25) which has previously been shown to give a good approximation of the response of the Wendling neural mass model (26) to node removal perturbations (20). A key assumption underlying this approximation is that the neural mass model is operating in the vicinity of a saddle node on invariant circle (SNIC) bifurcation, which has previously been used to model epileptiform dynamics (11, 26, 27). Nodes can display transitions between "normal activity" (stable fixed point) and "epileptiform dynamics" (stable limit cycle) through a saddle node on invariant circle (SNIC) bifurcation. The dynamics of node j ($j = 1, \ldots, N$, where N is the number of nodes in the network) is represented by its phase θ_j and obeys

$$\dot{\theta}_j(t) = \left(1 - \cos\theta_j(t)\right) + \left(1 + \cos\theta_j(t)\right) I_j(t) \quad (1)$$

where $I_j(t)$ is the input current that the node receives from the other nodes in the network,

$$I_j(t) = I_o + \xi_j(t) + \frac{K}{N}\sum_{i=1}^{N} a_{ij}\left[1 - \cos\left(\theta_i(t) - \theta_i^s(t)\right)\right]. \quad (2)$$

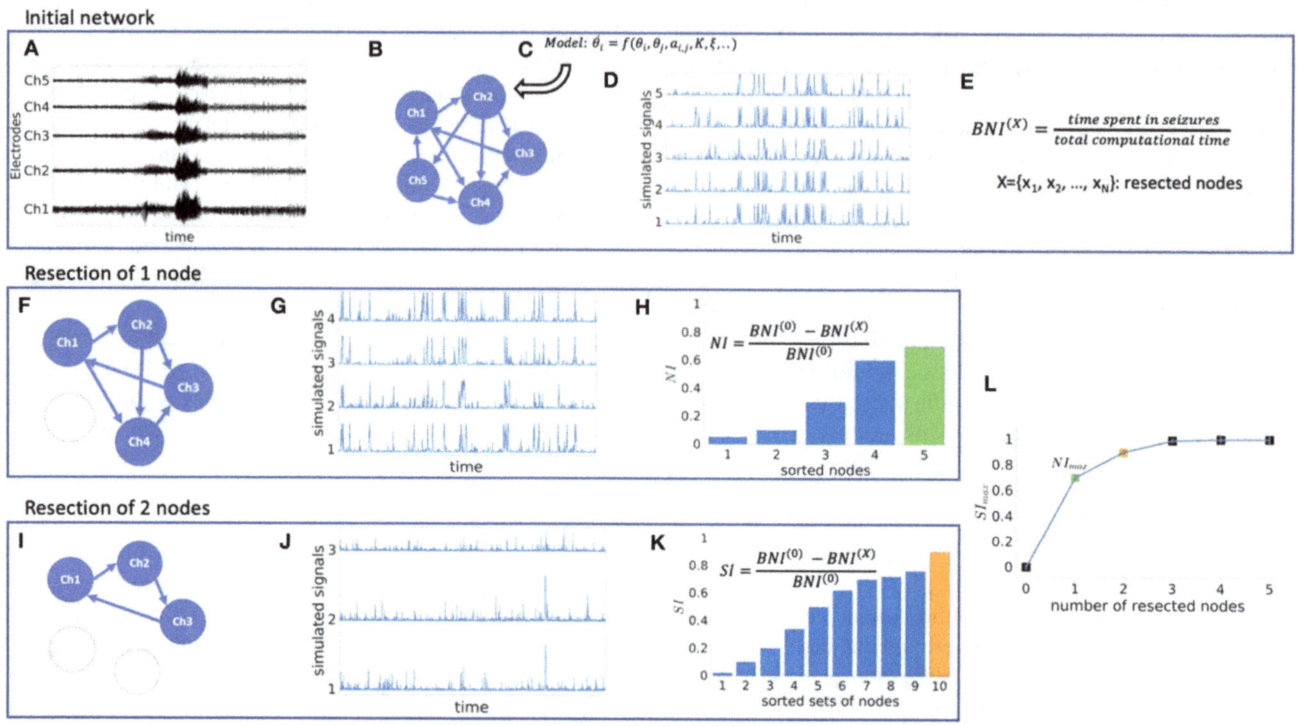

FIGURE 1 | Schematic representation of the mathematical framework. From intracranial recordings **(A)** we construct a functional network **(B)**. We then place a mathematical model on each node **(C)**, simulate signals from the model **(D)** and calculate brain network ictogenicity **(E)**. Then perturbations are applied to the network by removing individual nodes **(F)** or set of nodes **(I)**. Using the simulated signals from the perturbed networks **(G,J)**, Node Ictogenicity (*NI*) and Set Ictogenicity (*SI*) are calculated for all possible combinations of resected nodes [panels **(H,K)**, respectively]. Finally, for every number of resected nodes the set that contributes most to the seizure generation is the one with the maximum *SI* **(H,K,L)**. **(L)** Illustrates the *SI* of the most ictogenic sets split out by resection size.

In Equation (2) the term $I_o + \xi_j$ is white uncorrelated Gaussian noise with mean $I_o = -1.2$ and standard deviation 0.6, as used in previous studies (20). a_{ij} is the (i, j) th entry of the adjacency matrix (i.e., the weighted matrix that represents the functional network), K is a global scaling factor that scales the network interactions compared to the noise, and θ_i^s is the stable fixed point of node i ($\dot{\theta}_i = 0$ at $\xi_i = K = 0$). For the integration of Equation (1) we use the Euler-Maruyama method with step size 0.01.

Quantification of Ictogenicity

The theta model enables us to simulate brain dynamics on a network (**Figure 1D**). Low amplitude signals correspond to "normal activity" whilst high amplitude signals represent "epileptiform dynamics" (20). We use the quantity Brain Network Ictogenicity (*BNI*) (11, 15) to quantify the propensity of the network to generate seizures. In practice, *BNI* measures the average time that each node spends in epileptiform dynamics (t_i, $i = 1, \ldots, N$) over a sufficiently long computational time (we use 4×10^6 time steps),

$$BNI = \frac{1}{N} \sum_{i=1}^{N} \frac{t_i}{T}. \qquad (3)$$

BNI varies between zero (all nodes display "normal activity" all the time) and one (all nodes show "seizure activity" all the time). The change in *BNI* upon removal of individual nodes or a set of nodes allows us to quantify their ictogenicity. Here, removal of nodes is implemented by setting all incoming and outgoing connections from and to other nodes to zero (**Figures 1F–K**). To measure the impact of removing a set of nodes on *BNI*, we define Set Ictogenicity (*SI*) as

$$SI_X = \frac{BNI^{(0)} - BNI^{(X)}}{BNI^{(0)}} \qquad (4)$$

where $BNI^{(0)}$ is a reference value for the unperturbed network, and $BNI^{(X)}$ denotes the *BNI* value after the removal of all n nodes in the subset $X = \{x_1, .., x_n\}$. We tune the parameter K in the model such that $BNI^{(0)}$ equals 0.5 (11, 20) which means that on average the network spends half of the computational time in epileptiform dynamics. We consider this value as a useful reference because it enables us to study the result of network perturbations more efficiently (a realistic value of $BNI^{(0)}$ would be much smaller, and changes of *BNI* upon node removals would be more difficult to measure). Note that for $n = 1$ in Equation (4), SI_X is equivalent to the Node Ictogenicity (NI_X), previously introduced in Goodfellow et al. (11), which measures the effect of removing a single node in *BNI* (**Figures 1F–H**). SI_X is a succinct term for ΔBNI, which was introduced in Goodfellow et al. (11). Larger SI_X values denote greater contribution of the considered set X to seizure generation. SI_X takes a value of one when the removed set of nodes leads to elimination of epileptiform dynamics, whilst zero or negative values denote that removing those nodes did not reduce the network ictogenicity. In this study, we set all negative SI_X values to zero. More details about the calculation of *BNI* and *SI* are given in **Supplementary Text S2**.

Exemplar Networks and Topological Properties

In order to explore and understand the effect of perturbations in different network structures, we first study *SI* in exemplar networks. We consider both directed and undirected artificial networks with random and "scale-free" [i.e., generated by the Barabasi-Albert algorithm (28) and the static model (29)] topologies, comprising 20 and 40 nodes. Exemplar networks are provided in **Supplementary Figure 2**. The choice of these networks is motivated by the existence of many different methods to derive networks from clinical data, which could give rise to different types of networks, including weighted, unweighted, directed and undirected networks. We choose random networks to serve as a baseline and scale free networks to better represent real-world networks. For example, iEEG networks have previously been shown to contain rich clubs, or hubs (which are a characteristic of scale free networks), and an analysis of the patient data used herein shows around half of networks to have an approximately scale free distribution in the network weights (see **Supplementary Figure 3**). We note that in contrast to the weighted functional networks inferred from patient data (see section Patient Information and Data), we used binary artificial networks for simplicity. We further consider common graph theory measures, such as the degree, betweenness centrality, clustering coefficient and eigenvector centrality (30, 31) to study how *SI* relates to these topological properties (eigenvector centrality was only computed for undirected networks, because it is undefined for directed networks). Further details for the graph theory measures are provided in **Supplementary Text S3**.

Resection Strategies

In a network of N nodes there are $\binom{N}{n}$ distinct subsets of size n. Therefore, in order to evaluate how *SI* is distributed within a network of size N, and to definitively identify the set with the highest *SI*, one could use an exhaustive (or brute-force) search, which would require $\sum_{n=1}^{N}\binom{N}{n}$ calculations. We use such an approach herein to calculate the "ground truth" distribution of *SI*. For networks of size relevant for the study of the brain, the brute-force approach quickly becomes intractable. For example, a 40-node network exhaustive search would require $2^{40} - 1 \approx 10^{12}$ calculations. We therefore need to develop computationally tractable methods for studying *SI*. Previous studies (11, 20) have used heuristic methods based on recursively adding a single node to build up an optimal set. One method, which we refer to as "simple ordering" (11) calculates NI_X for all possible single node removals (i.e., N initial calculations). Nodes are ranked according to their NI_X values and added sequentially to the set. Each time a new node is added, the *SI* of the new set is calculated, with termination when *SI* is greater than 0.99. An extension to this method, which we refer to as "recurrent ordering" recalculates the distribution of *NI* after the removal of each node to ensure that in every iteration the node with the highest *NI* of the perturbed network is added.

In addition to these heuristics, we test a resection strategy based on optimizing *SI* with a genetic algorithm. Genetic algorithms are stochastic search methods based on mimicking natural selection, in which an evolving population of candidate problem solutions is used to find an optimal solution (17, 32, 33). A typical genetic algorithm (GA) starts with a population that comprises candidate solutions (called individuals). Each individual is evaluated by a fitness (objective) function which quantifies how successfully the individual solves the problem. Based on the fitness scores, the genetic algorithm creates a new population of individuals by performing a number of stochastic genetic operations (i.e. crossover, mutation, selection), and keeps the best solutions generated (those that minimize the objective function). This process continues for multiple iterations (called generations) until convergence to an optimum solution is achieved (see **Supplementary Figure 4**). Multi-objective genetic algorithms (MOGAs) optimize the given problem for more than one objective function, returning Pareto optimal solution sets which represent the optimal trade-off between the objectives (32, 33). Here, we use the Non-dominated Sorting Genetic Algorithm-II (NSGA-II) (32, 34). Particularly, we use the implementation of the algorithm included in the MATLAB Global Optimisation Toolbox (version R2017b) and follow the optimization protocol from Avramidis et al. (32). We note that the optimization algorithm and code was adapted from Avramidis and Akman (35). Given that our purpose is to find the smallest set with the largest *SI*, we use two objective functions that minimize the number of nodes removed as well as the quantity $1 - SI$. After multiple generations, the algorithm returns optimal sets of nodes with different resection sizes. Due to the stochastic nature of the genetic algorithm, we execute eight independent runs initialized from a uniformly distributed set of random points in each case, and then utilize the convergence metrics from Avramidis et al. [(32) and references therein] to assess whether the algorithm is robust and reliable at identifying optimal sets with respect to different population sizes and generation numbers (i.e., the MOGA hyperparameters). In short, the convergence metrics evaluate the spread of the optimal sets in the two-dimensional plane of the objective functions. For efficiency, we set the genetic algorithm to discard sets of nodes larger than half of the network size by attributing them arbitrarily large objective values. The final MOGA parameter setting implemented in this work yielded consistent solutions across multiple runs, as quantified by the convergence metrics.

All the aforementioned search methods were evaluated on 20-node networks. In 40-node networks we did not use the "ground truth" strategy, given that it is computationally intractable to calculate *SI* for $2^{40} - 1$ sets. We therefore introduce in this case an additional approach: a "random search" heuristic which picks at random a sample of sets of nodes for every resection size and takes as a solution the set with the maximum *SI*. For comparison purposes, we consider a sample size equal to the number of sets evaluated by the genetic algorithm across all generations. The number of samples per resection size was considered proportional to the logarithm of all possible sets of the respective size. This enabled a denser sampling at small resection sizes where the optimum solution is expected to be found.

Comparison Between Resection Strategies That Are Based on Node and Set Ictogenicity

The ground truth is the only strategy that guarantees the detection of the most ictogenic set, because it is the only one that has access to the *SI* of all sets of nodes (**Figures 1H,K,L**). Thus, for the 20-node networks we compare all strategies to the optimum solution found from the ground truth. In order to evaluate how close a given solution is to the highest *SI* observed in the ground truth, we compute the ΔSI,

$$\Delta SI = SI^{GT} - SI^{S}$$

where SI^{GT} is the highest *SI* observed in the ground truth and SI^{S} is the *SI* of the optimum solution detected by a strategy *S* (for a given resection size). Our aim is to find a strategy that may find SI^{GT} ($\Delta SI = 0$) while avoiding the inefficient and exhaustive search performed in the ground truth.

In the case of 40-node networks, we cannot calculate the ground truth and therefore we use the solution from the genetic algorithm (SI^{GA}) as a reference to compare with other strategies,

$$\Delta SI = SI^{GA} - SI^{s}.$$

Note that in this case the ΔSI could be negative, because the genetic algorithm might be outperformed by another strategy.

Patient Information and Data

We analyse intracranial electroencephalographic recordings from 20 patients (15 female, 5 male; median age 31 years, IQR 16 years, range 10–66 years) who underwent pre-surgical monitoring at Inselspital Bern. Thirteen of them were free from disabling seizures and auras for at least 1 year after surgery (Engel I), whereas the remaining seven did not show worthwhile improvement (Engel IV). Details regarding all patients included in this study are listed in **Table 1**. Before and after surgery, high resolution MRI images were acquired, as well as post-implantation CT images in order to identify the position of the implanted electrodes and the exact location of the resected brain tissue. Further details about this procedure can be found in Rummel et al. (10). An experienced epileptologist/electroencephalographer (K.S.) visually inspected all the recordings and identified the onset and termination of a representative seizure as well as any channels that had to be removed from the analysis due to the presence of permanent artifacts (<5% of channels). All signals were down-sampled to a sampling rate of 512 Hz, re-referenced against the median of all the artifact-free channels and band-pass filtered (forward and backward filtering to minimize phase distortion) between 0.5 and 150 Hz using a fourth-order Butterworth filter. All the patients gave written informed consent that their imaging and EEG data might be used for research purposes, and retrospective data analysis has been approved by the ethics committee of the Canton of Bern/Switzerland. In order to calculate functional networks using iEEG data we use a surrogate corrected version of mutual information (10, 24) which yields undirected networks (see **Supplementary Text S1** and **Supplementary Figure 1**).

RESULTS

The results section is arranged as follows. In order to better understand how sets of nodes within networks contribute to ictogenicity, we first study how *SI* is distributed across subnetworks of different sizes in artificially generated scale-free and random networks. We subsequently assess the relationship between *SI* and common graph theory metrics and test to what extent these metrics can predict the optimal set. We then apply a genetic algorithm and heuristics to the problem of finding the optimal set before finally testing the genetic algorithm on patient data.

Set Ictogenicity in Different Network Topologies

In a network of size *N*, for a given subset (collection) of *n* nodes, $X = \{x_1, .., x_n\}$, where $n < N$, we use SI_X to quantify the reduction in ictogenicity that is achieved by removing all nodes in *X* from the network. To gain insight into how seizures arise in networks, we first seek to uncover what the relationship is between the obtained reduction in ictogenicity (SI_X) and the number of nodes that are removed (*n*), and how this depends on network topology. For computational tractability we initially study 20-node artificially generated networks, considering the removal of up to ten nodes (i.e. up to half of the network). This network size is tractable for analysis using a brute-force approach and is relevant in the clinical context, where iEEG implantation schemes for some people may comprise around 20 electrodes, and investigations of standard clinical scalp EEG typically yields 19 channels.

Figures 2A,B,E,F demonstrate how *SI* is distributed in exemplar directed and undirected networks with scale-free and random topologies. We observe that the variance in *SI* is larger in the directed scale-free networks (**Figure 2A**) compared to random (**Figures 2B,F**) and undirected scale-free (**Figure 2E**) networks. **Figure 2A** shows that in the directed scale-free networks we studied, *SI* can take values between zero and one, depending on the set that is removed. Approximately 10% of sets do not reduce ictogenicity when removed. In addition, removal of 20% of the sets resulted in complete elimination of epileptiform dynamics (i.e., $SI_X = 0$). However, the effect of removal of the remaining sets is distributed approximately uniformly across *SI* values. In contrast, **Figures 2B,E,F** demonstrate that the *SI* distribution of random and scale-free undirected networks is more concentrated at high values, with very few sets having no effect on ictogenicity.

In **Figures 2C,D,G,H** *SI* is broken down by resection size. In all networks studied, the average *SI* increases as the size of the resected set increases. However, in the scale-free directed

TABLE 1 | Patient information.

Patient	Engel class	Age at surgery	Gender	Syndrome	Etiology/MRI/Histology	Number of iEEG channels	Number of resected iEEG channels
1	I	27	F	MTLE(R)	Non-lesional	64	20
2	I	58	F	MTLE(L)	Hippocampal sclerosis	64	13
3	I	27	M	LTLE(L)	Cluster of dysplastic neurons	56	5
4	I	36	M	PLE(L)	Low-grade glioma	74	13
5	I	19	F	MTLE(L)	Hippocampal sclerosis	42	11
6	I	25	F	FLE(R)	Non-lesional	98	11
7	I	27	M	TLE(L)	Non-lesional	60	11
8	I	27	F	PLE(R)	Non-lesional	68	13
9	I	10	F	MTLE(R)	Hippocampal sclerosis	37	9
10	I	20	M	MTLE(L)	Hippocampal atrophy	31	7
11	I	52	F	MTLE(R)	Hippocampal sclerosis	38	8
12	I	22	F	FLE(L)	Non-lesional	76	7
13	I	42	F	FTE(R)	Aneurysmal subarachnoid hemorrhage	80	6
14	IV	38	F	LTLE(L)	Dysplasia	59	2
15	IV	21	F	LTLE(L)	Meningitis	61	10
16	IV	59	F	MTLE(L)	Suspected amygdala dysplasia	49	8
17	IV	31	M	PLE(R)	Non-lesional	96	4
18	IV	31	F	FLE(R)	Tuberous sclerosis	36	3
19	IV	42	F	LTLE(L)	Temporo-basal dysplasia	24	6
20	IV	33	M	FLE(L)	Non-lesional	69	4

Every row corresponds to a different patient.
MTLE, medial temporal lobe epilepsy; LTLE, lateral temporal lobe epilepsy; PLE, parietal lobe epilepsy; FLE, frontal lobe epilepsy; TLE, temporal lobe epilepsy; FTE, fronto-temporal epilepsy; R, right; L, left.

networks (**Figure 2C**) we studied, the relationship between resection size and average *SI* is approximately linear, and in random (**Figures 2D,H**) and undirected scale-free networks (**Figure 2H**), large average *SI* values are reached more readily for small set (resection) sizes. Furthermore, whilst in the directed scale-free networks we studied there are few sets with very large *SI*, in random and undirected scale-free networks there are instead few low *SI* values. We observe that typically, small resections have on average greater impact (i.e., higher *SI*) in random networks, compared to equivalent resections in directed scale-free networks.

Set Ictogenicity and Graph Theory Measures

Figure 2 demonstrated that *SI* depends on network topology. To further understand this relationship, we investigated to what extent *SI* is related to common graph theoretic properties of nodes inside the sets selected for removal. We thus computed the Spearman's rank correlation between *SI* and the average degree, average betweenness centrality and average clustering coefficient of removed sets in directed scale-free and random networks. **Figure 3** shows that *SI* is correlated with average degree and average betweenness centrality (median correlation larger than 0.6 for most resection sizes, see **Figures 3A,B**), but not with the average clustering coefficient in both scale-free and random networks (directed and undirected, see **Supplementary Figure 7** for the latter). Analyzing different resection sizes we see that there are differences in correlation between directed scale-free networks and the other topologies we studied. In random networks, for example, the correlation between *SI* and average degree and betweenness centrality is high for small resection sizes but decreases for larger resections (**Figures 3D,E**). In contrast, correlation between degree and *SI* increases with resection size for directed scale-free networks (**Figure 3A**) and is relatively flat for betweenness centrality (**Figure 3B**). The low correlation for large resection sizes in random networks, particularly for betweenness centrality, is likely to be a consequence of the fact that most large sets have the same *SI* in random networks, as found in **Figure 2D**. Therefore, *SI* would be independent from measures of the constituent nodes.

Identifying Optimal Resections

Having explored properties of *SI* distributions, we now turn to the problem of finding the set that optimally reduces ictogenicity upon removal, which is analogous to identifying the optimal resection in epilepsy surgery. **Figure 3** demonstrated that the average degree and average betweenness centrality of removed sets are correlated with *SI*. This implies that these graph theory measures may potentially be used to find the sets with highest *SI*. We sought to test this by asking whether sets that produce maximum reductions in average degree or average betweenness centrality also produce maximal *SI* values. In order to identify maximal *SI* values, we calculated *SI* for all possible subsets of

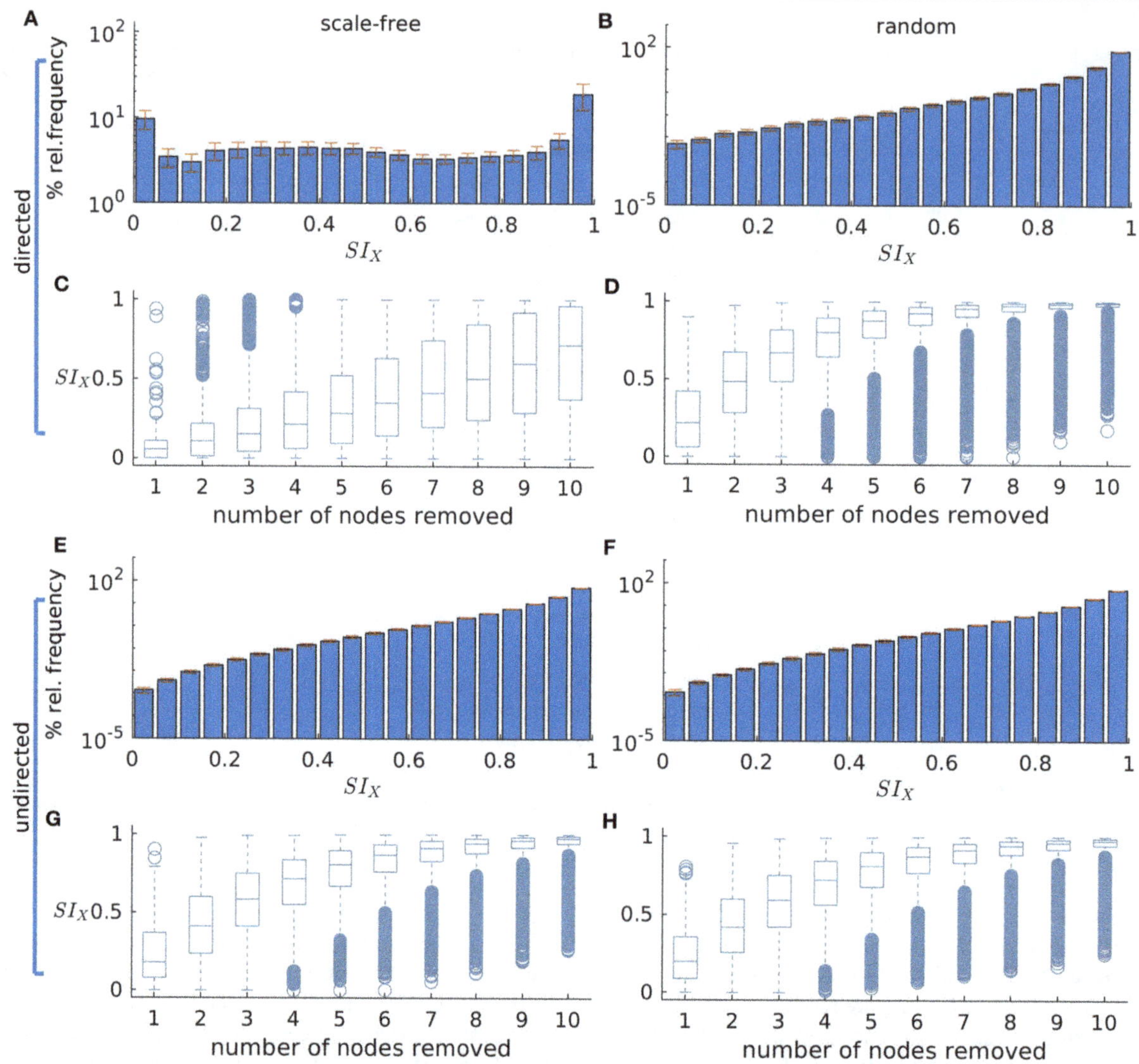

FIGURE 2 | The distribution of Set Ictogenicity (*SI*) depends on network topology and resection size. **(A,B)** display the average *SI* distribution for ten directed artificial scale-free **(A)** and random **(B)** networks, respectively. Error bars denote the standard error across the ten network realizations. **(C,D)** show *SI* distributions split out by resection size (i.e., number of nodes removed) for the networks of panels **(A)** and **(B)**, respectively. **(E–H)** are similar to **(A–D)**, but for undirected networks. Parameters: network size $N = 20$; in the directed networks the in and out degree is 2, whilst in the undirected the mean degree is 2; scale-free degree distribution exponent $\gamma = 3$. The horizontal line in each boxplot indicates the median, while the bottom and top edges of each box are the 25th and 75th percentiles, respectively. The whiskers denote the range and circles the outliers.

artificial networks with 20 nodes, which we refer to as the ground truth. Note that for a given network and resection size, there may exist multiple sets that produce maximal reductions in average degree or average betweenness centrality. We therefore calculated the average difference between the maximum *SI* (ground truth) and the *SI* of each set that yields maximum reduction of average degree and betweenness centrality (ΔSI). We henceforth denote sets that yield maximal reduction in average degree and average betweenness centrality as SI_{deg} and SI_{bet}, respectively.

Figure 4 shows the results of this analysis for directed scale-free (**Figures 4A,C**) and random (**Figures 4B,D**) networks. We observe that in both scale-free and random directed networks, sets corresponding to SI_{deg} and SI_{bet} can yield *SI* values close to the optimal *SI* as defined by the ground truth (i.e., $\Delta SI = 0$). In addition, the SI_{deg} and SI_{bet} sets always have lower ΔSI than the average *SI* from sets of the same size, which indicates that the reduction in average degree and average betweenness centrality are useful ways to find optimal sets (see the dashed line in the figure which represents the average ΔSI of every possible set of nodes). We also find that ΔSI gets smaller with increasing resection sizes, which is a consequence of how the distribution of *SI* changes with the resection size (i.e., as the number of nodes removed becomes large, *SI* becomes large in general, see **Figure 2**). However, we also observe that sets producing the same reduction in average degree or average betweenness centrality may have different *SI* values, as shown by the large error

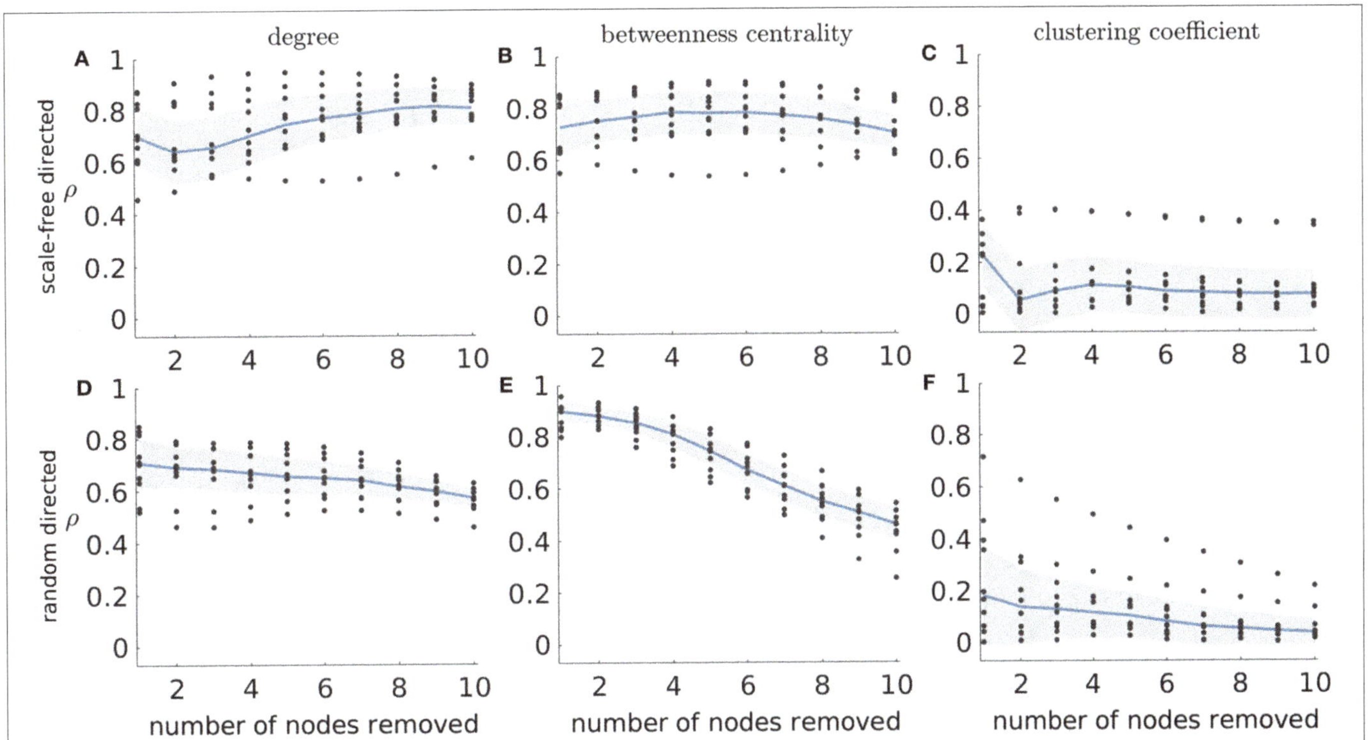

FIGURE 3 | Absolute Spearman's correlation (ρ) between *SI* and average graph theory measures of the nodes in removed sets. **(A–C)** correspond to scale-free directed networks while **(D–F)** represent random directed networks. Each column shows ρ between *SI* and a different network measure: **(A,D)** average degree; **(B,E)** average betweenness centrality; and **(C,F)** average clustering coefficient of removed nodes. Ten network realizations were considered per network topology, hence the 10 dots for each resection size (i.e., number of nodes removed). The blue line represents the median across the network realizations and the shaded area displays the median absolute deviation. The parameters were the same as in **Figure 2**.

bars in **Figures 4A,B**. This means that information regarding the degree or centrality alone is insufficient to identify the set with the largest *SI*, since we would need further information to identify which of the sets corresponding to $SI_{\deg}$ and SI_{bet} would have largest *SI*. Furthermore, ΔSI may be quite large for some realizations of directed scale-free networks (see the existence of outliers in **Figures 4A,B**). In contrast, in random directed networks average degree and average betweenness centrality more accurately identify sets with optimal *SI* (see **Figures 4C,D**), particularly at larger resections (which is to be expected given that most sets yield *SI* close to the highest at large resection sizes independent of their constituent nodes). Results for undirected networks are shown in **Supplementary Figure 8** where we also explored whether sets that produce maximum reduction in eigenvector centrality also produce maximal *SI* values. We also performed this analysis for clustering coefficient and found that the corresponding ΔSI values were very large which means that clustering coefficient was not able to identify the optimal set as defined by the ground truth.

Alternative Strategies for the Identification of the Most Ictogenic Sets

Figure 4 showed that graph theory measures may often be used to identify the most ictogenic set. However, they may not be reliable for certain network realizations, particularly in directed scale-free networks. Therefore, to find the set of nodes with maximal ictogenicity we should calculate *SI*. However, calculating the *SI* for all possible sets is challenging computationally due to the large number of possible sets, particularly in large networks. Hence, in order to study larger networks, and to find optimal resections in general for practical applications, efficient methods are required to find sets with optimal *SI*. Here, we study two previously used heuristics, along with the NSGA-II genetic algorithm (32, 34). The heuristics we use are the simple ordering (11) and recurrent ordering (20) methods, which are based on the contribution of individual nodes to seizure generation. In contrast to building pseudo-optimal sets recursively, the genetic algorithm makes stochastic searches in the space of all possible sets of nodes using natural selection criteria.

In **Figure 5** we compare these methods against the ground truth in 20-node directed networks. We find that whilst both simple and recurrent ordering are able to identify solutions close to the highest *SI*, the genetic algorithm is the only approach that uncovers the optimal solution in all cases [the red line overlaps with the green line in **Figure 5C**, and $\Delta SI = 0$ in panels (F) and (I)]. We further observe that in general the recurrent ordering provides better solutions than the simple ordering. These strategies performed differently for different network topologies, with scale-free directed networks being less

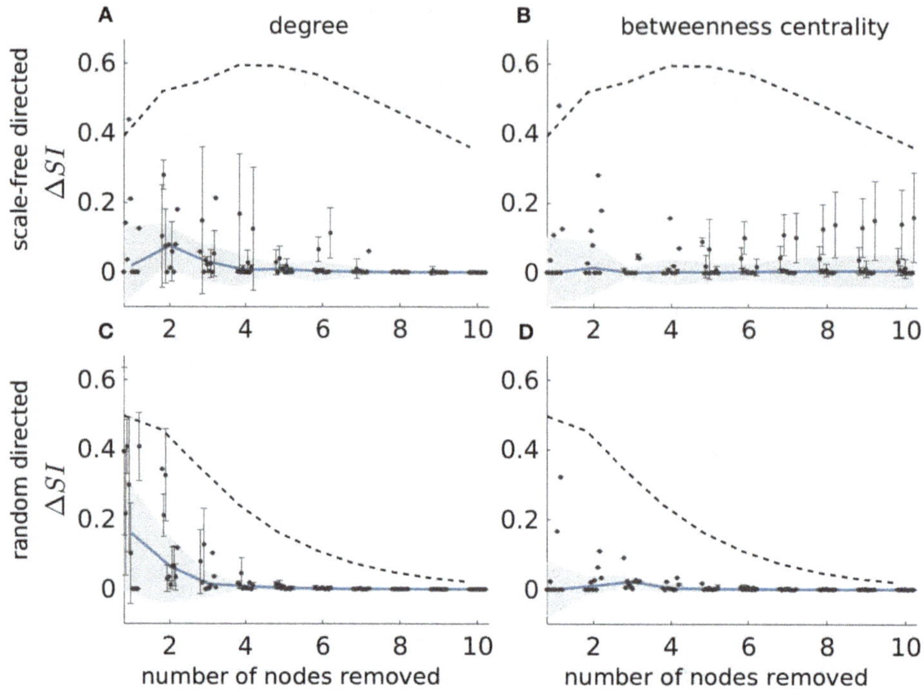

FIGURE 4 | Difference between the *SI* value of the most ictogenic set as identified from the ground truth and the average *SI* of the sets which caused a maximal reduction in average degree **(A,C)**, and average betweenness centrality **(B,D)**, i.e., ΔSI, as a function of resection size. Error bars denote the standard deviation of the ΔSI values across the different sets that yield the maximal reduction in average degree or betweenness centrality when removed. The blue curve describes the median of the ΔSI values across 10 network realizations (black dots) and the shaded area their median absolute deviation (the dots are slightly shifted in the x-axis for better visualization). **(A,B)** Correspond to scale-free directed networks, whilst panels **(C,D)** to random directed networks. The dashed line denotes the average ΔSI between the *SI* of the ground truth most ictogenic set and the *SI* of all other possible sets (also averaged over the 10 network realizations). Parameters are the same as in **Figure 2**.

amenable to the heuristic approaches than random networks [see the higher ΔSI values in **Figure 5** panels (D) and (E) compared to (G) and (H)]. In undirected networks we observe similar results, though in this case both the genetic algorithm and the recurrent ordering strategy are able to find the sets with highest *SI* (see **Supplementary Figure 9**). We note that the genetic algorithm and the recurrent ordering approaches perform better than the heuristics based on graph theory measures (compare, for example, **Figures 5E,H** with **Figure 4**), further motivating the benefit of calculating *SI*. For all considered network topologies of this study, we ensured that the genetic algorithm converged across multiple independent realizations. The *SI* values of the optimal sets across multiple runs as well as the convergence metrics for exemplar networks can be found in **Supplementary Figures 5, 6**. The analysis above showed that the genetic algorithm can identify sets with the largest *SI* in all of the 20-node networks considered. In addition, the recurrent ordering strategy also found solutions relatively close to the optimum *SI* (see **Figures 5E,H**). Therefore, we sought to explore whether these optimisation strategies may also achieve good performances on larger, 40-node networks. For these larger networks, we restricted our analysis to directed scale-free networks given that they proved to be the more difficult to approach in our analysis of 20-node networks. Scale-free networks are characterized by the presence of hubs, which have been shown to exist in analyses of functional brain networks (20, 31, 36) and therefore they are more relevant to the clinical setting. Indeed, an analysis of the patient networks studied herein demonstrates that many of them have an approximately scale free distribution of weights (**Supplementary Figure 3**). As explained in Methods, we do not compute the ground truth in 40-node networks, since the number of all possible sets of nodes is too large. Instead, we use the genetic algorithm as a proxy for the ground truth and compare this to the simple and recurrent ordering heuristics. In addition, we employ a random search heuristic that searches through a solution space whose size is equal to the one of the genetic algorithm in order to test the uplift in performance of the latter compared to a stratified random approach.

Figure 6 shows that in the 40-node scale-free directed networks we studied, the genetic algorithm clearly outperforms all the other strategies. Note that in this figure $\Delta SI > 0$ means that the genetic algorithm finds solutions with larger *SI* than the other approaches. We find that the uplift in performance of the genetic algorithm has a maximum at around sets of size 10 and then decreases for larger sets. This is due to larger resections being more likely to have $SI = 1$, as observed in our study of 20-node networks. This is further supported by

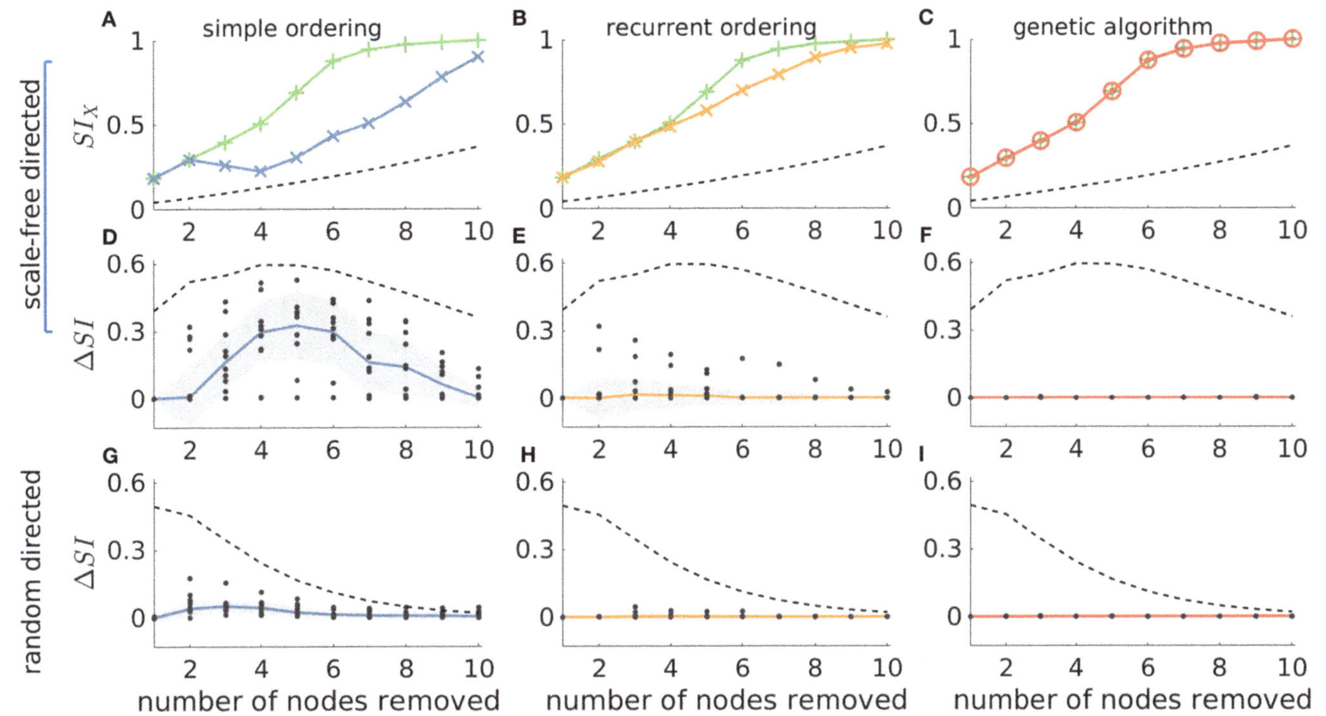

FIGURE 5 | The genetic algorithm is the only resection strategy that identifies the most ictogenic set in all considered networks. The ground truth is compared to simple ordering (first column), recurrent ordering (second column) and the genetic algorithm (third column). **(A–C)** display *SI* values over the number of resected nodes in an exemplar artificial 20-node scale-free directed network, where the green lines represent the ground truth (i.e., the most ictogenic sets), whilst the blue, orange, and red lines display the *SI* of the sets found by each of the search strategies. The second and third rows show the ΔSI between the *SI* value of the ground truth and the set identified by each search strategy in scale-free and random directed networks, respectively. The dashed line represents the average *SI* (or ΔSI) of all possible combinations of nodes for each resection size and serve as a reference for comparison. The dots in **(D–I)** correspond to ΔSI values obtained for 10 different network realizations, the solid lines depict the median of ΔSI values, and the shaded area represents the median absolute deviation. Parameters were the same as in **Figure 2**. Additionally, the genetic algorithm was run for 100 generations with a population size of 200.

the V-shaped dashed guideline curves corresponding to random removals which decrease for resection sizes larger than 15. In contrast, in undirected networks all approaches detect similar *SI* solutions (see **Supplementary Figure 10**).

Identifying Optimal Resections in Patient Data

Our analysis of artificial networks demonstrates that the genetic algorithm is a good strategy for identifying sets of nodes with the largest *SI*. We therefore sought to test the application of the genetic algorithm to networks inferred from a cohort of 20 people with pharmacoresistant epilepsy who underwent resective surgery (see Materials and Methods). Using iEEG recordings, we constructed a functional network for each patient (see **Supplementary Text S1** and **Supplementary Figure 1**) and used the genetic algorithm to identify the most ictogenic sets. Here, the network nodes correspond to iEEG channels, which in turn represent the brain tissue in the vicinity of the electrodes. Following (11) we defined the optimal set as the smallest set for which the *SI* exceeds 0.99. Note that as described in the Methods section, we executed multiple independent runs of the genetic algorithm, which is inherently stochastic, in order to obtain robust results. We observed that across the independent realizations we could obtain multiple optimal sets for a given patient (i.e., different sets of nodes with the same size and *SI* value).

In order to test the validity of predictions of the model, we compared them to the actual resections the patients underwent, and whether they were rendered seizure free as a result. Since the algorithm yielded multiple potential resections we calculated the overlap between the actual resected tissue and each of the optimal sets. **Figure 7** shows the largest overlap per patient (for the minimal overlap see **Supplementary Figure 11**), with individuals grouped by post-surgical outcome. The overlap indicates the portion of nodes (electrodes) in the model suggestion that belongs to the actual resected tissue. We found significantly larger overlaps (one-sided Wilcoxon rank sum test, $p = 0.003$) for individuals who had good post-surgical outcome (Engel I) compared to those who had poor outcome (Engel IV) (see **Figure 7A**). In addition, we found that three out of the seven patients with poor post-surgery outcome presented zero overlap, meaning that our methods suggested completely different resections compared to those that were performed. We also calculated the overlap between the actual resected tissue and equal size random sets of nodes. We found that this overlap (**Figure 7A**—unfilled triangles) was smaller than the overlap

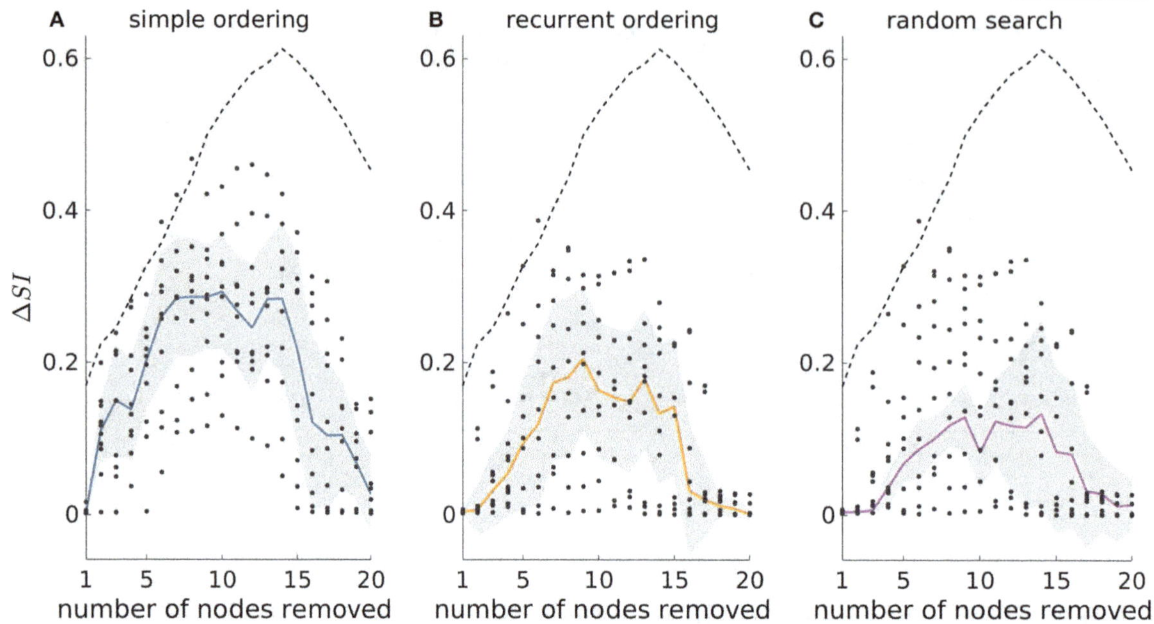

FIGURE 6 | The genetic algorithm outperforms both simple and recurrent ordering as well as the random search heuristic in 40-node scale-free directed networks. ΔSI denotes the difference between the SI value of the optimal set as detected by the genetic algorithm and the SI solution found by **(A)** simple ordering, **(B)** recurrent ordering, and **(C)** random search across different resection sizes. The solid lines depict the median of the dots which correspond to the ΔSI values across 10 network realizations, whilst the shaded area illustrates the median absolute deviation. The dashed line represents the difference between the optimal set as detected by the genetic algorithm and the average of 20,000 random sets for each resection size (for resections up to three nodes, we considered all possible sets, since there were fewer than 20,000). Parameters: mean in and out degree equal to 4; population size 200, number of generations equal to 150.

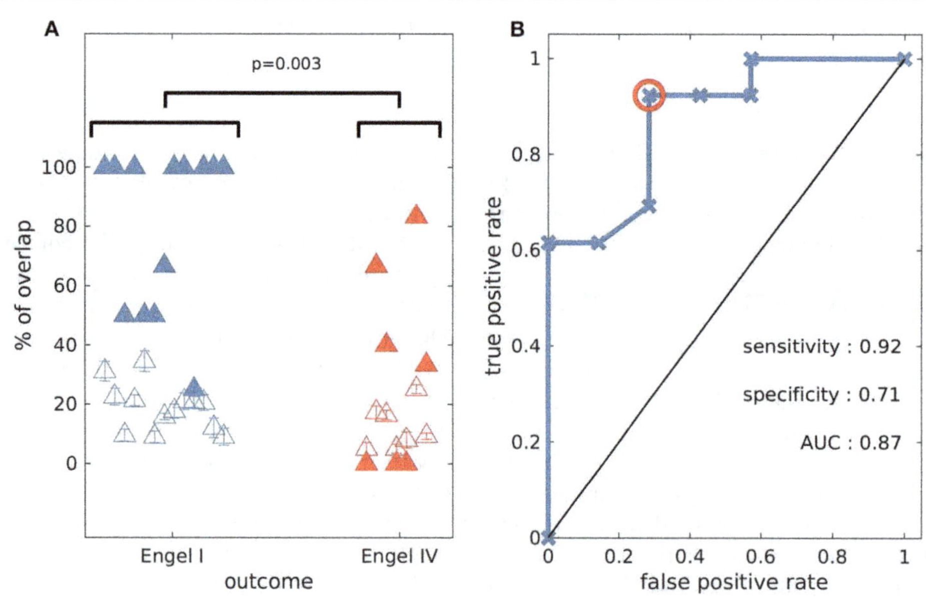

FIGURE 7 | The percentage overlap between actual resections and model predictions is higher for patients with good outcome compared to those who had poor post-surgical outcome (one-sided Wilcoxon rank sum test $p = 0.003$). **(A)** Percentage overlap vs. patient surgical outcome grouped by Engel class (filled triangles). The unfilled triangles correspond to an average overlap between actual resections and equal-size random resections (100 random samples, and the error bars denote the standard error). **(B)** Receiver operating characteristic (ROC) analysis for Engel I (seizure free patients) vs. Engel IV (non-seizure free patients) using the percentage overlap as the classifier. The red circle indicates the point that is used for the calculation of sensitivity and specificity. Parameter setting for the genetic algorithm: population size equal to 200 and number of generations equal to 150.

between the actual resected tissue and our model suggestions (**Figure 7A**—filled triangles). The only exceptions were again the three cases having zero overlap with our predictions. Using the overlap as a classifier we found a sensitivity of 0.92, a specificity of 0.71, and an area under the curve (AUC) of 0.87 (see **Figure 7B**), which suggests our methods are reliable for classifying into outcome classes at the individual level. Interestingly, using graph theory measures alone Engel class I and IV patients could not be separated (**Supplementary Figure 12**). However, we found that if *SI* and the genetic algorithm are used to calculate the optimal size of the resection as a first step, eigenvector centrality and strength were able to separate the two groups well, whereas betweenness centrality could not (**Supplementary Figure 13**).

Figure 8 illustrates the MRI and functional network of an Engel I patient (fourth of **Table 1**) where the optimal set suggested by the genetic algorithm belongs to the actual resected tissue. **Figure 9** demonstrates the MRI and functional network of an Engel IV patient (seventeenth of **Table 1**). In this case, the genetic algorithm revealed two alternative optimal sets (**Figures 9A,B,D,E**). Here we demonstrate a further advantage of the genetic algorithm: it facilitates the avoidance of removing a certain node or nodes. This can be achieved by setting the objective function to a high value if the node(s) that should be avoided appear in a solution during the execution of the algorithm. Here, we avoid the selection of a highly ictogenic node (**Figures 9C,F**) and consequently the genetic algorithm substitutes it with another one. This constrained strategy of the genetic algorithm may be clinically valuable given that there may exist network nodes that cannot be removed due to their overlap with eloquent cortex, blood vessels or other anatomically indispensable areas.

DISCUSSION

In this study we used computational modeling and evolutionary optimization to understand how sets of nodes within a network contribute to its seizure generating capability (i.e., its ictogenicity). To do this we used a quantity called Set Ictogenicity (*SI*), which is a model-based quantification of the effect that removing a set of nodes has on the capability of a network to transition between healthy and epileptiform dynamics. We demonstrated that the way in which *SI* varies for different sets of nodes depends upon network topology. Whilst in exemplar 20-node random directed networks most sets of nodes have similar and large *SI*, in exemplar directed networks generated using the Barabasi-Albert model (i.e., "scale-free" networks), we observed a V-shaped distribution of *SI*. In the latter case, most sets do not yield a large reduction in ictogenicity when removed from the network. This difference is in part explained by the observed high correlation between *SI* and degree: since nodes in scale-free networks have higher degree variability, this leads to higher *SI* variability across sets of nodes. We further observed that *SI* is correlated with betweenness centrality. These results build upon our previous findings in reference (20), where we analyzed the correlation between graph theory measures and the Node Ictogenicity (which is the reduction in ictogenicity obtained by removing a single node). Our results add further evidence that targeting hubs, which would be sets of nodes with high average degree and betweenness centrality, is likely to be a good strategy for epilepsy surgery (20, 36–38). However, we have also shown that using graph theory measures alone is not guaranteed to provide the optimal resection. The use of models to link network topology to epileptiform dynamics and global search methods applied to the dynamics could therefore be important in clinical settings.

Several other studies have advocated the use of ideas from network theory and modeling to understand the ictogenic network and the effects of epilepsy surgery. Burns et al. (39), for example, studied the evolution of brain networks before, during and after seizures using iEEG data. They found that during seizure onset a group of electrodes relating to the seizure onset zone disconnects from the remaining network. Studies, such as these can provide insight into the nature of the ictogenic network and how it evolves during changes of brain state. The use of computational models to understand data such as these can help to provide a mechanistic understanding and potentially provide additional information not apparent in static analyses of networks. For example, we showed that although *SI* correlates with graph theory metrics, sets of nodes which induce maximum reduction in average degree or centrality are not necessarily sets with *the highest SI.*

Complementary to our approach, Jirsa at al. (13) have used the simulation platform "The Virtual Brain" to construct person specific models of seizures with the aim to identify the epileptogenic zone prospectively. In their model, structural connectivity is combined with hypotheses regarding the location of the seizure onset zone and seizure propagation patterns are compared to patient data. In our approach, we work with networks derived from iEEG and use the output of a model to explore which resections would optimally reduce the occurrence of abnormal brain activity. This does not assume *a-priori* information regarding which brain region may be responsible for initiating seizures. That is, we do not assume we know where the seizure onset zone is, rather we let the network and the model tell us which nodes should be removed. Indeed, we have shown using models that there can be a complicated relationship between the seizure onset zone and the epileptogenic zone (40).

We developed a global optimization framework that can be deployed in general to find the optimal resection, given a network structure. Epilepsy surgery relies on the identification of brain regions that are responsible for the emergence of epileptiform activity, but wherever possible mitigating effects on normal brain function. We therefore studied two objectives: the *SI* and the size of the resection, using a multi-objective genetic algorithm. Genetic algorithms are optimization methods based upon the process of evolution and natural selection. They have been widely applied in neuroscience (32, 41–43) and it has been shown that they are a valuable tool to solve combinatorial type computational problems (16, 17). Here, we showed that in small networks our genetic algorithm was able to find minimal sets with highest ictogenicity. In larger networks, we compared the genetic algorithm with other heuristic approaches and demonstrated that the genetic algorithm was always at least

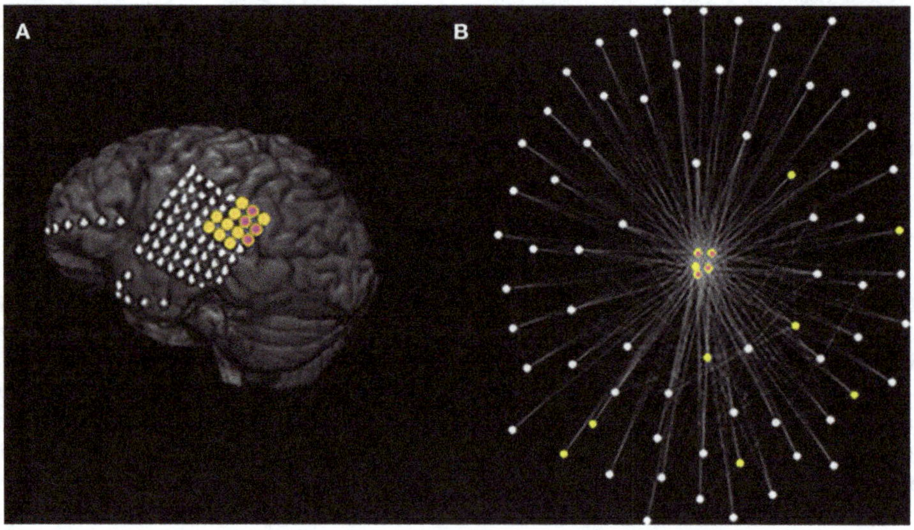

FIGURE 8 | Actual clinical resection together with model suggestion using data from a good outcome patient. **(A)** Illustrates the MRI of a patient (fourth of **Table 1**) with good post-surgical outcome. The yellow color denotes the actual resected tissue while the purple color denotes the nodes suggested by the Genetic Algorithm. **(B)** Demonstrates the functional network as determined using the surrogate corrected mutual information. The network visualization maps strength of connectivity to distance in the plane. Colors are the same as **(A)**. Parameters are the same as those in **Figure 7**.

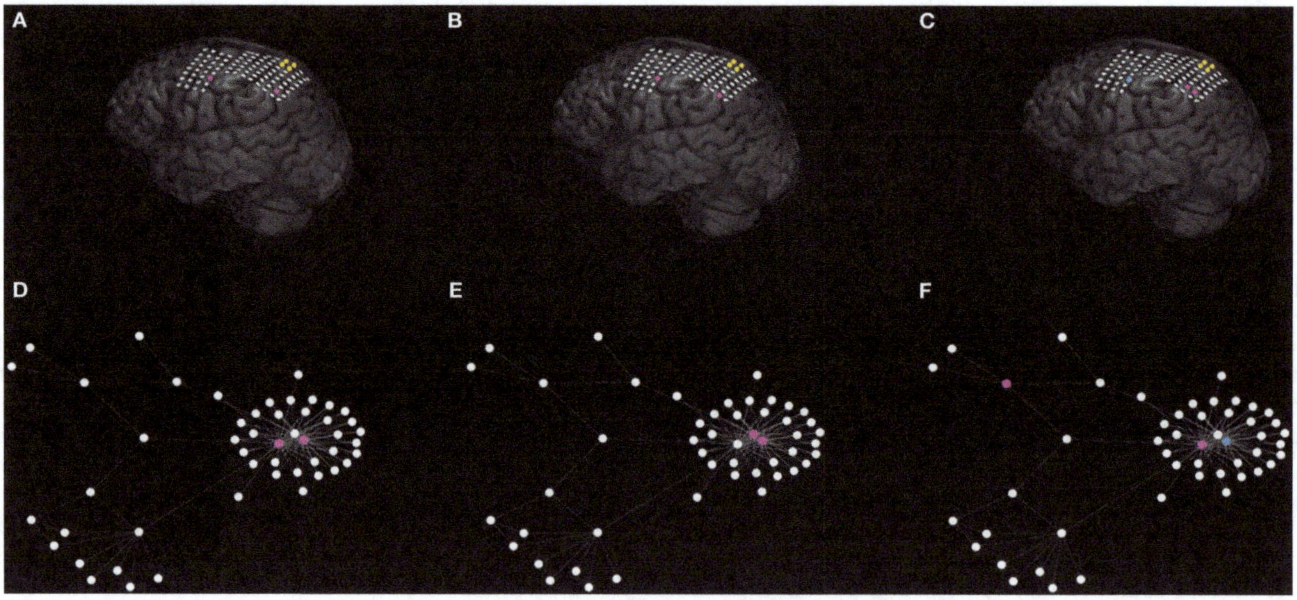

FIGURE 9 | The genetic algorithm suggests multiple optimal sets and may further provide alternative sets under given restrictions. **(A–C)** Illustrate the MRI of a patient (seventeenth of **Table 1**) with poor post-surgical outcome. The yellow color denotes the actual resected tissue. **(A,B)** Exemplify two different (unconstrained) optimal sets (in purple) suggested by the Genetic Algorithm. **(C)** Shows an additional alternative optimal set (in purple) when constraining the genetic algorithm to avoid selecting the blue node. **(D–F)** Illustrate the corresponding functional network as inferred from the surrogate corrected mutual information. For illustrative reasons we only display the largest connected component of the network and connections characterized by interrelations larger than 0.09. The network visualization maps strength of connectivity to distance in the plane. Color coding is the same as **(A–C)**. The actual clinical resection [yellow nodes of **(A–C)**] was not part of the displayed network component **(D–F)**. Parameters are the same as those in **Figure 7**.

as good or better than these heuristics at finding the sets with highest ictogenicity.

Brain networks may be studied at different spatial and temporal scales using different data modalities (44). In the context of epilepsy surgery, most studies have focused on large-scale brain networks inferred from iEEG (45, 46) and MRI (47, 48). Network topology has been shown to evolve during seizures (49, 50), with structures changing from random to more regular in seizures and increasing randomness after seizure termination (51). Furthermore, it has been shown that hubs may play a crucial role in the generation of seizures (20, 52, 53). That is why here we studied both random and scale-free networks to build understanding about the epileptic brain. We found that the *SI* distribution varies in networks with different topologies and is more heterogeneous in directed scale-free networks compared to directed random networks. The framework we introduced is flexible and can be applied to smaller spatial scales, e.g. neuronal networks or smaller sized regions of interest in whole brain models (54, 55). At the smaller scale, these methods could shed light on, for example, why hubs of granule cells in the dentate gyrus are responsible for the emergence of seizures after brain injury (56). Use of these methods combined with experimental testing of perturbations, for example using optogenetics (57), could open up new avenues for targeted treatment for seizures (58).

We demonstrated the potential applicability of the genetic algorithm by applying it to functional brain networks derived from iEEG recordings of 20 patients who had undergone epilepsy surgery. We found that the model-derived optimal set had larger overlap with actual resections in the case of patients who were ultimately seizure free. This is in line with previous studies that have used computational models and heuristic approaches, based on properties of individual nodes, to test potential alternative resections (11, 12, 20). Furthermore, our framework achieved a classification performance comparable to recent studies that used machine learning and quantitative EEG methods (59). Depending on the way in which ictogenic networks are constructed, it is possible that in epilepsy surgery multiple nodes from the brain network are removed. We therefore here aimed to identify the indispensable brain region for seizure generation by considering the ictogenicity of sets of nodes. A particular advantage of the genetic algorithm that we demonstrated is that it naturally suggests multiple optimal sets that suppress the epileptiform activity of the network, due to the random nature of the search. These are alternative sets that give rise to optimal *SI* (see **Figures 9A,B,D,E**). Furthermore, there are natural ways to implement constraints, for example on nodes that should not be removed because they are essential for healthy brain function (**Figures 9C,F**).

There are a number of caveats to the approaches we outlined and opportunities to enhance the methodologies in the future. We validated the approach by measuring the overlap of the optimal set with actual resections, taking into account post-operative seizure freedom. Although the results of **Figure 7** give confidence that the collection of nodes identified in the analysis were in fact ictogenic, it does not provide validation that the entire set itself is the optimal resection. Furthermore, the GA can provide multiple sets that are predicted to be effective in reducing seizures and these will be indistinguishable in our current model framework. In order to test these aspects further, we propose to work with experimental systems, whereby alternative resections can be performed (60).

We note that a large overlap between the model suggestion and the actual resected tissue was found in 2 cases in which outcome was Engel IV. In addition, in one Engel class I patient the overlap was small (see **Figure 7A**). Our approach assumes the existence of an ictogenic network and it has been shown that even focal epilepsies may involve widespread brain networks (46, 61–63). However, the electrodes are implanted in a designated brain region and the functional network that is inferred from them might not reflect the ictogenic network. Therefore, the initial placement of iEEG electrodes may be key here, and recent work has aimed to use modeling to uncover cases for which an alternative implantation scheme may be required (20). Future work should also aim to aid clinicians with regards to electrode implantation and to integrate different data modalities so that predictions may be more robust. We further note that although *SI* can be used to compare different resections, their actual values can be difficult to interpret. Linking *BNI* and *SI* to the rate of occurrence of epileptiform discharges in humans and experimental models will be an important avenue for future work that can aid the refinement of model predictions. We also note that the genetic algorithm is computationally more expensive than the other heuristics (see **Supplementary Text S4**), however, it may be further optimized in the future by making use of parallelization and GPUs (32), for example. In addition, employing a global search method allows one to incorporate constraints that may be useful in the clinical setting. For example, one could introduce a penalty for large spatial spread of nodes in the optimal set, therefore identifying optimal contiguous regions of tissue for resections in practice.

In conclusion we presented a computational approach that quantifies the contribution of brain regions to seizure generation. Our approach enhances the understanding of how perturbations in brain networks may lead to seizure freedom. It allows multiple surgical strategies to be tested *in silico* in order to find the optimal set that reduces the network ictogenicity. In addition, the genetic algorithm that we deployed finds the optimal trade-off between the size of the resected tissue and the reduction in network ictogenicity. Our results show promise that the computational approaches introduced herein have the potential to be incorporated into surgery decision pipelines in practice.

AUTHOR CONTRIBUTIONS

PL, MG, MR, KS, and CR: conceptualization. EAb, CR, and KS: data curation. PL and CR: formal analysis. MG: funding acquisition. PL, ML, MG, MM, CR, EAv, and OA: methodology. MG: project administration. PL, EAv, ML, MM, and CR: software. MG: supervision. PL, ML, and MG: writing-original draft preparation. PL, EAv, ML, EAb, MM, OA, MR, CR, KS, and MG: writing-review and editing.

FUNDING

MG, ML, and MR gratefully acknowledge funding from the Medical Research Council [grant number MR/K013998/1]. MG and MR received financial support from the EPSRC [grant number EP/N014391/1]. MG and PL received financial support from the EPSRC [grant number EP/P021417/1]. The contribution of MG was further generously supported by a

Wellcome Trust Institutional Strategic Support Award [grant number WT105618MA]. MR was also funded by the NIHR Biomedical Research Centre at South London and Maudsley NHS Trust and King's College London; and by the Medical Research Council Centre for Neurodevelopmental Disorders at King's College London [MR/N026063/1]. OA would like to acknowledge the financial support of the EPSRC [grant numbers EP/N017846/1 and EP/N014391/1]. CR and MM received support from the Swiss League Against Epilepsy. EAv acknowledges funding from EPSRC Tier-2 capital grant EP/P020259/1. EAb was funded by the European Union's Horizon 2020 research and innovation programme under the Marie Sklodowska-Curie grant agreement no. 75088.

ACKNOWLEDGMENTS

We would like to acknowledge Khulood Alyahya, Kevin Doherty, and Leandro Junges for fruitful discussions and comments. We also acknowledge Dr. Julian Tejada and Dr. Guilherme G. Podolsky-Gondim for helping to complete the review report.

REFERENCES

1. Brodie MJ. Road to refractory epilepsy: the Glasgow story. *Epilepsia.* (2013) 54:5–8. doi: 10.1111/epi.12175
2. Chen Z, Brodie MJ, Liew D, Kwan P. Treatment outcomes in patients with newly diagnosed epilepsy treated with established and new antiepileptic drugs: a 30-year longitudinal cohort study. *JAMA Neurol.* (2018) 75:279–86. doi: 10.1001/jamaneurol.2017.3949
3. Rosenow F, Lüders H. Presurgical evaluation of epilepsy. *Brain.* (2001) 124:1683–700. doi: 10.1093/brain/124.9.1683
4. Nowell M, Miserocchi A, McEvoy AW, Duncan JS. Advances in epilepsy surgery. *J Neurol Neurosurg Psychiatry.* (2014) 85:1273–9. doi: 10.1136/jnnp-2013-307069
5. De Tisi J, Bell GS, Peacock JL, McEvoy AW, Harkness WF, Sander JW, Duncan JS. The long-term outcome of adult epilepsy surgery, patterns of seizure remission, and relapse: a cohort study. *Lancet.* (2011) 378:1388–95. doi: 10.1016/S0140-6736(11)60890-8
6. Engel J, McDermott MP, Wiebe S, Langfitt JT, Stern JM, Dewar S, et al. Early Randomized Surgical Epilepsy Trial (ERSET) Study Group. Early surgical therapy for drug-resistant temporal lobe epilepsy: a randomized trial. *JAMA.* (2012) 307:922–30. doi: 10.1001/jama.2012.220
7. Fois C, Kovac S, Khalil A, Uzuner GT, Diehl B, Wehner T, et al. Predictors for being offered epilepsy surgery: 5-year experience of a tertiary referral centre. *J Neurol Neurosurg Psychiatry.* (2015) 87:209–11. doi: 10.1136/jnnp-2014-310148
8. Baud MO, Perneger T, Rácz A, Pensel MC, Elger C, Rydenhag B, et al. European trends in epilepsy surgery. *Neurology.* (2018) 91:96–106. doi: 10.1212/WNL.0000000000005776
9. Engel J. The current place of epilepsy surgery. *Curr Opin Neurol.* (2018) 31:192–7. doi: 10.1097/WCO.0000000000000528
10. Rummel C, Abela E, Andrzejak RG, Hauf M, Pollo C, Müller M, et al. Resected brain tissue, seizure onset zone and quantitative EEG measures: towards prediction of post-surgical seizure control. *PLoS ONE.* (2015) 10:0141023. doi: 10.1371/journal.pone.0141023
11. Goodfellow M, Rummel C, Abela E, Richardson MP, Schindler K, Terry JR. Estimation of brain network ictogenicity predicts outcome from epilepsy surgery. *Sci Rep.* (2016) 6:29215. doi: 10.1038/srep29215
12. Sinha N, Dauwels J, Kaiser M, Cash SS, Brandon Westover M, Wang Y, et al. Predicting neurosurgical outcomes in focal epilepsy patients using computational modelling. *Brain.* (2017) 140:319–32. doi: 10.1093/brain/aww299
13. Jirsa VK, Proix T, Perdikis D, Woodman MM, Wang H, Gonzalez-Martinez J, et al. The virtual epileptic patient: individualized whole-brain models of epilepsy spread. *Neuroimage.* (2017) 145:377–88. doi: 10.1016/j.neuroimage.2016.04.049
14. Steimer A, Müller M, Schindler K. Predictive modelling of EEG time series for evaluating surgery targets in epilepsy patients. *Hum Brain Mapp.* (2017) 38:2509–31. doi: 10.1002/hbm.23537
15. Petkov G, Goodfellow M, Richardson MP, Terry JR. A critical role for network structure in seizure onset: a computational modelling approach. *Front Neurol.* (2014) 5:261. doi: 10.3389/fneur.2014.00261
16. Hromkovič J. *Algorithmics for Hard Problems: Introduction to Combinatorial Optimization, Randomization, Approximation, and Heuristics.* Berlin; Heidelberg: Springer (2001).
17. Luque G, Alba E. *Parallel Genetic Algorithms: Theory and Real World Applications.* Boston, MA: Springer (2011).
18. Pearl J. *Heuristics: Intelligent Search Strategies for Computer Problem Solving.* Boston, MA: Addison-Wesley Longman (1984).
19. Branke J, Nguyen S, Pickardt CW, Zhang M. Automated design of production scheduling heuristics: a review. *IEEE Trans Evol Comput.* (2016) 20:110–24. doi: 10.1109/TEVC.2015.2429314
20. Lopes MA, Richardson MP, Abela E, Rummel C, Schindler K, Goodfellow M, et al. An optimal strategy for epilepsy surgery: disruption of the rich-club? *PLoS Comput Biol.* (2017) 13:1005637. doi: 10.1371/journal.pcbi.1005637
21. Van Laarhoven PJ, Aarts EH. Simulated annealing. In: Hazewinkel M, editor. *Simulated Annealing: Theory and Applications.* Dordrecht: Springer (1987). p. 7–15.
22. Beyer H-G, Schwefel H-P. Evolution strategies–a comprehensive introduction. *Nat Comput.* (2002) 1:3–52. doi: 10.1023/A:1015059928466
23. Kennedy J. Particle swarm optimization. In: Sammut C, Webb GI, editors. *Encyclopedia of Machine Learning.* Boston, MA: Springer (2010). p. 760–6.
24. Rummel C, Abela E, Müller M, Hauf M, Scheidegger O, Wiest R, et al. Uniform approach to linear and nonlinear interrelation patterns in multivariate time series. *Phys Rev E.* (2011) 83:066215. doi: 10.1103/PhysRevE.83.066215
25. Ermentrout GB, Kopell N. Parabolic bursting in an excitable system coupled with a slow oscillation. *SIAM J Appl Math.* (1986) 46:233–53. doi: 10.1137/0146017
26. Wendling F, Bartolomei F, Bellanger JJ, Chauvel P. Epileptic fast activity can be explained by a model of impaired GABAergic dendritic inhibition. *Eur J Neurosci.* (2002) 15:1499–508. doi: 10.1046/j.1460-9568.2002.01985.x
27. Goodfellow M, Schindler K, Baier G. Self-organised transients in a neural mass model of epileptogenic tissue dynamics. *Neuroimage.* (2012) 59:2644–60. doi: 10.1016/j.neuroimage.2011.08.060
28. Barabási AL, Albert R. Emergence of scaling in random networks. *Science.* (1999) 286:509–12. doi: 10.1126/science.286.5439.509
29. Goh KI, Kahng B, Kim D. Universal behavior of load distribution in scale-free networks. *Phys Rev Lett.* (2001) 87:278701. doi: 10.1103/PhysRevLett.87.278701
30. Newman MEJ. The mathematics of networks. New Palgrave Encycl Econ. (2007) 2: 1–12.
31. Rubinov M, Sporns O. Complex network measures of brain connectivity: uses and interpretations. *Neuroimage.* (2010) 52:1059–69. doi: 10.1016/j.neuroimage.2009.10.003
32. Avramidis E, Akman OE. Optimisation of an exemplar oculomotor model using multi-objective genetic algorithms executed on a GPU-CPU combination. *BMC Syst Biol.* (2017) 11:40. doi: 10.1186/s12918-017-0416-2
33. Zhou A, Qu B-Y, Li H, Zhao S-Z, Suganthan PN, Zhang Q. Multiobjective evolutionary algorithms: a survey of the state of the art. *Swarm Evol Comput.* (2011) 1:32–49. doi: 10.1016/j.swevo.2011.03.001
34. Deb K, Pratap A, Agarwal S, Meyarivan TA. M. T. A fast and elitist multiobjective genetic algorithm: NSGA-II. *IEEE Trans Evol Comput.* (2002) 6:182–97. doi: 10.1109/4235.996017
35. Avramidis E, Akman OE. Optimisation of an exemplar oculomotor model using multi-objective genetic algorithms executed on a GPU-CPU combination, v1.0, Zenodo,
36. Stam CJ. Epilepsy: what can we learn from modern network theories. *Epileptologie.* (2016) 33:38–43.

37. Van Diessen E, Hanemaaijer JI, Otte WM, Zelmann R, Jacobs J, Jansen FE, et al. Are high frequency oscillations associated with altered network topology in partial epilepsy? *Neuroimage.* (2013) 82:564–73. doi: 10.1016/j.neuroimage.2013.06.031
38. Zubler F, Gast H, Abela E, Rummel C, Hauf M, Wiest R, et al. Detecting functional hubs of ictogenic networks. *Brain Topogr.* (2015) 28:305–17. doi: 10.1007/s10548-014-0370-x
39. Burns SP, Santaniello S, Yaffe RB, Jouny CC, Crone NE, Bergey GK, et al. Network dynamics of the brain and influence of the epileptic seizure onset zone. *Proc Natl Acad Sci USA.* (2014) 111:5321–30. doi: 10.1073/pnas.1401752111
40. Lopes MA, Goodfellow M, Terry JR. A model-based assessment of the seizure onset zone predictive power to inform the epileptogenic zone. *Front Comput Neurosci.* (2019) 13:25. doi: 10.3389/fncom.2019.00025
41. Whitley D, Starkweather T, Bogart C. Genetic algorithms and neural networks: optimizing connections and connectivity. *Parallel Comput.* (1990) 14:347–61. doi: 10.1016/0167-8191(90)90086-O
42. Nevado-Holgado AJ, Marten F, Richardson MP, Terry JR. Characterising the dynamics of EEG waveforms as the path through parameter space of a neural mass model: application to epilepsy seizure evolution. *Neuroimage.* (2012) 59:2374–92. doi: 10.1016/j.neuroimage.2011.08.111
43. Wang HE, Friston KJ, Bénar CG, Woodman MM, Chauvel P, Jirsa V, et al. MULAN: evaluation and ensemble statistical inference for functional connectivity. *NeuroImage.* (2018) 166:167–84. doi: 10.1016/j.neuroimage.2017.10.036
44. Bassett DS, Zurn P, Gold JI. On the nature and use of models in network neuroscience. *Nat Rev Neurosci.* (2018) 19:566–78. doi: 10.1038/s41583-018-0038-8
45. Khambhati AN, Davis KA, Oommen BS, Chen SH, Lucas TH, Litt B, et al. (2015). Dynamic network drivers of seizure generation, propagation and termination in human neocortical epilepsy. *PLoS Comput Biol.* (2015) 11:1004608. doi: 10.1371/journal.pcbi.1004608
46. Bartolomei F, Lagarde S, Wendling F, McGonigal A, Jirsa V, Guye M, et al. Defining epileptogenic networks: contribution of SEEG and signal analysis. *Epilepsia.* (2017) 58:1131–47. doi: 10.1111/epi.13791
47. Proix T, Bartolomei F, Guye M, Jirsa VK. Individual brain structure and modelling predict seizure propagation. *Brain.* (2017) 140:641–54. doi: 10.1093/brain/awx004
48. Taylor PN, Sinha N, Wang Y, Vos SB, de Tisi J, Miserocchi A, et al. The impact of epilepsy surgery on the structural connectome and its relation to outcome. *NeuroImage Clin.* (2018) 18:202–14. doi: 10.1016/j.nicl.2018.01.028
49. Kramer MA, Eden UT, Kolaczyk ED, Zepeda R, Eskandar EN, Cash SS. Coalescence and fragmentation of cortical networks during focal seizures. *J Neurosci.* (2010) 30:10076–85. doi: 10.1523/JNEUROSCI.6309-09.2010
50. Lehnertz K, Ansmann G, Bialonski S, Dickten H, Geier C, Porz S. Evolving networks in the human epileptic brain. *Physica D.* (2014) 267:7–15. doi: 10.1016/j.physd.2013.06.009
51. Schindler KA, Bialonski S, Horstmann MT, Elger CE, Lehnertz K. Evolving functional network properties and synchronizability during human epileptic seizures. *Chaos.* (2008) 18:033119. doi: 10.1063/1.2966112
52. Wilke C, Worrell G, He B. Graph analysis of epileptogenic networks in human partial epilepsy. *Epilepsia.* (2011) 52:84–93. doi: 10.1111/j.1528-1167.2010.02785.x
53. Varotto G, Tassi L, Franceschetti S, Spreafico R, Panzica F. Epileptogenic networks of type II focal cortical dysplasia: a stereo-EEG study. *Neuroimage.* (2012) 61:591–8. doi: 10.1016/j.neuroimage.2012.03.090
54. Stead M, Bower M, Brinkmann BH, Lee K, Marsh WR, Meyer FB, et al. Microseizures and the spatiotemporal scales of human partial epilepsy. *Brain.* (2010) 133:2789–97. doi: 10.1093/brain/awq190
55. Smith EH, Liou JY, Davis TS, Merricks EM, Kellis SS, Weiss SA, et al. The ictal wavefront is the spatiotemporal source of discharges during spontaneous human seizures. *Nat Commun.* (2016) 7:11098. doi: 10.1038/ncomms11098
56. Morgan RJ, Soltesz I. Nonrandom connectivity of the epileptic dentate gyrus predicts a major role for neuronal hubs in seizures. *Proc Natl Acad Sci USA.* (2008) 105:6179–84. doi: 10.1073/pnas.0801372105
57. Chow BY, Boyden ES. Optogenetics and translational medicine. *Sci Transl Med.* (2013) 5:177. doi: 10.1126/scitranslmed.3003101
58. McGovern RA, Banks GP, McKhann GM. New techniques and progress in epilepsy surgery. *Curr Neurol Neurosci Rep.* (2016) 16:65. doi: 10.1007/s11910-016-0661-6
59. Müller M, Schindler K, Goodfellow M, Pollo C, Rummel C, Steimer A. Evaluating resective surgery targets in epilepsy patients: a comparison of quantitative EEG methods. *J Neurosci Methods.* (2018) 305:54–66. doi: 10.1016/j.jneumeth.2018.04.021
60. Sheybani L, Birot G, Contestabile A, Seeck M, Kiss JZ, Schaller K, et al. Electrophysiological evidence for the development of a self-sustained large-scale epileptic network in the kainate mouse model of temporal lobe epilepsy. *J Neurosci.* (2018) 38. 3776–91. doi: 10.1523/JNEUROSCI.2193-17.2018
61. Spencer SS. Neural networks in human epilepsy: evidence of and implications for treatment. *Epilepsia.* (2002) 43:219–27. doi: 10.1046/j.1528-1157.2002.26901.x
62. Richardson MP. Large scale brain models of epilepsy: dynamics meets connectomics. *J Neurol Neurosurg Psychiatry.* (2012) 83:1238–48. doi: 10.1136/jnnp-2011-301944
63. Besson P, Bandt SK, Proix T, Lagarde S, Jirsa VK, Ranjeva JP, et al. Anatomic consistencies across epilepsies: a stereotactic-EEG informed high-resolution structural connectivity study. *Brain.* (2017) 140:2639–52. doi: 10.1093/brain/awx181

21

Patients with Epilepsy Who Underwent Epilepsy Surgery During the COVID-19 Pandemic Showed Less Depressive Tendencies

Keiko Niimi, Ayataka Fujimoto, Keishiro Sato, Hideo Enoki and Tohru Okanishi*

Comprehensive Epilepsy Center, Seirei Hamamatsu General Hospital, Hamamatsu, Japan

***Correspondence:**
Ayataka Fujimoto
afujimotoscienceacademy@gmail.com

Introduction: Our hypothesis in this study was that differences might exist between patients with epilepsy (PWE) who underwent epilepsy surgery before and within the period of the coronavirus disease 2019 (COVID-19) pandemic. The purpose of this study was to compare results of the Zung Self-Rating Depression Scale (SDS) between PWE who underwent epilepsy surgery before and during the pandemic period.

Methods: Participants were PWE who underwent open cranial epilepsy surgery between February 2019 and February 2021 in our hospital. Patients who underwent surgery in the first half of this period, between February 2019 and January 2020, were defined as the pre-pandemic period group (pre-Group) and those treated in the second half, between February 2020 and February 2021, were categorized as the pandemic period group (within-Group). All patients completed the SDS before surgery, and scores were compared between groups.

Results: SDS score was significantly higher in the pre-Group than in the within-Group ($p = 0.037$). Other factors, including age ($p = 0.51$), sex ($p = 0.558$), epilepsy duration from onset to SDS score evaluation ($p = 0.190$), seizure frequency ($p = 0.794$), number of anti-seizure medications ($p = 0.787$), and intelligence quotient ($p = 0.871$) did not differ significantly between groups.

Conclusion: SDS score was higher in the pre-pandemic group than in the within-pandemic group, which may indicate that PWE with less-positive outlooks may be less likely to seek medical attention during stressful periods.

Keywords: Zung self-rating depression scale, pandemic, epilepsy surgery, COVID-19, SARS-CoV-2

HIGHLIGHTS

- PWE who underwent surgery during the pandemic period showed less depressive symptoms.
- PWE with depressive tendencies might be at risk during stressful periods.
- Technology might offer hope for PWE showing depressive tendencies.

INTRODUCTION

The coronavirus disease 2019 (COVID-19) pandemic caused by severe acute respiratory syndrome coronavirus 2 (SARS-CoV-2) started in 2019, and has shown three peaks in Japan since the beginning of 2020.

Previously, as pandemics in the 20th century, we experienced the Spanish flu, acquired immunodeficiency syndrome (AIDS) and highly pathogenic avian influenza viruses (1–4). However, in the 21st century, the frequency of epidemics seems to have increased markedly (5–9). Regardless of the cause, the possibility of pandemics occurring more frequently in the near future must naturally be considered.

Patients with epilepsy (PWE) are known to have been suffering during the calamity of COVID-19 due to anxiety and depression (10). In particular, PWE with surgically remediable epilepsy are known to be vulnerable to psychiatric disturbance before and after surgery, even when societal calamities are not present. Since the adequate treatment of psychiatric comorbidities increases the likelihood of seizure freedom and optimizes the psychosocial benefits afforded by epilepsy surgery (11), provision of psychological care to PWE must be a priority. At the same time, continuity of treatment for PWE is also necessary. The idea of continuing business functions in society has already been described in 2012 by the International Organization for Standardization (ISO) as ISO22301 (https://www.iso.org/standard/75106.html). This ISO standard describes how to continually manage business in an organization to protect against the occurrence of disruptive incidents. These underlying principles are also applicable to healthcare businesses and our hospital follows this standard.

We have already described a retrospective study showing the importance of local interdisciplinary care for PWE (12). We have also shown that SARS-CoV-2 did not influence the volume of epilepsy surgeries in our facility (13). From these efforts, approaches to the calamity from the healthcare perspective might improve such negative situations for PWE. However, in the real world, worsening of seizure frequency and postponement of medical examinations are commonplace experiences for many PWE during the COVID-19 pandemic (14). If many PWE postponed adequate medical treatments during the pandemic, psychological differences might exist between PWE who did not postpone treatments and underwent epilepsy surgery during the pandemic and PWE who underwent epilepsy surgery before the pandemic.

Our hypothesis for the present study was thus that psychological differences might exist between PWE who underwent epilepsy surgery before and during the COVID-19 pandemic. The purpose of this study was to compare results from a depression scale among PWE who underwent epilepsy surgery before and during the COVID-19 pandemic.

METHODS

Study Design and Ethics Approval

The ethics committee at Seirei Hamamatsu General Hospital, Japan, approved the protocol for this retrospective study (approval no. 3578), which was performed in accordance with the principles of the Declaration of Helsinki. Subjects in this study were identified from a review of the electronic medical records for patients who had undergone epilepsy surgery between February 2019 and February 2021 in the Comprehensive Epilepsy Center at Seirei Hamamatsu General Hospital.

Clinical Information

We collected information from patients who underwent epilepsy surgery between February 2019 and February 2021, as the first half of this period between February 2019 and January 2020 was pre-pandemic and the second half between February 2020 and February 2021 was just within the pandemic period in Japan. Patient age was recorded at the time of depression scale evaluation.

Data were obtained from all 32 patients who underwent open cranial epilepsy surgery for medically intractable epilepsy between February 2019 and February 2021 in our hospital. Among this population, inclusion criteria were: (1) age $\geq$18 years at evaluation, as the depression scale used was the Zung Self-Rating Depression Scale [SDS], which is adapted for individuals $\geq$18 years old (15); and (2) full intelligence quotient (IQ) $\geq$60. Among this population, exclusion criteria were: (1) patients who had undergone vagus nerve stimulation (VNS) therapy; and (2) patients who exhibited psychogenic non-epileptic seizures (PNES) (16) or other non-stereotypical activities.

As intellectual disorder and depression are sometime difficult to differentiate, such as in depressive cognitive disorders (17), patients with more than moderate intellectual disorder were allowed to enroll in this study. As VNS therapy has antidepressant effects (18), patients with VNS devices were excluded. All patients underwent long-term video electroencephalography and stereotypical epileptic seizures were captured. Based on the stereotypical seizure semiology, PWE who had experienced non-stereotypical activities were excluded because these non-stereotypical activities were regarded as possible PNES or non-epileptic events.

Depression Scale as the Primary Outcome Measurement

The SDS test is a 20-item self-reported questionnaire in common use as a screening tool, covering affective, psychological, and somatic symptoms associated with depression. The questionnaire takes 5–10 min to complete, and items are framed in terms of positive and negative statements. The total score is derived as the sum of scores for the individual item scores, ranging from 20 to 80. Patients who undergo epilepsy surgery in our institution undergo SDS before the surgery. We divided the enrolled patients into two groups: those who underwent surgery in the first half of the period, categorized as during the pre-pandemic period group between February 2019 and January 2020 (pre-Group); and those who underwent surgery in the second half of the period, categorized as during the pandemic period between February 2020 and February 2021 (within-Group). We compared SDS scores between these two groups.

Seizure Frequency, Duration From Epileptic Seizure Onset to SDS Score Evaluation, and Anti-seizure Medications as Secondary Outcome Measurements

We also compared seizure frequency, duration from onset to SDS score evaluation, and number of anti-seizure medications (ASMs) between the pre-Group and within-Group. Seizure

TABLE 1 | Clinical information and SDS scores.

	Pre-group ($n = 10$)	Within-group ($n = 9$)	p-value
Sex (female), n	3 (30%)	4 (44%)	0.558
Age at evaluation (years)	mean 30.7, SD 14.2, median 27	mean 34.7, SD 11.5, median 37	0.51
Type of epilepsy	7 TLE, 2 FLE, 1 OLE	7 TLE, 2 FLE	na
IQ	mean 85.8, SD 20.7, median 89.5	mean 84.3, SD 18.1, median 86	0.871
SDS score	mean 39.9, SD 6.4, median 41.5	mean 33.2, SD 6.45, median 32	0.037*
Seizure frequency	mean 2.6, SD 0.84, median 3.0	mean 2.67, SD 1.12, median 3	0.794
Duration from onset to SDS evaluation (m)	mean 115.5, SD 113.2, median 72	mean 193.3, SD 155.7, median 144	0.19
No. of ASMs	mean 2, SD 0.94, median 2	mean 1.89, SD 0.928, median 2	0.787

SD, standard deviation; SDS, self-rating depression scale; TLE, temporal lobe epilepsy; FLE, frontal lobe epilepsy; OLE, occipital lobe epilepsy; IQ, intelligence quotient; ASM, anti-seizure medication; m, months. Seizure frequency was classified as: (1) daily; (2) weekly; (3) monthly; or (4) yearly. *significant difference, $p < 0.05$.*

TABLE 2 | Use of ASMs.

	Pre-group							Within-group				
Anti seizure medications	LCM	LEV	PER	CBZ	CLB	TPM	LTG	LCM	LEV	PER	CBZ	CLB
No. of PWE	7	5	4	1	1	1	1	6	5	4	1	1

LCM, Lacosamide; LEV, Levetiracetam; PER, Perampanel; CBZ, Carbamazepine; CLB, Clobazam; TPM, Topiramate; LTG, Lamotrigine.

frequency was classified as: (1) daily; (2) weekly; (3) monthly; or (4) yearly. These secondary outcomes were chosen as factors potentially related to anxiety or depressive disorders (19).

Statistical Analyses

The Mann-Whitney U-test and Student's t-test were used in this study, as appropriate. Statistical significance was set at the level of $p < 0.05$. Analyses were conducted using Sigma plot (Systat Software, San Jose, CA, USA).

RESULTS

Clinical information and results of the SDS are shown in **Table 1**.

Seven female PWE and 12 male PWE (mean age at evaluation, 32.6 years; median age, 35.0 years; range, 18–59 years; standard deviation, 12.8 years; confidence interval of the mean, 6.16 years) fulfilled the inclusion criteria. None of the patients exhibited PNES. **Table 2** shows the ASMs used by the patients.

Primary Outcome Measurement

SDS scale score was significantly higher in the pre-Group than in the within-Group ($p = 0.037$). No other factors, including age ($p = 0.51$), sex ($p = 0.558$), or IQ ($p = 0.871$), showed significant differences between groups (**Table 1**).

Secondary Outcome Measurements

Epilepsy duration from onset to SDS score evaluation ($p = 0.190$), seizure frequency ($p = 0.794$), and number of ASMs ($p = 0.787$) all showed no significance differences between groups (**Table 1**).

DISCUSSION

SDS scale score was significantly higher in the pre-Group than in the within-Group. Even though scores were not within the diagnostic range for depression, the pre-Group was relatively closer to the range for depressive symptoms than the within-Group. This might be because PWE with a more positive outlook were less likely to put off epilepsy surgery even during the pandemic period.

Rayner and Wilson (11) reported that a less compromised psychiatric profile may contribute to better outcomes of epilepsy surgery. Even though we did not provide special treatments for psychiatric comorbidities for enrolled PWE, the fact that PWE with a less negative outlook underwent epilepsy surgery during the pandemic in this study might partially support this theory by Rayner and Wilson. Given the disaster-preparedness measures taken by our facility, the continuity plan might have worked. As Japan experiences relatively frequent disasters, such as earthquakes, typhoons, and floods, many facilities in Japan might prepare for such disruptive events. The other effort was that as our local interdisciplinary system for epilepsy treatment became established (13), the flow cycle for PWE among local general physicians and our epilepsy center was able to be maintained. Based on these approaches to the calamity that might be decreasing psychological stresses among surgical candidates, thereby improving such negative situations for PWE, epileptologists might not hesitate to perform epilepsy surgery even during a pandemic.

Conversely, about 30% of PWE are considered to have depressive symptoms (20). Many of these patients might be more strongly influenced by psychological factors than by the epilepsy itself (21). From our results and those of previous reports, the possibility should be considered that some PWE might neglect beneficial advanced medical care such as epilepsy surgery under disruptive situations.

As interventions in medical treatments, including for epilepsy, have a certain order of priority (22), some PWE might be classified as having non-urgent disorders (23), despite they might have severe conditions such as COVID-19-related status epilepticus (24). However, using advanced technologies such as telemetry (10, 25), home-video recordings (26) and tele-neuropsychology tests (27) should be implemented to maximize efficient provision of appropriate medical interventions.

A key limitation of this study was the small number of PWE in each group. However, the suggestion that some PWE might be neglected under various circumstances is important and worth exploring further in future work.

SDS scores obtained from multiple centers before and during the pandemic and other societal circumstances should be analyzed in future investigations.

CONCLUSION

SDS score was higher in the pre-pandemic group than in the within-pandemic group, which may indicate that PWE with less-positive outlooks may be less likely to seek medical attention during periods of societal or personal stress.

AUTHOR CONTRIBUTIONS

KN, AF, HE, KS, and TO: acquisition of data. AF, TO, and HE: analysis and interpretation of data. AF: epilepsy surgery. All authors contributed to the article and approved the submitted version.

REFERENCES

1. Landesman SH, Ginzburg HM, Weiss SH. The AIDS epidemic. *N Engl J Med.* (1985) 312:521–5. doi: 10.1056/NEJM198502213120829
2. Trilla A, Trilla G, Daer C. The 1918 "Spanish flu" in Spain. *Clin Infect Dis.* (2008) 47:668–73. doi: 10.1086/590567
3. Lai S, Qin Y, Cowling BJ, Ren X, Wardrop NA, Gilbert M, et al. Global epidemiology of avian influenza A H5N1 virus infection in humans, 1997-2015: a systematic review of individual case data. *Lancet Infect Dis.* (2016) 16:e108–18. doi: 10.1016/S1473-3099(16)00153-5
4. Aassve A, Alfani G, Gandolfi F, Le Moglie M. Epidemics and trust: the case of the spanish flu. *Health Econ.* (2021) 30:840–57. doi: 10.1002/hec4218
5. Dye C, Gay N. Modeling the SARS epidemic. *Science.* (2003) 300:1884–5. doi: 10.1126/science1086925
6. Fineberg HV. Preparing for avian influenza: lessons from the "swine flu affair". *J Infect Dis.* (2008) 197:S14–8. doi: 10.1086/524989
7. Fung IC-H, Tse ZTH, Cheung C-N, Miu AS, Fu K-W. Ebola and the social media. *Lancet.* (2014) 384:2207. doi: 10.1016/S0140-6736(14)62418-1
8. Lowe R, Rodo X, Barcellos C, Carvalho MS, Coelho CA, Bailey TC, et al. *Dengue Epidemic Early Warning System for* Brazil. UNISDR Scientific and Technical Advisory Group. (2015).
9. Basarab M, Bowman C, Aarons EJ, Cropley I. Zika virus. *BMJ.* (2016) 352. doi: 10.1136/bmj.i1049
10. Assenza G, Lanzone J, Brigo F, Coppola A, Di Gennaro G, Di Lazzaro V, et al. Epilepsy care in the time of COVID-19 pandemic in Italy: risk factors for seizure worsening. *Front Neurol.* (2020) 11:737. doi: 10.3389/fneur.202000737
11. Rayner G, Wilson SJ. Psychiatric care in epilepsy surgery: who needs it? *Epilepsy Curr.* (2012) 12:46–50. doi: 10.5698/1535-7511-12.246
12. Fujimoto A, Ichikawa N, Sato K, Nishimura M, Enoki H, Okanishi T. Inclusion of general physicians in the multidisciplinary treatment team for epilepsy may lead to an economic benefit. *Epilepsy Behav.* (2019) 95:56–60. doi: 10.1016/j.yebeh.2019.03041
13. Fujimoto A, Sato K, Enoki H. Change in patient flow in the epilepsy care network due to novel coronavirus infection: an opportunity to strengthen local interdisciplinary epilepsy care with general physicians. *Front Neurol.* (2020) 11:1467. doi: 10.3389/fneur.2020591423
14. Grande E, Tufo T, Ciavarro M, Di Muccio I, Fuggetta F, Silvestri M, et al. The impact of COVID-19 lockdown on people with epilepsy and vagal nerve stimulation. *Front Neurol..* (2021) 12:181. doi: 10.3389/fneur.2021640581
15. Zung WW. A self-rating depression scale. *Arch Gen Psychiatry.* (1965) 12:63–70. doi: 10.1001/archpsyc.196501720310065008
16. Anzellotti F, Dono F, Evangelista G, Di Pietro M, Carrarini C, Russo M, et al. Psychogenic non-epileptic seizures and pseudo-refractory epilepsy, a management challenge. *Front Neurol.* (2020) 11:461. doi: 10.3389/fneur.202000461
17. Sekhon S, Marwaha R. Depressive cognitive disorders. In: *StatPearls.* Treasure Island (FL): StatPearls Publishing Copyright © 2021, StatPearls Publishing LLC. (2021).
18. Assenza G, Tombini M, Lanzone J, Ricci L, Di Lazzaro V, Casciato S, et al. Antidepressant effect of vagal nerve stimulation in epilepsy patients: a systematic review. *Neurol Sci.* (2020) 41:3075–84. doi: 10.1007/s10072-020-04479-2
19. Dehn LB, Pfäfflin M, Brückner S, Lutz MT, Steinhoff BJ, Mayer T, et al. Relationships of depression and anxiety symptoms with seizure frequency: Results from a multicenter follow-up study. *Seizure.* (2017) 53:103–9. doi: 10.1016/j.seizure.2017.11008
20. Tombini M, Assenza G, Quintiliani L, Ricci L, Lanzone J, Ulivi M, et al. Depressive symptoms and difficulties in emotion regulation in adult patients with epilepsy: Association with quality of life and stigma. *Epilepsy Behav.* (2020) 107:107073. doi: 10.1016/j.yebeh.2020107073
21. Tombini M, Assenza G, Quintiliani L, Ricci L, Lanzone J, Di Lazzaro V. Epilepsy and quality of life: what does really matter? *Neurol Sci.* (2021). doi: 10.1007/s10072-020-04990-6
22. Grippo A, Assenza G, Scarpino M, Broglia L, Cilea R, Galimberti CA, et al. Electroencephalography during SARS-CoV-2 outbreak: practical recommendations from the task force of the Italian Society of Neurophysiology (SINC), the Italian League Against Epilepsy (LICE), and the Italian Association of Neurophysiology Technologists (AITN). *Neurol Sci.* (2020) 41:2345–51. doi: 10.1007/s10072-020-04585-1
23. Abokalawa F, Ahmad SF, Al-Hashel J, Hassan AM, Arabi M. The effects of coronavirus disease 2019 (COVID-19) pandemic on people with epilepsy (PwE): an online survey-based study. *Acta Neurol Belg.* (2021) 1–8. doi: 10.1007/s13760-021-01609-1
24. Dono F, Nucera B, Lanzone J, Evangelista G, Rinaldi F, Speranza R, et al. Status epilepticus and COVID-19: a systematic review. *Epilepsy Behav.* (2021) 118:107887. doi: 10.1016/j.yebeh.2021107887
25. Kuchenbuch M, D'Onofrio G, Wirrell E, Jiang Y, Dupont S, Grinspan ZM, et al. An accelerated shift in the use of remote systems in epilepsy due to the COVID-19 pandemic. *Epilepsy Behav.* (2020) 112:107376. doi: 10.1016/j.yebeh.2020107376
26. Ricci L, Boscarino M, Assenza G, Tombini M, Lanzone J, Di Lazzaro V, et al. Clinical utility of home videos for diagnosing epileptic seizures: a systematic review and practical recommendations for optimal and safe recording. *Neurol Sci.* (2021) 42:1301–9. doi: 10.1007/s10072-021-05040-5
27. Tailby C, Collins AJ, Vaughan DN, Abbott DF, O'Shea M, Helmstaedter C, et al. Teleneuropsychology in the time of COVID-19: the experience of The Australian Epilepsy Project. *Seizure.* (2020) 83:89–97. doi: 10.1016/j.seizure.2020.10005

Permissions

All chapters in this book were first published by Frontiers; hereby published with permission under the Creative Commons Attribution License or equivalent. Every chapter published in this book has been scrutinized by our experts. Their significance has been extensively debated. The topics covered herein carry significant findings which will fuel the growth of the discipline. They may even be implemented as practical applications or may be referred to as a beginning point for another development.

The contributors of this book come from diverse backgrounds, making this book a truly international effort. This book will bring forth new frontiers with its revolutionizing research information and detailed analysis of the nascent developments around the world.

We would like to thank all the contributing authors for lending their expertise to make the book truly unique. They have played a crucial role in the development of this book. Without their invaluable contributions this book wouldn't have been possible. They have made vital efforts to compile up to date information on the varied aspects of this subject to make this book a valuable addition to the collection of many professionals and students.

This book was conceptualized with the vision of imparting up-to-date information and advanced data in this field. To ensure the same, a matchless editorial board was set up. Every individual on the board went through rigorous rounds of assessment to prove their worth. After which they invested a large part of their time researching and compiling the most relevant data for our readers.

The editorial board has been involved in producing this book since its inception. They have spent rigorous hours researching and exploring the diverse topics which have resulted in the successful publishing of this book. They have passed on their knowledge of decades through this book. To expedite this challenging task, the publisher supported the team at every step. A small team of assistant editors was also appointed to further simplify the editing procedure and attain best results for the readers.

Apart from the editorial board, the designing team has also invested a significant amount of their time in understanding the subject and creating the most relevant covers. They scrutinized every image to scout for the most suitable representation of the subject and create an appropriate cover for the book.

The publishing team has been an ardent support to the editorial, designing and production team. Their endless efforts to recruit the best for this project, has resulted in the accomplishment of this book. They are a veteran in the field of academics and their pool of knowledge is as vast as their experience in printing. Their expertise and guidance has proved useful at every step. Their uncompromising quality standards have made this book an exceptional effort. Their encouragement from time to time has been an inspiration for everyone.

The publisher and the editorial board hope that this book will prove to be a valuable piece of knowledge for researchers, students, practitioners and scholars across the globe.

List of Contributors

Diem Kieu Tran, Frank Hsu and Sumeet Vadera
Department of Neurological Surgery, University of California, Irvine, Irvine, CA, United States

Demi Chi Tran, Lilit Mnatsakayan and Jack Lin
Department of Neurology, University of California, Irvine, Irvine, CA, United States

Patrick J. Karas, Nisha Giridharan, Jeffrey M. Treiber, Marc A. Prablek, A. Basit Khan, Ben Shofty and Sameer A. Sheth
Department of Neurosurgery, Baylor College of Medicine, Houston, TX, United States

Vaishnav Krishnan, Jennifer Chu, Paul C. Van Ness, Atul Maheshwari, Zulfi Haneef and Jay R. Gavvala
Department of Neurology, Comprehensive Epilepsy Center, Baylor College of Medicine, Houston, TX, United States

Masayoshi Oguri, Kaoru Ogo and Takashi Himoto
Department of Medical Technology, Kagawa Prefectural University of Health Sciences, Takamatsu, Japan

Yoshihiro Maegaki
Division of Child Neurology, Faculty of Medicine, Institute of Neurological Sciences, Tottori University, Yonago, Japan

Sotaro Kanai
Division of Child Neurology, Faculty of Medicine, Institute of Neurological Sciences, Tottori University, Yonago, Japan
Department of Child Neurology, Seirei-Hamamatsu General Hospital, Hamamatsu, Japan

Tohru Okanishi
Division of Child Neurology, Faculty of Medicine, Institute of Neurological Sciences, Tottori University, Yonago, Japan
Department of Child Neurology, Seirei-Hamamatsu General Hospital, Hamamatsu, Japan
Comprehensive Epilepsy Center, Seirei Hamamatsu General Hospital, Hamamatsu, Japan

Shimpei Baba
Department of Child Neurology, Seirei-Hamamatsu General Hospital, Hamamatsu, Japan

Hideo Enoki
Comprehensive Epilepsy Center, Seirei Hamamatsu General Hospital, Hamamatsu, Japan
Department of Child Neurology, Seirei-Hamamatsu General Hospital, Hamamatsu, Japan

Mitsuyo Nishimura
Department of Clinical Laboratory, University of Tsukuba Hospital, Tsukuba, Japan

Kazuo Okanari
Department of Pediatrics, Faculty of Medicine, Oita University, Yufu, Japan

Daniel L. Drane
Department of Neurology, Emory University School of Medicine, Atlanta, GA, United States
Emory Epilepsy Center, Atlanta, GA, United States
Department of Pediatrics, Emory University School of Medicine, Atlanta, GA, United States
Department of Neurology, University of Washington School of Medicine, Seattle, WA, United States

Cady Block, Adam S. Dickey and Abdulrahman Alwaki
Department of Neurology, Emory University School of Medicine, Atlanta, GA, United States

Ammar Kheder
Department of Neurology, Emory University School of Medicine, Atlanta, GA, United States
Department of Pediatrics, Emory University School of Medicine, Atlanta, GA, United States

Nigel P. Pedersen
Department of Neurology, Emory University School of Medicine, Atlanta, GA, United States
Emory Epilepsy Center, Atlanta, GA, United States, 3
Department of Pediatrics, Emory University School of Medicine, Atlanta, GA, United States
Department of Biomedical Engineering, Georgia Institute of Technology and Emory University, Atlanta, GA, United States

David S. Sabsevitz
Department of Psychology and Psychiatry, Mayo Clinic, Jacksonville, FL, United States
Department of Neurological Surgery, Mayo Clinic, Jacksonville, FL, United States

Yuguang Guan and Changqing Liu
Department of Functional Neurosurgery, Sanbo Brain Hospital, Capital Medical University, Beijing, China

Ranliang Hu
Department of Radiology, Emory University Hospital, Atlanta, GA, United States

Zhao Liu
Department of Functional Neurosurgery, Sanbo Brain Hospital, Capital Medical University, Beijing, China
Beijing Key Laboratory of Epilepsy, Epilepsy Center, Sanbo Brain Hospital, Capital Medical University, Beijing, China

Guoming Luan
Department of Functional Neurosurgery, Sanbo Brain Hospital, Capital Medical University, Beijing, China
Beijing Key Laboratory of Epilepsy, Epilepsy Center, Sanbo Brain Hospital, Capital Medical University, Beijing, China
Beijing Institute for Brain Disorders, Beijing, China

Chuanzuo Yang and Qingyun Wang
Department of Dynamics and Control, Beihang University, Beijing, China

Jing Wang and Mengyang Wang
Department of Neurology, Sanbo Brain Hospital, Capital Medical University, Beijing, China

Kunal Gupta
Department of Neurosurgery, Emory University Hospital, Atlanta, GA, United States
Department of Neurosurgery, Indiana University Health, Indianapolis, IN, United States

Edward Faught
Department of Neurology, Emory University Hospital, Atlanta, GA, United States

Jon T. Willie
Department of Neurosurgery, Emory University Hospital, Atlanta, GA, United States
Department of Neurological Surgery, Washington University School of Medicine, Washington, DC, United States

Manon Robert
University of Montreal Hospital Research Center (CRCHUM), University of Montreal, Montreal, QC, Canada

Bou Assi and Dang K. Nguyen
University of Montreal Hospital Research Center (CRCHUM), University of Montreal, Montreal, QC, Canada
Department of Neuroscience, University of Montreal, Montreal, QC, Canada

Younes Zerouali
University of Montreal Hospital Research Center (CRCHUM), University of Montreal, Montreal, QC, Canada
Institute of Biomedical Engineering, Polytechnique Montreal, Montreal, QC, Canada

Frederic Lesage and Philippe Pouliot
Institute of Biomedical Engineering, Polytechnique Montreal, Montreal, QC, Canada
Montreal Heart Institute, Montreal, QC, Canada

Fang Zhang, Yufang Yang, Kedi Xu and Yongte Zheng
Qiushi Academy for Advanced Studies, Zhejiang University, Hangzhou, China
Key Laboratory of Biomedical Engineering of Education Ministry, Department of Biomedical Engineering Zhejiang University, Hangzhou, China
Zhejiang Provincial Key Laboratory of Cardio-Cerebral Vascular Detection Technology and Medicinal Effectiveness Appraisal, Zhejiang University, Hangzhou, China

Ping Wang
Key Laboratory of Biomedical Engineering of Education Ministry, Department of Biomedical Engineering Zhejiang University, Hangzhou, China

Junming Zhu
Zhejiang Provincial Key Laboratory of Cardio-Cerebral Vascular Detection Technology and Medicinal Effectiveness Appraisal, Zhejiang University, Hangzhou, China
Epilepsy Center, School of Medicine, Second Affiliated Hospital, Zhejiang University, Hangzhou, China
Department of Neurosurgery, School of Medicine, Second Affiliated Hospital, Zhejiang University, Hangzhou, China

Vejay N. Vakharia, Anna Miserocchi, Andrew W. McEvoy and John S. Duncan
Department of Clinical and Experimental Epilepsy, University College London, London, United Kingdom
National Hospital for Neurology and Neurosurgery, London, United Kingdom
Chalfont Centre for Epilepsy, London, United Kingdom

Rachel E. Sparks, Alejandro Granados and Sebastien Ourselin
School of Biomedical Engineering and Imaging Sciences, King's College London, London, United Kingdom

Kanupriya Gupta
University of Pittsburgh School of Medicine, Pittsburgh, PA, United States
Department of Neurological Surgery, University of Pittsburgh, Pittsburgh, PA, United States

Pulkit Grover
Center for the Neural Basis of Cognition, Carnegie Mellon University/University of Pittsburgh, Pittsburgh, PA, United States
Department of Electrical and Computer Engineering, Carnegie Mellon University, Pittsburgh, PA, United States

Taylor J. Abel
University of Pittsburgh School of Medicine, Pittsburgh, PA, United States
Department of Neurological Surgery, University of Pittsburgh, Pittsburgh, PA, United States
Center for the Neural Basis of Cognition, Carnegie Mellon University/University of Pittsburgh, Pittsburgh, PA, United States
Department of Bioengineering, University of Pittsburgh, Pittsburgh, PA, United States

Golnoosh Kamali
Neuromedical Control Systems Laboratory, Department of Electrical and Computer Engineering, Institute of Computational Medicine, Johns Hopkins University, Baltimore, MD, United States

Rachel June Smith
Neuromedical Control Systems Laboratory, Department of Biomedical Engineering, Institute of Computational Medicine, Johns Hopkins University, Baltimore, MD, United States

Sridevi V. Sarma
Neuromedical Control Systems Laboratory, Department of Electrical and Computer Engineering, Institute of Computational Medicine, Johns Hopkins University, Baltimore, MD, United States
Neuromedical Control Systems Laboratory, Department of Biomedical Engineering, Institute of Computational Medicine, Johns Hopkins University, Baltimore, MD, United States

Mark Hays
Cognitive Research, Online Neuroengineering and Electrophysiology Laboratory, Department of Biomedical Engineering, Johns Hopkins University, Baltimore, MD, United States

Christopher Coogan and Nathan E. Crone
Cognitive Research, Online Neuroengineering and Electrophysiology Laboratory, Department of Neurology-Epilepsy, Johns Hopkins School of Medicine, Baltimore, MD, United States

Joon Y. Kang
Department of Neurology-Epilepsy, Johns Hopkins School of Medicine, Baltimore, MD, United States

Patrick Greene and Adam Li
Neuromedical Control Systems Lab, Institute for Computational Medicine, Biomedical Engineering, Johns Hopkins University, Baltimore, MD, United States

Jorge González-Martínez
Neurosurgery, Cleveland Clinic, Cleveland, OH, United States

Amaury De Barros
Department of Neurosurgery, Toulouse University Hospital, Toulouse, France

Julien Francisco Zaldivar-Jolissaint, Dominique Hoffmann, Emmanuel De Schlichting and Stephan Chabardès
CHU Grenoble Alpes, Clinical University of Neurosurgery, Grenoble, France

Anne-Sophie Job-Chapron, Lorella Minotti and Philippe Kahane
CHU Grenoble Alpes, Clinical University of Neurology, Grenoble, France

Elaine Keiko Fujisao, Karen Fernanda Alves, Thais O. P. Rezende and Luiz Eduardo Betting
Departamento de Neurologia, Psiquiatria e Psicologia, Faculdade de Medicina de Botucatu, UNESP - Universidade Estadual Paulista, Botucatu, Brazil

Amir H. Faraji
Department of Neurological Surgery, Houston Methodist Hospital, Houston, TX, United States
Department of Neurological Surgery, University of Pittsburgh, Pittsburgh, PA, United States

Madison Remick
Department of Neurological Surgery, University of Pittsburgh, Pittsburgh, PA, United States

Yi Guo
Department of General Practice, School of Medicine, Second Affiliated Hospital, Zhejiang University, Hangzhou, China
Epilepsy Center, School of Medicine, Second Affiliated Hospital, Zhejiang University, Hangzhou, China

Yushan Liu and Yang Chen
School of Computer Science, Fudan University, Shanghai, China

Wenjie Ming, Zhongjin Wang, Meiping Ding and Chunhong Shen
Epilepsy Center, School of Medicine, Second Affiliated Hospital, Zhejiang University, Hangzhou, China
Department of Neurology, School of Medicine, Second Affiliated Hospital, Zhejiang University, Hangzhou, China

Lijun Yao
Shanghai Pudong New Area Mental Health Center, Tongji University School of Medicine, Shanghai, China

Gaëtan Frusque and Paulo Gonçalves
Univ Lyon, Inria, CNRS, ENS de Lyon, UCB Lyon 1, LIP UMR 5668, Lyon, France

Pierre Borgnat
Univ Lyon, CNRS, ENS de Lyon, UCB Lyon 1, Laboratoire de Physique, UMR 5672, Lyon, France

Julien Jung
National Institute of Health and Medical Research U1028/National Center for Scientific Research, Mixed Unit of Research 5292, Lyon Neuroscience Research Center, Lyon, France
Department of Functional Neurology and Epileptology, Member of the ERN EpiCARE Lyon University Hospital and Lyon 1 University, Lyon, France

C. Constantino
Brain Modulation Lab, Department of Neurological Surgery, University of Pittsburgh School of Medicine, Pittsburgh, PA, United States

Nathaniel D. Sisterson
Department of Neurosurgery, Massachusetts General Hospital, Boston, MA, United States

Naoir Zaher and Alexandra Urban
Department of Neurology, University of Pittsburgh School of Medicine, Pittsburgh, PA, United States
University of Pittsburgh Comprehensive Epilepsy Center, Pittsburgh, PA, United States

R. Mark Richardson and Vasileios Kokkinos
Department of Neurosurgery, Massachusetts General Hospital, Boston, MA, United States
Harvard Medical School, Boston, MA, United States

Richard Drexler, Lasse Dührsen, Franz L. Ricklefs and Manfred Westphal
Department of Neurosurgery, University Medical Center Hamburg-Eppendorf, Hamburg, Germany

Sharona Ben-Haim
Department of Neurosurgery, University of California San Diego, San Diego, CA, United States

Christian G. Bien
Epilepsy Centre Bethel, Krankenhaus Mara, Bielefeld, Germany

Valeri Borger
Department of Neurosurgery, University Hospital Bonn, Bonn, Germany

Francesco Cardinale
"C. Munari" Epilepsy Surgery Center, Niguarda Hospital, Milan, Italy

Alexandre Carpentier and Bertrand Mathon
Department of Neurosurgery, Pitié-Salpêtrière Hospital, Paris, France

Fernando Cendes
Department of Neurology, University of Campinas, Campinas, Brazil

Sarat Chandra and Manjari Tripathi
Department of Neurosurgery, AIIMS, New Delhi, India

Hans Clusmann and Daniel Delev
Department of Neurosurgery, University Hospital RWTH Aachen, Aachen, Germany

Albert Colon
School for Mental Health and Neuroscience (MHeNS), University Maastricht (UM), Maastricht, Netherlands

Marco de Curtis, Giuseppe Didato and Thomas Sauvigny
Epilepsy Unit, IRCCS "C. Besta" Neurological Institute Foundation, Milan, Italy

Jibril Osman Farah
The Walton Centre NHS Foundation Trust, Liverpool, United Kingdom

Marc Guenot and Claire Haegelen
Department of Functional Neurosurgery, P. Wertheimer Hospital, Hospices Civils de Lyon, Lyon, France
Department for Neurosurgery, University of Lyon, Lyon, France

Saadi Ghatan and Fedor Panov
Department of Neurosurgery, Icahn School of Medicine at Mount Sinai, New York, United States

Hajo Hamer and Johannes Lang
Epilepsy Center, Department of Neurology, University of Erlangen-Nürnberg, Erlangen, Germany

Jason S. Hauptmann
Department of Neurosurgery, University of Washington, Seattle, WA, United States

Rosalind L. Jeffree
Department of Neurosurgery, Royal Brisbane and Womens Hospital, Brisbane, QLD, Australia
Herston Clinical School, University of Queensland, Brisbane, QLD, Australia

Thilo Kalbhenn
Department of Neurosurgery (Evangelisches Klinikum Bethel), Bielefeld University, Medical School, Bielefeld, Germany

Josua Kegele and Georgios Naros
Department of Neurology and Epileptology, Hertie Institute of Clinical Brain Research, University of Tubingen, Tubingen, Germany

Niklaus Krayenbühl
Division of Pediatric Neurosurgery, University Children's Hospital Zurich, University of Zurich, Zurich, Switzerland

Julia Onken and Ulf C. Schneider
Department of Neurosurgery, Universitätsmedizin Charité-Berlin, Berlin, Germany

Christian Raftopoulos and José Géraldo Ribero Vaz
Department of Neurosurgery, University Hospital St-Luc, Université Catholique de Louvain (UCL), Brussels, Belgium

Kim Rijkers
Department of Neurosurgery, Academic Center for Epileptology UMC Maastricht, Maastricht, Netherlands

Michele Rizzi
Department of Neurosurgery, Fondazione IRCCS Istituto Neurologico Carlo Besta, Milan, Italy

Karl Rössler
Department of Neurosurgery, Medical University Vienna, Vienna, Austria

Olaf Schijns
Department of Neurosurgery, Academic Center for Epileptology UMC Maastricht, Maastricht, Netherlands
School for Mental Health and Neuroscience (MHeNS), University Maastricht (UM), Maastricht, Netherlands

Andrea Spyrantis and Adam Strzelczyk
Department of Neurosurgery and Epilepsy Center Frankfurt Rhine-Main, Center of Neurology and Neurosurgery, Goethe-University Frankfurt, Frankfurt, Germany

Stefan Stodieck
Hamburg Epilepsy Center, Protestant Hospital Alsterdorf, Department of Neurology and Epileptology, Hamburg, Germany

Mario A. Alonso-Vanegas
National Institute of Neurology and Neurosurgery, Manuel Velasco Suarez, Mexico City, Mexico

Jörg Wellmer and Tim Wehner
Ruhr - Epileptology, Department of Neurology, University Hospital Knappschafts-Krankenhaus, Ruhr - University Bochum, Bochum, Germany

Petroula Laiou
Living Systems Institute, University of Exeter, Exeter, United Kingdom
EPSRC Centre for Predictive Modelling in Healthcare, University of Exeter, Exeter, United Kingdom
College of Engineering, Mathematics and Physical Sciences, University of Exeter, Exeter, United Kingdom

Ozgur E. Akman
College of Engineering, Mathematics and Physical Sciences, University of Exeter, Exeter, United Kingdom

Eleftherios Avramidis
Research Computing Services, University of Cambridge, Cambridge, United Kingdom

Marinho A. Lopes and Marc Goodfellow
Living Systems Institute, University of Exeter, Exeter, United Kingdom
EPSRC Centre for Predictive Modelling in Healthcare, University of Exeter, Exeter, United Kingdom
College of Engineering, Mathematics and Physical Sciences, University of Exeter, Exeter, United Kingdom
Wellcome Trust Centre for Biomedical Modelling and Analysis, University of Exeter, Exeter, United Kingdom

Eugenio Abela and Mark P. Richardson
Institute of Psychiatry, Psychology and Neuroscience, King's College London, London, United Kingdom

Michael Müller
Support Center for Advanced Neuroimaging, University Institute for Diagnostic and Interventional Neuroradiology, Inselspital, Bern University Hospital, University of Bern, Bern, Switzerland
Department of Neurology, Inselspital, University Hospital Bern, Bern, Switzerland

Christian Rummel
Support Center for Advanced Neuroimaging, University Institute for Diagnostic and Interventional Neuroradiology, Inselspital, Bern University Hospital, University of Bern, Bern, Switzerland

Kaspar Schindler
Department of Neurology, Inselspital, University Hospital Bern, Bern, Switzerland

Keiko Niimi, Ayataka Fujimoto and Keishiro Sato
Comprehensive Epilepsy Center, Seirei Hamamatsu General Hospital, Hamamatsu, Japan

Index

www.ingramcontent.com/pod-product-compliance
Lightning Source LLC
LaVergne TN
LVHW082148200926
848484LV00008B/2120